Cardiothoracic Trauma

Cardiothoracic Trauma

Edited by

Stephen Westaby BSc FRCS MS
Oxford Heart Centre, UK

John A Odell MBChB FRCS
Mayo Clinic Jacksonville, Florida, USA

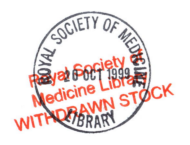

ARNOLD

A member of the Hodder Headline Group
LONDON • SYDNEY • AUCKLAND
Co-published in the USA by Oxford University Press, Inc., New York

First published in Great Britain in 1999
by Arnold, a member of the Hodder Headline Group,
338 Euston Road, London NWI 3BH
http://www.arnoldpublishers.com

Co-published in the United States of America by
Oxford University Press, Inc.,
198 Madison Avenue, New York, NY 10016
Oxford is a registered trademark of Oxford University Press

British Library Cataloguing in Publication Data
A catalogue record for this book is available from the British Library

Library of Congress Cataloging-in-Publication Data
A catalog record for this book is available from the Library of
Congress

ISBN 0 340 57320 1

Publisher: Nick Dunton
Project Editor: Melissa Morton
Production Editor: James Rabson
Production Controller: Helen Whitehorn
Cover design: Mouse Mat Design

Typeset in 10/12 pt Minion by
Scribe Design, Gillingham, Kent
Colour Separation by
Tenon & Polert Colour Scanning Ltd
Printed in China

Contents

Contributors

Bridget L Atkins MRCP MRCPath
Senior Registrar, Clinical Microbiology, Department of
Microbiology, Public Health Laboratory, Headington, Oxford,
UK

Emile A Bacha MD
Chief Resident, Cardiothoracic Surgery, Massachusetts
General Hospital, Boston, Massachusetts, USA

Stephen James Beningfield MBChB FFRad
Chief Specialist and Chairman, Department of Radiology,
Groote Schuur Hospital, Cape Town, South Africa

Farooq A Chaudhry MD
Department of Cardiology, Hahnemann University Hospital,
Philadelphia, Pennsylvania, USA

John M Cho MD
Major, United States Army Medical Corps; Chief Resident in
Thoracic Surgery, Walter Reed Army Medical Center,
Washington, DC; Assistant Professor of Surgery, Uniformed
Services University of the Health Sciences, Bethesda,
Maryland, USA

Derek W M Crook MB BCh
Consultant, Clinical Microbiology, John Radcliffe Hospital,
Headington, Oxford, UK

K Mark De Groot MD FRCSC
Associate Professor, Department of Cardiothoracic Surgery,
Groote Schuur Hospital, Cape Town, South Africa

James O Fulton MB BCh FCS
Department of Cardiothoracic Surgery,
University of Cape Town, Cape Town, South Africa

Hillel Tuvia Goodman MBChB MPraxMed MFGP FFRad FRCR
Associate Professor, University of Cape Town; Principal
Specialist, Department of Radiology, Groote Schuur
Hospital, Cape Town, South Africa

Geoffrey M Graeber MD FACS
Professor of Surgery; Director of Surgical Research,
Department of Surgery, Section of Cardiovascular and
Thoracic Surgery, West Virginia University School of
Medicine, Morgantown, West Virginia, USA

Hermes C Grillo MD
Visiting Surgeon, General Thoracic Surgical Unit,
Massachusetts General Hospital; Professor of Surgery,
Harvard Medical School, Boston, Massachusetts, USA

Michael J Joyner MD
Associate Professor of Anesthesiology and of Physiology and
Biophysics, Department of Anesthesiology, Mayo Clinic and
Foundation, Rochester, Minnesota, USA

Dean G Karalis MD
Cardiology Consultant, Department of Cardiology,
Hahnemann University Hospital, Philadelphia, Pennsylvania,
USA

John D Knottenbelt MRCP FRCS FFAEM
Consultant in Accident and Emergency, Northwick Park
Hospital, Harrow, UK

Tim J Lamer MD
Chair, Department of Anesthesiology, Chair, Division of Pain
Services, Mayo Clinic Jacksonville, Jacksonville, Florida, USA

Scott A LeMaire MD
Instructor in Surgery, Resident in Thoracic Surgery,
Department of Surgery, Baylor College of Medicine,
Houston, Texas, USA

Jeffrey Lipman MB BCh DA FFA
Associate Professor & Director, Intensive Care Facility, Royal
Brisbane Hospital, University of Queensland, Brisbane,
Australia

Douglas J Mathisen MD
Chief, General Thoracic Surgery Unit, Massachusetts General
Hospital, Boston, Massachusetts, USA

Kenneth L Mattox MD
Professor and Vice Chairman, Department of Surgery,
Baylor College of Medicine; Chief of Staff/Chief of Surgery,
Ben Taub General Hospital, Houston, Texas, USA

David J J Muckart FRCS
Senior Lecturer, Department of Surgery, University of Natal
Medical School, Durban, South Africa

Gregory A Nuttall MD
Assistant Professor of Anesthesiology, Department of
Anesthesiology, Mayo Clinic and Foundation, Rochester,
Minnesota, USA

John A Odell MB ChB FRCS
Professor of Surgery, Mayo Medical School; Section of
Thoracic and Cardiovascular Surgery, Mayo Clinic
Jacksonville, Jacksonville, Florida, USA

Steve G Peters MD
Associate Professor of Medicine, Division of Pulmonary and
Critical Care, Mayo Clinic and Mayo Foundation, Rochester,
Minnesota, USA

John V Robbs ChM FRCS FRCPS
Head, Metropolitan Vascular Service, Head, Division of
Surgery, University of Natal, Durban, South Africa

John J Ross Jr RCVT RDCS
Department of Cardiology, Hahnemann University Hospital,
Philadelphia, Pennsylvania, USA

Paul Roux MB ChB MD FCP(Paed) DCH
Senior Lecturer and Senior Paediatrician, Department of
Paediatrics and Child Health, Paediatric Service, Groote
Schuur Hospital, Cape Town, South Africa

Roger Saadia BA MD FRCS
Professor of Surgery, University of the Witwatersrand, Chief
Surgeon, Baragwanath Hospital, Johannesburg, South Africa

Ulrich O Von Oppell MB BCh FCS PhD
Chris Barnard Professor of Cardiothoracic Surgery, University
of Cape Town; Head, Department of Cardiothoracic Surgery,
Groote Schuur Hospital & Red Cross War
Memorial Children's Hospital, Cape Town, South Africa

Robert B Wagner MD
Clinical Associate Professor of Surgery, Uniformed Services
University of the Health Sciences, Bethesda, Maryland;
Consultant in Thoracic Surgery, Walter Reed Army Medical
Center, Washington, DC; United States Naval Hospital &
National Institutes of Health, Bethesda, Maryland, USA

Matthew J Wall Jr MD
Associate Professor, Department of Surgery, Baylor College
of Medicine; Deputy Chief of Surgery, Chief of General
Surgery, Director of Trauma & Critical Care, Ben Taub
General Hospital, Houston, Texas, USA

Stephen Westaby BSc FRCS MS
Consultant Cardiothoracic Surgeon, Oxford Heart Centre, UK

Cameron D Wright MD
Associate Visiting Surgeon, General Thoracic Surgical Unit,
Massachusetts General Hospital; Assistant Professor of
Surgery, Harvard Medical School, Boston, Massachusetts,
USA

part 1

Resuscitation and assessment

The pathophysiology of chest trauma

STEPHEN WESTABY

The cause of traumatic injury to the chest varies greatly in different parts of the world. In large American cities and parts of South Africa, black males have a one in twenty chance of being fatally shot or stabbed before the age of 30 years. Although terrorism and civilian violence are on the increase throughout Europe, the absolute numbers of victims remain small in comparison. In England and Wales, the annual death rate from stabbing and gunshot wounds is fewer than 200. Britain and Europe, nevertheless, have increasing figures for road casualties. England and Wales have more than 60 000 hospital admissions per year after road traffic accidents whilst London and south-east England has 57 fatal or serious road traffic accidents per 100 km of road.

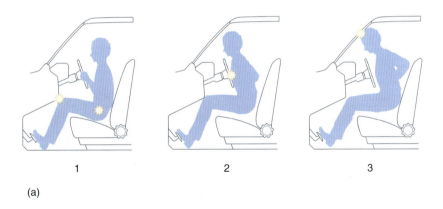

1 2 3

(a)

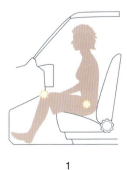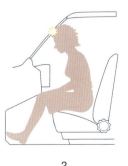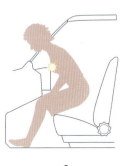

1 2 3

(b)

Figure 1.1 *Mechanism of the injuries sustained by motor vehicle driver and front seat passenger. (a) Sequence of impact of the unrestrained motor vehicle driver with: 1, dashboard; 2, steering wheel; and 3, windscreen. (b) Sequence of impact of the unrestrained front seat passenger with: 1, dashboard (initial impact); 2, windscreen; and 3, dashboard.*

AETIOLOGY OF BLUNT THORACIC INJURIES

Blunt thoracic injury is almost exclusively caused by rapid deceleration or crushing in motor vehicle collisions. In Europe, approximately 60% of thoracic injuries are sustained in road traffic accidents, and 60% of these occur in the driver or passengers in the vehicle (Fig 1.1). Motor cyclists account for less than 10% of blunt chest trauma victims but have the highest mortality (30%). The remaining 40% of injuries are sustained during industrial accidents (15%), domestic incidents (10%), sport (10%), or during interpersonal conflict or suicide (5%).

Of those patients with a primary diagnosis of thoracic trauma, about 10% have a penetrating wound, 35% have major chest wall damage and 10–15% have a visceral lesion without chest wall damage. Of patients who reach hospital, 4–6% have an aortic transection and 45% die subsequently. The average mortality of all chest injuries is 18–20%. For blunt thoracic trauma victims, 70% have multiple injuries including long bone fractures in 46% (24% mortality), skull fracture with cerebral contusion in 42% (26% mortality), or abdominal injury in 32% (31% mortality). The anatomical distribution of injuries sustained by motor vehicle occupants is shown in Fig 1.2.

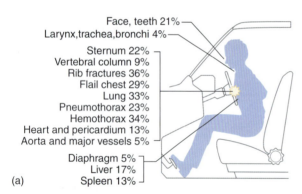

Face, teeth 21%
Larynx, trachea, bronchi 4%
Sternum 22%
Vertebral column 9%
Rib fractures 36%
Flail chest 29%
Lung 33%
Pneumothorax 23%
Hemothorax 34%
Heart and pericardium 13%
Aorta and major vessels 5%
Diaphragm 5%
Liver 17%
Spleen 13%

(a)

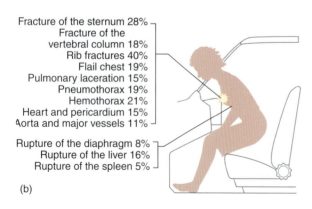

Fracture of the sternum 28%
Fracture of the vertebral column 18%
Rib fractures 40%
Flail chest 19%
Pulmonary laceration 15%
Pneumothorax 19%
Hemothorax 21%
Heart and pericardium 15%
Aorta and major vessels 11%
Rupture of the diaphragm 8%
Rupture of the liver 16%
Rupture of the spleen 5%

(b)

Figure 1.2 *Incidence of different types of injury in unrestrained motor vehicle occupants: (a) driver; (b) front seat passenger.*

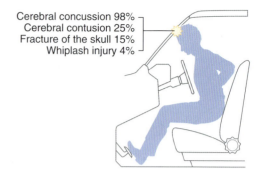

Cerebral concussion 98%
Cerebral contusion 25%
Fracture of the skull 15%
Whiplash injury 4%

(b)   (55% of drivers are affected)

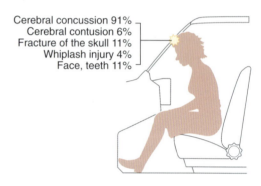

Cerebral concussion 91%
Cerebral contusion 6%
Fracture of the skull 11%
Whiplash injury 4%
Face, teeth 11%

(a)   (70% of passengers are affected)

Figure 1.3 *Injuries sustained to the head and neck during impact with the windscreen (unrestrained, no airbag): (a) driver; (b) front seat passenger.*

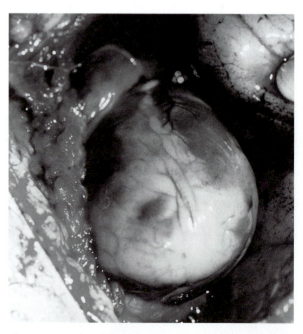

Figure 1.4 *Pericardial laceration with herniation of the heart discovered during emergency thoracotomy for electromechanical dissociation after deceleration blunt chest injury. This injury is associated with blunt cardiac contusion and occasionally laceration of the pulmonary veins (the Princess Diana injury).*

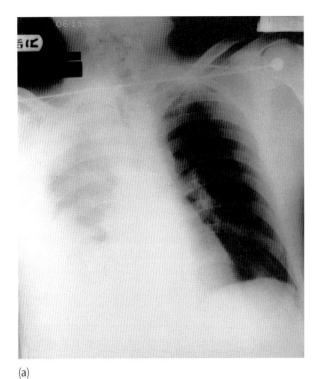

(a)

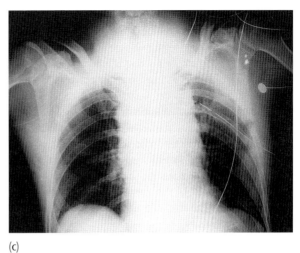

(c)

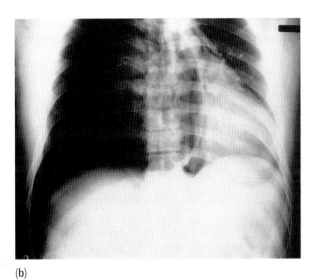

(b)

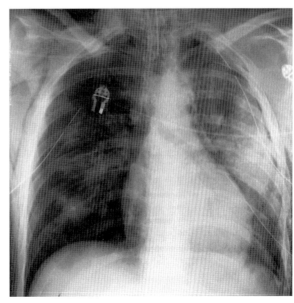

(d)

Figure 1.5 *Chest radiograph appearances of injuries commonly sustained during deceleration blunt chest trauma. (a) Extensive right hemothorax. (b) Tension right pneumothorax with severe mediastinal displacement to the left chest causing circulatory arrest. (c) The typical widened mediastinum of aortic transection. There is an intercostal drain in the left pleural cavity. (d) Ruptured left hemidiaphragm with stomach in the left chest and left hemothorax. (e) Severe blunt chest injury with bilateral pulmonary contusion and subcutaneous emphysema through barotrauma. Intercostal drains evacuated a pneumothorax on both sides. There was severe blunt cardiac trauma with right ventricular contusion, tricuspid regurgitation and first degree heart block.*

(e)

The type and severity of injury depends basically on the velocity of impact, the design of the vehicle, where the patient was sitting in the vehicle and whether or not a safety belt or inflatable air bag was in use at the time (Fig 1.3). Two-thirds of head-on car crash victims are male. During a head-on collision, an unrestrained driver is thrown heavily against the steering wheel in 90% of cases. The impact between the central portion of the steering wheel and the lower sternum is often particularly violent and followed a fraction of a second later by impact of the rim of the steering wheel on the face and abdomen. If the rim breaks or buckles, the force of the blow to the sternum becomes correspondingly more damaging.

The pattern of injury sustained may include a fracture of the sternum or vertebral column, anterior flail chest with cardiac and pulmonary contusion, rupture of the liver, spleen, diaphragm, or aorta and, on occasions, pericardial laceration with herniation of the heart (Fig 1.4). Approximately 35% sustain hemothorax, 25% pneumothorax, 5% transected aorta, 5% ruptured diaphragm and 15% blunt cardiac trauma (Fig 1.5). Associated rupture of the liver or spleen occurs in 15–20% of patients; 55% of drivers and 70% of passengers sustain injuries to the brain, skull, face or cervical

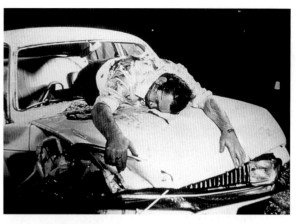

Figure 1.7 *Unrestrained passenger propelled against the dashboard and through the windscreen during deceleration road traffic accident. The patient died at the site of injury from traumatic aortic rupture.*

vertebrae after impact with the windscreen or dashboard (Fig 1.6). Instead of hitting the steering wheel, a front seat passenger hits the dashboard with his trunk after the head hits the windscreen (Fig 1.7). Knee, hip and pelvic fractures occur through impact with the dashboard. Impact of the neck with steering wheel or dashboard may cause injury to the larynx or trachea (Fig 1.8).

BALLISTIC INJURY TO THE CHEST

Approximately 15% of combat injuries sustained during conventional land warfare involve the chest. One-third of patients have concomitant injuries to the head, abdomen or limbs, but for the remaining two-thirds the thoracic wound is the principal injury. Ten percent of chest wounds are restricted to the superficial tissues and are minor in surgical terms. Those that penetrate the thoracic cavity are classified into two populations of roughly equal distribution. The first have missile wounds involving the mediastinum. Injuries to the heart, great vessels or pulmonary hilum usually prove fatal on the battlefield though a small number do survive to reach a field station or hospital. The remainder have wounds of the pulmonary parenchyma and survive with appropriate treatment. For these patients, the pathophysiological processes causing death (if untreated) are shock and hypoxia from blood loss, hemopneumothorax and interference with the mechanics of breathing (Fig 1.9).

It is unusual for combat casualties or disaster victims to survive and present for treatment after massive intrathoracic bleeding. By contrast, most patients with injuries limited to the lungs or chest wall can be stabilized in the field by judicious chest tube insertion and drainage. It is a mistake to initiate fluid

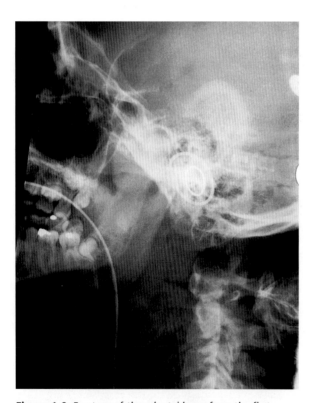

Figure 1.6 *Fracture of the odontoid peg from the first cervical vertebrae and extensive disruption of the spinal canal. There is a large prevertebral hematoma pushing the esophagus and trachea forward. This is demonstrated by the greatly increased separation between endotracheal tube and vertebral bodies.*

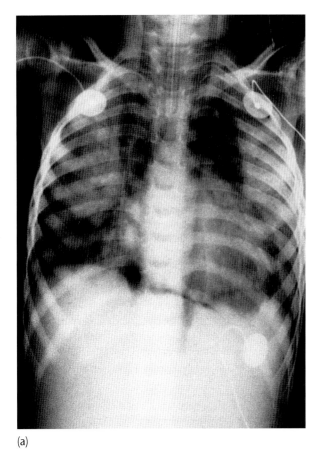

(a)

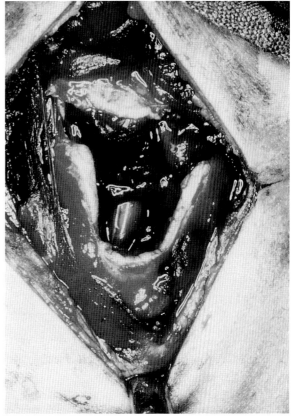

(c)

(b)

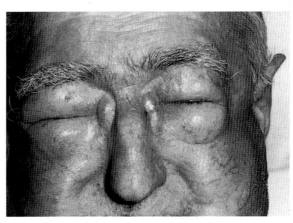

(d)

Figure 1.8 *Major airways injury through blunt impact on the neck. (a) Plain chest radiograph showing gross mediastinal emphysema and air beneath the deep cervical fascia. There is bilateral pulmonary contusion. This patient suffered transection of the trachea during impact of the thoracic inlet with the dashboard. (b) Lateral neck x-ray showing severe disruption of the airways. This patient sustained direct impact of the larynx with the rim of the steering wheel. (c) Exposure of the transected larynx at operation. The laryngeal cartilages are fractured and there is extensive edema within the larynx. The endotrachael tube enters the airway through disruption in the anterior pharyngeal wall. (d) Subcutaneous emphysema of the face through penetrating major airways injury. Air has a predilection for the periorbital tissues.*

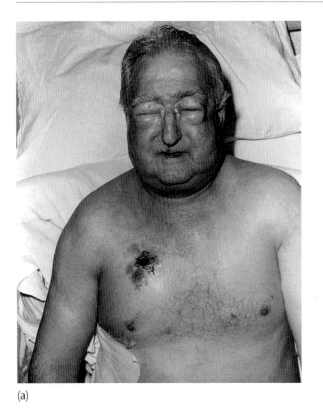

(a)

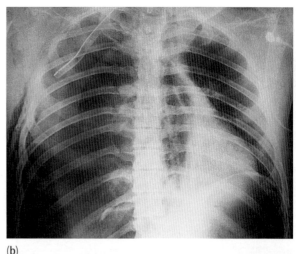

(b)

Figure 1.9 *(a) Low velocity bullet wound to the right chest from close range with powder burns around the wound and extensive subcutaneous emphysema from injury to the right upper lobe bronchus. (b) Plain chest radiograph on admission shows a tension pneumothorax secondary to the bronchial injury. A poorly placed chest drain did not enter the pleural cavity.*

replacement away from surgical facilities in patients with penetrating vascular injuries. A fall in blood pressure allows local mechanisms to arrest bleeding. An upswing in pulse pressure disrupts the blood clot, causing a potentially fatal rebleed.

The efficiency of energy transfer from a bullet or bomb fragment is determined by the flight pattern and physical characteristics of the missile (Fig 1.10) and by specific features of the tissue and organs encountered. The specific gravity of a tissue determines to a large extent its susceptibility to ballistic injury. The greater the tissue's specific gravity the more efficient a ballistic barrier it becomes as it absorbs missile energy. Bone and muscle in the chest wall have higher specific gravities than lung and are more susceptible to injury. In contrast to solid organs such as liver and brain, the lung parenchyma is relatively immune to missile trauma because of its very low specific gravity.

Low energy transfer missiles in the chest usually adopt an erratic course after penetrating the skin. They dissect along soft tissue planes, deflect from bony structures and follow the path of least resistance. Consequently, accurate prediction of damage from the site of entry or exit wounds is difficult. By contrast, missiles entering the body at high velocity often follow a predictable course and may produce profound tissue damage by laceration and cavitation following significant energy transfer. High velocity wounds are compounded by the generation of secondary missiles, including shards of bone, missile fragments and disrupted soft tissue elements generated after missile

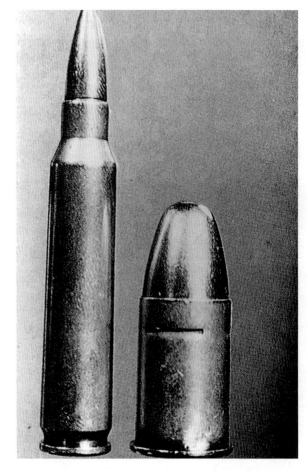

Figure 1.10 *High velocity rifle bullet and low velocity hand gun bullet.*

Table 1.1 *Mechanisms and patterns of blunt thoracic trauma*

Mechanisms of injury	Chest wall injury	Possible thoracic visceral injuries	Common associated injuries
High velocity impact (deceleration)	Chest wall is often intact *or* fractured sternum *or* bilateral rib fractures with anterior flail (steering wheel)	Ruptured aorta Cardiac contusion Major airways injury Ruptured diaphragm	Head and faciomaxillary injuries Fractured cervical spine Lacerated liver or spleen Long bone fractures
Low velocity impact (direct blow)	Lateral: Unilateral fractured ribs	Pulmonary contusion	Lacerated liver or spleen if ribs 6–12 are involved
	Anterior: Fractured sternum	Cardiac contusion	Faciomaxillary injuries
Crush injury	Anteroposterior: Bilateral rib fractures ± anterior flail	Ruptured bronchus Cardiac contusion	Fractured thoracic spine Lacerated liver or spleen
	Lateral: Ipsilateral fractures ± flail Possible contralateral fractures	Pulmonary contusion	Lacerated liver or spleen

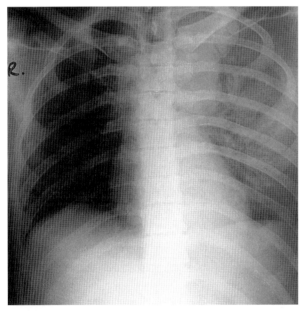

(a)

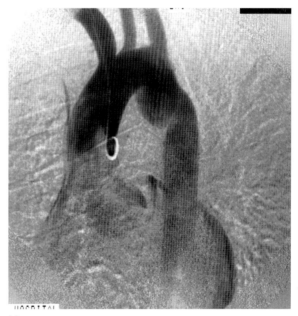

(c)

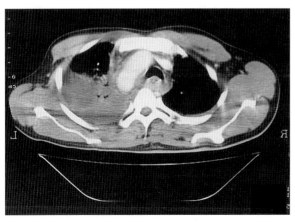

(b)

Figure 1.11 *A plain anteroposterior chest radiograph following high speed deceleration trauma. There is a left hemothorax and hematoma in the upper mediastinam. Whilst the appearances are less dramatic than in Figure 1.5(c), they nevertheless suggest an aortic injury. (b) Because the patient had a fractured sternum and was in a district general hospital without cardiac surgery, a CT scan was performed to differentiate between anterior mediastinal hematoma and the likelihood of aortic rupture. The CT scan shows hematoma around the proximal descending thoracic aorta. (c) The patient was transferred to a cardiac center where an aortogram confirmed the aortic injury. This patient was operated on 9 hours after the accident. Major trauma centers conveyed the benefit of speed in investigation and treatment.*

impact. Few victims survive high velocity wounds to the heart, great vessels or pulmonary hilum. Many high velocity injuries of the chest also involve vital structures in the abdomen or root of the neck, with fatal consequences.

PATHOPHYSIOLOGICAL PROCESSES IN THORACIC TRAUMA

Though less than 15% of patients with chest trauma require surgical intervention, many needless deaths occur through inadequate or delayed treatment of an easily remediable injury. The possibility of serious visceral injury can usually be predicted from knowledge of the type of accident (Table 1.1) and should be confirmed or excluded by the appropriate investigation such as plain chest radiography, ultrasound, or CT scan

(Fig 1.11). Sudden profound deceleration produces the so-called intrathoracic bell clanger effect. The chest wall suffers direct impact and the aorta, a heavy column of blood with inertia, swings like the clanger of a bell within the thorax, producing severe shear forces. These forces may tear the vessel at its fixed points, usually at the posterior chest wall, causing transection. The main bronchi situated beneath the aortic arch are subject to similar forces and may rupture (Fig 1.12). Impact of the neck may transect the trachea (Fig 1.8a) and compression of the abdominal viscera may rupture the diaphragm the spleen or the liver (Fig 1.13).

In life-threatening high velocity injuries there may be little or no injury to the bony chest wall though bilateral clavicular fractures or a fractured sternum should arouse suspicion. Anterior chest wall contusion is an indicator of underlying myocardial injury. In the absence of severe deceleration trauma, low velocity impact is unlikely to cause vascular injury but produces

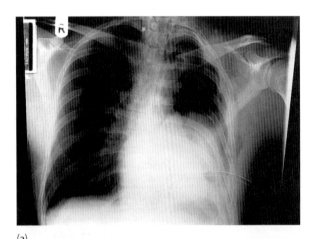

(a)

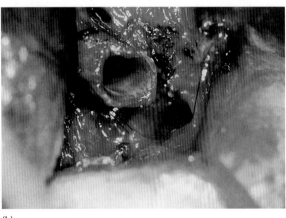

(b)

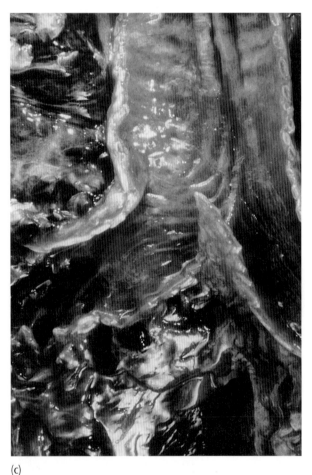

(c)

Figure 1.12 *Plain chest radiograph in a patient with complete transection of the left main bronchus. Tension pneumothorax has been relieved by the intercostal drain. Deprived of bronchial support, the airless left lung falls to the diaphragm in this semi-erect anteroposterior radiograph. There are multiple rib fractures on the left and subcutaneous emphysema. (b) The completely separated edges of the bronchus at operation. (c) Postmortem finding in a patient who died from traumatic aortic transection and right-sided tension pneumothorax. The right main bronchus (left of the picture) is transected though the mucosa remains intact.*

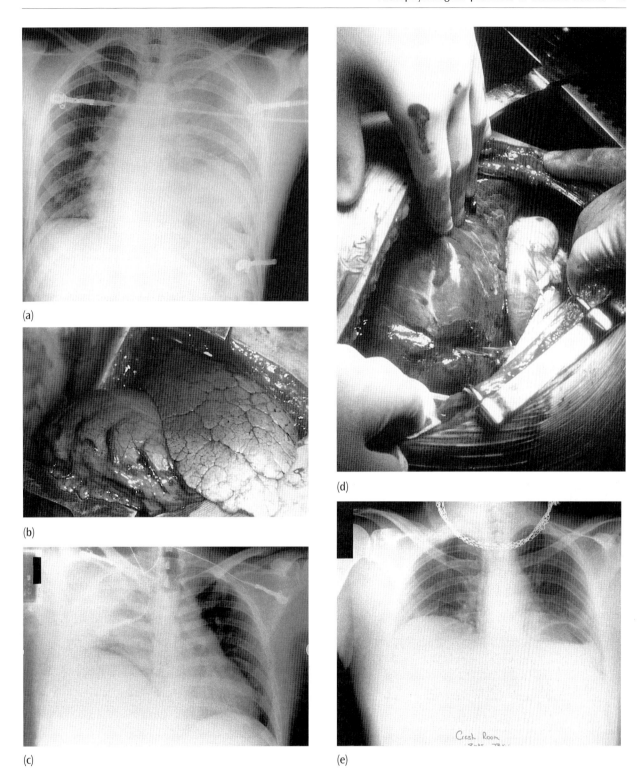

Figure 1.13 *(a) Plain chest radiograph after deceleration injury. The mediastinum is deviated to the right. There is a left-sided hemothorax. The left diaphragm cannot be seen but there is gas and a mass (the ruptured spleen) in the chest. The appearances are those of ruptured left hemidiaphragm and splenic rupture. (b) Left thoracotomy showing stomach herniated through the diaphragm and prolapsing into the wound. (c) Plain chest radiograph after a direct severe blow to the right side. The mediastinum is displaced to the left. There is an extensive right hemithorax and the appearance of a raised right hemidiaphragm. This appearance is due to right diaphragmatic rupture with herniation of the liver into the right pleural cavity. (d) Right thoracotomy showing a lacerated liver and a loop of ileum prolapsing through the bisected right hemidiaphragm. (e) Plain anteroposterior chest radiograph after fall from a great height. Both hemidiaphragms appear elevated but symmetrical with a large gas bubble in the stomach. In fact, both hemidiaphragms were ruptured with herniation of the stomach on the left and the liver on the right. The diagnosis was made only after failure to wean from the ventilator 10 days after the accident.*

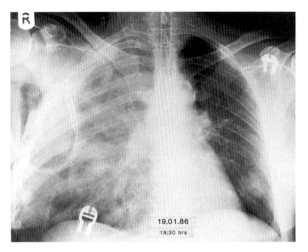

Figure 1.14 *Low velocity blow to the right hemithorax resulting in multiple rib fractures and right hemothorax.*

direct damage to the bony thorax with or without contusion of the underlying lungs or myocardium (Fig 1.14). Low velocity blows do not usually create stress or compression forces sufficient to damage the bronchi or diaphragm though the liver and spleen may be ruptured by a strategic blow over the lower part of the thoracic cage. Low velocity crush injuries may cause multiple bilateral rib fractures and the sternum may be forced backwards to touch the spine. With acute widening of the transverse diameter of the chest, the lateral motion pulls the two lungs apart, producing traction on the trachea at the carina. Bronchial rupture occurs when the elasticity of the tracheobronchial tree is exceeded. If the glottis is closed at the moment of impact, intrathoracic and intrabronchial pressure may rise suddenly.

The greatest tension develops in the larger bronchi and promotes the tendency to rupture.

Effective treatment of those who survive a major thoracic injury depends on an understanding of the pathophysiological processes which cause morbidity and potential mortality.

TRAUMA TO THE LUNGS AND CHEST WALL

Chest injuries adversely affect pulmonary function by three separate mechanisms: altered mechanics of breathing, ventilation/perfusion imbalance, and impaired gas transfer.

Altered mechanics of breathing

Even relatively minor injuries with fractured ribs but no underlying pulmonary contusion may cause sufficient pain to cause hypoventilation, atelectasis, failure to clear secretions, pneumonia, respiratory failure and even death in an elderly or bronchitic patient. Blunt trauma with multiple rib fractures and penetrating injuries that enter the pleural cavity cause severe impairment of the mechanics of breathing through pneumothorax (particularly tension pneumothorax), hemothorax, ruptured diaphragm, chest wall derangement, or injury to the major airways. The most extensive disruption to the chest wall tends to occur with crush injuries where multiple bilateral rib fractures, ruptured diaphragm, or fracture of the spine or sternum coexist. A single rib fracture causes blood loss of about 150 ml. Multiple

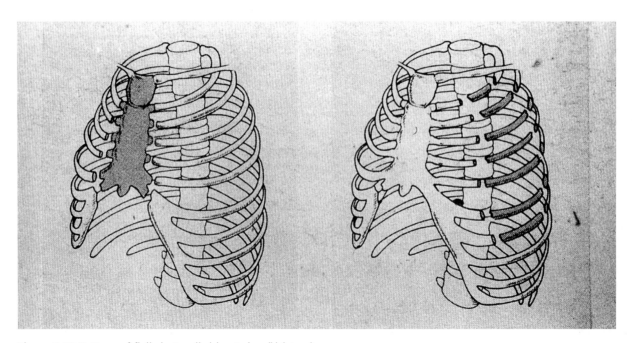

Figure 1.15 *Patterns of flail chest wall: (a) anterior; (b) lateral.*

fractures may cause substantial hemorrhage into the chest wall and pleural cavity and this is increased by laceration of the underlying lung by sharp edges.

There are two main types of chest wall derangement: a functionally important traumatic defect (sucking chest wound) and a flail segment. The latter may be unilateral with double fractures of three or more ribs, or anterior with fractures of three or more ribs on both sides of the sternum (Fig 1.15). Some fractures may occur through the costochondral junctions not visible on the plain chest radiograph. An unstable segment moves inwards on inspiration (paradoxical movement) and compromises ventilation by reducing tidal volume. Blood or air in the underlying pleural cavity may cause complete unilateral pulmonary collapse, arteriovenous shunt and hypoxia. Traumatic diaphragmatic rupture may have the same effect when the abdominal contents are sucked into the chest on inspiration. A ruptured liver or spleen then bleeds into the pleural cavity, causing further pulmonary atelectasis. Injuries to the major airways or inhalation of foreign material (teeth, windscreen glass, or stomach contents) may physically occlude the large or small airways, thereby obstructing air entry.

The patient with impaired mechanics of breathing may be brought in hypoxic and cyanosed with respiratory distress. Tension pneumothorax may be so pronounced as to impair contralateral ventilation and venous drainage through distortion of the venae cavae (Fig 1.5b). Prompt action is required on the basis of clinical examination and should not always wait for radiological confirmation. Intercostal drainage and pressure stabilization of an unstable segment are usually sufficient to improve ventilatory mechanics and gas exchange pending radiology and problem-orientated treatment.

Ventilation/perfusion imbalance

Oxygenation of the blood and elimination of carbon dioxide depends on the balance between ventilation of the lung and its blood supply. Chest injuries compromise ventilation/perfusion balance through mechanisms such as lobar collapse or mechanical obstruction of the airway. Distribution of inspired air in the lung is influenced by regional variations in airway resistance and lung compliance. The latter is governed by gravity-dependent intrapleural pressure gradients so that gas distribution in the lung is uneven during normal resting tidal ventilation. In the lower, more dependent pleural space the pressure is closest to atmospheric (least negative) and it becomes increasingly negative towards the apex of the lung. When a normal inspiration is taken from end-expiration, expansion of the initially smaller dependent alveoli is governed by the steep portion of the compliance curve. Consequently, basal alveoli expand

more for each unit of pressure change than do those at the apices which are influenced by the upper flatter portion of the curve. These differences result in preferential distribution of inspired gases to the areas of greater expansion in the basal segments of the lungs. However, if terminal air spaces collapse due to hemopneumothorax, inspiration results in preferential distribution to expanded areas as determined by the compliance curve. The maldistribution of ventilation is worsened by airflow obstruction in terminal airways due to external compression, elevated intrapleural pressure or interstitial edema fluid. When a whole lobe or lung eventually collapses, there is perfusion of non-ventilated lung and a venoarterial shunt. Impaired oxygenation of the venous blood is reflected by widening of the arteriolar–arterial oxygen gradient and systemic hypoxia.

Blood flow through the lungs is also influenced by gravity and the pressure gradient between the pulmonary arteries and left atrium. Blood is normally directed preferentially to the dependent parts of normal lung where ventilation is most efficient. After injury, perfusion may be impaired by vascular thrombosis in contused lung or widespread microembolism by fat, bone marrow, or platelet/neutrophil microemboli in patients with disseminated intravascular coagulation or adult respiratory distress syndrome (ARDS) (Fig 1.16). Even after relatively minor chest trauma the effects of ventilation/perfusion mismatch may lead to unexpectedly severe hypoxia seldom recognized without blood gas analysis. Pulmonary contusion, intrapulmonary hemorrhage and hemo- or pneumothorax are often associated with serious deterioration in pulmonary function (Fig 1.17). In turn, hypoxia has a profoundly negative effect on cardiac function and the ability of the brain to tolerate injury.

Impairment of gas transfer

Passive diffusion of gas across the alveolar–capillary barrier is dependent on the surface area available, the width of the membrane, certain plasma and erythrocyte enzymatic factors, and the partial pressure gradient between the alveolar and vascular spaces. After chest injury a number of factors may damage the alveolar–capillary barrier. These include direct injury to the pulmonary parenchyma by contusion, inhalation of gastric contents or smoke, impaired cardiac output, and interstitial pulmonary edema due to overtransfusion (elevated left atrial pressure). ARDS primarily impairs gas transfer after triggering of the humeral cascades complement, coagulation, kallikrein, and plasminogen. This process results in activation of neutrophils with trapping in the pulmonary microvasculature. The trapped neutrophils release protease enzymes and oxygen free radicals with the potential to damage the alveolar–capillary membrane. When ARDS occurs in a

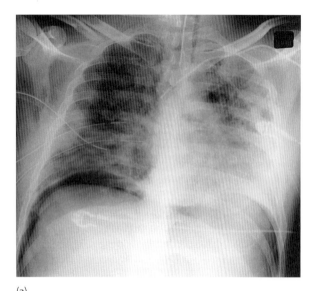

(a)

Figure 1.16 *Patient with multiple injuries who developed the adult respiratory distress syndrome (ARDS). High ventilation pressure through impaired pulmonary compliance resulted in barotrauma with bilateral pneumothoraces (three chest drains on the right) and air beneath both diaphragms. (b) Lung histology showing severe intra-alveoli hemorrhage and white cell trapping in the pulmonary microvasculature. (c) Electron micrograph showing trapped neutrophils (G) in the alveolar septae.*

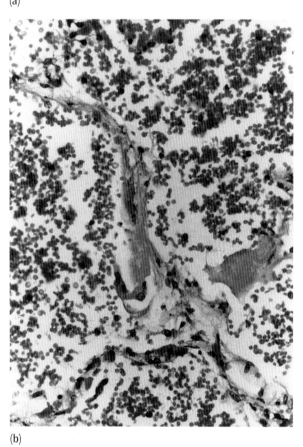

(b)

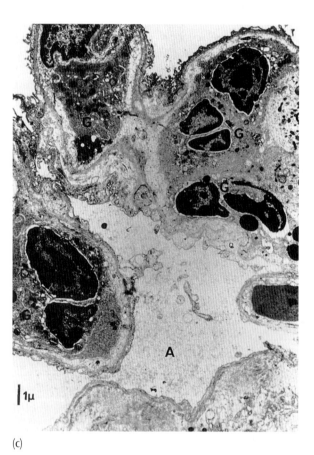

1μ

(c)

patient with thoracic trauma and multiple injuries, the chances of survival decrease markedly. Gas exchange is impaired by widening of the diffusion pathway with hyaline membrane and edema fluid in the alveoli. Terminal air-space collapse and closure of capillary channels further reduce the surface for diffusion. Hypoxia and hypercapnia then cause acid–base shifts in erythrocyte enzyme kinetics. Pulmonary hypertension develops through hypoxic vasoconstriction. Resistance to flow in small vessels is worsened by increased inter-

stitial fluid pressure. Disseminated intravascular coagulation may exacerbate these problems and further contribute to ventilation/perfusion mismatch.

Hypoxia is the first objective sign and cardinal index of progression of ARDS. Carbon dioxide retention develops at a later stage with consequent disturbances of acid–base balance. Unless blood gases are monitored continuously, respiratory insufficiency will be reflected first by deterioration in cardiovascular or cerebral function.

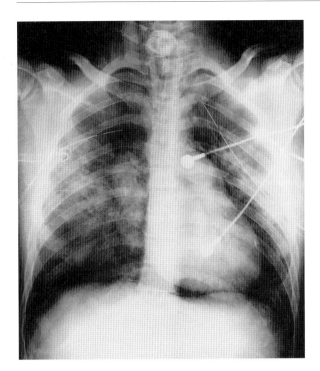

Figure 1.17 *Severe direct pulmonary contusion associated with myocardial contusion which required intra-aortic balloon pump support.*

HEMORRHAGIC SHOCK

Bleeding may be obvious because it reaches the exterior (in penetrating wounds), or may be internal and concealed. In this case hemorrhage is diagnosed from indirect evidence. Intrathoracic bleeding may be from arteries, veins or capillaries. Arterial bleeding is usually more rapid than venous because of the greater pressure, though retraction of smaller arteries can arrest bleeding. Venous bleeding is not stemmed by vessel constriction but may be arrested by tamponade as intravenous pressure falls. Bleeding from small subpleural vessels is usually self-limiting when clotting is normal.

When hemorrhage is unchecked and untreated it causes the clinical syndrome of shock. Shock is a generalized reduction in tissue perfusion with oxygenated blood. The critical aspect of circulatory physiology in hemorrhagic shock is reduced venous return to the heart. The smaller volume of blood in the capacitance vessels on the venous side of the circulation results in reduced right and left atrial filling pressures. The resulting decrease in stroke volume causes a reduction in cardiac output. Lowered pressure on both the venous and arterial sides of the circulation causes reflex baroreceptor responses which autoregulate the blood pressure. The baroreceptors are situated in the carotid sinuses and the arch of the aorta. Their afferent nerve fibers pass via the glossopharyngeal and vagus nerves to the cardiovascular center in the medulla of the brain. There are also baroreceptors on the venous side of the circulation in the superior and inferior vena cavae and within the atria themselves. Impulses generated in the baroreceptors stimulate parasympathetic activity and inhibit the sympathetic vasoconstrictor nerves to the systemic arteries and veins. A fall in blood pressure decreases the inhibitory discharge in the afferent nerves arising from the baroreceptors. The parasympathetic discharge from the cardiovascular center is then diminished so the vagal regulatory effect on the heart is reduced and heart rate increases. Sympathetic discharge from the cardiovascular center is increased, thereby elevating heart rate and force of contraction. Smooth muscle tone in the walls of arterioles and veins increases, causing increased peripheral vascular resistance by closure of precapillary sphincters.

The net effect is a tendency to restore arterial blood pressure towards normal. In turn, decreased capillary pressure results in recruitment of water and electrolytes from the interstitial space through greater oncotic pressure at the venous end of the capillaries. In acute aortic dissection or traumatic transection the baroreceptors are separated from the aortic lumen by blood clot, leading to inappropriate elevation of afterload and blood pressure.

The clinical syndrome of hemorrhagic shock

The clinical features of shock emanate from increased sympathetic discharge. They include tachycardia, sweating, pallor, coldness of the skin, especially at the periphery, and venospasm, which may cause difficulty in venous cannulation. Overextraction of oxygen from stagnant or sluggish blood in the capillary circulation causes peripheral cyanosis.

Hemorrhage causing 10% loss of the blood volume in a fit young subject is well tolerated. The right atrial stretch receptors and low pressure baroreceptors in the great veins relay their information to the vasomotor center and blood pressure is maintained at a normal level. Fluid efflux to the interstitial space is minimized through reduced pressure at the arterial end of the capillary and decreased renal perfusion causes sodium and water retention. A 10% blood loss is restored by compensatory mechanisms within 24 hours. An increase of water and electrolytes in the extracellular and intravascular compartments is balanced by plasma proteins from the liver in 3–4 days. Red cell mass is restored over a week by the bone marrow.

Systemic arterial pressure is generally maintained until 20% of the blood volume is lost. Sympathetic hyperactivity and peripheral vasoconstriction maintain pressure but not cardiac output, though cerebral and coronary blood flow is preserved by autoregulation at the expense of other organs and tissues. The brain is

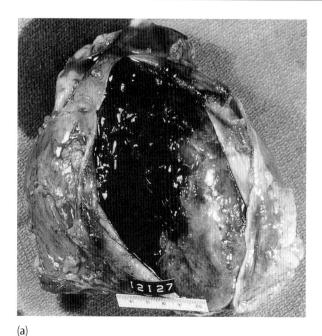

(a)

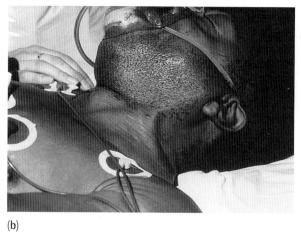

(b)

Figure 1.18 *Cardiac tamponade. (a) Distended pericardial sac full of blood clot at autopsy following death from tamponade. (b) Distended neck veins in a cardiac stab wound patient. Venous pressure is raised despite blood loss.*

most sensitive to shock because there is no cushion of anaerobic metabolism against the effects of hypoxia. Despite cerebral autoregulation, one of the first clinical signs of shock is agitation and restlessness. When blood volume loss exceeds 30%, the peripheral circulation shuts down, causing ischemia and acidosis. Prolonged hypovolemic shock results in permanent tissue injury through inadequate perfusion or during reperfusion. In severe shock, neutrophils accumulate in the lungs, capillary permeability increases and the alveoli fill with protein-rich exudate (Fig 1.16). Hypoperfusion of the gut releases endotoxin and, because the Kupffer cells and other elements of the reticuloendothelial system are inactivated in the hypoxic liver, the metabolism of toxic metabolites is compromised.

HEMOTHORAX

Blood volume loss is difficult to assess in both pleural and peritoneal cavities. The classical signs of tachycardia, low blood pressure, pallor, sweating and air hunger may occur in respiratory distress as well as blood loss. Cardiac tamponade may cause plethora with raised jugular venous pressure as opposed to pallor with imperceptible venous pulse wave (Fig 1.18). Traumatic aortic laceration with a mediastinal hematoma separates the baroreceptors from the adventitia of the aortic lumen, causing hypertension despite blood loss. Consequently, the hemodynamic status in chest trauma should always be determined by invasive arterial and venous pressure monitoring and transcutaneous oxygen saturation measurements. Failure to monitor venous pressure or diagnose cardiac tamponade may result in death during fluid resuscitation.

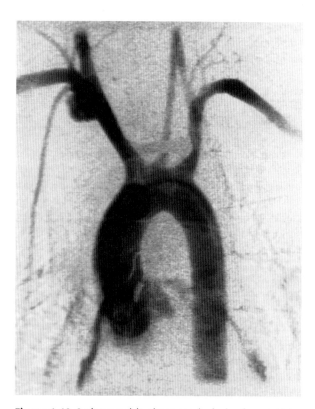

Figure 1.19 *Stab wound in the supraclavicular fossa which lacerated the innominate artery. Aortogram shows a false aneurysm. The patient was kept hypotensive (80 mmHg) before direct surgical access was obtained.*

Penetrating injuries of the aorta and brachiocephalic vessels usually cause torrential hemorrhage and death (Table 1.2) before hospital admission (Fig 1.19). Lacerations of the main pulmonary arteries or vena cavae may also prove fatal if they communicate with the

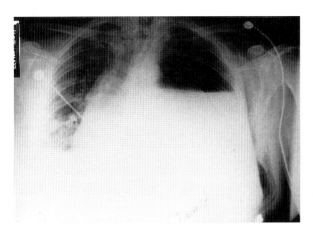

Figure 1.20 *Extensive hemothorax with fluid level after a gun shot wound which transected the right main bronchus and pulmonary artery.*

Table 1.2 *Is the patient dead or alive?*

Pulseless but warm with reactive pupils	Resuscitate vigorously until good reason to stop
Pulseless and cool with fixed dilated pupil	Do not resuscitate
Pulse present but pupils fixed and dilated	Resuscitate first. Decisions later*

*Remember that organ donation may restore active life to several other patients.

pleural cavity. Laceration of the great veins may also cause death if the patient takes a deep breath and entrains sufficient air to cause an air lock in the right atrium or jugular venous system. In some cases the tamponade effect of hematoma constrained by overlying pleura may prevent exsanguination unless overenthusiastic resuscitation tips the balance in favor of renewed bleeding. In major vascular injuries (diagnosed or suspected) a systolic pressure of 70–80 mmHg is sufficient to sustain life until direct surgical access to the injury is obtained.

Survival after traumatic aortic rupture relies on the local tamponade effect. The natural history of blunt aortic rupture is immediate death in 82% of patients whilst most of the remainder die within 2 weeks. The classical findings in aortic transection are of normal or elevated blood pressure, sometimes with lower pulse pressure or absent pulses in the legs through a coarctation effect. Urine flow is often decreased or absent. There may be asymmetry of the arm pulses if the root of the left subclavian artery is involved. Often there may be no chest wall injuries. The classical chest radographic appearance of a widened superior mediastinum is usually the first clue to aortic injury and, once seen, the blood pressure must be kept below 100 mmHg.

There are now both experimental and clinical data to reinforce the overwhelming impression that early aggressive volume replacement is harmful for many patients with chest injury. A vascular injury should be predicted or diagnosed from a brief history, the physical signs and plain chest radiograph. On the basis of this information (obtainable within 10 minutes of admission), full intravenous fluid resuscitation can either proceed or be restricted pending aortography or emergency surgery. Elevation of arterial pulse pressure will reopen a vascular injury and cause further blood loss. Ongoing resuscitation then replaces oxygen carrying capacity (blood) with cold clear fluid, causing severe

acid–base derangement and myocardial depression. Chances of survival then decrease markedly. Herein lies the danger of blind prehospital fluid resuscitation.

The sources of hemothorax include lacerated intercostal vessels, superficial pulmonary injuries, cardiac or great vessel lesions or hemorrhage from an abdominal viscus through a ruptured diaphragm. Without pleural drainage it is difficult to assess the volume of blood in a hemothorax. A large athletic male hemothorax may contain 4000 ml of blood with little pulmonary compression (Fig 1.20) whilst a 1000 ml hemothorax in a frail elderly female may produce massive tension. For a 70 kg man, a hemothorax that fills the costophrenic angle in an upright plain chest radiograph is greater than 300 ml. A hemothorax that separates the convexity of the lung from the chest wall by 1 cm usually measures between 1000 and 1500 ml. In hemopneumothorax with a fluid level 5 cm above the diaphragm, the pleural cavity usually contains at least 1000 ml of blood. Massive hemothorax (greater than 2000 ml) is twice as common on the left side and may signify aortic rupture. Intercostal drainage with a high volume suction pump serves to relieve dyspnea and cyanosis and serves to identify ongoing bleeding and the need for thoracotomy. When initial chest drain insertion yields more than 1250 ml of blood (or more than 1000 ml plus 250 ml in the first hour), or if 500 ml is drained in three consecutive hours with no decreasing trend, surgical exploration is indicated.

PENETRATING CARDIAC WOUNDS

Approximately 80% of patients with penetrating cardiac wounds are dead before hospital admission. Consequently, major intracardiac injuries such as valve disruption, coronary artery transection, or septal defects are rare in patients but more frequent in autopsy series. Those patients who reach hospital alive are a self-selected group who survive through arrest of bleeding (by cardiac tamponade), or who are conveyed rapidly with bleeding from potentially fatal injuries (Fig 1.21). Cardiac wounds consequently present with one of two distinct syndromes, either pericardial tamponade or hemorrhagic shock.

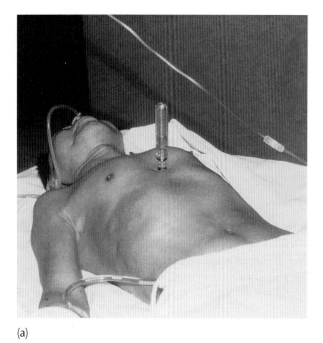

(a)

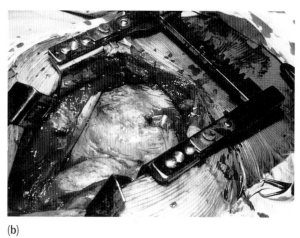

(b)

Figure 1.21 *(a) Precordial stab wound with a screwdriver left in place. The patient had elevated jugular venous pressure and a normal systemic blood pressure. He was conveyed directly to the operating room. (b) Median sternotomy was performed initially with the screwdriver in place. With access to the pericardium and site of injury, the screwdriver was withdrawn and the hole in the right ventricle closed with a single Teflon pledgeted mattress suture. The patient did not require fluid resuscitation or blood transfusion at any stage.*

The key to successful management is immediate resuscitation and repair. In penetrating trauma the triad of a mediastinal entrance wound, evidence of cardiac tamponade and profound systemic hypotension are pathognomonic of important cardiac injury. Though a posterior, subxiphoid, or subcostal penetrating wound may also produce cardiac injury, a mediastinal penetration site is responsible for 85% of cases. The diagnosis is made rapidly from the clinical overview and should seldom await diagnostic studies other than the plain chest radiograph or two-dimensional echocardiography in equivocal stable cases with tamponade (Fig 1.22). Many patients are admitted lifeless but have not sustained irreversible brain damage. The first question is whether the patient is dead or alive and should attempts at resuscitation proceed (Table 1.2)?

Hemorrhagic shock follows cardiac wounding when the pericardial laceration is large enough to allow free exit of blood so that tamponade cannot occur. Those patients who arrive moribund should undergo immediate thoracotomy on the side of the injury with the objective of controlling bleeding from the cardiac wound, then restoring blood volume and acid–base status afterwards (Fig 1.23). Unmatched type-specific or non-specific universal donor blood is given as soon as surgical control is obtained. Arterial pH and blood gas measurements are taken early and bicarbonate administered to correct profound acidosis. A small number of patients who survive laceration of a major coronary artery or valve disruption may require further repair or cardiopulmonary bypass after urgent thoracotomy.

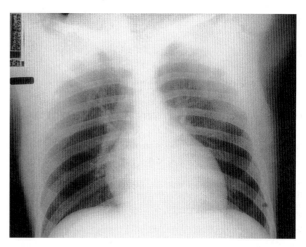

Figure 1.22 *Anteroposterior chest radiograph in a patient with a precordial stab wound and cardiac tamponade. The cardiac ratio is only slightly increased but a heart shadow has an abnormal globular appearance for a young man. The pericardium contained about 500 ml of clotted blood.*

Most patients who respond to treatment are then transferred to an operating room for formal exploration and wound closure.

Reviews of large series of patients undergoing emergency room thoracotomy in the USA demonstrate two groups with clear prognostic differences. Patients who suffer circulatory arrest more than 4 minutes prior to admission and who are unresponsive on arrival rarely survive. Those patients who are admitted warm with

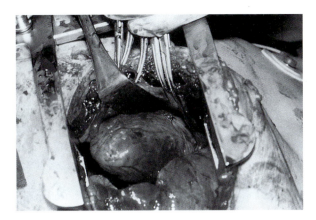

Figure 1.23 *Emergency room thoracotomy through the fifth anterolateral interspace for exanguinating hemorrhage from a cardiac stab wound.*

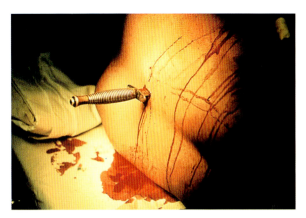

Figure 1.24 *Deep paraspinal stab wound with the knife in place. This prevented exsanguination since the blade passed through both left and right atria. Thorocotomy was performed, providing direct access to these structures before the knife was removed.*

some signs of life have a better prognosis. Survival correlates well with neurological status immediately after resuscitation. Those patients who show early improvement in neurological status with resuscitation usually have a satisfactory outcome. Young age, only brief cerebral hypoxia, and absence of major intracardiac structural injury are good prognostic features. Factors associated with a high mortality include gunshot wounds (versus stab wounds), left ventricular injury and unconsciousness and the absence of measurable blood pressure on arrival.

Cardiac tamponade occurs when blood accumulates within the pericardial sac and clots, thereby arresting hemorrhage. Tamponade is recognized by the combination of a precordial entrance wound, hypotension and tachycardia with distended neck veins despite bleeding (Fig 1.18b). The majority of these patients are conscious but anxious, cold, sweating and cerebrally obtunded. The cardiac wound is usually small and bleeding stops when the intracardiac pressures fall. The distended pericardium usually contains blood clot equivalent to between 500 and 1500 ml of blood. Bleeding of this volume may not lower the blood pressure and the patient's overall condition may not suggest a cardiac wound. In tamponade the cardiac shadow is typically globular in shape (Fig 1.22). Two-dimensional echocardiography shows a pericardial effusion with compression of the cardiac chambers and abnormal ventricular filling. Patients who survive the journey to hospital can usually survive the transfer to an operating room as long as fluid resuscitation is withheld. Most centers that treat sufficient numbers of penetrating cardiac wounds have abandoned needle pericardiocentesis in favor of early thoracotomy since the pericardial blood has usually clotted. Some advocate transdiaphragmatic pericardotomy through a small subxiphoid incision to produce temporary clinical improvement until median sternotomy or thoracotomy can be carried out. However, it may also disturb the blood clot in a

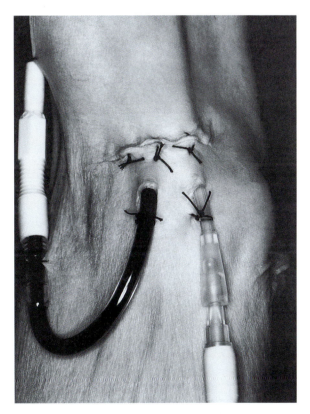

Figure 1.25 *Antecubital cutdown to insert nasogastric tubes as intravenous cannulae anticipating blood loss from a major vascular injury.*

cardiac wound and precipitate fatal hemorrhage before surgical access is possible. If the knife or wounding implement is still in place, it is important not to withdraw this until exposure of the damaged structures has been obtained (Fig 1.24). The best policy is to convey the patient directly to the operating room and insert large bore intravenous cannulae in preparation for anesthesia (Fig 1.25). The patient is anesthetized on

Table 1.3 *Conduct of surgery for penetrating cardiac wounds*

- Insert large bore peripheral and central venous lines under local anesthetic.
- Keep systemic and filling pressures down.
- Connect internal defibrillator paddles and fibrillator.
- Have two large suckers for the pericardium.
- Anesthetize and intubate on the operating table prepared for sternotomy.
- Give muscle relaxant when the sternum is split.
- Transfuse as the pericardium is opened.
- Occlude cardiac laceration with a finger and close with Teflon pledgeted Prolene mattress sutures.
- Temporarily fibrillate if necessary.
- Inspect the rest of the heart carefully for exit wound.

the operating table, which invariably causes a precipitous fall in blood pressure in the tamponade patient. The sternotomy or thoracotomy is then performed rapidly to gain access to the injury (Table 1.3).

FREE AIR IN THE CHEST

Simple closed pneumothorax occurs when gas escapes into the pleural cavity. The inherent elasticity of the lung causes collapse of about 20% lung volume with impairment of the mechanics of breathing. Pneumothorax remains uncomplicated in approximately 85% of the cases. Tension pneumothorax (Fig 1.5b) is found in 15% and results from ongoing air leak from a pulmonary laceration, ruptured trachea or main bronchus, or rarely from injury to the esophagus. One-third of patients have concomitant hemothorax and a quarter have subcutaneous free air. Pneumopericardium occurs during barotrauma or tension pneumothorax with a pericardial laceration (Fig 1.26). Both simple and tension pneumothoraces are more frequent on the left side than the right. Bilateral pneumothoraces occur in about 15% of patients. Whilst pneumothorax alone is rarely fatal, the risks increase if the patient is mechanically ventilated. The pleural cavity should always be drained in pneumothorax before positive pressure ventilation is instituted, but prophylactic chest drains should not be used for ventilated patients if no hemopneumothorax exists. This policy prevents lung penetration in the 10–15% of patients with an obliterated pleural space (Fig 1.27).

The clinical signs of pneumothorax are tachypnea, hyper-resonance on the affected side and depressed breath sounds. In tension pneumothorax there is deviation of the trachea away from the affected side. Coughing, shouting or glottic spasm may promote tension in a simple pneumothorax. As intrapleural pressure increases, systemic venous return is progressively reduced as the affected lung collapses. The mediastinum is displaced towards the ventilated side and cardiac output falls. The life-threatening problem is rapidly resolved by intercostal drainage.

Open or communicating pneumothorax through a chest wall defect is referred to as a sucking wound. The

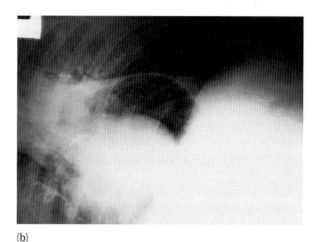

(b)

Figure 1.26 *Pneumopericardium after blunt chest injury. (a) Anteroposterior chest film showing a halo of air around the cardiac silhouette. (b) A lateral decubitous view confirms that the air is within the pericardium and not beneath the mediastinal pleura.*

(a)

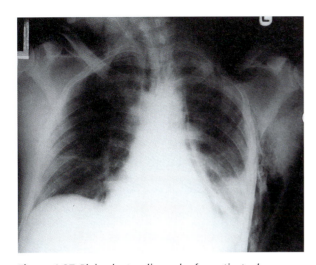

Figure 1.27 *Plain chest radiograph of a patient who presented with subcutaneous emphysema over the left chest wall after blunt trauma. An intercostal drain was inserted despite the absence of hemopneumothorax. The patient had a pleural space previously obliterated by inflammatory adhesions and the drain passed through the lung parenchyma, causing intrapulmonary bleeding.*

pleural cavity communicates with the atmosphere so that virtually complete pulmonary collapse occurs unless there is adhesion between visceral and parietal pleura due to previous inflammation. Open pneumothorax is usually caused by either stab or gunshot wounds or a transfixion injury. When the chest wound is smaller than the glottis the pneumothorax is usually small (20%) and ventilation is preserved. When the wound is larger than the glottis the lung collapses even in the absence of tension. Paradoxical motion of the mediastinum occurs as it swings from side to side with the phase of respiration. During inspiration, air is more easily aspirated through the chest wall defect than through the glottis. The mediastinum is drawn towards the partially inflated healthy lung, thereby increasing the pneumothorax. During expiration, air escapes more rapidly through the wound than through the glottis, so the mediastinum shifts in the other direction. Mediastinal instability is aggravated by increased dead space in the airway. During inspiration, desaturated air passes from the collapsed lung to the intact lung whilst on expiration air from the ventilated lung is rebreathed

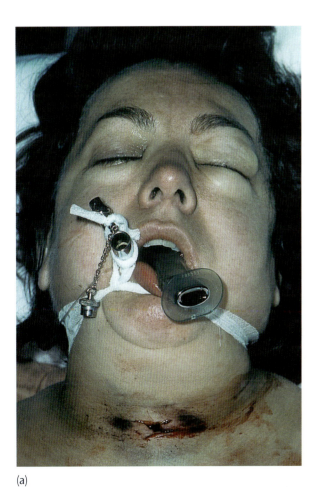

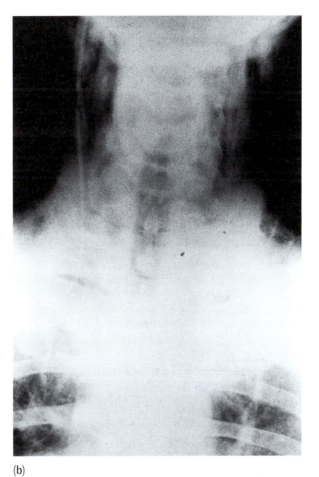

(a)   (b)

Figure 1.28 *Female patient with a stab wound to the neck which penetrated the trachea. The neck, face and eyelids are swollen with subcutaneous air. (b) Plain radiograph of the thoracic inlet shows extensive free air beneath the deep cervical fascia. An internal jugular line can be seen on the right.*

into the partially collapsed lung. This, together with cyclical torsion of the great veins, may prove fatal. The condition is stabilized by covering the chest wall defect.

Subcutaneous emphysema occurs when air penetrates the subcutaneous tissues (Fig 1.28). It is crepitant to the touch and finger pressure leaves an imprint. With a continued subcutaneous air leak, swelling can spread to the neck, face, abdomen and scrotum. Air may also originate from the major airways and spread throughout the mediastinum. In more than 50% of patients, the air originates from a pneumothorax or lacerated visceral pleural surface in a pleural space obliterated by adhesions. About 25% of cases have no detectable cause, whilst the remainder occur through more sinister laryngeal, tracheal, bronchial, or esophageal injury (Fig 1.29). With careful examination subcutaneous emphysema is found in about 15% of chest injury patients. When the pleura is torn, air from a pneumothorax or injured airway infiltrates the tissues of the thoracic wall, spreads through the muscles and reaches the subcutaneous tissues. There are no barriers to spread upwards to the neck and face or downwards into the abdominal wall. Air accumulates in areas where the subcutaneous tissue is less dense, producing a bloated appearance in the eyelids, face, chest wall, neck and scrotum. The forehead and scalp are usually unaffected. Patients with pulmonary emphysema, chronic obstructive airways disease or an obliterated pleural cavity may have extensive subcutaneous emphysema even in the absence of tracheobronchial injury. Crepitus in the chest wall or supraclavicular foci is common in patients with rib fractures. When more extensive, the possibility of major airways or esophageal injury must be ruled out. Laryngeal, tracheal and proximal injuries to the bronchi release air into the mediastinum without pneumothorax. Penetrating wounds to the esophagus often communicate with the pleural cavity, producing mediastinal emphysema and spilling gastric contents into the plural cavity. Endotracheal intubation and positive pressure ventilation rapidly aggravate subcutaneous emphysema, particularly in the presence of tracheobronchial injury. Whilst the presence of mediastinal emphysema should initiate a routine search for tracheobronchial injury or esophageal perforation, mediastinal emphysema may also occur through propagation of subcutaneous emphysema, a direct air leak from tension pneumothorax through a tear in the mediastinal pleura, a direct air leak from pulmonary laceration in patients with an

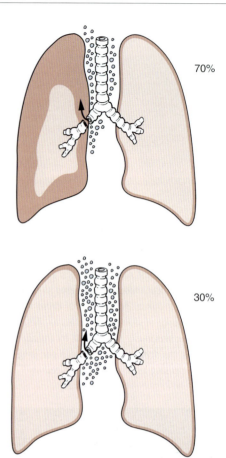

70%

30%

Figure 1.29 *The origin of mediastinal and deep cervical air in bronchial rupture. In 70% of cases the lacerated bronchus communicates with the pleural cavity, producing a pneumothorax. In 30% the injury occurs proximal to the pleural sheath so that air escapes into the mediastinal tissues with no pneumothorax.*

obliterated pleural cavity or from an interstitial pulmonary air leak that spreads along the bronchial sheath and pulmonary vessels after barotrauma.

Except for the anxiety and discomfort of the patient, subcutaneous emphysema has little clinical significance except as a warning sign for potential major airways injury in a minority of patients. The swelling and skin crepitation usually disappear 3 or 4 days after the air leak subsides as gas is absorbed by the tissues. In very severe cases when the whole body is affected and the eyes are closed, a number of cutaneous skin cuts will promote deflation.

2

Logistics of chest trauma management

JOHN KNOTTENBELT

Chest injuries may be life-threatening or result in prolonged morbidity, especially if treatment is suboptimal. Detailed preparation and planning is essential if those managing patients with chest trauma are to apply their skills in an unimpeded fashion. This involves those managing the patient prior to hospitalization (Fig 2.1), as well as those in trauma reception and the hospital. This chapter provides guidelines on how to prepare ahead to ensure an organized environment for the resuscitation and management of chest trauma patients.

PREHOSPITAL LOGISTICS

Table 2.1 gives the four phases of the prehospital response. All will need attention if the patient is to reach the hospital in the best possible condition.

Table 2.1 *Phases of the prehospital response*

- Notification of the injury
- Despatch of prehospital personnel (encompasses paramedical, ambulance crews and nursing teams) and transport
- On-scene assessment and interventions
- Transport to the trauma facility

Notification and despatch

The call for help is most often directed to an ambulance service. It is essential that the person receiving the call determines whether a life-threatening injury is present or not, and gathers enough details to pass on to the prehospital team and receiving hospital. It is, of course, vital to take the caller's name and telephone number so that communication can be re-established if it is lost. A

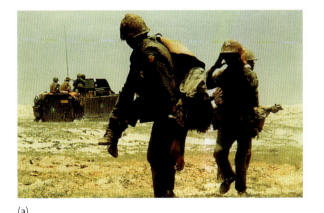

(a)

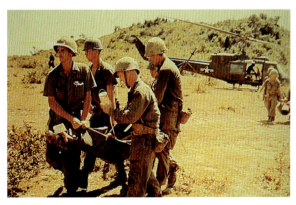

(b)

Figure 2.1 *(a, b) The concept of triage was refined during the Vietnam war. Injured soldiers were carried from the battlefield and transported by helicopter to mobile surgical hospitals away from the fighting. Specialist surgeons were available to treat the injured, beginning with those likely to survive. (Stephen Westaby Trauma Collection; SWTC.)*

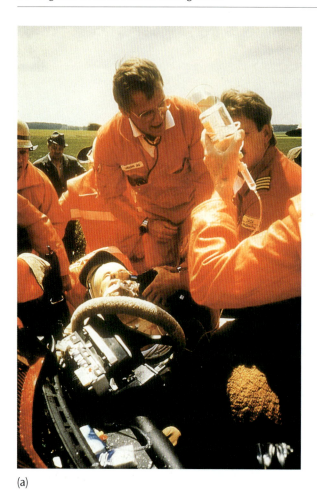

(a)

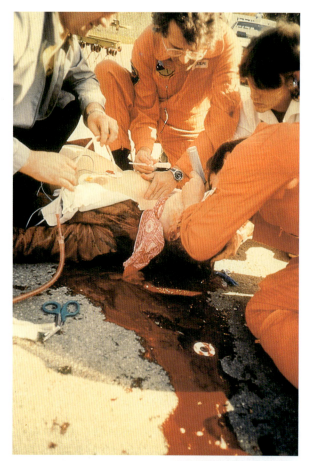

(b)

Figure 2.2 *(a–c) Current prehospital care by paramedics or mobile medical teams allows resuscitation at the site of injury and rapid transportation by helicopter to a trauma center. (SWTC.)*

suggested list of questions to ask is given below, with action points and urgency assessment for each.

WHAT HAPPENED?

Blunt injury to the chest from road accidents or falls from a height will usually require on-scene stabilization and management of other injuries such as head injury or fractured limbs. Attendance by the prehospital team in an ambulance or helicopter may be necessary.

Penetrating injuries from stab or gunshot wounds are usually best served by removal to the nearest trauma facility by whatever means is available, e.g. police transport or private car.

WHO IS/ARE THE PATIENT(S)?

The number of patients is important, especially if they are going to need ambulance or air transport. If there are multiple casualties, a major incident plan should be invoked to ensure adequate on-scene support and

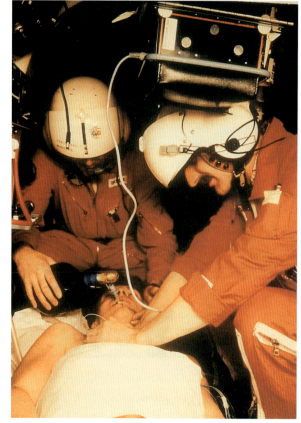

(c)

proper distribution of cases. If the patients include young children this may well influence destination.

WHAT IS THE PATIENT'S CONDITION?

Signs of urgency are unconsciousness, difficulty in breathing and pallor or cyanosis. Pain in the chest after blunt injury, which is worse on breathing or coughing, suggests fractured ribs. A patient who is comfortable, talking and who has a warm skin is unlikely to be suffering major chest injury.

WHERE IS THE SCENE?

An accurate location is vital so that the prehospital team can make their way there without waste of time. Accessibility may determine the type of transport and composition of the prehospital team. Knowledge of the location will also allow an informed decision as to which hospital will be asked to receive the casualty. Clearly, the nearest hospital with adequate facilities and available personnel to complete the life-saving interventions is the best to use.

WHAT ASSISTANCE IS AVAILABLE ON-SCENE?

It may be that the police or others with readily available high speed transport are present, and will be able to bring a casualty with penetrating chest injury to the nearest hospital immediately. If a medically qualified person is on-scene, then it is often best to speak to him/her directly to get an assessment of the patient's condition and give directions as to what to do until the team gets there. Lay-persons often mis-assess the problem.

The first response personnel and facilities

Since chest injuries may threaten cardiorespiratory function, with death by hypoxia or shock, a fast response is critical. The main determinant of survival (other than the injury itself) is delay in implementation of life-saving measures such as airway management and chest or pericardial decompression. The ideal situation is to have a team arrive within minutes who can recognize the danger signs and intubate, ventilate and decompress the pleural cavity effectively, and then monitor the patient to detect further problems while en route to a trauma facility (Fig 2.2). The team may consist of doctors, paramedics, or both, but at least two suitably trained persons should be present. The skills and equipment required are listed in Tables 2.2 and 2.3. These lists are intended only as guidance and are not exhaustive. They may need modification for compliance with local guidelines and paramedic skills. However, it is better to be overequipped rather than underequipped

Table 2.2 *Skills in the prehospital management of chest injury*

Clinical recognition of:
- Compromised or inadequate airway
- Ventilatory inadequacy
- Shock
- Tension pneumothorax
- Cardiac tamponade

Interventions
- Endotracheal intubation and manual ventilation
- Cricothyroidotomy (needle)
- Surgical airway
- Needle decompression of the pleural cavity
- Tube drainage of the pleural cavity (air transport)
- Closure of open pneumothorax
- Intravenous cannulation

Table 2.3 *Equipment required in the prehospital management of chest injury*

Interventions
- Oxygen supply and face mask
- Laryngoscope
- Portable suction
- Range of endotracheal tubes for adults and children
- Bag and reservoir for hand ventilation
- Cricothyroidotomy and chest decompression needles
- Artery forceps (for stabilizing decompression needles)
- Chest tubes and non-return valve kit (e.g. Heimlich's)
- Intravenous cannulae (range)
- Intravenous fluids (e.g. saline or Ringer's lactate/Hartmann's)
- Adequate lighting
- Polyurethane adhesive film for closure of open chest wounds

Monitoring
- Pulse oximeter
- Expiratory capnograph
- Sphygmomanometer (manual and automatic non-invasive)
- Electrocardiographic monitor (3-lead)
- Thermometer (low reading electronic, e.g. tympanic)

as medically qualified bystanders are surprisingly often present at accidents, but are powerless without suitable equipment to hand.

Paramedic training should be taken very seriously if advanced techniques are to be allowed, with regular practices and review of cases. Again, it is better to overtrain paramedics so that they can undertake interventions authorized by a doctor in the control center. This is particularly important if air transport is contemplated, as even a small pneumothorax requires decompression before ascending to altitude.

EMERGENCY ROOM LOGISTICS

Layout of department, planning

Common mistakes in emergency department design are to insist on the resuscitation room being at the front door, and to allow inadequate space for the trauma team. A short stretcher ride within the department will seldom compromise a patient's survival, and will allow for adequate proximity to x-ray and operating room facilities, while making it more awkward for the curious bystander to get in the way. Overhead-mounted x-ray machines are desirable if funds and space allow, but should not compromise lighting in the resuscitation room. This should be sufficient to allow emergency thoracotomy if necessary (Fig 2.3). A portable x-ray machine is a minimum requirement. Access to operating rooms, laboratory services, blood bank, vascular imaging and CT scanning are all important and independence from lifts is highly desirable (Fig 2.4). Communication between reception staff and resuscita-

tion room is essential so that a record folder and patient labels can be obtained very soon after arrival. This will minimize difficulties in obtaining blood for transfusion where delay in establishing a unique identity or hospital number can be crucial.

Clinical personnel

Ideally, information concerning patients with chest injury should have been communicated to the emergency department (ED) prior to arrival. The level of preparation will depend on the adequacy of assessment by the prehospital team. If the patient is known to have impaired vital signs in the field, a precordial wound, or multiple injuries in addition to a chest injury, it is important to have the trauma team waiting for the patient. The minimum trauma team consists of a general surgeon, an anesthetist, an emergency department doctor and two nurses. The general surgeon should have experience in emergency room thoracotomy and be competent to open the pericardium and perform open cardiac massage (Fig 2.5).

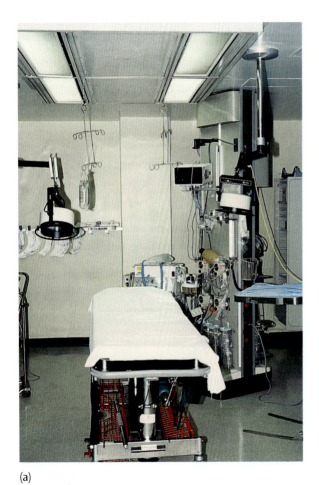

(a)

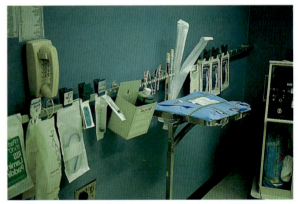

(b)

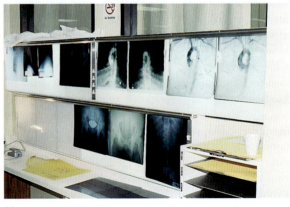

(c)

Figure 2.3 *Reception area at a major trauma center. (a) Reception bay with overhead x-ray equipment, operating lights and anesthetic equipment. (b) Intravenous cannulae, endotracheal tubes and thoracotomy set easily available from a rack on the wall. (c) Nearby x-ray screens for rapid review of radiological investigations. (SWTC.)*

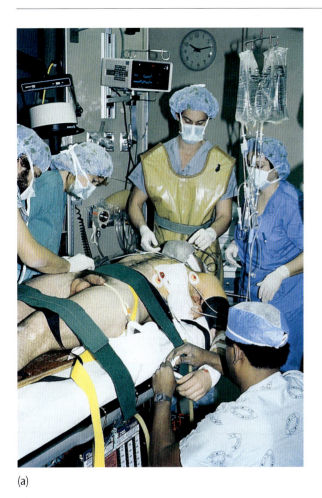

(a)

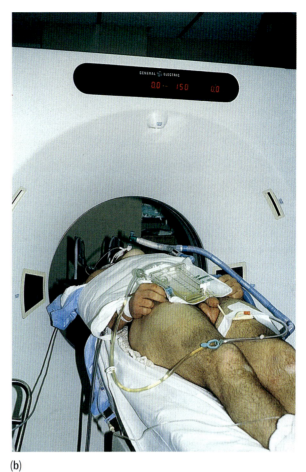

(b)

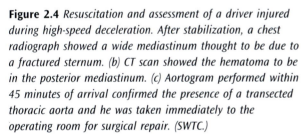

Figure 2.4 *Resuscitation and assessment of a driver injured during high-speed deceleration. After stabilization, a chest radiograph showed a wide mediastinum thought to be due to a fractured sternum. (b) CT scan showed the hematoma to be in the posterior mediastinum. (c) Aortogram performed within 45 minutes of arrival confirmed the presence of a transected thoracic aorta and he was taken immediately to the operating room for surgical repair. (SWTC.)*

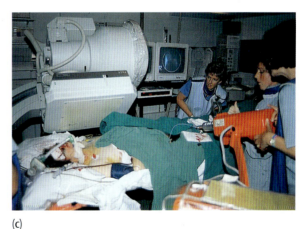

(c)

An orthopedic surgeon should normally be present if blunt injury is the problem but otherwise need not be called. When the patient is stable, with no difficulty in breathing or shock in the prehospital phase (Fig 2.6), initial assessment can be carried out by a doctor trained in the ATLS approach, and the relevant team called if necessary. Dedicated portering staff should be available for the resuscitation area.

Equipment in the ED

All the equipment specified in Table 2.3 should be readily available, with the additional items specified in Table 2.4. If volume of chest trauma is high, arrangements should be made for the recycling of sterile supplies after-hours and at weekends so that multiple casualties can be dealt with.

Support services for ED evaluation and management of chest trauma

RADIOLOGY

Chest radiography, and preferably real-time ultra-sound/echocardiography should be available in the

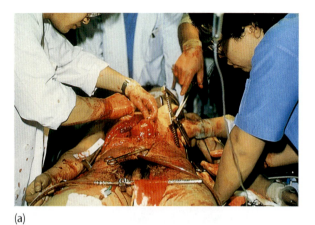

(a)

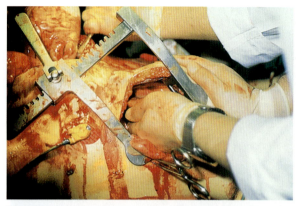

(b)

Figure 2.5 *Immediate surgical resuscitation for a patient with exsanguinating abdominal trauma and cardiac arrest. (a) Left thoracotomy was performed to cross-clamp the descending aorta and arrest hemorrhage from abdominal vessels. (b) Internal cardiac massage was then used to restore blood flow to the brain and coronary arteries. After initial stabilization, the patient was transferred to the operating room for splenectomy and partial hepatectomy (c). (SWTC.)*

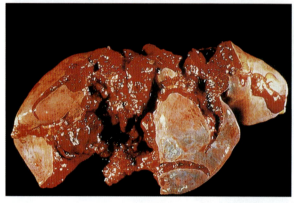

(c)

resuscitation room. The CT scanner and angiography suite should be nearby and suitably equipped for the ongoing monitoring of patients undergoing imaging after chest trauma. The radiology service must be available on a 24-hour basis, 365 days a year. Radiographers

and technical personnel to operate the relevant apparatus should also be available on an instant access basis.

BLOOD TRANSFUSION SERVICE

Transfusion requirements are often very high, and the blood should be as fresh as possible. The blood transfusion service should be staffed on a 24-hour instant access basis. Communication with the blood bank

Table 2.4 *Special equipment for ED management of chest trauma*

Interventions
- Items as specified in Table 2.3
- Volume-cycled ventilator
- Double lumen (Carlens) endotracheal tubes
- High flow intravenous cannula conversion kits
- Blood warming apparatus and pressure infusors for high flow transfusion
- Autotransfusion apparatus (Sorenson and/or cell salvage)
- Central line insertion kit and manometer apparatus
- Defibrillator with internal paddles
- Underwater seal chest drainage equipment and tubes (28F–32F), with facilities for applying high volume/low pressure suction
- Constant positive airway pressure apparatus
- Tracheostomy tray
- Emergency thoracotomy instrument pack (see Table 2.5), with high pressure air line if necessary for sternal saw

Diagnostic and monitoring
- Items as specified in Table 2.3
- X-ray apparatus – overhead or portable
- Portable ultrasound imaging
- Arterial blood gas machine
- Urinary catheterization tray
- Flexible and rigid bronchoscopes

Table 2.5 *Emergency thoracotomy pack*

- General surgical set with long artery and dissecting forceps
- Sterile drapes
- Scalpel with no. 20 blade (or equivalent)
- Gigli saw and/or manual sternotomy chisel set
- Oscillating sternotomy saw set, preferably air-powered
- Rib/sternal self-retaining retractors
- Lung retractor
- Selection of non-crushing vascular clamps, straight and angled (e.g. Satinsky)
- Skin staples
- Teflon felt pledgets for supporting cardiac sutures (double armed needles)
- Thoracotomy/sternotomy closure equipment and sutures
- Fogarty balloon catheters for intravascular control

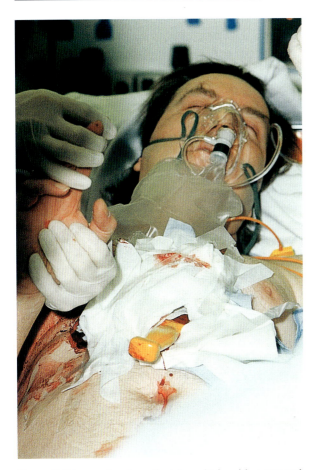

Figure 2.6 *Young female patient brought in with a serrated bread knife sticking out of her lower chest and covered in bloodstained dressings. Despite the dramatic appearance, this self-inflicted knife wound had not entered the chest or abdominal cavity. (SWTC.)*

should be excellent and airtube transmission of samples may save much time. Rarely should there be a need for more than 2 units of group O universal donor blood, and type-specific blood should be available within 5 minutes. Platelet packs and fresh frozen plasma products must be stocked as a routine in hospitals receiving chest trauma. Cell-saver autologous transfusion apparatus is safe and can be extremely useful, but requires a technician to operate, while the Sorenson apparatus is easier but has drawbacks if large volumes are retransfused.

Post-resuscitation facilities

OPERATING ROOM

Every effort should be made to perform major chest operations in a fully equipped operating room if possible, preferably by a thoracic surgeon used to dealing with traumatic problems. Facilities for heparinless left heart bypass to allow repair of aortic rupture are neces-

sary in a trauma center. As the abdomen may well be involved in a multitrauma patient, laparotomy equipment, as well as a general surgical team, should always be on standby. The anesthetist should be senior and experienced as these patients are often extremely unstable. However, transfer to the main operating room will not always be possible and an emergency room thoracotomy may be necessary. Even then it may be best to transfer the patient who has been stabilized by emergency room personnel for formal re-exploration and revision in the main operating room, while still under anesthetic.

INTENSIVE CARE

Every hospital receiving chest trauma must have an intensive care unit (ICU) and personnel capable of delivering advanced critical care, with invasive monitoring, in the postoperative period. Patients who have been shocked for a long time are often hypothermic and adequate warming apparatus must be available.

ANCILLARY SERVICES

Treatment by physiotherapists familiar with the management of patients with rib fractures and chest drains can make a big difference to levels of morbidity from these causes. Pain control is essential and either the attending doctors or a pain-control team should ensure adequate analgesia so that the physiotherapy is effective. Self-administration of opiate analgesics by the intravenous or intranasal route requires only simple apparatus and minimal additional monitoring. Intrapleural anesthesia with bupivacaine can be instilled through a chest tube; the bed should be capable of tilting head down. If epidural analgesia is given, it is usually recommended that the patient is kept in a high dependency area.

Rehabilitation

The patient who recovers from major chest trauma will often require rehabilitation services to restore normal activity. The provision of these services is beyond the scope of this text, but adequate and comprehensive follow-up arrangements must never be overlooked.

FURTHER READING

Alexander RH, Proctor HJ. *Advanced Trauma Life Support for Physicians.* Chicago, IL: American College of Surgeons, 1993; Chapter 4.

The Joint Colleges Ambulance Liaison Committee. *Ambulance Service Paramedic Training.* Bristol: NHS

Training Directorate, 1993; Sections 3 and 4.

Riggs L (ed.). *Emergency Department Design.* Dallas, TX: American College of Emergency Physicians, 1993.

Wilson RF. Thoracic trauma. In: Tintinalli JE, Ruiz E, Krome RL (eds). *Emergency Medicine.* New York: McGraw-Hill, 1996; 1156–82.

3

Imaging of chest trauma

HILLEL TUVIA GOODMAN AND STEPHEN JAMES BENINGFIELD

A brief review of the relevant anatomy is followed by the description of a practical approach to the radiological diagnosis of important injuries resulting from thoracic trauma. Strong emphasis is placed on the value of the plain chest radiograph.

ANATOMY OF THE CHEST

The chest wall

THE SOFT TISSUES

Muscle, fat and skin, and the breasts in women, constitute the bulk of these soft tissues. Narrow soft tissue 'companion shadows' often parallel the inner borders of the upper ribs. Prominent extrapleural fat can resemble pleural fluid or pleural thickening (Fig 3.1). The serratus anterior muscle bundles may cause bilaterally symmetrical, low density opacities crossing the lower ribs. Breast shadows vary widely in configuration, and some asymmetry is often present. High, sharply angulated axillary folds are often seen following mastectomy. The opacity of the breasts may obscure, or falsely suggest, lung pathology. Nipple shadows usually have clearer lateral than medial borders, and are usually found at or close to the levels of the ninth posterior ribs in males. Nipple markers usually clarify the nature of such rounded opacities.

BONES

Spine

The lower cervical and thoracic spine lies posteriorly in the neck and thorax, protecting the spinal cord. The cervical transverse processes point inferolaterally, whilst

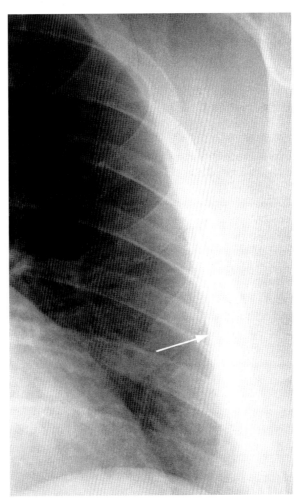

Figure 3.1 *Localized view of a chest radiograph showing the left chest wall with prominent extrapleural fat (arrow) which can simulate pleural fluid. This appearance was present bilaterally.*

those of the upper thoracic spine project superolaterally. The transverse processes are seen as 'thumbprint-like' opacities and may create composite densities where they cross the posteromedial rib. Covering part of the transverse processes with a finger can assist in deciding whether these apparent lesions are real or composite. On the lateral radiograph the cervicothoracic junction region is poorly seen.

Important radiographic features of the thoracic spine[1,2] include the following.

- On the lateral view, the cortical edges of each vertebra should be complete and well defined, except for the posterior borders which are frequently interrupted in a characteristic fashion.
- Lines drawn through the anterior and posterior borders of the thoracic vertebral bodies should form smooth curves.
- The posterior vertebral body height should not exceed the anterior height by more than 2 mm.[1]
- The vertebral bodies and disc spaces should have similar heights from level to level.
- On the frontal view the interpediculate distances of adjacent thoracic vertebrae should not vary by more than 2 mm, and should not exceed the larger of the interpediculate distances of either of the contiguous vertebrae.[3]

The paravertebral (or paraspinal) stripes

The paravertebral soft tissues form linear interfaces with the medial posterior lungs (Fig 3.2).[4-6] The right paravertebral stripe is infrequently seen unless displaced by osteophytes. It is usually less than 4 mm wide, but can occasionally be up to 10 mm thick.[5] The more constant left paravertebral stripe usually measures less than 12 mm across.[7] We use a maximum width of less than half that of the descending aorta from the lateral vertebral margin, except inferiorly. This stripe does not normally extend above the 4th thoracic vertebral body (T4).[6] The paravertebral stripe has the visual illusion of a white edge, while the subclavian artery and descending aorta appear to have black margins. These appearances both arise because of the Mach effect, a visual deception (Fig 3.2). Localized bulging, uniform widening or partial obliteration of the paravertebral stripes occur with aortic, mediastinal or vertebral injuries.

Ribs

The curvature of the ribs hinders their clear visualization on frontal views. They also slope steeply downward. Costal cartilages are only seen radiographically if calcified.

Clavicles

The clavicles articulate medially with the superolateral margins of the manubrium, anterosuperior to the first ribs at the level of T4 or T5. The inferiorly located

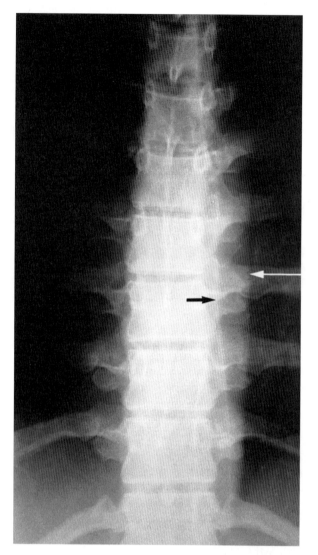

Figure 3.2 *A penetrated, collimated view of the thoracic spine demonstrating the positive Mach effect of the left paravertebral stripe producing a white margin (long arrow). The descending aortic interface with its negative Mach effect produces a black line (short arrow). The left paravertebral stripe starts superiorly at the level of the aortic arch and should be less than half the distance away from the vertebral edge than the width of the descending aorta. Notice the absence of the right paravertebral stripe.*

deltoid fossa of the medial clavicle may simulate a pathological lucency.

Sternum

The sternum is poorly seen on frontal radiographs. It is better visualized on lateral or oblique views, or tomography.

Scapulae

The scapulae are poorly visualized on chest radiographs. They may create apparent lesions on both frontal and lateral radiographs. The straight medial edge can

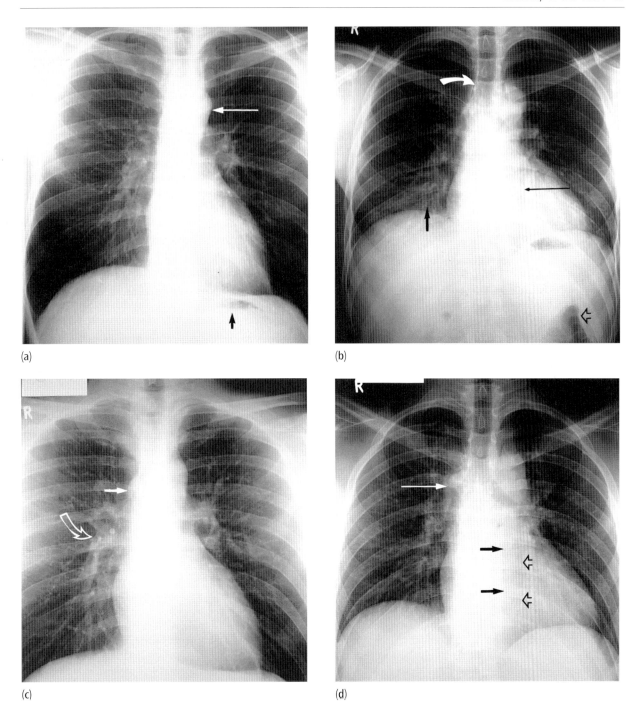

Figure 3.3 (a) A normal deep inspiratory erect frontal chest radiograph displaying a clearly defined lateral edge of aortic arch (long thin arrow), also known as the aortic knob or knuckle. At least six anterior ribs are seen above the dome of the diaphragm. Note the normal contour of hemidiaphragms. Also observe the more lucent left hemithorax due to the patient's rotation to the left. The pulmonary vessels are seen below the domes of the diaphragm. The stomach bubble (arrow) is in a normal position less than 20 mm from the left lung. (b) A normal expiratory erect frontal chest radiograph showing apparent cardiomegaly and increased basal lung markings which may simulate pathology, best seen on the right (arrow). Also note the splenic flexure of the colon indented (open arrow) by normal spleen. Note how the descending aortic outline (thin arrow) has shifted to the left compared with the inspiratory film (Fig 3.3a). The right paratracheal stripe is also demonstrated (curved arrow). (c) Normal well inspired supine chest radiograph showing a prominent azygous arch (arrow), the similar size of upper and lower lobe vessels and the even distribution of translucency. The right hilar point is well shown (open curved arrow). (d) Supine expiratory chest radiograph with widening of the superior mediastinum. The left paravertebral stripe (arrows) is well defined, commencing superiorly at the level of the aortic arch. The edge of the descending aorta (open arrows) is less clearly seen. Also note the prominent azygos vein (long arrow). Vessel size remains equal in upper and lower lungs. The heart appears larger than it does on either the supine inspiratory radiograph or the erect expiratory film. The carinal angle is widened.

simulate the pleural line of a pneumothorax on the frontal radiograph. On the lateral view, the straight anterior borders may run parallel to the trachea and suggest an air-containing tube. The bulbous inferior ends of the scapulae may simulate lung lesions on either frontal or lateral views.

The thoracic inlet/outlet

The thoracic inlet is encircled by a bony rim and slopes steeply anteroinferiorly. Enclosed anteriorly by the superior manubrium and medial clavicles, laterally by the first ribs and posteriorly by T1 vertebral body, it is narrow in an anteroposterior diameter and wide transversely. The lung apices bulge superior to the inlet. The sternocleidomastoid muscles extend obliquely across the thoracic inlet. The trachea, esophagus, subclavian vessels, common carotid and vertebral arteries, internal jugular and subclavian veins all pass through the inlet. The external jugular veins course laterally over the sternocleidomastoid muscles. The brachial plexuses, both phrenic and vagal nerves and the thoracic duct also traverse this space. Large muscle groups occupy the paravertebral space.

The mediastinum

THE SUPERIOR MEDIASTINUM

The superior mediastinum lies above the aortic arch and between the lungs (Fig 3.3). The anterior brachiocephalic veins pass in front of the brachiocephalic arteries and the centrally placed trachea and esophagus. The systemic vessels chiefly determine the width of the vascular pedicle.[8] This width is measured between the lateral margin of the origin of the left subclavian artery from the aortic arch, and the right edge of the superior vena cava (SVC) where it crosses the right main bronchus (Fig 3.3).[8] This width should be less than 58 mm on an erect posteroanterior (PA) chest radiograph, but can increase on average by 20% on a supine view.[9] The 2–4 mm thick superior esophageal stripes that are occasionally seen through the trachea represent the esophageal walls outlined by air.

THE AIRWAYS

The trachea starts at the fifth cervical vertebra (C5) and initially widens over a short distance as it descends. It enters the thorax in the midline opposite T3, overlying the spinous processes. It is then frequently deviated to the right by the aortic arch, ending approximately opposite T5 or T6 where it divides into the right and left main bronchi (Fig 3.3). The right paratracheal stripe should be less than 5 mm wide,[10,11] and be visible down to the azygos arch.

The airways may be difficult to visualize.

Delineation of the airways is improved by holding the radiograph at a vertical angle away from the viewing box.

The right main bronchus runs inferiorly at approximately 20° from the vertical; the left between 40 and 50°.[12] The right upper lobe bronchus passes superolaterally and the bronchus intermedius inferolaterally (Fig 3.3d). The longer left main bronchus is concave upwards as it runs laterally into the upper lobe bronchi, and continues inferiorly into the lower lobe bronchi.

On the lateral radiograph the posterior wall of the trachea is continuous with those of the bronchus intermedius and right lower lobe bronchus, and measures less than 4 mm. The slightly anteriorly curved left main bronchus is frequently just posterior to its right counterpart.

THE HEART

The right chambers of the heart occupy the right and anterior portion of the cardiac shadow; the left chambers are located to the left and posteriorly. Extrapericardial (also known as pericardial) fat pads are often present inferiorly. The right cardiac border is formed by the right atrium and abuts the middle lobe. The left border is constituted mainly by the left ventricle and lies against the lingula segment.

Both lateral cardiac borders should be clearly defined.

The main pulmonary artery, which is crossed by the left pulmonary artery, creates the left mediastinal interface leading up to the aortopulmonary window below the aortic arch. The normal left atrium may occasionally be seen on a frontal radiograph as an oval density inferior to the carina. The anteriorly situated cardiac shadow is frequently seen extending below the left diaphragmatic silhouette.

The cardiothoracic ratio is the ratio of the sum of the two maximum distances to which the heart projects from the midline, divided by the maximum transverse distance across the inner aspects of the ribs. The traditional upper limit of 50% on an adequately expanded PA chest in an adult, and 60% in young children, may be less valuable than is generally held.[7] In the supine position the horizontal displacement of the heart and the radiographic magnification of the anteroposterior (AP) projection increase the accepted upper limit (Fig 3.3c).

On the lateral radiograph (Fig 3.4) the posterior cardiac interface is formed superiorly by the left atrium

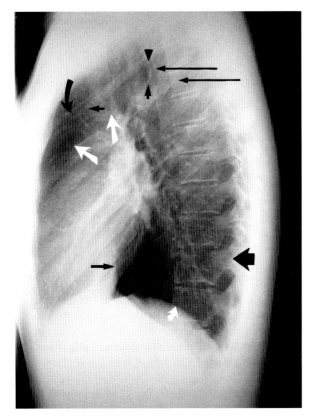

Figure 3.4 *Lateral chest radiograph illustrating anatomical features. Note the three lucent triangles which should be visible. These are the retrosternal triangle (curved arrow), the retrocardiac triangle (broad arrow) and the retrotracheal triangle (arrowhead). The vertebral bodies should become increasingly dark inferiorly. The posterior wall of the IVC (arrow) is seen. Also note the positions of the pulmonary artery (oblique arrows) and the ascending aorta and aortic arch (small arrows). The left hemidiaphragm (small curved arrow) is seen curving anteriorly where it is effaced by the heart shadow. The anterior edges of both scapulae are also visible (long thin arrows).*

and inferiorly by the left ventricle. The pulmonary artery forms the inferior part of the anterosuperior supracardiac border, with the anterior ascending aorta superior to it. Left ventricular enlargement is indicated by posterior displacement of cardiac border beyond the IVC of more than 18 mm at a point 2 cm superior to the level at which the IVC crosses the cardiac border.[13] Anterosuperior extension of the heart into the retrosternal space suggests right ventricular enlargement.

THE SYSTEMIC VESSELS

The aorta arises centrally in the mediastinum opposite the third anterior intercostal space. It initially runs anterosuperiorly and to the right. It is not usually visualized on the frontal radiograph, but may form a separate interface from that of the SVC. On the lateral radiograph the ascending aorta runs cephalad to the main pulmonary artery (Fig 3.4). After crossing anteriorly to the trachea, it turns posteroinferiorly, forming the visible part of the aortic arch to the left of T5.

> The margins of the aortic arch and the descending aorta should be clearly seen down to the diaphragm on adequately penetrated radiographs (Fig 3.3).

The inferiorly concave left subclavian artery interface curves superolaterally, disappearing at the level of the clavicle where it is surrounded by soft tissue (Fig 3.3c). The descending aorta normally veers slightly to the right as it descends.

The SVC is seen just to the right of the vertebral column, inferior to the clavicles. The right brachiocephalic vein may be seen merging with it superiorly (Fig 3.3c). On the lateral radiograph the SVC forms a broad pretracheal band. The azygous arch curves anteriorly in the right mediastinum to enter the posterior aspect of the SVC just inferior to the level of the aortic arch. There it forms an oval opacity at the lower end of the right paratracheal stripe in the tracheobronchial angle (Fig 3.3c). Its transverse diameter should not exceed 10 mm in an erect patient, or 16 mm in the supine position (Fig 3.3c).[7]

On the frontal radiograph, the right border of the inferior vena cava (IVC) can be seen ascending to join the right atrium, and overlying the cardiac shadow. On the lateral view, the posterior wall of the IVC is seen above the right hemidiaphragm and through the superimposed left ventricle (Fig 3.4).

THE ESOPHAGUS

This posterior structure is not visible radiographically unless it contains air or contrast. It deviates to the left as it approaches the esophagogastric junction, where it lies close to the left mediastinal pleura.

THE THORACIC DUCT

The thoracic duct passes upwards through the aortic hiatus in the diaphragm and runs up the right posterior mediastinum between the aorta and the azygos vein. At the level of T7 it crosses to ascend in the left mediastinum. It usually arches to enter the left subclavian vein close to its junction with the left internal jugular vein.

The lungs and pleura

THE HILA AND HILAR POINTS

The pulmonary arteries and veins are the main constituents of the hila opacities. The radiographic hila points are specifically defined radiographic loci that aid in the detection of lung volume alterations that displace or rotate the hila. The right superior pulmonary vein crossing the intermediate pulmonary artery defines the right hilar point (Fig 3.3c). The horizontal fissure approaches but does not cross this site. The left hilar point is at the convergence of the pulmonary arteries (Fig 3.3c). We find a location 6–8 mm above the concave upper margin of the left main bronchus more useful. The left hilum and hilar point are 15–25 mm superior to the right hilum and hilar point, as the left pulmonary artery unlike its right counterpart runs above its associated bronchus (Fig 3.3c).

THE SMALLER BRONCHI

The segmental airways are occasionally seen as 'pencil-thin' circles radiographically when viewed end on.

THE SEGMENTAL AND PERIPHERAL PULMONARY VESSELS

The pulmonary vessels produce nearly all the markings on the normal chest radiograph. Pulmonary arteries and veins are often difficult to distinguish, but are usually similarly affected by hemodynamic alterations. This diminishes the importance of making this distinction.

> The pulmonary vessels are normally clearly delineated.

They should extend to within 20–25 mm of the periphery of the lungs but this may not be clear on suboptimal radiographs. They should be visible below the diaphragmatic interfaces on adequately penetrated radiographs. The vessels are fairly evenly distributed throughout the lung and often have gently curving courses.[14] In the erect position the upper lobe vessels have a lesser diameter than do the lower lobe vessels at points equidistant from the hilum (Fig 3.3a).[15] On the supine radiograph these diameters approximate each other (Fig 3.3c, d).[14]

THE LUNGS

Both hemithoraces are of similar size and the lungs are equally translucent (Fig 3.3c). The lucency increases caudally on erect radiographs. This is well seen on the lateral radiograph where the lower thoracic vertebrae in the inferior retrocardiac triangle become increasingly dark inferiorly (Fig 3.4). The superior retrosternal area (Fig 3.4), when not covered by soft tissue, has a similar lucency to that of the inferior retrocardiac triangle. A further small lucent triangle is seen superior to the aortic arch, posterior to the trachea and anterior to the

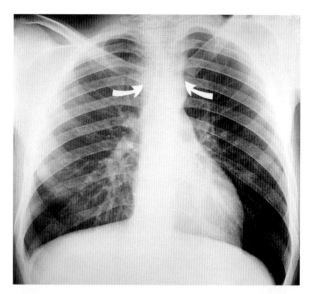

Figure 3.5 *A frontal chest radiograph demonstrating the effect of patient rotation on the difference in lucency of the two hemithoraces. The position of the medial end of each clavicle (curved arrows) shows that the left clavicle is further away from the midline than its right counterpart. The left hemithorax is consequently more lucent than the right. Viewing the left lung with a bright light reveals normal lung vasculature.*

vertebrae (Fig 3.4). On the supine radiograph, the lower lungs should be at least as lucent as the remainder of the lungs. A portion of the posterior right lung protrudes medially against the azygos vein and the esophagus, forming the azygoesophageal recess.

On the frontal radiograph, patient rotation can cause a difference in the lucency of the hemithoraces (Fig 3.5). The side on which the medial end of the clavicle is further away from the vertebral spinous process is the more lucent.

THE PLEURA

The two pleural layers encasing the lungs are not normally seen radiographically. The lateral costophrenic (CP) angles are acute, with inferiorly directed 'V' shapes (Fig 3.3a, d). These angles can be shallow in teenagers or in patients with hyperinflation. The medial cardiophrenic angles are more variable (Fig 3.3a).

On the lateral radiograph, the posterior CP angles should be acute and deep (Fig 3.4). The anterior sternophrenic and CP angles vary, but are often less acute and may be poorly defined. The CP recesses are fairly constantly related to the eighth rib in the midclavicular line, the 10th rib in the midaxillary line and the 12th rib posteriorly, with the inferior lung edges located a few centimeters superiorly. This distance depends on the degree of lung inflation.

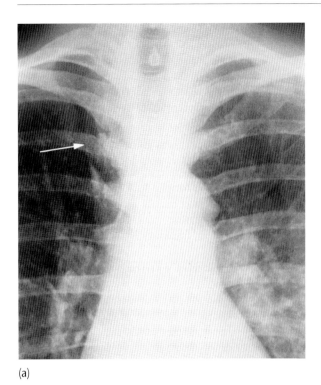

(a)

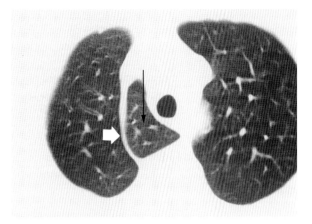

(b)

Figure 3.6 (a) A close-up view of the upper zones of the lung on a frontal chest radiograph showing an azygous fissure (arrow), causing a slightly veiled appearance to the medially located azygous lobe. (b) A CT scan through the upper chest demonstrating the azygous fissure (broad arrow) and the posteromedially positioned lobe (long thin arrow).

THE FISSURES

The horizontal fissure between the right upper and middle lobes is usually seen on both frontal and lateral radiographs. Starting medially at the bronchus intermedius, it extends laterally, crossing the anterior aspect of the fourth rib. It may deviate superiorly or inferiorly by up to 15° and is often not seen along its entire length. The fissure may appear duplicated as it undulates along its course. On the lateral radiograph it may appear to extend posterior to the oblique fissures.

The oblique fissures separate the right upper and middle lobes from the right lower lobe, and the left upper lobe and lingula from the lower lobe. They are usually only seen on the lateral radiograph. The oblique fissures commence superiorly at the level of T4 or T5. On computed tomography (CT) scanning, the left oblique fissure is usually seen superiorly at the level of the aortic arch. Inferiorly, the right fissure tends to be anterior to the left. Both fissures join the hemidiaphragm a few centimeters posterior to the sternophrenic junction.[16] These fissures may appear to be surprisingly posteriorly situated, falsely suggesting lower lobe volume loss. However, supporting evidence of volume loss, such as hilar displacement or rotation and compensatory hyperinflation, should be sought. The oblique fissures may also appear duplicated because of their undulating nature.

The azygous lobe fissure curves down from the apex of the right lung to the 'tear drop' of the azygous arch (Fig 3.6). It is usually easy to recognize. It may cause veiling of the azygous lobe, suggesting a pathological process.

The hemidiaphragms

The hemidiaphragms separate the thoracic contents from those of the abdomen. The right hemidiaphragm is usually 15–25 mm higher than the left. Each hemidiaphragm commonly peaks in the medial two-thirds of the hemithorax. Centrally the diaphragm is often flattened. The lateral halves descend fairly abruptly. The medial aspect of the left hemidiaphragm abuts the inferior cardiac surface and therefore is often not seen throughout its length.

On the lateral radiograph, the hemidiaphragms have anterior peaks with prominent posterior descents. The left hemidiaphragm is effaced anteriorly by the heart. Diaphragmatic configurations vary widely on both frontal and lateral radiographs.

> The hemidiaphragms should be crisp and clearly defined.

Overinflation of the lung can depress the hemidiaphragm and may produce a serrated appearance.

THE CHEST RADIOGRAPH IN TRAUMA: GENERAL PRINCIPLES

Importance

Although radiology plays a critical role in the investigation of patients with chest trauma, clinical evaluation and resuscitation take precedence in the patient's initial management. In dire emergencies radiology may have to be delayed, but thereafter is crucial for optimal planning and prioritization of treatment.

High and low velocity penetrating injuries, and blunt injuries have different imaging features and management considerations. Associated inhalation, aspiration and iatrogenic injuries should always be considered. Chest radiography is essential in injured patients in whom no clinical history is available. It can also reveal pulmonary conditions resulting from extrathoracic trauma.

Technique

The most commonly performed radiological examination in injured patients is the chest radiograph. The erect patient faces directly towards (PA) or away (AP) from the film for the routine frontal radiograph, which is taken in arrested deep inspiration. The PA radiograph places the anteriorly positioned heart close to the radiograph, thereby reducing the magnifying effect of the diverging x-ray beams and revealing the maximum area of the lungs.

In many injured patients only supine AP chest radiographs are obtainable. These may be of inferior quality to PA erect films. A lateral radiograph is also difficult to obtain in this situation, but may be very beneficial in diagnostic problems. The patient may be restless, unable to cooperate or to take a deep inspiration. Radiopaque supporting and immobilizing devices which may be superimposed on the radiograph should, wherever possible, be moved out of the region of interest. Potential medicolegal evidence should be retained and recorded.[17]

The suboptimal radiographs sometimes obtained may encourage a tendency to look only for prominent radiological abnormality.

The tendency to seek only gross changes on suboptimal films should be strongly resisted.

Assessment

A methodical and complete evaluation of each radiograph is essential.

The chest radiograph should be examined in a positive and analytical manner.

Once a regular system of examination has been developed and is consistently followed, such a routine does not take significantly longer than a haphazard, random and potentially incomplete approach. A personal mental 'tick list' of the aspects to be examined on each radiograph should be individually developed, refined and adhered to. Repeatedly examining the entire radiograph in a predetermined fixed order reinforces the habit and familiarizes one with the normal range of appearances. This routine is especially important when examining the radiograph under stressful conditions. Should a thorough initial examination of the radiographs not be performed because of urgent patient management needs, a complete re-examination should be performed at the first available opportunity. The suggested order of examination is as follows.

VERIFICATION OF THE RADIOGRAPH

The patient's name, identity number, the date and time of examination, and the labeling of the radiograph are verified. Permanent marker labels should indicate the left or right side of the radiograph. Marking the film after the exposure should be avoided, as conditions such as situs inversus and cardiomediastinal shift can lead to incorrect labeling.

EXAMINATION OF PREVIOUS RADIOGRAPHS

Ensuring that previous radiographs are available and are examined greatly aids the recognition of chronic disease which may otherwise be mistaken for an acute process (Fig 3.7), and allows for comparison of any alterations between radiographs.

ASSESSMENT OF THE QUALITY OF THE RADIOGRAPH

Six anterior and nine posterior ribs should be seen above the midpoint of the right hemidiaphragm on an adequately inspired radiograph. This is less likely to be achieved in the supine position. A poorly inspired radiograph may either obscure disease, or falsely suggest basal lung pathology because of vessel crowding and increased opacification (Fig 3.3b, d).

Patient rotation is assessed by comparing the distance of the medial end of each clavicle from the spinous process (Fig 3.5). In children, the relative lengths of the anterior ribs is a more useful guide. Rotation may affect lung lucency and produce apparent mediastinal shift, especially of anterior structures. Mediastinal and vascular configuration can also be altered. The SVC and the ascending aorta may appear displaced towards the right with apparent widening of the vascular pedicle in right-sided rotation.[8] Left-sided rotation may cause the left hilum to be obscured by the left cardiopulmonary opacity.

The outline of the thoracic spine should normally just be visible without the disc spaces being seen (Fig

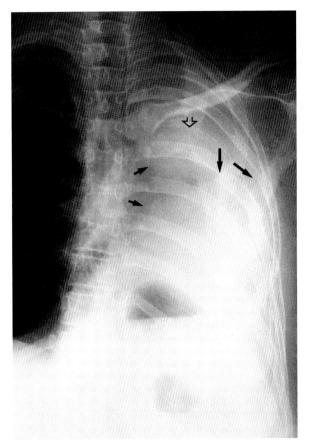

Figure 3.7 *An erect frontal expiratory chest radiograph revealing fresh rib fractures (long arrows), some of which are segmental, in a patient with a previous left pneumonectomy. Note the postsurgical rib changes (open arrow) and marked leftward mediastinal shift with no visible cardiac shadow. The stomach bubble is considerably raised from its expected position. Note the extension of the right lung across the midline (short arrows).*

3.5). However, more penetrated views are usually of greater value in the trauma setting (Fig 3.3d).

EXAMINATION OF THE CHEST RADIOGRAPH

> Each region of the radiograph should be examined with a focused awareness of the likely injuries in that area. Certain easily missed chest injuries may have serious consequences.

One should therefore specifically search for evidence of:

- A tension pneumothorax.
- Aortic and major vessel injuries.
- Tracheal and bronchial compromise.
- Cardiac and pericardial damage.
- Lung contusion.
- Diaphragmatic disruption.
- Sternal, vertebral or flail rib fractures.

The following anatomical areas need to be examined:

- The chest wall: the soft tissues including the inner chest wall; the bones.
- The mediastinum: the superior mediastinum, the right paratracheal stripe, the paravertebral stripes and the esophagus; the trachea and central bronchi; the cardiac shadow; the central systemic vessels including the descending aorta, and the aortopulmonary window.
- The lungs: the hila; the segmental bronchi; the pulmonary vessels; the lung parenchyma including the apices; the pleura; the fissures; the costophrenic and cardiophrenic angles.
- The hemidiaphragms.
- Adjacent regions: the neck; the subdiaphragmatic space.

Review areas

'Blind areas', including the lung apices and the retrocardiac and subphrenic regions should be reviewed. One should also specifically reassess the areas in which the serious conditions listed above may occur.

Radiopaque foreign bodies, central venous lines, nasogastric tubes, endotracheal tubes and surgical drains should always be sought and their positions carefully assessed.

The regions of the lateral radiograph are examined in a similar sequence to the frontal film, with the following specific additions:

- The thoracic vertebrae.
- The trachea and the posterior tracheal stripe.
- The retrotracheal triangle.
- The retrosternal area.
- The retrocardiac region.
- The area covered by the heart.

> Intrathoracic damage is frequently associated with concurrent injury to other regions of the body.

- Intrathoracic injury may arise from trauma below the diaphragm or above the thoracic inlet.
- Detecting damage to one intrathoracic organ does not preclude damage to another.
- Chest disease may follow from distant organ injury.
- Chest injury may cause distant organ involvement.

Specific examination of the trauma radiograph

CHEST WALL

Soft tissues

Attention is given to any distortions of normal outlines, to extrapleural bulges, localized soft tissue swellings, air

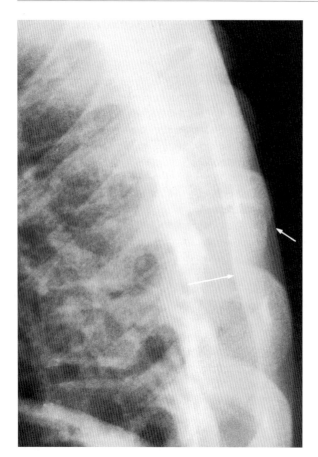

Figure 3.8 *A localized view of a lateral chest radiograph with a rib fracture (short arrow) and a small associated extrapleural hematoma (long thin arrow).*

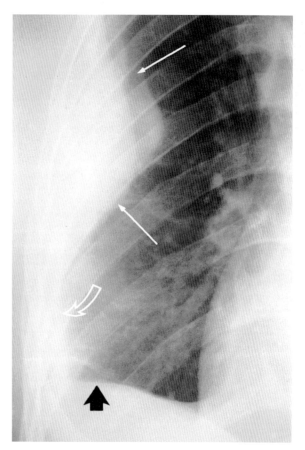

Figure 3.9 *The patient was stabbed in the chest. The typical appearance of lateral extrapleural hematoma (thin long arrows) is seen on this collimated frontal chest radiograph. Also note evidence of pleural fluid (curved open arrow). The lateral peak (broad arrow) of the right hemidiaphragm is a feature of subpulmonic fluid. The fluid was confirmed on a left-side-down decubitus view (not shown).*

in the tissue (surgical emphysema) or radiopaque foreign material. Focal change in a chest wall may be associated with a rib fracture (Figs 3.8, 3.9). Surgical emphysema indicates a breach of skin, lung, airway or hollow viscus and occasionally, gas-producing infection. This air is usually easily recognizable as lucent striations or loculations tracking along muscular planes (Fig 3.10), but it may be subtle. It is important to ensure that this is not air trapped under a breast, by bandages or in a wound. Increasing surgical emphysema may indicate a misplaced chest drain. A diffuse increase in chest wall width may result from intravascular fluid overload.

Bones

The important lower cervical vertebral region, although difficult to see, should be meticulously studied. The cervicothoracic junction is vulnerable to injury which is easily overlooked. Penetrated 'flying angel' or 'swimmer's' radiographs should be liberally used for this area, followed by tomography or CT scanning as needed.

The thoracic paravertebral stripes must be carefully examined.

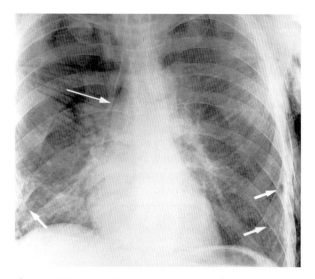

Figure 3.10 *An erect frontal chest radiograph with extensive surgical emphysema associated with bilateral rib fractures (short arrows) making detection of the bilateral pneumothoraces difficult. Note the normal right paratracheal stripe (long arrow).*

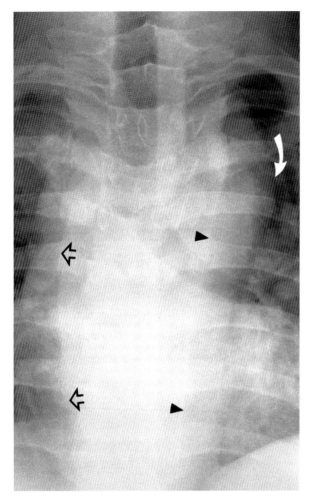

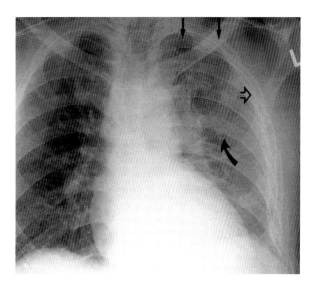

Figure 3.12 *Hemothorax. A supine frontal chest radiograph revealing multiple left lateral rib fractures (short arrows). Ribs 4–10 were found to be fractured at autopsy. A left hemothorax is causing diffuse left lung opacification (curved arrow). This was confirmed on the decubitus view. Note the preserved lung vessels on the left. Also note the abnormal left hemidiaphragmatic elevation, which should prompt consideration of diaphragmatic injury. There is also increased left retrocardiac density in keeping with the hemothorax. Pleural fluid is noted (open arrow).*

Figure 3.11 *A localized view of a supine frontal chest radiograph demonstrating the paravertebral stripes in a patient following severe crushing chest injury. The radiograph shows a markedly widened mediastinum measuring 97 mm. The left paravertebral stripe (arrowheads) is straight and just more than half the width of the descending aorta at T6, but appears to continue superior to the aortic arch. The aortic arch (curved arrow) is abnormally shaped and the aortopulmonary window and right paratracheal stripes are not defined. The right paravertebral stripe (open arrows) is displaced. The arch aortogram was entirely normal. The patient had suffered fractures of the third, fourth and fifth vertebral bodies and of both scapulae.*

- Vertebral fractures are frequently at multiple levels and can involve non-contiguous vertebrae. CT scanning may be of great benefit.[2]

Rib fractures are frequently not detected and their number underestimated. The cortical lines of the posterior, anterior and lateral portions of each rib need individual evaluation. The inferior edges of the medial sixth to eighth posterior ribs are often poorly defined. Ribs commonly fracture laterally. This is an area easily overlooked (Fig 3.12).

Any blurring or displacement of these stripes could indicate injury to adjacent structures.[2] A paravertebral hematoma following vertebral injury has many radiological features in common with a mediastinal hematoma (Fig 3.11).

- Dedicated spinal views are essential if any deviation from the normal spinal radiological anatomy is seen, or if a fracture is suspected clinically.

Examining the chest radiograph with the long axis of the spine in a horizontal orientation allows the ribs to be more easily followed. This maneuver highlights any rib abnormality.

If clinically indicated, oblique and collimated radiographs may be necessary to detect rib fractures (Fig 3.13). One should carefully exclude an associated pneumothorax. Lower rib fractures are often better seen on abdominal (Fig 3.14) or penetrated localized radiographs and may be associated with upper abdominal visceral injuries. Clinical evaluation and radiography are both important where a flail chest injury, defined as segmental fractures of three or more ribs, is suspected (Figs 3.7, 3.12, 3.15, 3.16).

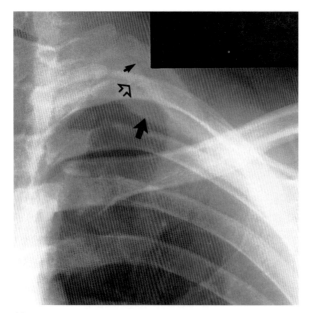

(a)

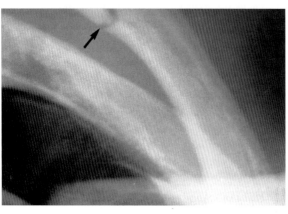

(b)

Figure 3.13 (a) Localized view of left lung apex demonstrating extrapleural hematoma (broad arrow) associated with first rib fracture (open and small arrows). (b) The apical oblique view demonstrates the inferior aspect of the fracture (arrow) more clearly. Note the radiographic errors: the patient's identity label partly covers the first rib on (a), and on (b) the rib is only partially included on the film.

The humeral head may erroneously appear superiorly displaced on a frontal chest radiograph. This should be clarified by clinical assessment. Fractures of the clavicles and especially the scapulae are easily overlooked on frontal radiographs, and commonly require special views for their diagnosis.

Sternal fractures are often subtle on frontal radiographs and not noticed on lateral views. Collimated lateral (Fig 3.17) or oblique radiographs and tomography or CT examinations are more helpful. An associated hematoma may simulate mediastinal widening on the frontal radiograph.

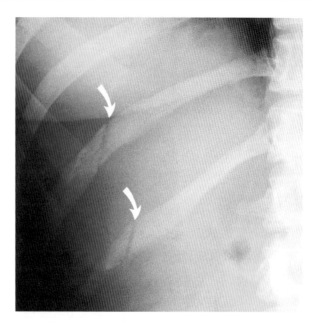

Figure 3.14 This localized view of an abdominal radiograph demonstrates oblique rib fractures of the 11th and 12th ribs (curved arrows). Underlying visceral injury should be suspected in association with these fractures. Lower rib fractures are often better seen on penetrated localized lower chest views or abdominal radiographs. These fractures were not visible on the chest radiograph (not shown).

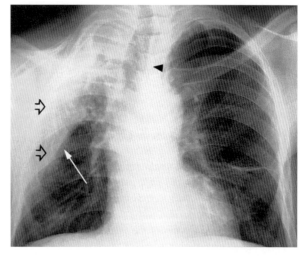

Figure 3.15 This frontal chest radiograph demonstrates a flail rib injury (open arrows) of the right hemithorax. Also note the associated extrapleural hematoma (long arrow). There is tracheal shift (arrowhead) to the right due to previous tuberculosis with right upper lobe fibrosis and volume loss.

Fractures of the scapulae, sternum and the upper three ribs may indicate considerable applied force, and are therefore markers of potential organ damage.

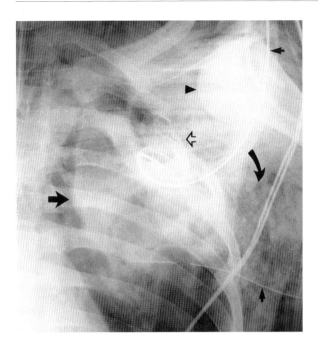

Figure 3.16 *A frontal supine chest radiograph revealing first and second left rib fractures with a free floating segment of second rib (open arrow). Underlying lung contusion and/or hematoma (broad arrow) is present – note the clear outline of the opacity. A dislocated left humeral head (arrowhead) is also shown. Surgical emphysema (curved arrow) and chest drains (small arrows) are present.*

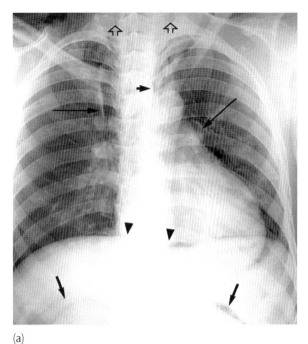

(a)

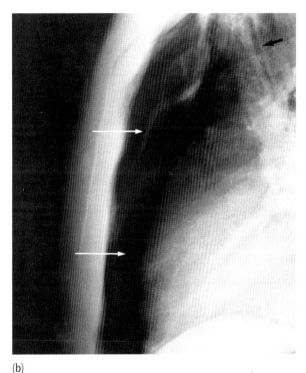

(b)

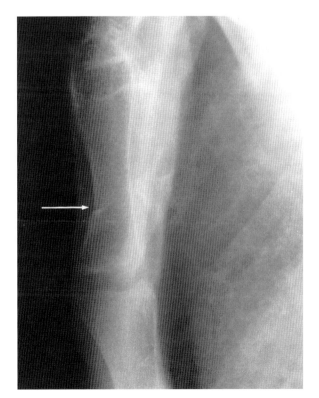

Figure 3.17 *Lateral radiograph of the manubrium showing an impacted fracture (long thin arrow). Underlying visceral injury should be suspected in association with sternal fractures.*

Figure 3.18 *This patient was stabbed in the neck, with a consequent anterior tracheal injury. (a) A frontal chest radiograph demonstrates perinephric retroperitoneal air (medium arrows). It also exhibits the 'continuous diaphragm' sign (arrowheads), the bilaterally displaced parietal pleural layers (long thin arrows), mediastinal lucency (short arrow) and well delineated aorta indicating a pneumomediastinum. Surgical emphysema is present in the lower neck (open arrows). (b) A localized view of the lateral chest radiograph performed 4 hours later reveals the retrosternal air associated with a pneumomediastinum (long arrows) and surgical emphysema (short arrow).*

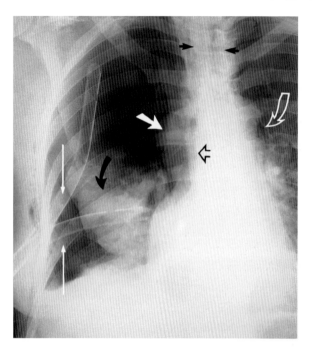

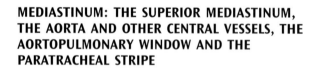

Figure 3.19 *Tracheal stab repaired at thoracotomy. An erect frontal chest radiograph of a patient rotated to the right, showing a large pneumothorax with two chest drains (long thin arrows) present. The opacified right middle and lower lobes (closed curved arrow) are located unusually inferiorly and laterally, simulating a 'fallen lung' suggesting a bronchial disruption. The right upper lobe appears to have collapsed against the mediastinum (oblique arrow). Notice the superior mediastinal air (small arrows) and the left mediastinal air, demonstrating the medial pleura (or periaortic fascia) (open curved arrow). The ascending aorta (open arrow) is unusually clearly defined. There is loss of clarity of the right hemidiaphragm with adjacent partially collapsed lung. A left pneumothorax was also present but is not demonstrated here.*

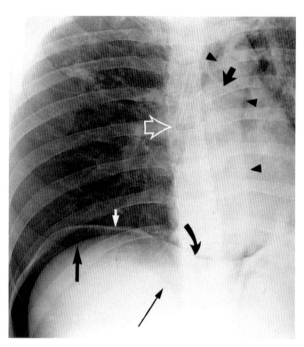

Figure 3.20 *Pneumomediastinum and pneumoperitoneum. The patient was stabbed in the neck. His trachea was transected. He then suffered a cardiac arrest and was vigorously resuscitated. This supine chest radiograph exhibits free subphrenic air (medium arrow) under the right hemidiaphragm (short arrow). Note the thickness of the right hemidiaphragm as compared with the pleural thickness in Figure 3.52. The endotracheal tube ends in the right main bronchus (open arrow). Note the clearly delineated aorta (arrowheads), both edges of the superior border of the left main bronchus (broad arrow) and the 'continuous diaphragm' sign (curved arrow) denoting the presence of a pneumomediastinum. There is also pleural air in the anterior cardiophrenic recess (long arrow). Also shown are bilateral upper lobe lung nodules with an elevated horizontal fissure. There is slight mediastinal shift to the left due to left-side volume loss, possibly as a result of the misplaced*

MEDIASTINUM: THE SUPERIOR MEDIASTINUM, THE AORTA AND OTHER CENTRAL VESSELS, THE AORTOPULMONARY WINDOW AND THE PARATRACHEAL STRIPE

Pneumomediastinum

Extraluminal air in the mediastinum can reach this site from the mouth, the esophagus, the trachea (Figs 3.18, 3.19), the bronchi, or from below the diaphragm. It commonly results from alveolar rupture and central tracking of air along the airways, the Macklin effect (Fig 3.20). A pneumomediastinum[1,18] should not arise from an uncomplicated pneumothorax.[19]

The appearance may be typical, with multiple linear lucencies (Fig 3.21), commonly extending into the retropharyngeal space (Fig 3.22). These linear mediastinal streaks are often well seen in the retrosternal area

on the lateral radiograph (Figs 3.18, 3.23). Delineation of the left border of the SVC (Fig 3.21), the brachiocephalic vessels, the azygos vein, the pulmonary artery and the ascending aorta (Figs 3.20, 3.21) may be seen.[20] A thin white line, the mediastinal or central parietal pleura, is frequently seen close to the left side of the heart (Figs 3.21, 3.23).

It may be difficult on occasions to distinguish a pneumomediastinum from a pneumothorax or pneumopericardium. The 'continuous diaphragm sign'[21] of a pneumomediastinum in which the superior aspect of the diaphragm is outlined by mediastinal air, is helpful if present (Figs 3.18, 3.20, 3.21), although this could theoretically occur in a large pneumopericardium. Pericardial air is limited superiorly by the confines of the superior pericardial recess, which only extends up to the level of the aortic arch. Decubitus

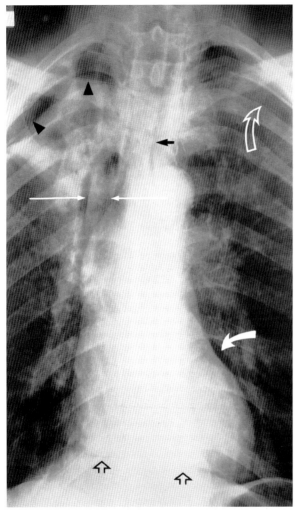

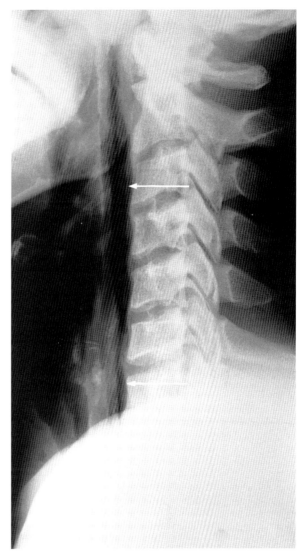

Figure 3.21 *A localized view of a frontal chest radiograph demonstrating a pneumomediastinum with linear lucencies in the mediastinum (short arrow) extending into the neck, the continuous diaphragm sign (open arrows) and air outlining the SVC (long arrows) and trachea (short arrow). The left paracardiac parietal pleura is seen (curved arrow). A small right apical pneumothorax (arrowheads) with adjacent consolidated lung is present, and is more easily seen than the left pneumothorax (open curved arrow).*

Figure 3.22 *A lateral radiograph of the neck showing superior extension of mediastinal air into the retropharynx (long arrows) in a patient following chest trauma.*

radiographs may assist by showing free movement of air within the pericardium, or a shift in the position of pleural air, whilst air in a pneumomediastinum should not change position. Clearly air can coexist in these different anatomical planes. A CT examination will show the presence of air and its location clearly, and can be used if clinically important.

Mediastinal hematoma and acute aortic injury

The patient with a blunt injury of the aorta may appear remarkably well. If the patient is markedly unstable, radiological investigations will be bypassed for urgent surgery. Coexistent damage, such as a ruptured

diaphragm or pelvic fractures,[22] may be present (Figs 3.24, 3.25).

The mediastinum widens in the supine position (Fig 3.3c, d), with poor inspiration, unfolded vessels, intravascular fluid overload, and mediastinal pathology. The width, and more specifically, the overall appearance of the superior mediastinum are of cardinal significance in the acutely injured patient, primarily because mediastinal hematoma is a marker of possible acute traumatic aortic injury. The mediastinal hematoma associated with aortic injury is not usually from the aorta itself, but from other mediastinal vessels.[6] The measurement of the width of the superior mediastinum is made just superior to the aortic arch from the left side of the origin of the left subclavian artery, to the right of the SVC. In a young patient, on an erect PA radiograph the superior mediastinum should not be significantly

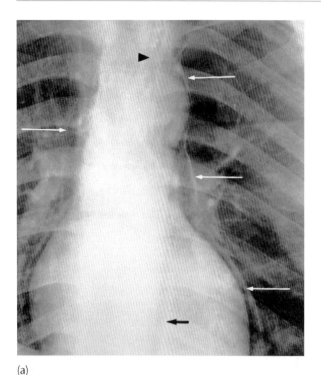

(a)

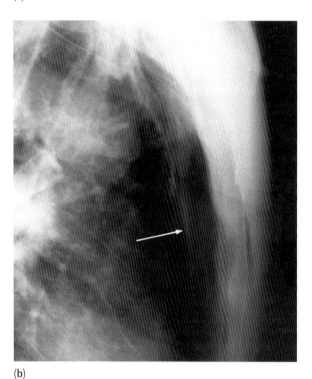

(b)

Figure 3.23 *This patient was involved in a motor vehicle accident. (a) A frontal supine chest radiograph demonstrates features of a pneumomediastinum. Notice bilateral mediastinal pleura outlined by mediastinal air extending above the aortic arch (long thin arrows) and the streaky linear lucencies in the mediastinum (arrowhead). The descending aortic parietal pleura is elevated by air (arrow). (b) A part of the lateral view reveals the retrosternal linear lucencies (long thin arrow) characteristic of a pneumomediastinum.*

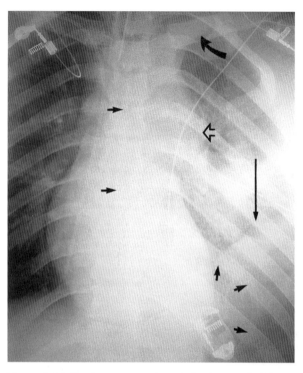

Figure 3.24 *Simultaneous aortic and diaphragmatic injury. Regional view of supine frontal chest radiograph showing part of an abnormal left hemidiaphragm (long thin arrow), homogenous left thoracic opacification as a result of a left hemothorax, and a nasogastric tube which passes superior to the expected level of the hemidiaphragm (small arrows). Note also the superior mediastinal abnormalities: an apical cap (curved arrow), indistinct and abnormal aortic arch contour (open arrow), filled-in aortopulmonary window, and loss of definition of the right paratracheal stripe in this patient. ECG leads and a central line in the right atrium are seen.*

wider than the underlying vertebral body. On a supine radiograph exposed at 100 cm, however, a width of 8 cm is usually accepted as the upper limit.[23]

More accurate predictors of a mediastinal hematoma than mediastinal widening are thought to be:[24]

- Loss of clarity, loss of continuity or abnormal configuration of the aortic arch (Figs 3.24–3.27), the descending aortic contour (Fig 3.26), or the aortopulmonary window (Figs 3.24, 3.25, 3.27).
- Widening or loss of clarity of the right paratracheal stripe (Figs 3.24–3.28) or of the paravertebral stripes (Figs 3.24, 3.26, 3.27, 3.29).[25]
- The extension of the left paravertebral stripe above the level of the aortic arch.[6]

The margins of the aortic arch and descending aorta should be clearly seen. A well penetrated exposure is essential.[24,26]

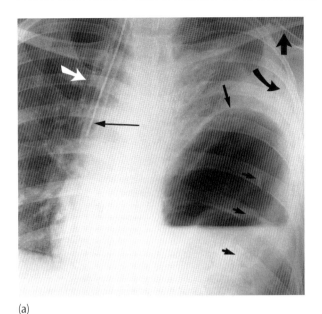

(a)

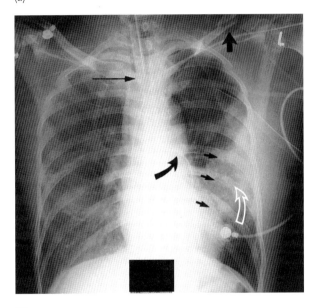

(b)

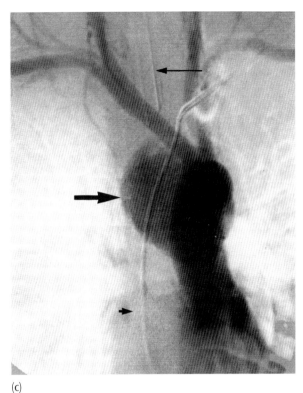

(c)

Figure 3.25 *Ruptured left hemidiaphragm and aortic injury following a motor vehicle accident. (a) A rupture of the left hemidiaphragm with herniation of stomach and colon (medium arrow) into the left chest is seen on the chest radiograph. The mediastinum is displaced to the right. The endotracheal tube (long arrow) is in the right bronchus. Rib fractures (short arrows) and a peripheral left extrapleural or pleural hematoma (curved arrow) are present. The left side of the superior mediastinum, the aortopulmonary window and the aortic arch are obscured. The right paratracheal stripe (oblique arrow) is indistinct and measures 4 mm across, which is just within the limits of normality. A left clavicular fracture (broad arrow) is also evident. (b) A mobile supine chest radiograph performed 2 days after repair of the ruptured left diaphragm shows a uniform increase in density of the right hemithorax, indicating probable pleural fluid. Lung contusion is present in the left lung (open curved arrow). The vessel outlines are preserved on the right and obscured on the left. The left clavicular fracture (broad arrow) and the rib fractures (short arrows) are again evident. A pulmonary artery catheter (closed curved arrow) and an endotracheal tube (long arrow) can also be seen. The right paravertebral stripe is difficult to define. There is filling in of the aortopulmonary window and a double outline is present. The descending aortic outline and the right paratracheal stripe are not well defined, but there is increased density in the area. (c) A frontal view of an intravenous digital subtraction aortogram demonstrating a large false aneurysm (arrow) projecting from a ruptured aortic arch. Partially subtracted endotracheal tube (long thin arrow) and venous catheter (short arrow) extending into the right atrium can be seen.*

It is relatively easy to miss a loss of continuity of any interface. The natural tendency appears to be to 'close the gap' between two ends of an interrupted line and thus to overlook the discontinuity.

A useful maneuver, perhaps best termed the 'two-finger test', can be employed to counteract the tendency to overlook any interruption.

The index and middle fingers are placed about 20 mm apart on the line or interface being examined, and are then moved along the interface while concentrating on the integrity and continuity of the exposed portion between one's fingers. This may also be applied to other

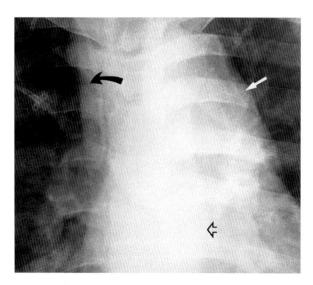

Figure 3.26 *False aneurysm and AV fistula. An erect frontal chest radiograph in a patient who had suffered a chest stab wound. Note the very abnormal contour of the aortic arch (arrow), the wide superior mediastinum and the abnormal bulge (open arrow) of the left paravertebral stripe. The right paratracheal stripe is not seen. A central venous catheter is also shown in the SVC (curved arrow).*

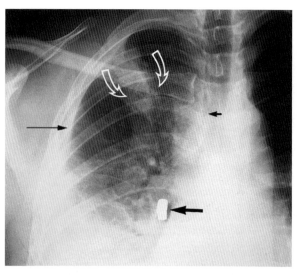

Figure 3.28 *A frontal chest radiograph in a patient who sustained a gunshot injury to the right upper chest. Notice the bullet (arrow), which has created a band of opacification (open curved arrows), caused by lung laceration and hemorrhage along its course through the lung. Note also the right lateral pleural blood (long arrow), apparently widened right mediastinum and loss of clarity of the lower right paratracheal stripe (short arrow).*

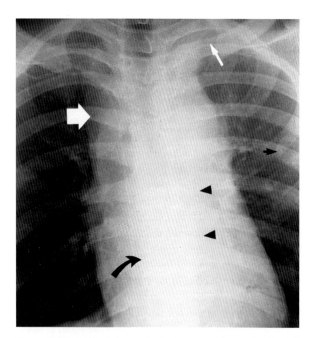

Figure 3.27 *Aortic stab, repaired at surgery. The supine frontal chest radiograph demonstrating an abnormal and wide superior mediastinum, measuring 8.5 cm in width. A small left apical cap (medium arrow) is noticed extending superior to the medial left clavicle. The aortic arch is partially concealed, with the left paravertebral stripe (arrowheads) visible. The aortopulmonary window is hidden and filled in. The inferior right paratracheal stripe is obscured. The SVC interface is displaced and irregular (broad arrow). A central venous catheter (curved arrow) is incidentally noticed in the right atrium where it may provoke arrhythmias or cause a perforation. A small granuloma is seen peripherally in the left upper lung (small arrow).*

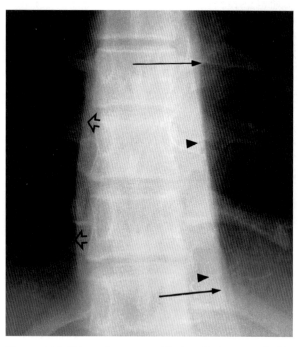

Figure 3.29 *This patient was stabbed, suffering a small chip fracture of the T12 vertebral body and an aortic laceration which was later surgically repaired. A collimated frontal radiograph of the thoracic spine exhibits the 7 mm wide right (open arrows) and 17 mm wide left (arrowheads) paravertebral stripes. Note the varying widths of the stripes, and that the left stripe is superimposed on that of the descending aorta (long arrows), indicating abnormality. Note that the left paravertebral stripe does not extend above the aortic arch.*

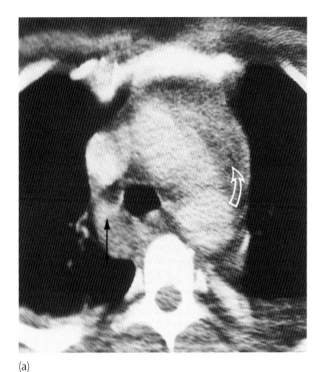

(a)

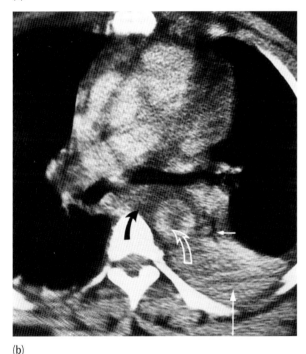

(b)

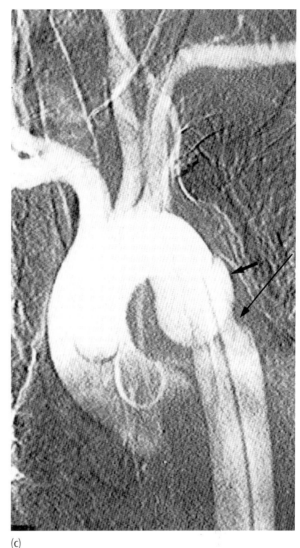

(c)

Figure 3.30 *The patient was involved in a motor vehicle accident. Chest radiograph (not shown) suggested a mediastinal hematoma. (a) CT scan with intravenous contrast medium at the level of aortic arch demonstrates periaortic hematoma (open curved arrow). The hematoma in the right paratracheal area (long arrow) shows how the paratracheal stripe can be effaced or widened by a mediastinal hematoma. (b) A section through the descending aorta reveals further hematoma anteromedial to the aorta (closed curved arrow). Also seen are a rounded lucency (open curved arrow) in the lumen of the descending aorta, high density pleural fluid (long thin arrow) and adjacent lung atelectasis with an air bronchogram (short arrow). (c) The patient had an absent right femoral pulse and a weak left femoral pulse. A digital subtraction arch aortogram performed by a femoral approach demonstrates a false aneurysm (medium arrow) and focal narrowing (long arrow) at the aortic isthmus. These features are those of an acutely acquired traumatic aortic coarctation. The lucency on the CT scan (b) (open curved arrow) was felt to represent a cross-section through the narrowed aortic wall projecting into the aortic lumen.*

continuous radiological lines or interfaces such as the two hemidiaphragms, the paravertebral stripes and the cardiac borders.

Interruption of the aortic interface may arise from contiguous hematoma, hemothorax or medial pleural fluid, or from pulmonary collapse, contusion or consolidation.

Other described radiological signs suggestive of aortic injury which we find of less practical assistance include:

- A shift of the trachea or esophagus (as delineated by a nasogastric tube) to the right of the T4 spinous process.
- A left apical cap (Figs 3.24, 3.27).
- Left pleural fluid.
- Depression of the left main bronchus.

In addition, an interruption of linear aortic wall calcification has been described as a sign of aortic injury.[27]

If uncertainty about the normality of the superior mediastinum exists, and the patient is able to stand or sit upright, a well penetrated PA[28] and possibly a lateral erect radiograph should be obtained. These may demonstrate a normal mediastinum, or a hematoma associated with sternal or vertebral fractures simulating mediastinal widening. Unless these radiographs show an entirely normal mediastinum, further investigation is indicated. Even with a normal chest radiograph, if there is a very strong clinical suspicion of an aortic injury, angiography may be required.[26,29]

If the superior mediastinum is abnormal on the erect radiograph, thoracic aortography is indicated. Approximately one in 10 angiograms will demonstrate aortic injury using the radiological criteria mentioned above. If the appearance of the mediastinum is equivocal and there is a low clinical suspicion of injury to the aorta, a CT examination may be performed to exclude a mediastinal hematoma (Fig 3.30).[29-37] This would especially be indicated if the patient is already undergoing a CT examination.

CT changes that suggest aortic injury include a mediastinal hematoma, a change in the contour and diameter of the aorta and an intimal flap (Fig 3.30).

Mirvis et al. state that mediastinal hematomas seen on CT always extend to the paravertebral area or to the superior or middle mediastinum and do not involve the anterior or posterior mediastinum in isolation.[33] Helical CT scanning improves the detection of aortic injury, particularly with CT arteriography (CTA).[32] If the mediastinum is normal on CT, an angiogram would not usually be undertaken. If a mediastinal hematoma is present, aortography is indicated (Fig 3.30). Should there be doubt concerning the presence of a hematoma, a repeat CT study with intravenous contrast medium may be helpful. One should, however, bear in mind the effect of the added contrast medium in these compromised patients.

Any focal bulge, obscuration or widening of the mediastinal contours after a penetrating injury is an indication for angiography.

Linear calcification of the aortic arch which is displaced from the aortic edge, and especially if this distance has increased since a previous radiographic examination, should suggest the possibility of aortic dissection.

TRACHEA AND CENTRAL BRONCHI

> The trachea and bronchi need careful inspection throughout their entire length.

The trachea and bronchi should be followed individually, searching for any foreign body, lumenal opacification, narrowing or occlusion.

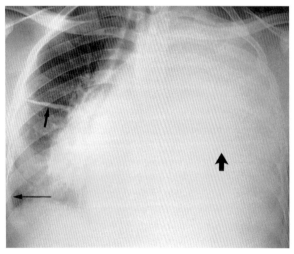

(a)

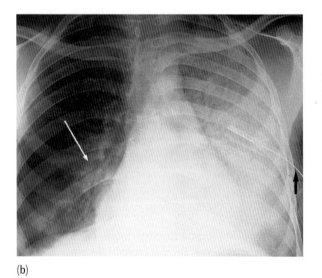

(b)

Figure 3.31 (a) A frontal chest radiograph revealing a large left chylothorax (broad arrow) causing marked mediastinal shift to the right. A small peripheral pleural effusion (thin long arrow) and a thickened horizontal fissure (medium arrow) are also shown on the right. The right juxtacardiac lung appears compressed. Radiologically chylothorax does not differ from other pleural fluid collections. (b) An erect chest radiograph taken 3.5 hours later, after drainage, exhibits diffuse left lung opacification probably due to re-expansion pulmonary edema. The heart has shifted back from the right. There is still middle lobe opacification (long thin arrow). The left chest drain is also shown (medium arrow).

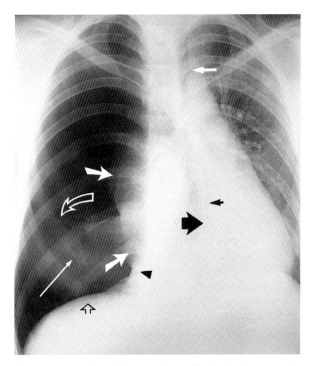

Figure 3.32 *A frontal chest radiograph showing features of a right tension pneumothorax. There is marked mediastinal shift to the left, as shown by tracheal shift (medium arrow) and displacement of the azygoesophageal recess (short arrow). Note the expansion of the right hemithorax and depression of the right hemidiaphragm, (open arrow), displacement and compression of right cardiac contour, and collapsed right upper and lower lung lobes (oblique arrows). The right middle lobe (open curved arrow) is tethered laterally by adhesions and is only partially collapsed. Note the prominent left lung vessels due to shunting of blood to the left lung. The IVC (arrowhead) is outlined by air. The nipple shadow on the right (long arrow) is also shown.*

Radiographically dense structures such as the aortic arch and vertebral pedicles frequently may appear to indent the trachea falsely, but on careful inspection the tracheal wall will usually be seen crossing these structures.

Linear tomography and CT scanning delineate the airways, extraluminal air and hematomas well.

Thoracic scoliosis and patient rotation may cause apparent shift of the trachea from the midline. Lung fibrosis (Fig 3.15) and volume loss (Figs 3.7, 3.20) pull the trachea towards the diseased hemithorax, whilst the airway may be pushed away by space-demanding lesions such as a hemothorax, hydrothorax (Fig 3.31) or tension pneumothorax (Fig 3.32).

The trachea and bronchi can be disrupted by blunt[38–41] or penetrating[41] injury. Penetrating injuries can occur anywhere along their lengths, whereas blunt trauma usually affects either the subglottic area directly, or the regions just above or below the carina. There may be no radiological signs, or the signs of injury may be delayed.

Extraluminal mediastinal air should specifically be sought.

The signs of airway injury include[39]:

- A pneumomediastinum (Figs 3.18, 3.19), occasionally forming a cuff of air around the airway.
- Deep cervical air (Fig 3.18).
- Surgical emphysema.
- Unilateral or bilateral pneumothoraces (Fig 3.19). These can occur with or without a pneumomediastinum. They may be massive, under tension and resistant to tube drainage, but can also be small and resolve with drainage.[39]
- Lung collapse.
- A widened or indistinct mediastinum.
- Occasionally, if a bronchus is transected, the lung may fall away from the hilum producing the 'fallen lung' sign.[42]

Additional signs include:

- An overdistended endotracheal (ET) cuff of over 25 mm diameter.[38] This may also be seen with esophageal intubation.
- An ET cuff which bulges beyond the outline of the tracheal wall.
- An ET cuff within 15 mm of the distal end of the ET tube.[38]
- A misplaced ET tube.
- Angulation or truncation of the airway.

A CT examination may demonstrate these signs with increased sensitivity. Vascular and esophageal injuries may occur together with airway injury.

It is essential to examine the important right paratracheal stripe described in the anatomy section. This may occasionally be difficult to define clearly.

On an adequately penetrated film, widening or blurring of the right paratracheal stripe indicates a possible mediastinal injury.

HEART[17,18]

The cardiac borders should be carefully traced and fully examined. Exposing small sections of the interface using the 'two-finger test' described above in the mediastinal section, is very useful. Loss of continuity of the cardiac interface can signify adjacent lung contusion, collapse or consolidation, or a large or anteriorly positioned pleural collection. The presence of focal bulging should raise the possibility of a pericardial injury or defect with associated hematoma or cardiac herniation (Fig 3.33).

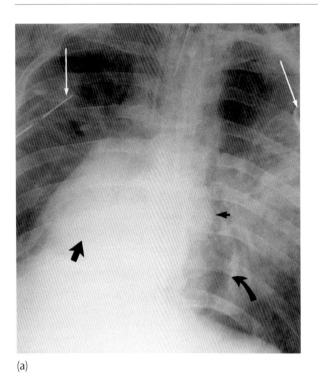

(a)

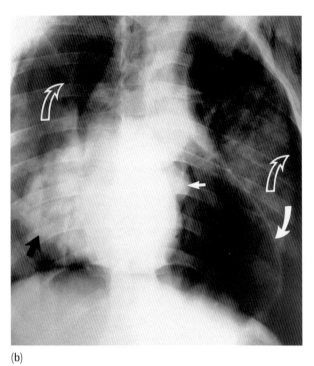

(b)

Figure 3.33 *Motor vehicle accident. The patient developed a tension pneumothorax. Regional view of (a) a supine frontal and (b) a right-side-down decubitus radiograph done on the same day. A right-sided cardiac dislocation (broad arrow), which occurred through a pericardial defect, simulates dextrocardia. An opacity to the left of the spine (arrow) is possibly the left atrial appendage. The pneumopericardium (closed curved arrow) is more distinct on the decubitus view, which also accentuates the pneumothoraces (open curved arrows), which are well seen because of adjacent lung contusion. Bilateral chest drains (long arrows) are noted. Rib fractures (not shown) were also present. The lung changes suggest contusion.*

> The densities of the left and right sides of the heart shadow should be similar.

Apart from the vascular structures seen through the heart, no other opacities should be visible (Figs 3.12, 3.34–3.36).

Cardiac contusion, infarction and hemopericardium[43] should always be considered in the appropriate clinical setting. Acute intrapericardial hemorrhage does not necessarily expand the pericardium (Fig 3.36).[43]

> Cardiac tamponade can occur with little alteration in cardiac size or configuration (Fig 3.36).

The presence and quantity of pericardial fluid can usually be reliably demonstrated by an ultrasound (US) examination (Fig 3.37). Cardiac tamponade can cause distension of the azygos vein (Fig 3.36), the IVC, the hepatic and renal veins and periportal edema.[18] If US visualization is limited by overlying bandages or

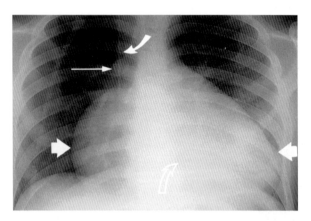

Figure 3.34 *A supine frontal chest radiograph demonstrating a globular cardiac shadow (broad arrows) as the result of a hemopericardium following a precordial stab 15 days previously. The size of the pericardial shadow suggests a gradual accumulation of blood. Note the distended azygos vein (long arrow) and the central venous catheter (curved arrow) which just extends into the right atrium. The increased left retrocardiac opacity (curved open arrow) and the diffuse increase in left lower lung opacification probably represent encysted pleural fluid or lung collapse/consolidation, possibly resulting from pressure on the left bronchus. The lungs are relatively clear with well defined vessels, suggesting chronic cardiac disease is unlikely.*

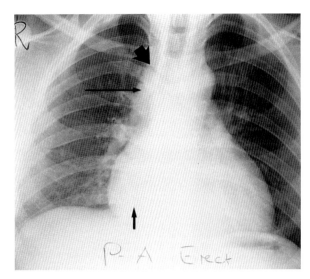

Figure 3.35 *Patient clinically suspected of cardiac tamponade following a chest stab. PA erect frontal chest radiograph showing a large globular cardiac shadow with increased right retrocardiac opacity (arrow). Note the clear cardiac outline and the prominent azygos vein (long arrow) and SVC (broad arrow). The difference in lucency between the two hemothoraces may be due to patient rotation. An ultrasound examination (not shown) confirmed fluid and clot in the pericardium. A hemopericardium and a sealed injury of the right ventricle were found at surgery.*

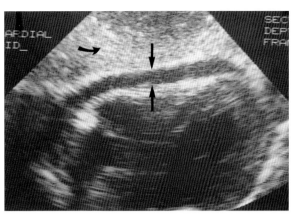

Figure 3.37 *This patient was stabbed in the left parasternal area. The chest radiograph revealed a slightly enlarged cardiac shadow and prominent upper lobe vessels. Transverse epigastric ultrasound revealing a moderate size hemopericardium (arrows). The left lobe of liver (curved arrow) lies superficial to the pericardium; the left and right ventricles lie deep to the pericardial space. This patient subsequently developed an aortopulmonary fistula.*

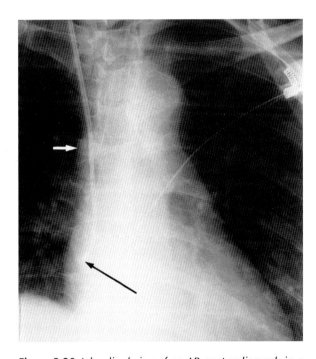

Figure 3.36 *A localized view of an AP erect radiograph in a patient who had recently undergone a liver transplant. During the postsurgical period she collapsed. A pericardial effusion was demonstrated, which at surgery consisted of 300 ml of parenteral nutrition fluid. The tip of the central catheter (long thin arrow) had perforated the right atrium. The azygos vein (arrow) is prominent in keeping with pericardial tamponade.*

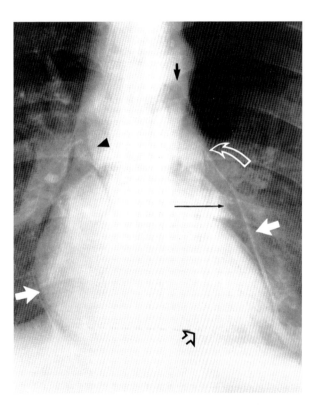

Figure 3.38 *An erect frontal chest radiograph showing a pneumopericardium limited by the superior pericardial recess above (small arrow), with the pleuropericardial lines well seen (broad arrows). Note the difference in thickness between the two sides. Within the pericardium the left atrial appendage (long arrow), the pulmonary artery (curved open arrow) and the ascending aorta (arrowhead) are clearly outlined by air. A left pneumothorax is also present. The surgical staples of the precordial stab wound are faintly seen (open arrow).*

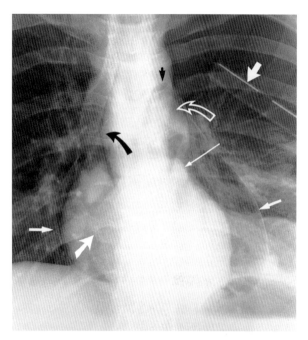

Figure 3.39 *A localized part of an erect frontal chest radiograph demonstrating a pneumopericardium with the thin pleuropericardial line well seen (medium arrows). Within the pericardium the left atrium (oblique arrow) and its appendage (long arrow), the pulmonary artery (open curved arrow) and the ascending aorta (curved arrow) are clearly outlined by air. Note how far superiorly the superior pericardial recess extends (small arrow). A left chest drain is present (broad arrow). The heart appears compressed. A left pneumothorax is present, not shown on this radiograph. Left lung contusion was suspected. The left basal changes suggest the presence of left pleural fluid.*

Figure 3.40 *A 1-year-old child with an iatrogenic esophageal rupture. (a) The supine frontal chest radiograph reveals a right tension pneumothorax and right middle and lower lobe collapse (broad arrow), with mediastinal shift despite two right chest drains (medium arrow). Note also the nasogastric tube (long arrow) and the left retrocardiac consolidation (open arrow). Naclerio's 'V' sign (arrowhead and small arrow) associated with lower esophageal rupture is also shown. (b) A close-up view showing air bronchograms in the left retrocardiac area (open arrow) and Naclerio's 'V' sign produced by mediastinal (short arrows) and extrapleural supradiaphragmatic air in the left cardiophrenic angle (arrowheads), indicating an esophageal leak. (c) A CT scan revealing a drain (arrow) lying either within lung parenchyma or a fissure, and possibly entering the mediastinum. Note also the pneumothorax (long arrow), pleural fluid (short arrow) and air locules (open arrows) in the pleural space. A nasogastric tube (arrowhead) is present.*

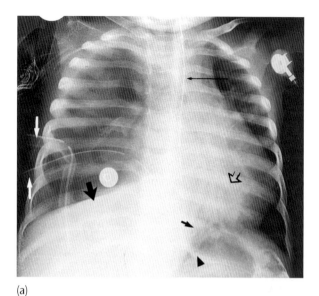

(a)

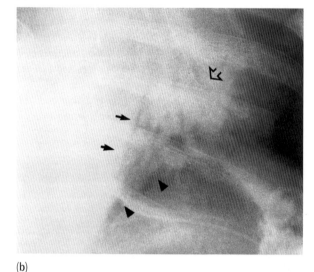

(b)

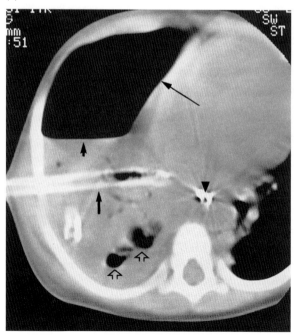

(c)

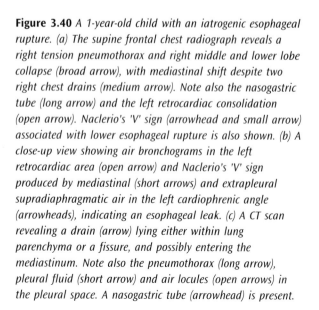

subcutaneous air, a CT or transesophageal echocardiogram (TEE) examination is recommended.

A pneumopericardium is usually readily recognized if the combined pleura and pericardium is thicker than normal pleura on its own, and if it has an irregular inner edge (Figs 3.38, 3.39). The intrapericardial structures may be outlined by air. Pericardial air can be bilateral, and is limited superiorly by the superior pericardial recess just below the aortic arch (Figs 3.38, 3.39). It may be difficult to differentiate from a medial pneumothorax or pneumomediastinum when the combined pericardial and pleural layer is thin (Figs 3.38, 3.39). A decubitus radiograph can be helpful in showing shift of air to the opposite side of the pericardium.

Air fluid levels close to the heart are not necessarily horizontal, as cardiac contractions can cause motion in the fluid.

ESOPHAGUS

A ruptured or lacerated esophagus may present with very little radiological change. However, the following signs may be present[18]:

- A pleural effusion.
- A pneumothorax (Fig 3.40).
- A hydropneumothorax.
- A pneumomediastinum (Fig 3.41), which may be localized.
- Swelling and loss of clarity of the mediastinal structures.
- Displacement of the trachea.
- A widened paratracheal stripe.
- Naclerio's 'V' sign[44]

Naclerio's 'V' sign in the left cardiomediastinal angle is produced by the junction of two layers of air, one in the mediastinum, and the other extrapleural above the left hemidiaphragm (Fig 3.40). It is strongly suggestive of a ruptured lower esophagus.

In esophageal injuries the air leak is frequently localized. This is well seen on CT.

An esophagogram should be performed in four orthogonal views, first using Gastrografin [meglumine and sodium diatrizoate (Schering)], and if necessary, a dilute barium suspension thereafter (Fig 3.41).

LUNG

The hila
The normal direction of the bronchi and hilar vessels should be confirmed. Displacement or rotation of the radiological hila usually indicates loss of lung volume (Fig 3.42). The hilar vessels should be well defined. Loss of clarity implies an adjacent pathological process in the adjacent lung. In patients with a large pleural effusion, the main bronchus may spuriously appear to be occluded.

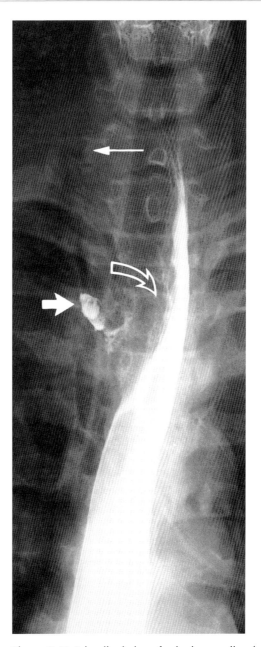

Figure 3.41 *A localized view of a barium swallow in a patient with a central chest stab demonstrating a leak of contrast agent at the site of the esophageal injury (broad arrow). Also note the compression of the esophagus by an adjacent hematoma (open arrow). The pneumomediastinum and surgical emphysema in the lower neck (thin arrow) are also seen.*

The segmental and subsegmental bronchi
The bronchi are not usually seen beyond their main segmental divisions. On occasions when the normal left upper lobe bronchus is poorly seen, the visible left lower lobe bronchus may deceptively suggest left bronchus depression (see Fig 3.3d).

The bronchi may be truncated by disruption, by intraluminal material, or by compressive hematoma. The main features of the associated lobar collapse are

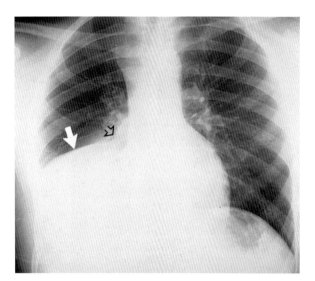

Figure 3.42 *Frontal chest radiograph showing right middle and lower lobe collapse (broad arrow) and compensatory shift of the mediastinum towards the right. The right hemithorax is smaller than its left counterpart with rib crowding. The right interlobar artery (open arrow) can be seen entering the collapsed lobes.*

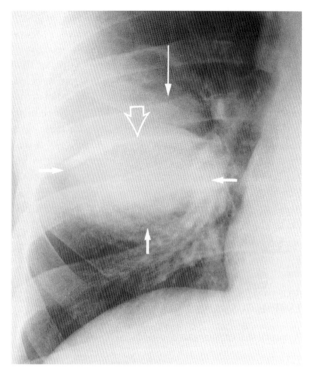

(a)

displacement of the fissures, trachea, mediastinum, hila and the hemidiaphragm (Figs 3.15, 3.42). The normal positions of these structures should be established by the regular, systematic scrutiny of all radiographs.

As with the trachea, bronchi can be 'pushed' or 'pulled' (Fig 3.15) by a pathological process. A medially or posteriorly situated pleural effusion can cause deviation of the associated bronchus and pulmonary vessels away from the opacity. In consolidation or collapse, the bronchus and vessel may enter the posteromedial opacity (Fig 3.42). This can be difficult to assess on the lateral radiograph because of the overlying vessels from the other side.

The bronchial walls may be thickened by fluid in cardiac failure or intravascular volume overload, or by cellular infiltrate in bronchial inflammatory airways diseases.

Lung parenchyma, including lung contusion

Skin bandages, soft tissue swelling or pleural fluid can increase the hemithorax density, simulating lung disease. A lateral radiograph may be helpful in demonstrating these conditions, especially when the cause is extrapulmonary. It may be difficult to decide on the acuteness or chronicity of lung opacification if previous radiographs are not available. Acute traumatic changes superimposed on chronically diseased lung may produce unusual appearances.

Multiple regions of the thorax may be injured during the same traumatic event.

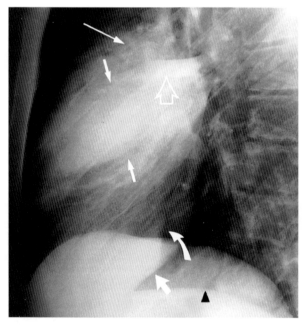

(b)

Figure 3.43 *(a) Frontal and (b) lateral chest radiographs of a large, fairly well defined intrapulmonary hematoma (medium arrows), with an overlying layer of blood in the horizontal fissure (open arrow) and contusion superiorly (long arrow). Note also the posterior wall of the IVC (curved arrow). Note how the heart obliterates the anterior border of the left hemidiaphragm (arrowhead) on the lateral view. The triangular area (broad arrow) created by overlap of the right hemidiaphragm and inferior aspect of the heart should not be mistaken for an abnormal opacity.*

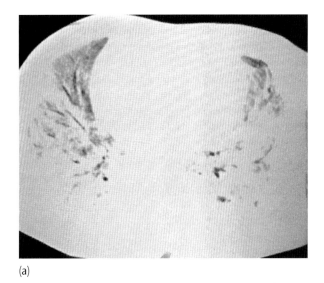

(a)

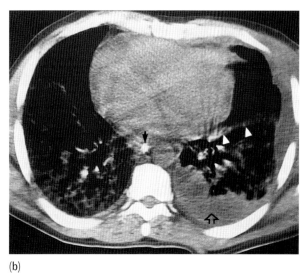

(b)

Figure 3.44 *The patient was stabbed 10 days previously with chest, diaphragm and stomach injuries. Gastric content entered the left thoracic cavity, resulting in septic shock. (a) CT scan on lung settings showing the diffuse consolidation of ARDS. (b) At the same level on different settings, a left posterolateral encysted pleural fluid collection is seen (open arrow). Fluid is present in the oblique fissure (arrowheads). The extent of the lung opacification is not as clearly revealed as in (a). A nasogastric tube (small arrow) is present.*

Significant lung contusion[45,46] may give rise to hypoxemia. The opacification is often peripheral and related to the ribs; it is usually evident within 6 hours of the injury (Figs 3.16, 3.33, 3.43). It commonly spreads across anatomical boundaries. Air bronchograms are seldom present. The areas of opacification may coalesce for up to 48 hours, and often start clearing after 48–72 hours. The opacification usually resolves by 7–10 days.[45]

Intrapulmonary hematomas are usually more dense and are fairly well defined, except where abutted by contused lung (Figs 3.16, 3.43).

Abnormalities are easily overlooked in the periphery and apices of the chest because of the number of distracting normal structures present, including the ribs, clavicles, scapulae and soft tissues. Holding the radiograph at an angle to the viewing box improves visualization of the periphery. A lordotic view helps to clear the apex of overlying bony structures.

Lung lacerations may be caused by penetrating objects such as knives, bullets, fractured ribs or chest drains. The affected lung can be relatively opaque if associated with bleeding (Fig 3.28), or exhibit a hypolucent track.

Acute diffuse post-traumatic lung opacification may be caused by aspiration, consolidation or severe lung volume loss (Fig 3.42). Air bronchograms indicate a parenchymal process and are most frequently seen in lung consolidation. Consolidation occurs when alveoli fill with water, pus, blood, gastric content, tumor cells or, rarely, eosinophils. Pulmonary edema (Fig 3.31b) may be due to raised capillary hydrostatic pressure, as in fluid overload or cardiac failure. It may also result from capillary leakage, such as after brain injury, inhala-

tion of noxious gases, or in adult respiratory distress syndrome (ARDS) (Fig 3.44), which may follow blood transfusions, fat embolism or sepsis. It can be difficult to differentiate these types of edema radiologically. ARDS commonly only manifests after 12–24 hours. The earliest sign of a diffuse pulmonary process may be loss of clarity of the intrapulmonary vessels. Steam or smoke inhalation usually damages the airways to a greater extent than it does the lungs.

> Acute pulmonary edema without cardiac enlargement raises the possibility of pericardial or cardiac injury.

CT examination is very useful in localizing and characterizing intrathoracic conditions such as lung contusion.

The pleura

Pleural fluid Pleural fluid[47,48] may consist of transudate, exudate (Fig 3.45), blood (Fig 3.46), pus (Figs 3.47, 3.48), bowel content, or chyle (Fig 3.31). In the erect position, free-flowing fluid gravitates to the inferior cardiophrenic recesses. If lung markings can be seen below the hemidiaphragm on an erect, adequately penetrated radiograph, a significant pleural effusion is unlikely. A larger pleural effusion is usually situated laterally and posteriorly but can extend anteriorly or medially. It can obscure the hemidiaphragms. A free-flowing pleural effusion of more than 125–275 ml fills

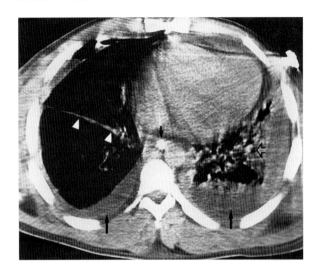

Figure 3.45 *This patient suffered a gunshot injury to his chest and abdomen 5 days previously. He had bilateral pneumothoraces, bilaterally injured hemi-diaphragms, liver lacerations, a ruptured spleen and a perforated stomach. CT was requested to explain ongoing clinical features of sepsis. CT scan demonstrates bilateral pleural fluid collections (arrows) and fluid in the oblique fissure (arrowheads). Lung consolidation with suspected breakdown is also present (open arrow). The nasogastric tube is also shown (small arrow).*

the CP angle,[49] producing a concave upper border on the erect radiograph, extending higher laterally than medially. In fact this is a radiographic illusion; the fluid extends upwards to the same extent around all free pleural surfaces.[47] The fissures are often accentuated

(Figs 3.31, 3.46). A 'step' into the horizontal fissure can sometimes be seen. An 'affected side down' decubitus radiograph will demonstrate movement of free pleural fluid to the lateral chest wall and is helpful in differentiating between pleural fluid and long-standing pleural

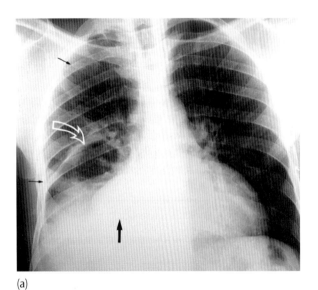

(a)

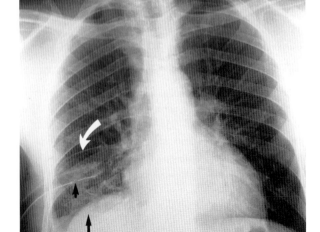

(b)

(c)

Figure 3.46 *All radiographs from the same patient on the day of presentation revealing a hemothorax following a chest stab 3 weeks previously. (a) The frontal film exhibits an apparently enlarged heart with the right side (medium arrow) denser than the left, loss of the right diaphragm and pleural fluid peripherally (small arrows) and in the horizontal fissure (open curved arrow). (b) A right-side-down decubitus chest radiograph demonstrates a moderately large right pleural fluid component (arrow) layered out against the lateral chest wall and tracking into the horizontal fissure (curved arrow) (c). This frontal film after drainage shows clearing of the retrocardiac fluid with residual prominence of the horizontal fissure (curved arrow). The right hemidiaphragm (arrow) has an abnormal configuration. The chest drain is noted (short arrow).*

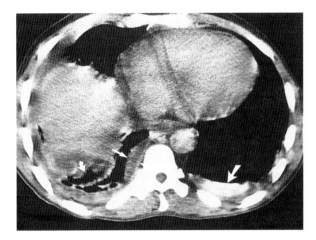

Figure 3.47 *This patient suffered blunt abdominal trauma with multiple surgical procedures, and recently developed pyrexia and leukocytosis. This CT scan after intravenous contrast medium through the lower chest demonstrates suspected breakdown (small curved arrow) of a right lower lobe pneumonic process with an enhancing pleural layer (short arrows) in keeping with an empyema. The high attenuation area (oblique arrow) in the left thorax was thought to be due to subsegmental atelectasis anterior to a small amount of pleural fluid.*

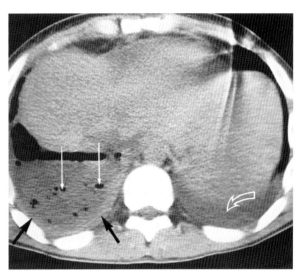

Figure 3.48 *A CT scan performed without intravenous contrast medium through the lower chest demonstrates gas locules (thin arrows) in an infected pleural collection (medium arrows) with associated left pleural fluid (curved open arrow).*

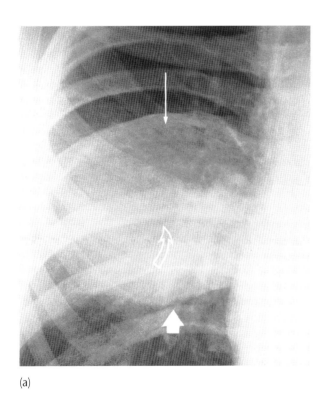

(a)

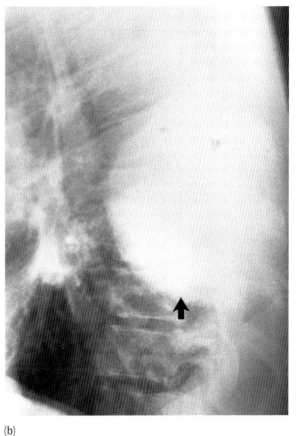

(b)

Figure 3.49 *A pleural hydatid cyst masquerading as an encysted effusion or extrapleural hematoma. Localized views of (a) frontal and (b) lateral chest radiographs in a patient with recent blunt right chest trauma showing a rounded opacity (broad arrow) with a poorly seen superior aspect in the right hemithorax. The lateral view exhibits a typical 'D'-shaped opacity (broad arrow), usually associated with an encysted effusion or extrapleural hematoma. However, on the frontal view the rib narrowing (thin arrow), cortical thickening (open curved arrow) and rib separation indicate chronicity.*

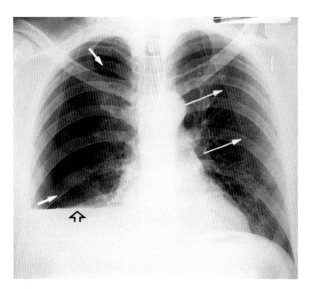

Figure 3.50 *A frontal erect chest radiograph demonstrating a large right hemopneumothorax with a clearly visible pleural line (short arrows) and a fluid level (open arrow) extending peripherally in the hemithorax. Notice how the medial edge of left scapula (long arrows) can simulate the pleural line of a pneumothorax at first sight. Note also the normal distance between the stomach bubble and left lung.*

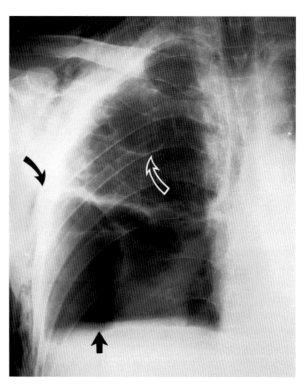

Figure 3.51 *The patient was stabbed in the chest. A frontal AP erect chest radiograph reveals bullous disease (open curved arrow) and adhesions in the right upper lobe, together with the fluid level of a hemopneumothorax (broad arrow) in the lower chest. Volume loss in the middle and lower lobes is seen. Surgical emphysema is also present (curved arrow).*

thickening, loculated fluid or clotted blood. The opposite decubitus view is useful in examining the underlying lung.

> Pleural and pulmonary pathological processes may coexist. CT scanning helps substantially in determining the extent of the two processes.

A large pleural effusion usually displaces the mediastinum to the opposite side (Fig 3.31), whereas lung collapse causes mediastinal shift toward the diseased hemithorax.

Pleural adhesions can significantly alter the appearances of pleural fluid. Loculated pleural fluid, blood or pus often has a typical 'D' shape on the lateral radiograph. It is usually posteriorly situated with an obtuse superior angle. On the frontal film, the superior border frequently fades out gradually. The CP angles may be clear with encysted pleural fluid. Other disease processes can simulate pleural or extrapleural collections (Fig 3.49).

Posteromedially situated pleural fluid may produce a triangular opacity along the vertebral border (Fig 3.46), obliterating the descending aortic interface on the left. It is seen posteriorly on a lateral radiograph. The position of the relevant bronchus and pulmonary artery may be useful in differentiating between a pleural effusion and collapse/consolidation, as described in the lung section. Fluid may also be seen medially adjacent to the cardiac shadow, or above the hemidiaphragm in a subpulmonic (or infrapulmonic) location.[50,51]

On an erect radiograph, a hemopneumothorax (Figs 3.50–3.52) or hydropneumothorax is recognized by an air fluid level which extends to the periphery of the hemithorax (Fig 3.50). This level is usually longer on one projection than on the orthogonal view.

On a supine radiograph, the posterior distribution of pleural blood or fluid will cause diffuse opacification (Figs 3.12, 3.24, 3.46). This posterior opacification does not efface the pulmonary vascular outlines (Fig 3.12), nor does it produce air bronchograms. It can extend to the apex, forming a cap-like opacity.[49,52] It may also spread medially, causing apparent widening of the mediastinum.[20] It often extends into the fissures, emphasizing these structures (Fig 3.31). Fluid can easily be overlooked in the supine position, particularly if it is bilateral or associated with lung contusion or other lung opacification.

US examination is an excellent method for confirming and localizing pleural fluid.

Subpulmonic fluid[47,50,51] In the erect chest radiograph, the distance between the superior part of the gastric air bubble and the left lung base should be less than 20 mm (Figs 3.3, 3.50).[53]

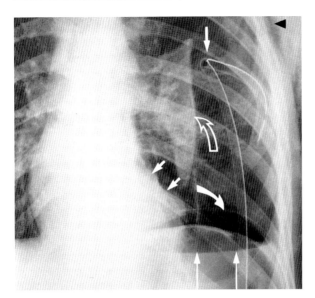

Figure 3.52 *Subpulmonic hemopneumothorax. An erect frontal chest radiograph showing a left chest drain with acute angulation at the skin entry site (medium arrow). Note the angular opacity representing a large shard of intrathoracic glass (curved open arrow). Note also the subpulmonic hemopneumothorax with a clearly seen air/fluid level (long arrows) and the thin superior visceral pleura (curved solid arrow). A left apical pneumothorax was also present but is not shown. Surgical emphysema is present (arrowhead). Left lower lung collapse/consolidation (short arrows) is suspected.*

Subpulmonic fluid collections cause:

- Widening of this gastric to pulmonary distance (Fig 3.53).
- Lateral peaking of the apparent diaphragm (Fig 3.9, 3.53), which may be well seen on an expiratory frontal film.[50]
- A deep, preserved CP angle.
- Loss of visibility of the vessels behind the diaphragm.[51]
- An associated small lateral pleural fluid collection.
- An elevated CP angle.
- On the lateral projection, an elevated apparent diaphragm with a straight anterior component appearing to end abruptly at the inferior aspect of the oblique fissure, which may be thickened.[50]

Lateral flow of fluid on a decubitus radiograph confirms the presence of a hydrothorax or hemothorax (Figs 3.53, 3.54). Interestingly, pleural fluid may remain localized to the subpulmonic space in the supine position.

Pneumothorax A special effort must be made to detect a pneumothorax. The use of a bright light is recommended.

> Even small pneumothoraces can become tension pneumothoraces, especially when the patient is ventilated.[1,54]

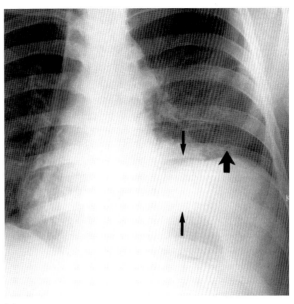

(a)

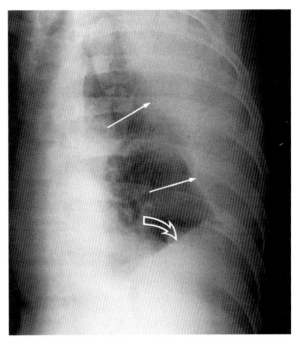

(b)

Figure 3.53 *This patient suffered blunt trauma. (a) The erect chest radiograph demonstrates elevation and a lateral peak of the apparent left diaphragmatic (broad arrow) and an increased distance from the gastric air bubble to lung (arrows). All these features strongly suggest a left subpulmonic fluid collection. There is increased soft tissue density in the left upper quadrant. The patient is rotated, accounting for the apparent displacement of the heart to the right. (b) The left-side-down decubitus film confirms the large pleural fluid component (long arrows) and also displays the abnormal contour of the left hemidiaphragm (open curved arrow) more clearly. The fullness and density of the left upper quadrant persist. At surgery a rupture of the left hemidiaphragm and the spleen were confirmed.*

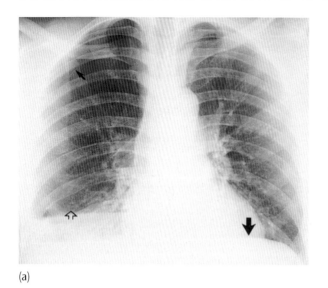

(a)

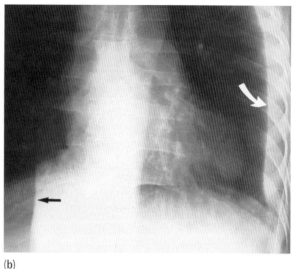

(b)

Figure 3.54 *This patient was stabbed on both sides of the chest. (a) An erect chest radiograph clearly shows a right pneumothorax (short arrow) and the fluid level of a hemothorax (open arrow). The left subpulmonic fluid collection (broad arrow) may be overlooked.[76] (b) A left-side decubitus radiograph reveals the left pleural fluid (curved arrow). On the right, an air fluid level (arrow) interrupted by lung is visible, confirming the hemopneumothorax.*

To diagnose a pneumothorax, a sharply defined, uniformly thin white pleural line measuring less than 1 mm wide should be seen between the lung with normal markings and the lucent pneumothorax without lung markings (Fig 3.50, 3.52). In the erect position, pleural air is commonly situated apically and superolaterally (see Fig 3.21). Although recognition is easy in most cases, overlying surgical emphysema may make this difficult (see Fig 3.10). Pleural air is occasionally found medially alongside the cardiac border or in a subpulmonic location (Figs 3.55–3.57). An expiratory radiograph can accentuate a small pneumothorax because, although the lung deflates, the pneumothorax does not. Adjacent lung opacification also enhances the detection of a pneumothorax by accentuating the lucency of this area (see Fig 3.21).

Difficulty can arise in the presence of pleural adhesions, where the pneumothorax is situated anterior or posterior to the adherent lung. Lung markings may then extend to the periphery. Usually, however, the pneumothorax extends superior or inferior to the area of adhesion (Fig 3.51).

It may occasionally be difficult to distinguish bullous lung disease from a pneumothorax. The walls of bullae are usually more acutely curved and thinner than the pleural line of a pneumothorax. Bullous disease does, however, predispose to the development of pneumo-thoraces. CT imaging is often helpful in differentiating these two conditions, but may on occasions fail to solve the conundrum.

Malpositioned chest drains may not function adequately and can create significant iatrogenic problems. Above the diaphragm, the drain could be improperly positioned (Fig 3.58), placed directly into

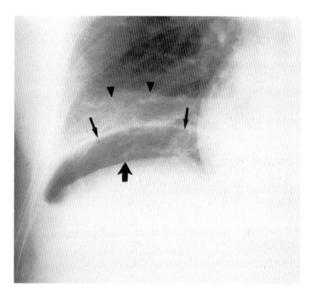

Figure 3.55 *Localized view of an erect chest radiograph showing a large subpulmonic pneumothorax (broad arrow) with slightly thickened pleura (medium arrows) and small associated posteriorly loculated hemopneumothorax (arrowheads) confirmed on the lateral film (not shown). A subpulmonic pneumothorax may on occasion simulate subphrenic free air. The pleura in this case is thought to have been thickened by the fluid.*

lung parenchyma (Fig 3.59), into a fissure (Fig 3.60) into mediastinal structures (Fig 3.40) or a herniated viscus. Intrafissural drains often function normally and do not necessarily require replacement. Low placements may lead to perforations of the spleen, liver (Fig 3.61) or other subphrenic (Fig 3.62) viscera. Some chest drains may appear to be surprisingly low when they are,

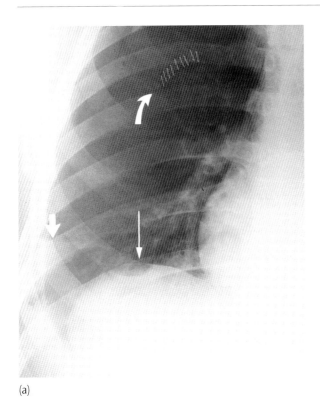

(a)

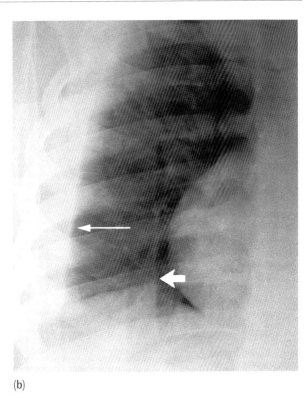

(b)

Figure 3.56 *Subpulmonic pleural collection. (a) Close-up view of an erect frontal chest radiograph showing a focal bulge in the outline of the apparent right hemidiaphragm, suggesting liver herniating through the diaphragmatic defect. Air is present at the apex of opacity with a thin border. The site of the stab is indicated by the surgical staples (curved arrow). A hemopneumothorax with a fluid level (broad arrow) and subpulmonic component (long thin arrow) are present. (b) A localized view of a right-side-down decubitus radiograph confirms the hemothorax (thin arrow). An air fluid level is present (broad arrow). Compare Fig 3.56a with Fig 3.65.*

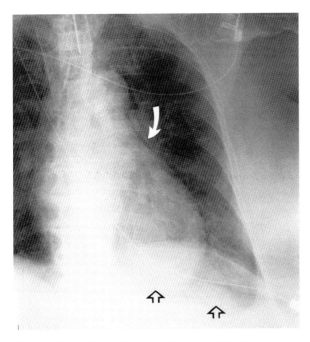

Figure 3.57 *Supine radiograph following difficulty in attempted introduction of tracheostomy tube (arrow). Note the double diaphragm sign of a pneumothorax in the supine position (open arrows). Also note the mediastinal pleura (curved arrow) lifted by mediastinal air.*

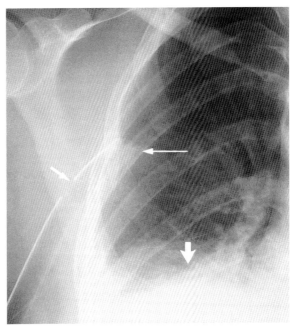

Figure 3.58 *Erect chest radiograph demonstrating incorrectly sited right chest drain with side hole (short arrow) in the chest wall. Small area of opacification in the adjacent right lung (long arrow) may have occurred during attempted drain placement. Basal pleural fluid is present (broad arrow).*

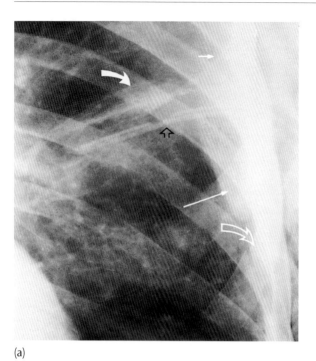
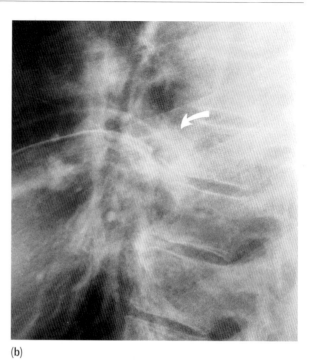

(a)   (b)

Figure 3.59 *Localized views of (a) frontal and (b) lateral chest radiographs showing lung hemorrhage (curved arrow) surrounding a chest drain (open arrow) inadvertently placed into lung parenchyma. A pneumothorax (short arrow) and subcutaneous emphysema are also present. A fractured rib (curved open arrow) and associated extrapleural hematoma (long arrow) can also be seen.*

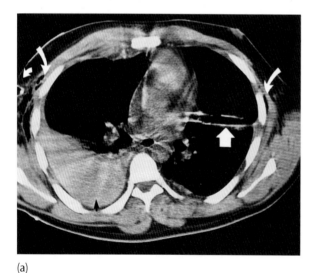

(a)

Figure 3.60 *(a) A CT scan at the level of T8 revealing a chest drain (broad arrow) placed in the left oblique fissure. A large right pleural fluid collection (small arrow) is present. A right chest drain is seen passing through the chest wall (small curved arrow). Note also the bilateral chest wall surgical emphysema (large curved arrows), possibly related to the chest drain placements. (b) A localized view on lung settings demonstrates the straight posterior edge of the oblique fissure (long arrow) and surgical emphysema (curved arrow).*

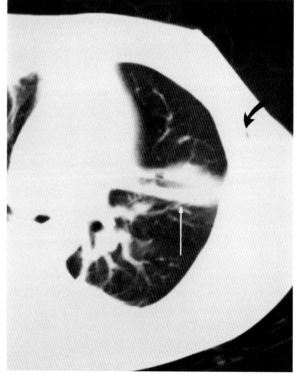

(b)

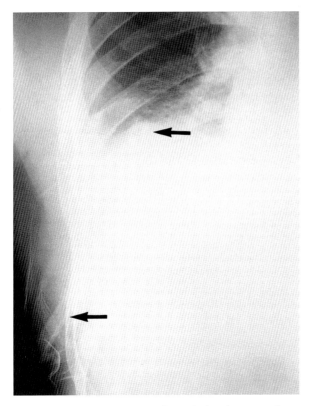

Figure 3.61 *A frontal chest radiograph showing a very low right chest drain placement (arrows). At surgery this was found to have passed through the liver and right hemidiaphragm to enter the right hemithorax.*

in fact, entirely intrapleural. This is because of the low location of the CP angle recesses.

An anteromedial pneumothorax does not produce a typical peripheral pleural line unless it is fairly large. A small centrally and anteriorly located pneumothorax can be especially difficult to see on the supine film.

Signs of a pneumothorax on a supine radiograph include:[55,56]

- A sometimes subtle lucency over the lower medial hemithorax and upper quadrant (Figs 3.57, 3.63).[56] The superior surface of the diaphragm may be crisply delineated.[20]
- A wide, deep and clear lateral CP angle (Fig 3.63).[57]
- An apparent double diaphragm where both the inferior limit of the anterior descent of the diaphragm and the dome of the diaphragm are seen as separate contours (Fig 3.57).[56]
- Clear delineation of the pericardial fat pads, the heart,[56] the IVC and the upper mediastinal structures such as the SVC, azygos vein and left subclavian artery.[20]

If fully erect films are not possible, semi-erect or decubitus (Fig 3.33) radiographs with the abnormal side uppermost are preferred to supine horizontal beam 'shoot-through' radiographs to demonstrate a pneumothorax.

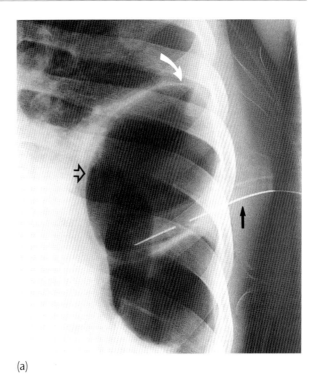

(a)

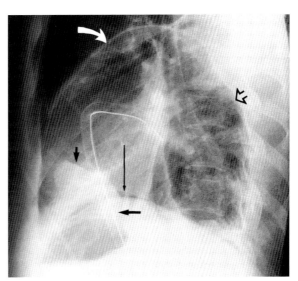

(b)

Figure 3.62 *Herniation of bowel following a stab wound. Views of (a) frontal and (b) lateral chest radiographs demonstrating a low insertion site for an intercostal drain (medium arrow) in the presence of a ruptured left hemidiaphragm and colonic herniation (open arrow). This illustrates the need for obtaining a chest radiograph before inserting a chest drain, although the large bowel may have been misinterpreted as a loculated pneumothorax. In this instance the bowel was not damaged. The mediastinum is displaced to the right. The thin crescent of air seen on the lateral view (thin arrow) is part of a loop of bowel. Note the non-visualization of the left hemidiaphragm and the thin, acutely bulging visceral wall (curved arrow). The anterior well defined opacity on the lateral view may represent a hematoma (short arrow).*

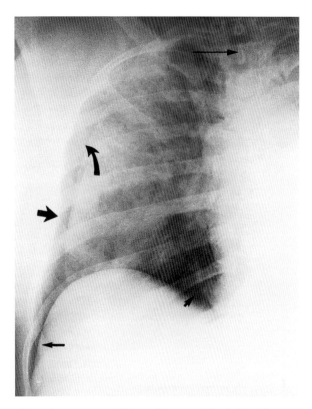

Figure 3.63 *Motor vehicle accident. Localized view of a supine frontal chest radiograph demonstrating features of a supine hemopneumothorax: (a) the deep sulcus sign (medium arrow); (b) the relative lucency in the right cardiophrenic area (small arrow). The hemothorax has spread in the pleural space, reducing the lucency of the pneumothorax (curved arrow). A pneumomediastinum (long arrow) and small extrapleural hematoma (broad arrow) are present.*

In a supine hemopneumothorax the pleural blood may diminish the anticipated peripheral lucency of a pneumothorax alone (Fig 3.63).

A CT examination can demonstrate a very small amount of pleural air. All injured patients subjected to abdominal or head CT should have limited lower chest scans, which need to be inspected on lung settings to exclude coexisting pneumothoraces.[54]

Tension pneumothorax The clinical evaluation is critical in this condition. Radiographic interpretation can be misleading in either falsely suggesting or overlooking a tension pneumothorax.

Radiographic signs suggestive of a tension pneumothorax (see Fig 3.32) include:

- Marked loss of lung volume on the side of the pneumothorax. The stiff lungs in patients with ARDS or chronic obstructive airways disease can

prevent this anticipated lung volume loss, yet the patient may suffer respiratory compromise.
- Flattening, depression and especially inversion of the hemidiaphragm.
- Shift of the mediastinum or azygoesophageal recess away from the affected hemithorax (Fig 3.32).
- Flattening of the SVC and the right side of the heart are particularly serious signs (Fig 3.32).

Pseudopneumothorax The companion shadows inside the posterior upper ribs do not usually cause diagnostic difficulty. They may occasionally suggest pleural thickening or a small localized effusion. If a thin lucent line of fat separates them from the ribs (Fig 3.64), they become more suggestive of pneumothoraces, but are usually bilateral, poorly defined inferiorly and do not continue to the lateral hemithorax.

A pseudopneumothorax may also be created by skin folds over the chest wall, especially in young and old patients. Clues to this origin include:

- The folds extending beyond the thoracic outline.
- The absence of two clearly delineated lucent areas sharply abutting a well defined clear white line. Instead, a gradually increasing opacification up to one aspect of the skin fold is seen.
- Lung markings seen peripheral to the fold.
- A multiplicity of folds.
- The folds may not run parallel to the chest wall.

Bowel herniated into the left chest may also occasionally simulate a pneumothorax (Figs 3.25, 3.62). This is important to recognize before any proposed pleural drainage.

The fissures

Change in position of the fissures is generally a sensitive indicator of regionally altered lung volume (Figs

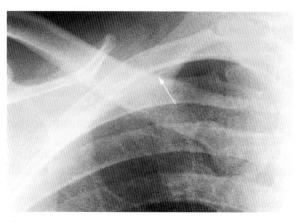

Figure 3.64 *A close-up view of the right apex of a frontal chest radiograph demonstrating the appearance of a 'companion shadow' (long thin arrow) slightly separated from the rib edge. This could be incorrectly interpreted as a pneumothorax, but is usually bilateral, as it was here.*

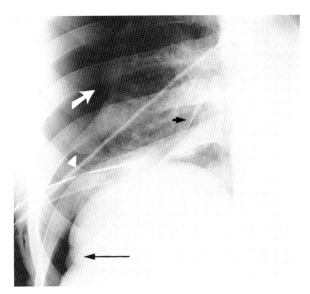

Figure 3.65 *Ruptured right diaphragm with herniated liver. The contour of the right diaphragm is markedly abnormal with a focal bulge medially and a lobulated, waist-like defect laterally (long arrow). Note the large right pneumothorax with mediastinal shift to the left. The oblique fissure is prominent (short arrow). There is considerable loss of volume (oblique arrow). Note the pseudo-lesion created by the inferior portion of the scapula (arrowhead). Compare with Fig 3.56.*

3.42, 3.65). Any thoracic opacification bounded by a fissure strongly suggests an intrapulmonary process (Fig 3.42). Loculated intrafissural fluid can simulate a tumor, often with a characteristic biconvex shape and tapering extensions.

The costophrenic angles

On an erect radiograph, blunting or filling in of these angles occurs most commonly as a result of pleural fluid. An overlying anterior rib can simulate a lateral pleural effusion but does not efface the hemidiaphragm.

The hemidiaphragms

Diaphragmatic injury may be caused by blunt or penetrating injury.[58,59]

> The hemidiaphragms require careful scrutiny, not only in the immediate post-trauma situation but also on subsequent radiography.[60]

Small diaphragmatic defects may be missed unless the superior contours of both hemidiaphragms are conscientiously examined. Examining the radiograph with the long axis of the spine in a horizontal orientation assists this evaluation, as does the 'two finger test' described in the mediastinum section. Requesting a post-extubation chest radiograph is strongly recom-

mended in any patient with the possibility of diaphragmatic injury.[60]

> Any deviation from the normal delineation, configuration or position of the hemidiaphragms should evoke a high degree of suspicion of the possibility of a rupture.

Plain chest radiological signs of a ruptured diaphragm (Figs 3.66, 3.67) include:[18]

- Inability to delineate the full extent of the hemidiaphragm.
- An apparently elevated diaphragm (Figs 3.24, 3.53, 3.65–3.67).
- Gas or air fluid levels in the lower chest. These can occasionally resemble a tension pneumothorax or a hemopneumothorax (Figs 3.24, 3.25, 3.62).
- An abrupt upward bulge of the hemidiaphragm which does not extend across the entire hemithorax

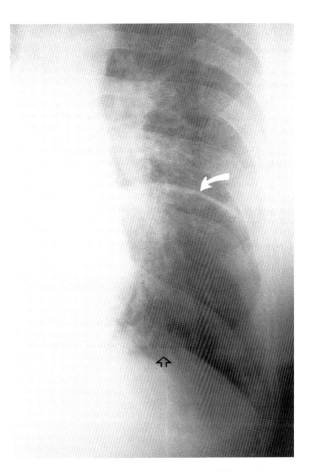

Figure 3.66 *Ruptured diaphragm. Motor vehicle accident. Localized view of a supine frontal radiograph. The medial portion of the left diaphragm (open arrow) is not visualized. The operative notes record a diaphragmatic rupture but do not describe herniated viscera. The presumed herniated viscus (curved arrow) may have been reduced as a result of operative ventilation. Compare with Figs 3.69 and 3.70.*

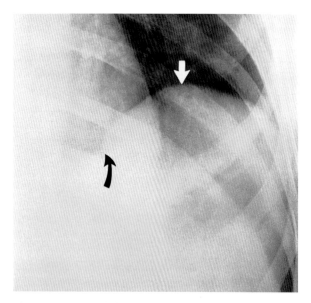

Figure 3.67 *Blunt injury, ruptured diaphragm. The abnormal left diaphragmatic contour on a localized view of a frontal supine chest radiograph shows a focal bulge (broad arrow) with the abrupt change in direction (curved arrow) of this ruptured diaphragm. The visibility of the bulge through the cardiac shadow indicates that it is posteriorly located.*

on either the frontal of lateral views (Figs 3.62, 3.65, 3.67). This sign is particularly helpful.
- Any radiological change above the hemidiaphragm, including basal soft tissue opacification, apparent or real pleural effusions or basal atelectasis (Figs 3.53, 3.62).
- Mediastinal displacement (Figs 3.24, 3.25, 3.65).[61]
- A nasogastric tube which descends through the esophagogastric junction and then ascends above the normal diaphragmatic position (Fig 3.24).[62] This can also occur with other causes of diaphragmatic elevation.

A non-ruptured elevated hemidiaphragm may on occasions simulate this condition (Fig 3.68).

Diaphragmatic herniation occurs more commonly on the left. On the right the liver both protects the diaphragmatic defect and hides the diagnosis. Blunt traumatic diaphragmatic injuries have a very high association with liver, spleen (Fig 3.53) and other organ injury (Figs 3.24, 3.25),[61,63] fractured pelvis[6,64] and posterior dislocation of the hip.

Intraperitoneal air in a patient stabbed above the diaphragm usually indicates diaphragmatic penetration.[59] These penetrating injuries are often small, frequently preventing early herniation of abdominal content, and thus delaying the diagnosis.[59]

An upper and/or lower gastrointestinal contrast examination in the head-down position may demonstrate herniation of viscus through a diaphragmatic defect. Gastrografin should be used if bowel perforation is suspected, and can be added to a dilute barium

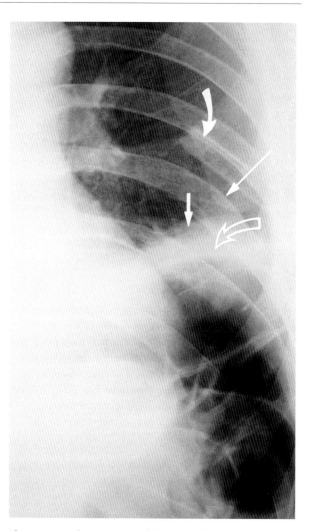

Figure 3.68 *Blunt trauma with pseudo-diaphragmatic rupture. The frontal chest radiograph of a patient following blunt thoracic trauma, with a left pneumothorax and loss of volume of the left lung. Note the indistinct and elevated 'apparent' left diaphragm (arrow) with clearly seen bowel loops (open curved arrow), suggesting a rupture of the diaphragm with bowel herniation. Chest drain (closed curved arrow) and a rib fracture (long arrow) are also present. An intact diaphragm was demonstrated on further evaluation.*

suspension to hasten the passage of barium through the bowel. With a small diaphragmatic defect, a characteristic constriction of herniated bowel may be seen (Figs 3.69–3.71). This constriction is not seen with a diaphragmatic eventration or paralyzed hemidiaphragm. Bowel constriction may prevent contrast material from entering the herniated segments, producing the 'amputated fundus' sign[59] of the stomach (Fig 3.70), an equivalent colonic 'amputation', or barium retention in the herniated segment. It is unusual for small bowel to herniate without accompanying stomach or colon.[59]

Ultrasonography may show a diaphragmatic defect and a waist in the liver bulging through this defect. This

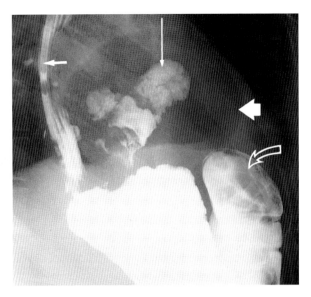

Figure 3.69 *Motor vehicle accident, ruptured diaphragm. A limited part of an upper gastrointestinal barium series demonstrating the distended gastric fundus (broad arrow) herniating superiorly through a narrow diaphragmatic defect. This defect only allows a small amount of barium (thin arrow) to pass into the gas-filled fundus. This demonstrates how the 'amputated fundus' sign could arise, and how the residual stomach can then be incorrectly interpreted as normal. Note the nasogastric tube (arrow), and the barium present in the splenic flexure of the colon (open curved arrow) from a concomitant examination. Diaphragmatic defects following blunt trauma can also be small.*

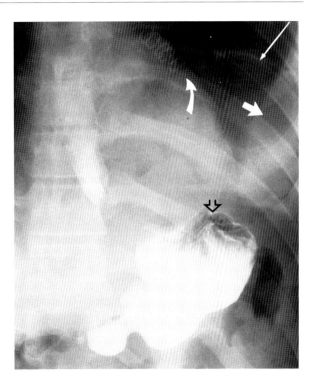

Figure 3.70 *A barium study of the stomach showing the 'amputated fundus' (open arrow), where the gastric fundus has herniated through the short diaphragmatic defect and does not fill with barium. The residual stomach could falsely be interpreted as normal. The large rounded lucency (long arrow) in the left hemithorax represents the distended herniated gastric fundus. A long air fluid level was noticed within this structure on another radiograph (not shown). A left hemothorax (broad arrow) and surgical staples (curved arrow) are also present.*

waist is also occasionally seen radiographically (Fig 3.65).

CT scans[65–67] may demonstrate:

- Interruption of the diaphragmatic crus (Fig 3.72).
- An absent hemidiaphragm (Fig 3.72).
- Bowel or mesenteric fat herniation (Fig 3.72).
- Constriction of herniated bowel.

Interruption of the crura can occur normally, usually in patients over 40 years of age.[68]

Sagittal and coronal views from reconstructed helical CT scans and magnetic resonance imaging (MRI) are also effective ways of demonstrating a herniated viscus. Thoracoscopy and laparoscopy have greatly facilitated this diagnosis.[69,70]

Always consider a rupture of the diaphragm in the appropriate clinical setting.[64,66]

ADJACENT REGIONS

A left upper quadrant mass causing gastric or colonic displacement or a wide lateral properitoneal stripe suggesting splenic injury should be deliberately sought (see Fig 3.53).

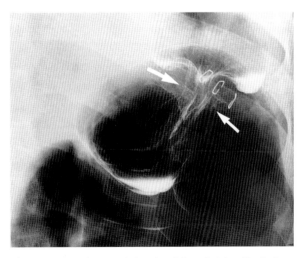

Figure 3.71 *Stab wound, herniated bowel. A localized view of a barium enema demonstrating herniated large bowel passing through a defect in the left hemidiaphragm. The constriction (arrows) of the large bowel as it passes through the diaphragmatic defect is well shown. This is in keeping with the short rent in the diaphragm associated with penetrating injuries. Surgical staples in the stab wound are noted.*

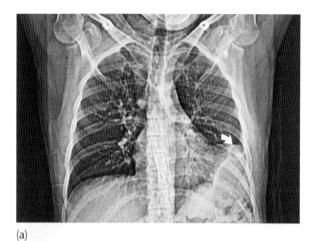

(a)

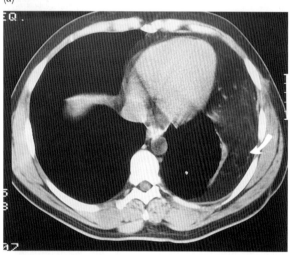

(b)

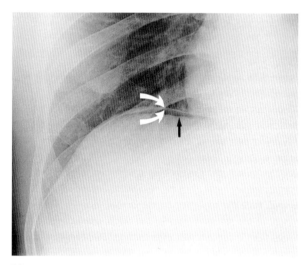

(a)

Splenic injury can lead to widening of the space between the left lung and the top of the stomach bubble to over 20 mm.

> Extraluminal upper abdominal air should always be excluded.

Subphrenic free air may arise from above or below the diaphragm, or from a gas-producing infection. On the erect view, intraperitoneal free air is usually easily seen as a crescentic subphrenic lucency (Fig 3.73). A

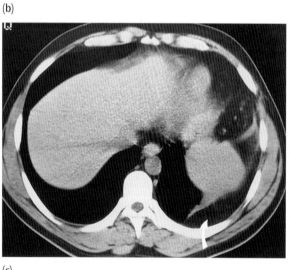

(c)

Figure 3.72 *Ruptured left diaphragm confirmed surgically. (a) The abnormal contour of the left diaphragm is seen on a CT planning view. Note the well defined opacity (curved arrow) located superior to the lateral left hemidiaphragm. The relatively low density of this tissue suggests fatty tissue. (b and c) CT sections through the left diaphragm showing fatty omentum (curved arrow) herniating through an interrupted diaphragm to lie posterolaterally in the costophrenic recess.*

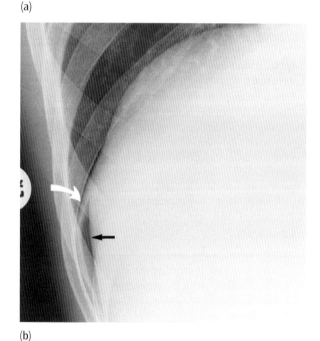

(b)

Figure 3.73 *(a) Localized view of an erect posteroanterior chest radiograph and (b) collimated view of a left decubitus radiograph exhibiting the typical appearance of free subphrenic intraperitoneal air (arrow). Note the thickness of the diaphragm (curved arrows).*

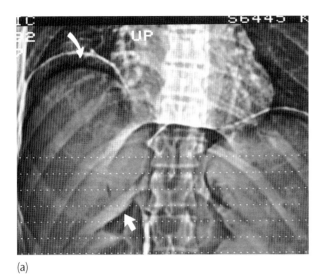

(a)

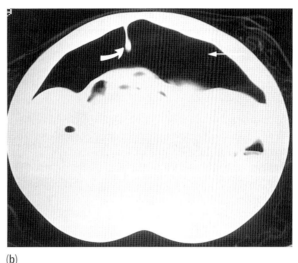

(b)

Figure 3.74 *CT scan revealing the features of a supine pneumoperitoneum. (a) The planning view demonstrates the subphrenic air (curved arrow) clearly, with increased lucency overlying the central abdomen delineating the inferior surface of the liver (broad arrow). (b) A CT scan through the upper abdomen shows the large pneumoperitoneum (long arrow) with the falciform ligament containing the obliterated umbilical vein (curved arrow) in its free edge.*

thin diaphragm can make the distinction between pneumoperitoneum and subpulmonic pneumothorax difficult. Free peritoneal air is occasionally seen as small locules anterior to the right liver or in the hepatorenal fossa. Small amounts are best detected on erect chest radiographs (Fig 3.73a) or a left decubitus upper abdominal film (Fig 3.73b). Peridiaphragmatic fat can simulate free air, but is less lucent and has less distinct edges than air.

Signs of free air on the supine radiograph (Fig 3.74) can be subtle, but include detection of:

• Triangular extraluminal air collections trapped between bowel loops.
• Both inner and outer borders of bowel loops.
• A lucency in the upper abdomen overlying the liver (Fig 3.74).
• The falciform ligament, seen as a linear opacity within a lucency.
• The inferior edge of liver (Fig 3.74).
• The medial diaphragm defined by free air.

The distinction between retroperitoneal and intraperitoneal air can occasionally also be perplexing. Visualization of the renal outlines (see Fig 3.18a) or psoas muscle edges indicate retroperitoneal air. CT scanning shows the presence and location of small amounts of extraluminal air clearly, and can be useful in equivocal cases.

Need for repeated radiographs

Further radiographs are important during continued management of the trauma victim. The frequency of these radiographs depends on the nature of the patient's initial injury and the subsequent progress.

> Identifying a pneumothorax before surgery or positive pressure ventilation is very important.

Radiographs are essential following chest drain or catheter placement to ensure their correct positioning, to exclude complications and to confirm the desired effect. Increasing pleural fluid or soft tissue opacification may indicate continuing hemorrhage. Increasing surgical emphysema suggests chest drain malposition.

The appearance of delayed mediastinal air or soft tissue changes, or pleural fluid may be the first indication of airway or esophageal injuries. Delayed changes in the diaphragmatic contour can indicate a ruptured hemidiaphragm.[60,61] Newly detected subphrenic air may indicate bowel compromise. In the days following trauma, an indistinct or 'shaggy' diaphragm suggests subphrenic infection, and may require an US or CT examination for elucidation.

Follow-up films are important in a patient with potential pulmonary contusion to evaluate the development and extent of the injury and to detect complications. Delayed chest radiographs are valuable in pulmonary conditions such as ARDS which usually shows radiological change after 12–24 hours. After pericardial injury, altered heart size and configuration may be evident after some delay (see Fig 3.34).

In cases of diagnostic difficulty, it is often worth performing the follow-up radiograph in different projections, such as a lateral or decubitus views.

OTHER IMAGING

Contrast studies (see Fig 3.41)

ESOPHAGUS

The radiological clues to esophageal injury have been described above. Endoscopy and contrast swallows offer alternatives for further evaluation. Esophograms may identify, localize and define the size of the injury. The study should be performed in multiple projections, in both supine and prone positions.

OTHER

The use of contrast agents to detect bowel herniation through diaphragmatic ruptures has been referred to above. Iodinated contrast material may occasionally be introduced into catheters or drains to define their positions, patency and the spaces with which they communicate.

Angiography

Angiography remains the gold standard for the evaluation of aortic and arterial trauma. It is critical to evaluate the entire arch and its branches, together with the descending aorta to the diaphragm, in patients with suspected blunt vascular injuries. Contrast medium extravasation, false aneurysms (Figs 3.30c, 3.75), arteriovenous fistulae (Fig 3.76) and occlusions may all be encountered. Associated cardiac injuries may also be present. Ductus diverticulae, atherosclerotic plaques and existing aneurysms can all simulate aortic injury. Examinations may be falsely interpreted as normal if an inadequate number of views are performed or if small injuries are overlooked or disregarded.

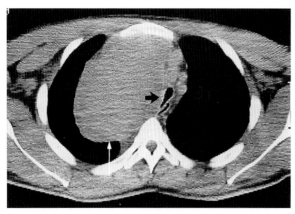

(a)

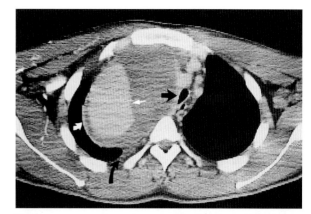

(b)

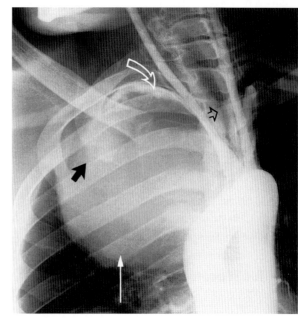

(c)

Figure 3.75 *CT scans (a) before and (b) after intravenous contrast medium administration above the level of the aortic arch demonstrate a large right apical soft tissue opacity (long arrow) with enhancing central (short arrow) and peripheral (curved arrow) components. These features suggest a subclavian artery false aneurysm. Note also the tracheal (broad arrow) and mediastinal compression and displacement to the left. A small focal pleural fluid collection is seen posteriorly (large curved arrow). (c) An arch angiogram in the same patient demonstrates a large, partially clotted false aneurysm (thin arrow) arising from the right subclavian artery (curved open arrow) with contrast medium entering its lumen (broad arrow). Note again the tracheal narrowing and its displacement to the left (open arrow).*

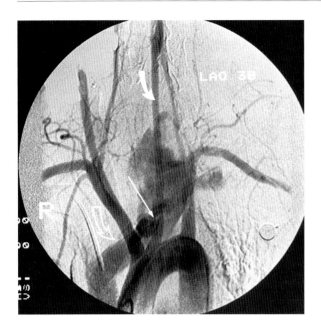

Figure 3.76 *Digital subtraction arch aortogram showing a large arteriovenous fistula (long arrow) from the left common carotid artery (curved closed arrow) into the left brachiocephalic vein (curved open arrow). The patient was stabbed in his neck, with a widened mediastinum on the chest radiograph (not shown).*

The procedure does take a moderate amount of time, and usually entails removal of the patient from the trauma unit for this period. Infrequent, specific complications include the aggravation of the aortic or arterial injury by catheter or guidewire manipulations, or by the contrast medium injection.

Computed tomography (CT)

CT examination (see Figs 3.6, 3.40, 3.60, 3.74, 3.75) has a role in patients with suspected aortic arch injury (Fig 3.30),[29–36] ruptured diaphragm (Fig 3.72),[67] airway injury, pleural (Figs 3.47, 3.48) or pericardial fluid,[43] pulmonary disease including lung contusion (Figs. 3.44, 3.45),[46,71] or pneumothorax.[54] A CT examination clarifies the extent of each process where there is coexisting lung and pleural disease. Hemothoraces may have a density of approximately 30 Hounsfield Units (HU).[43] A limited CT examination of the lower thorax added to a head or body CT scan may detect a pneumothorax. This is likely to require the introduction of a chest drain (Figs 3.40, 3.60).[54] CT scanning is also useful for determining the positions of chest drains.[72] Spinal injuries and sternoclavicular dislocation[72] are also well shown by CT scanning.

A CT study may require patient transfer and a moderate amount of time to complete. Various patient support and monitoring devices may cause artifacts and should be repositioned if this is clinically acceptable. Scan quality on slower scanners can be detrimentally affected by the rapid respiratory rates and inability of some trauma patients to cooperate.

Magnetic resonance imaging (MRI)

Despite its multiplanar capabilities and unique imaging information, MRI has minimal application in thoracic trauma. It has no major role in diagnosing acute aortic injury. Diaphragmatic herniation of liver, bowel or omentum have been well demonstrated in sagittal and coronal MRI scans.[73] Intrapulmonary hematoma can have a characteristic hyperintensity.[74] Airway injuries can also be diagnosed and evaluated.

Specific problems include the limited access for active resuscitation and the incompatibility of some life support systems.

Ultrasound (US)

US readily makes the diagnosis of a hemopericardium (Fig 3.37). Some chest wall, pleural, lung, lower neck and subphrenic collections can be identified, localized, aspirated and drained under ultrasound guidance.

Difficulties include patient tenderness, the limited access because of patient immobility and surgical wounds, drains and dressings.

Color Doppler examination offers promise in the detection of brachiocephalic vascular injuries.

ECHOCARDIOGRAPHY AND TRANSESOPHAGEAL ECHOCARDIOGRAPHY (TEE)

TEE offers better cardiac and thoracic aortic visualization than does standard echocardiography.[1,75] It can be performed in the trauma unit but requires trained staff and sometimes patient sedation. Valve injuries, cardiac contusion and infarction can be identified. The aortic isthmus is well seen by TEE, and periaortic hematoma and aortic injuries can be confidently identified. However, the brachiocephalic arteries and pretracheal aortic arch are not seen. This severely limits its role.

INTRAVASCULAR ULTRASOUND

Intravascular ultrasound[1] is able to demonstrate aortic injuries well, but also suffers from a limited depth of view and does not routinely show the brachiocephalic vessels. It is more difficult and invasive than TEE.

Nuclear medicine imaging

Post-traumatic myocardial infarction and subsequent cardiac dysfunction can be evaluated by isotope-labeled compounds, but use in myocardial contusion is limited.[76] Bone scans can detect radiologically occult rib fractures.[77] Diaphragmatic injury may be detected by demonstrating a 'waisted' bulge of herniating liver or spleen. CT scanning has largely supplanted the diagnostic use of isotopes in solid organ injuries.

Interventional radiology

Percutaneous catheter drainage of pleural, intrapulmonary, mediastinal or subphrenic collections is well established. Transcatheter embolization of arterial sources of hemorrhage with steel coils or other agents provides a useful alternative to surgery. Whereas embolization is restricted to smaller branch arteries, the recent use of covered expandable metal stents for injuries to larger arteries such as the aortic arch[78] holds promise for the future.

A close working relationship between the clinician and the radiologist optimizes the benefits of imaging to the patient with thoracic trauma.

ACKNOWLEDGEMENTS

The authors would like to thank the current and past staff of the Groote Schuur Hospital Trauma Unit for providing much of the radiographic material in this chapter, and for the productive clinical interaction we enjoy. Thanks to Miss B. Neumann for secretarial assistance in the preparation of this chapter.

REFERENCES

1. Groskin SA. Selected topics in chest trauma. *Semin Ultrasound CT MRI* 1996; **17(2):** 119–41.
2. Meyer S. Thoracic spine trauma. *Semin Roentgenol* 1992; **27(4):** 254–61.
3. Martijn A, Veldhuis EFM. The diagnostic value of interpediculate distance assessment on plain films in thoracic and lumbar spine injuries. *J Trauma* 1991; **31(10):** 1393–5.
4. Garland LH. The postero-mesial pleural line. *Radiology* 1943; **41:** 29–33.
5. Lien HH, Kolbenstvedt A. The thoracic paraspinal shadow: normal appearances. *Clin Radiol* 1982; **33:** 31–5.
6. Harris JH, Harris WH, Novelline RA. Chest. In: Harris JH, Harris WH, Novelline RA. *The Radiology of Emergency Medicine*, 3rd edn. Baltimore: Williams & Wilkins, 1993; 469–622.
7. Fraser RG, Pare JAP, Pare PD, Fraser RS, Genereux GP. The normal chest. In: Fraser RG, Pare JAP, Pare PD, Fraser RS, Genereux GP. *Diagnosis of Diseases of the Chest*, 3rd edn. Philadelphia: WB Saunders, 1988; 1–314.
8. Milne ENC, Pistolesi M, Miniati M, Giuntini C. The vascular pedicle of the heart and the vena azygous. Part 1. The normal subject. *Radiology* 1984; **152:** 1–8.
9. Milne ENC, Pistolesi M. Assessing systemic intra- and extravascular water. In: Milne ENC, Pistolesi M. *Reading the Chest Radiograph: a Physiologic Approach*. St Louis: Mosby, 1993; 80–119.
10. Savoca CJ, Austin JHM, Goldberg HI. The right paratracheal stripe. *Radiology* 1977; **122:** 295–301.
11. Woodring JH, Pulmano CM, Stevens RK. The right paratracheal stripe in blunt chest trauma. *Radiology* 1982; **143:** 605–8.
12. Meschan I. The respiratory system. In: Meschan I. *An Atlas of Anatomy Basic to Radiology*. Philadelphia: WB Saunders, 1975; 581–658.
13. Meschan I. The heart and major blood vessels. In: Meschan I. *An Atlas of Anatomy Basic to Radiology*. Philadelphia: WB Saunders, 1975; 692–761.
14. Milne ENC, Pistolesi M. Quantification of pulmonary blood volume, flow, and pressure: principles. In: Milne ENC, Pistolesi M. *Reading the Chest Radiograph: a Physiologic Approach*. St Louis: Mosby, 1993; 164–241.
15. Groskin SA. *Heitzman's the Lung. Radiologic–Pathologic Correlations*, 3rd edn. St Louis: Mosby, 1993; 156.
16. Wilson AG. Pleura and pleural disorders. In: Armstrong P, Wilson AG, Dee P, Hansell DM (eds). *Imaging of Diseases of the Chest*, 2nd edn. St Louis: Mosby, 1995; 641–716.
17. Calhoon JH, Grover FL, Trinkle JK. Chest trauma. Approach and management. *Clin Chest Med* 1992; **13(1):** 55–67.
18. Mirvis SE, Templeton P. Imaging in acute thoracic trauma. *Semin Roentgenol* 1992; **27(3):** 184–210.
19. Heitzman ER. The mediastinum. In: *Radiological Correlations with Anatomy and Pathology*. St Louis: Mosby, 1977; 48.
20. Tocino I. Abnormal air and pleural fluid collections. In: Goodman LR, Putman CE (eds). *Critical Care Imaging*, 3rd edn. Philadelphia: WB Saunders, 1992; 137–60.
21. Levin B. The continuous diaphragm sign. A newly-recognized sign of pneumomediastinum. *Clin Radiol* 1973; **24:** 337–8.
22. Ochsner MG, Champion HR, Chambers RJ, Harviel JD. Pelvic fracture as an indicator of increased risk of thoracic aortic rupture. *J Trauma* 1989; **29(10):** 1376–9.
23. Marsh DG, Sturm JT. Traumatic aortic rupture: roentgenographic indications for angiography. *Ann Thorac Surg* 1976; **21(4):** 337–40.
24. White CS, Mirvis SE. Pictorial review: imaging of traumatic aortic injury. *Clin Radiol* 1995; **50:** 281–7.
25. Peters DR, Gamsu G. Displacement of the right paraspinous interface: a radiographic sign of acute traumatic rupture of the thoracic aorta. *Radiology* 1980; **134:** 599–603.
26. Miller GL, Hansen ME. Emergency evaluation of vascular

injuries. In: Redman HC, Purdy PD, Miller GL, Rollins NK (eds). *Emergency Radiology*. Philadelphia: WB Saunders, 1993; 451–514.

27. Perchinsky MJ, Long WB, Urman S, Borzotta A. 'The broken halo sign': a fractured calcified ring as an unusual sign of traumatic rupture of the thoracic aorta. *Injury* 1994; **25(10):** 649–52.

28. Ayella RJ, Hankins JR, Turney SZ, Cowley RA. Ruptured thoracic aorta due to blunt trauma. *J Trauma* 1977; **17(3):** 199–205.

29. Brasel KJ, Weigelt JA. Blunt thoracic aortic trauma: a cost-utility approach for injury detection. *Arch Surg* 1996; **131:** 619–26.

30. Agee CK, Metzler MH, Churchill RJ, Mitchell FL. Computed tomographic evaluation to exclude traumatic aortic disruption. *J Trauma* 1992; **33(5):** 876–81.

31. Durham RM, Zuckerman D, Wolverson M, *et al.* Computed tomography as a screening exam in patients with suspected blunt aortic injury. *Ann Surg* 1994; **220(5):** 699–704.

32. Gavant ML, Flick P, Menke P, Gold RE. CT aortography of thoracic aortic rupture. *Am J Roentgenol* 1996; **166:** 955–61.

33. Mirvis SE, Shanmuganathan K, Miller BH, White CS, Turney SZ. Traumatic aortic injury: diagnosis with contrast-enhanced thoracic CT – five year experience at a major trauma center. *Radiology* 1996; **200:** 413–22.

34. Morgan PW, Goodman LR, Aprahamain C, Foley WD, Lipchik EO. Evaluation of traumatic aortic injury: does dynamic contrast-enhanced CT play a role? *Radiology* 1992; **182:** 661–6.

35. Raptopoulos V. Chest CT for aortic injury: maybe not for everyone. *Am J Roentgenol* 1994; **162:** 1053–5.

36. Raptopoulos V, Sheiman RG, Phillips DA, Davidoff A, Silva WE. Traumatic aortic tear: screening with chest CT. *Radiology* 1992; **182:** 667–73.

37. Cohen AM, Crass JR. Traumatic aortic injuries: current concepts. *Semin Ultrasound CT MRI* 1993; **14(2):** 71–84.

38. Rollins RJ, Tocino I. Early radiographic signs of tracheal rupture. *Am J Roentgenol* 1987; **148:** 695–8.

39. Roxborgh JC. Rupture of the tracheobronchial tree. *Thorax* 1987; **42:** 681–8.

40. Unger JM, Schuchmann GG, Grossman JE, Pellett JR. Tears of the trachea and main bronchi caused by blunt trauma: radiologic findings. *Am J Roentgenol* 1989; **153:** 1175–80.

41. Wiot JF. Tracheobronchial trauma. *Semin Roentgenol* 1983; **271(1):** 15–22.

42. Oh KS, Fleischner FG, Wyman SM. Characteristic pulmonary finding in traumatic complete transection of a main-stem bronchus. *Radiology* 1969; **92:** 371–2.

43. Stern EJ, Frank MS. Acute traumatic hemopericardium. *Am J Roentgenol* 1994; **162:** 1305–6.

44. Naclerio EA. The 'V sign' in the diagnosis of spontaneous rupture of the esophagous (an early Roentgen clue). *Am J Surg* 1957; **93:** 291–8.

45. Stevens E, Templeton AW. Traumatic nonpenetrating lung contusion. *Radiology* 1965; **85:** 247–52.

46. Wagner RB, Crawford WO, Schimpf PP. Classification of parenchymal injuries of the lung. *Radiology* 1988; **167:** 77–82.

47. Raasch BN, Carsky EW, Lane EJ, O'Callaghan JP, Heitzman ER. Pleural effusion: explanation of some typical appearances. *Am J Roentgenol* 1982; **139:** 899–904.

48. Rudikoff JC. Early detection of pleural fluid. *Chest* 1980; **77(1):** 109–11.

49. Woodring JH. Recognition of pleural effusion on supine radiographs: how much fluid is required? *Am J Roentgenol* 1984; **142:** 59–64.

50. Bryk D. Infrapulmonary effusion. Effect of expiration on the pseudiaphragmatic contour. *Radiology* 1976; **120:** 33–6.

51. Schwartz MI, Marmorstein BL. A new radiologic sign of subpulmonic effusion. *Chest* 1975; **67(2):** 176–8.

52. Ruskin JA, Gurney JW, Thorsen MK, Goodman LR. Detection of pleural effusions on supine chest radiographs. *Am J Roentgenol* 1987; **148:** 681–3.

53. Felson B. Chest Roentgenology. Philadelphia: WB Saunders, 1973; 424.

54. Tocino IM, Miller MH, Frederick PR, Bahr AL, Thomas F. CT detection of occult pneumothorax in head trauma. *Am J Roentgenol* 1984; **143:** 987–90.

55. Tocino IM, Miller MH, Fairfax WR. Distribution of pneumothorax in the supine and semirecumbent critically ill adult. *Am J Roentgenol* 1985; **144:** 901–5.

56. Ziter FMH, Westcott JL. Supine subpulmonary pneumothorax. *Am J Roentgenol* 1981; **137:** 699–701.

57. Gordon R. The deep sulcus sign. *Radiology* 1980; **136:** 25–7.

58. Wiencek RG, Wilson RF, Steiger Z. Acute injuries of the diaphragm. An analysis of 165 cases. *J Thorac Cardiovasc Surg* 1986; **92:** 989–93.

59. Fataar S, Schulman A. Diagnosis of diaphragmatic tears. *Br J Radiol* 1979; **52:** 375–81.

60. Shapiro MJ, Heiberg E, Durham RM, Luchtefeld W, Mazuski JE. The unreliability of CT scans and initial chest radiographs in evaluating blunt trauma induced diaphragmatic rupture. *Clin Radiol* 1996; **51:** 27–30.

61. Shah R, Sabanathan S, Mearns AJ, Choudhury AK. Traumatic rupture of diaphragm. *Ann Thorac Surg* 1995; **60:** 1444–9.

62. Perlman SJ, Rogers LF, Mintzer RA, Mueller CF. Abnormal course of the nasogastric tube in traumatic rupture of left hemidiaphragm. *Am J Roentgenol* 1984; **142:** 85–8.

63. Meyers BF, McCabe CJ. Traumatic diaphragmatic hernia. Occult marker of serious injury. *Ann Surg* 1993; **218(6):** 783–90.

64. Guth AA, Pachter HL, Kim U. Pitfalls in the diagnosis of blunt diaphragmatic injury. *Am J Surg* 1995; **170:** 5–9.

65. Murray JG, Caoili E, Gruden JF, Evans SJJ, Halvorsen RA, Mackersie RC. Acute rupture of the diaphragm due to

blunt trauma: diagnostic sensitivity and specificity of CT. *Am J Roentgenol* 1996; **166:** 1035–9.

66. Pagliarello G, Carter J. Traumatic injury to the diaphragm: timely diagnosis and treatment. *J Trauma* 1992; **33(2):** 194–7.

67. Worthy SA, Kang EY, Hartman TE, Kwong JS, Mayo JR, Muller NL. Diaphragmatic rupture: CT findings in 11 patients. *Radiology* 1995; **194:** 885–8.

68. Caskey CI, Zerhouini EA, Fishman EK, Rahmouni AD. Aging of the diaphragm: a CT study. *Radiology* 1989; **171:** 385–9.

69. Nel JHT, Warren BL. Thoracoscopic evaluation of the diaphragm in patients with knife wounds of the left lower chest. *Br J Surg* 1994; **81:** 713–14.

70. Ochsner MG, Rozycki GS, Lucente F, Wherry DC, Champion HR. Prospective evaluation of thoracoscopy for diagnosing diaphragmatic injury in thoraco-abdominal trauma: a preliminary report. *J Trauma* 1993; **34(5):** 704–10.

71. Kang E-Y, Muller NL. CT in blunt chest trauma: pulmonary, tracheobronchial, and diaphragmatic injuries. *Semin Ultrasound CT MRI* 1996; **17(2):** 114–18.

72. Kerns SR, Gay SB. CT of blunt chest trauma. *Am J Roentgenol* 1990; **154:** 55–60.

73. Shanmuganathan K, Mirvis SE, White CS, Pomerantz SM. MR imaging evaluation of hemidiaphragms in acute blunt trauma: experience with 16 patients. *Am J Roentgenol* 1996; **167:** 397–402.

74. Takahashi N, Murakami J, Murayama S, Sakai S, Masuda K, Ishida T. Case report: MR evaluation of intrapulmonary hematoma. *J Computer Assist Tomogr* 1995; **19(1):** 125–7.

75. Brooks SW, Young JC, Cmolik B, *et al.* The use of transesophageal echocardiography in the evaluation of chest trauma. *J Trauma* 1992; **32(6):** 761–8.

76. Hendel RC, Cohn S, Aurigemma G, *et al.* Focal myocardial injury following blunt chest trauma: a comparison of indium-111 antimyosin scintigraphy and other noninvasive methods. *Am Heart J* 1992; **123:** 1208–15.

77. LaBan MM, Siegel CB, Schutz LK, Taylor RS. Occult radiographic fractures of the chest wall identified by nuclear scan imaging: report of seven cases. *Arch Phys Med Rehabil* 1994; **75(3):** 353–4.

78. Mitchell RS, Dake MD, Semba CP, *et al.* Endovascular stent-graft repair of thoracic aortic aneurysms. *J Thorac Cardiovasc Surg* 1996; **111:** 1054–62.

FURTHER READING

Calhoon JH, Grover FL, Trinkle JK. Chest trauma. Approach and management. *Clin Chest Med* 1992; **13(1):** 55–67.

Cohen AM, Crass JR. Traumatic aortic injuries: current concepts. *Semin Ultrasound CT MRI* 1993; **14(2):** 71–84.

Groskin SA. Selected topics in chest trauma. *Semin Ultrasound CT MRI* 1996; **17(2):** 119–41.

Harris JH, Harris WH, Novelline RA. Chest. In: Harris JH, Harris WH, Novelline RA. *The Radiology of Emergency Medicine*, 3rd edn. Baltimore: Williams & Wilkins, 1993; 469–622.

Mirvis SE, Templeton P. Imaging in acute thoracic trauma. *Semin Roentgenol* 1992; **27(3):** 184–210.

Raasch BN, Carsky EW, Lane EJ, O'Callaghan JP, Heitzman ER. Pleural effusion: explanation of some typical appearances. *Am J Roentgenol* 1982; **139:** 899–904.

Tocino I. Abnormal air and pleural fluid collections. In: Goodman LR, Putman CE (eds). *Critical Care Imaging*, 3rd edn. Philadelphia: WB Saunders, 1992; 137–60.

Wiencek RG, Wilson RF, Steiger Z. Acute injuries of the diaphragm. An analysis of 165 cases. *J Thorac Cardiovasc Surg* 1986; **92:** 989–93.

4

Fluid resuscitation in the patient with chest trauma

KENNETH L MATTOX, MATTHEW J WALL JR AND SCOTT A LEMAIRE

EPIDEMIOLOGICAL CONSIDERATIONS

The epidemiology of chest injury is covered in many chapters of this book. Seven percent of all homicide deaths are the direct result of chest injury. Each year, 20% (16 000) of the trauma deaths in the USA are attributable to chest trauma.[1] Among chest injury patients, approximately 85% have relatively 'minor' injuries that can be managed by observation, tube thoracostomy, or pain management alone. In this group, the outcome is favorable unless fluid resuscitation is overly aggressive and/or complications occur. Among trauma patients in general, 92–94% have injuries which do not result in hypotension, in that intravascular volume loss is less than 30% of the total blood volume.[1-4] Among the 6–8% of trauma patients with hypotension, 2–3% (33% of the hypotensive patients) are initially 'unstable' and have injury which results in a fatal outcome, even with the most aggressive therapy, including operation. In another 2–3% (33% of the hypotensive patients) the injury is relatively minor, and the hypotension is secondary to pre-existing conditions, gastric dilatation, pneumothorax, presence of alcohol or drugs in the bloodstream, or other conditions such as pneumothorax. In this group of patients, compensation is rapid, and the outcomes are identical whether or not fluid resuscitation is accomplished. In 2–3% of trauma patients (33% of the hypotensive cohort) a significant injury exists, but normal compensation mechanisms result in adequate cardiac output and a 'compensated' blood pressure, possibly 80/– to 90/–. In this group of patients, aggressive crystalloid resuscitation has been demonstrated to increase the rate of 'new' precontrol bleeding, pulmonary complications, coagulopathies, and compartment syndromes. Thus, aggressive fluid resuscitation in patients with chest trauma is not supported by currently available epidemiological data.[1-4]

HISTORIC APPROACHES TO VOLUME RESUSCITATION IN TRAUMA

During the early part of this century, limited crystalloid resuscitation in chest trauma patients was the rule. Following a series of 'controlled hemorrhage shock model' experiments, the recommendations for replacement with 3 ml of crystalloid for each 1 ml of estimated blood volume loss became a 'standard' approach for the operative management of patients with hemorrhage during the late 1950s and early 1960s. This was a time when the specialty of emergency medicine and emergency medical services (EMS) did not functionally exist. This '3:1 rule' became a standard policy without prospective, randomized, controlled, human evaluations. During the late 1960s and early 1970s, when emergency medicine became a discipline and prehospital EMS began to extend resuscitation, it was logical to 'start IVs' in the ambulance and attempt aggressive resuscitation.[5-9] This was often started prior to a surgeon's presence and without physician supervision. Protocols were developed which included devices capable of 'rapid infusion' of fluids in the ambulance, emergency center (EC), operating room and the intensive care unit (ICU). Even the advanced trauma life support (ATLS) course of the American College of Surgeon's Committee on Trauma initially recommended two 'large bore' intravenous sites to rapidly infuse crystalloid fluids at the '3:1' rate. Often, fluids were administered at even greater rates. For patients with chest injury, especially blunt chest trauma and pulmonary contusion, this aggressive volume resuscitation often resulted in pulmonary insufficiency and systemic inflammatory response syndromes (SIRS) with its pulmonary manifestation [adult respiratory distress syndrome (ARDS)].[10–15] The goal of field and EC resuscitation was often elevation of the blood pressure to normal or super normal levels, rather than to an appropriate life-sustaining level.

TYPES OF RESUSCITATIVE FLUID

Around the world, many 'resuscitative' fluids are available – normal saline, balanced salt solutions, hypertonic solutions including hypertonic saline, dextrans, various starches, and albumin, as well as blood and blood products. Each of these products has its champions and its detractors. Some are readily available and regionally accepted, whereas others are strongly condemned by detractors. The fact there is such an international variation is a reflection that the 'ideal' resuscitative fluid or philosophy has yet to be conceived.

Ringer's lactate and other balanced salt solutions and normal saline

Balanced salt solutions and normal saline were used during the 1950s and 1960s in controlled hemorrhage models to establish the '3:1' resuscitation rule. With equal distribution of fluid volumes in both interstitial and intravascular spaces, expanded blood and interstitial fluid during resuscitation resulted in considerable edema and weight gain. With moderate resuscitation, complications of ARDS were infrequent, but dilutional coagulopathy and dilutional anemia were common.[10–15] Such expanded fluid volumes did elevate blood pressure toward and even above normal. Renal blood flow was increased acutely, compared to controls. In the USA, these solutions became the resuscitative fluid of choice well into the 1990s.

Hypertonic saline

For the past 10 years, animal and clinical studies have evaluated 3.5–7.5% NaCl, with and without additional dextran.[16–24] The philosophy for use of hypertonic saline was that this solution would 'recruit' water from the interstitial and intracellular spaces. Although hypertonic saline has some theoretical benefit in patients with head injury, any incremental benefit compared to standard isotonic fluids (or even no fluid resuscitation) in patients with thoracic injury has not been demonstrated. One theoretical advantage of hypertonic saline as a resuscitative fluid is that it does not appear to activate cytokines, in opposition to balanced salt solutions.

Blood

In patients with severe thoracic injuries and blood loss exceeding 30% (class 3 hemorrhagic shock), blood transfusion can provide an immediate physiological benefit.[25] Additionally, many trauma surgeons prefer using blood as the principal resuscitative fluid in patients with pulmonary contusions or established ARDS. Allogenic blood transfusion, however, poses numerous risks, including transmission of infectious disease, transfusion reactions and immunosuppression (Table 4.1). These risks must be weighed carefully against any potential benefits.

Although the risk of transfusion-transmitted infection is declining, this complication remains a major concern. The transmission of viruses, bacteria and parasites continues to result in significant early and late morbidity. Transfusion-related viral hepatitis, caused by the hepatitis C virus in more than 90% of cases, leads to chronic liver disease in up to one-third of cases.[26]

Compared to elective blood transfusion, the use of blood products in the emergency treatment of a critically injured patient creates a situation that makes severe transfusion reactions not only more likely to occur, but also more difficult to detect. The administration of incompatible blood due to clerical error remains the most common cause of fatal hemolytic transfusion reaction.[26] The potentially chaotic atmosphere during resuscitation of an unstable trauma victim must be avoided to prevent such disasters. The manifestations of

Table 4.1 Risks associated with allogenic blood transfusion[2]

Complication	Risk
Transfusion reactions	
Minor allergic reaction	1:100
Hemolytic reaction	1:6000
Anaphylactic shock	1:500 000
Fatal hemolytic reaction	1:600 000
Infection	
Viral hepatitis	1:5000
HIV infection	1:420 000
HTLV I/II infection	1:200 000
Immunomodulation	
Immunosuppression	?
Systemic inflammatory response syndrome	?

Table 4.2 *Manifestations and management of suspected transfusion reaction*[6]

Manifestations	Management
Symptoms	**Treatment**
Pain	Discontinue transfusion immediately
Infusion site (burning)	Hemodynamic and respiratory support
Severe headache	Intravenous epinephrine (adrenaline) (10 ml of 1:10 000)
Back, flank, or joints	Change tubing of involved intravenous line
Restlessness	Maintain brisk urine output via volume expansion
Dyspnea	and administration of diuretics [furosemide (frusemide) and mannitol]
Chills	
Signs	**Investigation**
Fever	Send involved unit of blood and sample of patient's blood to blood bank for repeat type- and cross-match
Hypotension	Send patient blood sample for CBC, haptoglobin, free hemoglobin, bilirubin, BUN, creatinine and electrolytes; send urine for hemoglobin assay
Hemoglobinuria	
Coagulopathy (DIC)	
Respiratory failure	

hemolytic or anaphylactic transfusion reactions (Table 4.2) are likely to be masked by, and attributed to, the patient's injuries. A high degree of suspicion is, therefore, critical in any patient who develops sudden deterioration after receiving blood products. Management of a suspected severe transfusion reaction includes immediate cessation of the transfusion, aggressive physiological support, and prompt diagnostic investigation (Table 4.2).

Immunomodulation is the most recently recognized, and perhaps most significant, complication of blood transfusion in trauma patients. With regard to immunosuppression, multiple prospective randomized studies have demonstrated an increased incidence of postoperative infections in patients who received allogenic blood transfusion.[26] Recent studies with multiple regression analyses have identified blood transfusion as an independent predictor of infectious complications and multiple organ failure in trauma patients.[27,28] In addition to an apparent immunosuppresive effect, a transfusion-induced systemic inflammatory mediator storm with neutrophil activation may play a role in the development of multiple organ failure.[28,29] Large cohort studies with carefully stratified and well matched groups of trauma patients are needed to clarify these issues.

Type-specific blood replacement has considerable physiological benefit, especially if not overused or for a less than 30% blood loss. Blood, however, possesses numerous risks, especially viral risks, from hepatitis or HIV. In patients with pulmonary contusion or established ARDS, many trauma surgeons prefer using blood as the principal resuscitative fluid.[30,31]

Artificial blood

Currently under investigation but not available for clinical use are a variety of hemoglobin solutions to aid in oxygen transport, and some preliminary 'success' in general surgery patients has been reported.[32–35] These solutions currently possess vasoactive properties, which might be undesirable in the patient with thoracic trauma. As oxygen consumption will undoubtedly become a metric of monitoring the adequacy of perfusion (as opposed to a blood pressure target) level, solutions that increase oxygen transport will become a greater focus of fluid resuscitation in the future. Resuscitation oxygen-carrying solutions of the future may be entirely different from the current focus on stroma-free hemoglobin solutions.

Autotransfused blood

Autotransfusion has some of its greatest utility in thoracic surgery. Scavenged hemothorax blood can be reinfused via a variety of devices.[36,37] Reinfusion of blood which has been in contact with the pleural or pericardial surfaces for greater than 1 hour is not recommended, as the blood contains thrombolysins, which tend to increase the rate of bleeding and contribute to coagulopathies. Devices used in ECs and some ICUs contain a sterile blood collection device (some which mix anticoagulants with the collected blood) in series with the suction device. The collected blood can be reinfused directly. Operating room autotransfusion devices usually collect blood and, using a centrifuge, concentrate and wash the collected red blood cells prior to reinfusion. Autotransfusion is especially helpful in instances of thoracic great vessel injury, particularly injury to the aorta, pulmonary arteries and veins, intrathoracic vena cava, and thoracic outlet vascular injury.

LOCATION OF RESUSCITATION

It is logical to assume that triage, evaluation, resuscitation, staged definitive procedures and rehabilitation are continua of the same treatment. This process begins at the instant of injury. Many times, it is just as important not to compound the injury or physiological complications as it is to exercise good judgment in administering care. Such is particularly true with regard to fluid resuscitation of the thoracic trauma victim.

Prehospital

Since the late 1960s, prehospital care services have grown around the world, and in many areas even include air ambulance services. The more sophisticated the transportation service, such as helicopter air ambulance services, the greater the skill and educational level of the ambulance personnel. Often, there is a tendency for the ambulance attendant to 'do something', including administering aggressive fluid resuscitation via 'large bore' intravenous portals. Additionally, other interventions directed at elevating the blood pressure are often added.[1-9,38-45] Current evidence suggests that air ambulance resources are beneficial for wilderness, off shore, and high rise rescue, but are *not* beneficial for transport of trauma patients within a metropolitan area or for distances of less than 40 miles from a trauma center. Some recent data even suggest that patients with penetrating chest trauma within a major city have better survival if transported to a trauma center by private car rather than by advanced life support vehicles.[46] For victims of penetrating thoracic trauma, administration of prehospital resuscitation fluids has a detrimental effect, compared with delaying fluid resuscitation until skin incision.[47] These data appear to also be true for blunt chest trauma, but the data are not as compelling as they have been for penetrating trauma.[38,48-52]

Emergency center (EC)

The EC is where emergency physicians often aggressively administer crystalloid balanced salt solutions to victims of trauma, especially hypotensive patients. The 1997 version of the ATLS course, however, significantly downplays fluid resuscitation until *after* bleeding has been stopped. In patients with blunt chest trauma and a propensity for pulmonary contusion, aggressive fluid resuscitation often results in heightened pulmonary insufficiency and progressive hypoxemia. In patients with multiple rib fractures, the syndrome of 'flail chest' is not clinically evident until *after* more than 1500 ml of crystalloid resuscitative fluid have been administered, often 30 minutes to 2 hours *after* the patient has arrived in the EC. Trinkle[53] recommended, almost two decades ago, that crystalloid fluid resuscitation in the patient with a potential for flail chest be limited to less than 1000 ml/24 hours.

The restriction of resuscitative crystalloid fluids in the EC must be an active process. Large volumes of fluid via multiple ports tend to be administered because attention is directed to the primary and secondary surveys and the exact volume of crystalloid tends to get out of hand. In the EC, fluid resuscitation should not be the primary objective in patients with thoracic trauma. Limited and moderate volume restoration with a balanced salt solution, such as Ringer's lactate, is recommended. Monitoring parameters such as cerebral activity, urinary output, oxygen consumption and acidosis are undoubtedly more important than using predefined levels of blood pressure and pulse as indicators of the adequacy of perfusion. Recently developed transthoracic bioelectric impedance and transcutaneous oxygen monitors allow non-invasive monitoring of cardiac output and tissue oxygen delivery, respectively, shortly after arrival in the EC.[54]

Preoperative holding area

While patients with thoracic injuries are awaiting definitive surgical control of hemorrhage, permissive hypovolemia provides physiological control of hemorrhage. When bleeding is contained by fresh clot or surrounding tissues, aggressive volume replacement can raise blood pressure and disrupt the containing boundary. The dilution of platelets and coagulation factors is equally undesirable in the preoperative setting.

For a patient with planned surgery for truncal trauma, whether trauma is in the chest, abdomen, groin, or neck, the fluid resuscitation philosophy in the preoperative holding area should be the same as or more conservative than that in the EC. Specifically, the preoperative holding area (and the operating room prior to skin incision) should not be used as an opportunity to 'volume load' a patient who has chest trauma. If anything, this is a time to consciously restrict the crystalloid fluid volume load because of the numerous complications associated with aggressive fluid volume resuscitation.

Operating room

In the operating room, 'aggressive' administration of crystalloid resuscitative fluids, blood and blood products, including autotransfusion, has become the 'norm'. Especially for anesthesiologists trained during the last 15 years, this aggressive volume loading and fluid administration has become more common than judicious volume resuscitation. In most operating rooms devices are available which allow for the rapid infusion of very large volumes of fluid (often with the added ability to warm the infused solutions).

In the patient with chest injury with either blunt or penetrating trauma to the lung, such aggressive fluid administration results in increased lung water, consolidation and increased intrapulmonary shunting. The surgeon, often diverted by technical challenges, may be unaware of this aggressive volume resuscitation, which very often exceeds estimated losses. In addition, the choice of fluids is often not discussed with the surgeon, although the surgeon is responsible for managing this patient's pulmonary insufficiency in the ICU. In such patients, most surgeons strongly oppose the use of albumin and other colloidal solution, which leave the intravascular space, increase interstitial edema, and further compromise an already compromised pulmonary status. In all trauma patients, especially those with chest injury, it is extremely important neither to under- nor to over-fluid resuscitate. As in all other areas where personnel from multiple disciplines interact to join talents in the care of an extremely sick patient with complex problems, honest and open communication is imperative. This is especially important in the patient with a chest injury who is in need of fluid administration. The type, route, rate and reason for that particular fluid should be openly discussed and not become an authority or turf issue.

Intensive care unit (ICU)

In the ICU, fluid therapy of patients with chest injury should be focused on 'maintenance and replacement', rather than continued 'resuscitation'. Although Shoemaker[54] has recommended 'super-resuscitation' for trauma patients in the ICU, most of the patients were not thoracic trauma victims. This suggested super-resuscitation is guided by very careful hemodynamic monitoring of pulmonary artery and systemic pressures as well as cardiac output, urinary output, peripheral vascular resistance, and base deficit. In addition to greater than normal volumes of crystalloid fluids being 'pushed', drugs to increase cardiac contractility and manipulation of peripheral vasoconstriction are also administered. Most trauma surgeons do not aggressively continue crystalloid resuscitation in the ICU. For patients with pulmonary contusion, pulmonary hematomas, or flail chest, crystalloid fluid in the ICU should be limited to less than 1000 ml/24 hours, if possible.[53] Should volume expansion be required, colloid solutions such as blood are recommended, rather than crystalloids. In patients with blunt cardiac injury and cardiac decompensation, or in patients with penetrating trauma and right heart failure, fluid administration must be very carefully managed, sometimes considering pulmonary artery vasodilatation and systemic use of vasoconstrictive drugs, and even use of a hemoconcentration device to remove intravascular water. In rare instances, one might consider use of a right ventricular assist device, although such devices in patients with chest trauma have infrequently been successful.

ADJUNCTS TO THORACIC TRAUMA RESUSCITATION

Consideration for vascular access

Effective vascular access obviously requires an intact vascular conduit between the access site and the heart. Therefore, patients with potential injuries to the superior vena cava, subclavian veins, or the innominate vein should have large bore (16 gauge or larger) intravenous access established in the lower extremities whenever possible. Access can rapidly be accomplished via the saphenous vein, which can be cannulated percutaneously or via cutdown at the ankle or groin. When a saphenous vein cutdown is performed, sterile intravenous extension tubing directly into the vein provides excellent large bore access.

Percutaneous cannulation of the femoral vein is another option for establishing rapid intravenous access; associated infectious and thrombotic complications pose some concerns. In the absence of a palpable femoral pulse, the femoral vein can be reliably located by inserting the cannula below the inguinal ligament at the midpoint between the anterior superior iliac spine and the symphysis pubis. To prevent potential infectious and thrombotic complications, early removal of femoral lines after the patient has stabilized and other access sites have been obtained is recommended.

When a subclavian venous catheter is required in a patient with suspected subclavian vascular injury, the contralateral subclavian vein should be used for insertion. Placing the catheter on the side of an existing chest tube also minimizes the potential pneumothorax complication associated with subclavian vein cannulation. Should an injury to the innominate vein or aortic arch be suspected, a left subclavian venous line should not be inserted, as it might be clamped and divided should innominate vein division be required.

Finally, for patients undergoing emergency thoracotomy, a right atrial line can be placed in those with inadequate venous access. A Foley catheter is inserted through a right atriotomy. After inflating the balloon with saline, the catheter is secured with a polypropylene purse string suture or heavy silk tie placed around the atriotomy. After aspirating air from the catheter, large bore blood tubing can be inserted into the end of the Foley catheter, allowing for rapid fluid administration.

Tube thoracostomy

Following chest trauma, hemothorax and/or pneumothorax is the most common occurrence. Simple (and single) intercostal tube thoracostomy through the fourth or fifth interspace provides not only a release of hemo/pneumothorax, but also is an important monitoring mechanism as well as a guide to volume replacement. Autotransfusion of acute hemothorax blood loss (less than 1 hour's contact with the pleural or peritoneal surface) is an ideal application of this technology. This should be placed in the mid-axillary line. The chest should be entered only with the finger as 15% of patients have a pleural symphysis. In addition, the operating surgeon should digitally explore the chest, feeling for tamponade or a diaphragmatic injury. Finally, the chest tube removal is an underrated procedure and carries its own set of complications.

EC thoracotomy

Thoracotomy in the EC is an important resuscitative adjunct to consider in dying, not irreversible and/or obviously dead patients.[55,56] Most applicable in patients with penetrating (especially stab) wounds to the heart, EC thoracotomy also has been successful in resuscitating patients with a wide variety of etiologies, including selected patients with blunt trauma. During this operation, performed in the EC by surgeons, large volumes of crystalloid and blood replacement are usually required.

Hemoconcentration devices

Devices designed to remove fluid volume, especially water, are often indicated in trauma patients. Trauma patients are often given excessively large volumes of fluid prehospital, in the EC and in the operating room. In patients with thoracic injury, especially blunt injury to the heart or lungs, and in patients with a 'mediator storm,' secondary pulmonary capillary leak makes additional crystalloid administration a compounding factor to any existing pulmonary insufficiency. Diuretics are often ineffectual in removing excessive lung and intravascular water. In such instances, extracorporal devices, such as hemoconcentrators and dialysis equipment, both peritoneal and hemo-access, are sometimes indicated.

Mechanical assist devices

Although not used in fluid resuscitation, ventricular assist devices are occasionally used in the trauma patient. Right ventricular failure is increasingly being recognized, secondary to either direct injury to the myocardium or secondary right ventricular failure resulting from volume overload or increased pulmonary vascular resistance. In such instances, the ventricular assist device allows the heart to 'rest' for a few days and provides time for removal of fluid or recovery of a depressed myocardium. Patients with massive thoracic trauma often develop cardiac

failure. Early efforts to use cardiopulmonary bypass were abandoned due to the need for systemic heparinization. Recent advances with heparin-bonded tubing, centrifugal pumps and selective ventricular support may result in a resurgence of interest in these adjuncts. Regardless, due to the complexity of these injuries, mechanical assist may never become a practical reality.

Compared to limited fluid administration, the use of cardiopulmonary life support devices in trauma lies at the opposite extreme of the resuscitation spectrum. Patients with massive thoracic trauma often develop cardiac failure due either to direct myocardial injury, or secondary to volume overload or increased vascular resistance.[57–59]

Autotransfusion devices

Cited throughout this chapter are references to the use of autotransfusion to aid in resuscitation in thoracic trauma. In the EC, operating room and surgical ICU, autotransfusion is an integral part of resuscitation for chest trauma. Devices are available which directly reinfuse anticoagulated blood from a pleural collection container as well as concentrate, wash and reinfuse the processed scavenged blood. Both types should be readily and easily set up and operated by both surgeons and nurses in a trauma center.

RESEARCH IN HYPOVOLEMIC FLUID RESUSCITATION

Basic science

Basic science research is currently directed to further elucidating the physiology of hypotension, shock and resuscitation. Cytokine production and the downregulation of lymphocytes does not occur with hypotension alone, but is activated after resuscitation is begun. Cytokine activation does not appear to occur with whole blood or hypertonic saline fluid resuscitation, but is activated with all other current solutions, including Ringer's lactate. Uncontrolled hemorrhagic shock models have demonstrated that limited resuscitation carries an acute mortality less than that which occurs with aggressive fluid resuscitation. Aggressive fluid resuscitation in this uncontrolled model results in a renewed and increased rate of bleeding. Furthermore, as in the clinical studies, an acute alteration in the clotting tests (including platelet counts) occurs even with moderate crystalloid resuscitation. Currently, additional research, relating to the value of hypothermia as a 'protective' mechanism in post-traumatic hypotension, is ongoing.

Military

Future warfare will undoubtedly be different from the major wars of the twentieth century (WWI, WWII, Korea and Vietnam). Military campaigns will occur rather quickly, require rapid dispatch of troops, be accompanied by many special operations, and possibly be over within a few days or a few weeks. There will not be time for an orderly build-up of troops and supportive medical facilities. Furthermore, there will be no time to develop a 'learning curve' for injuries of the 'new' warfare. Current military medical and concept research and development are directed toward portable facilities, directed personnel, as well as use of new technology in imaging, monitoring, communications, hemorrhage control techniques and streamlined equipment.[60] In addition, in the USA, innovative military/civilian trauma education and research initiatives have been proposed from Congress, special panels, Joint Chiefs of Staff and the civilian trauma leadership. Thus, the military medical research is directed in basic science, clinical applications and systems development. In the area of acute trauma resuscitation, including chest injury, the current US military recommendations for the future parallel those from major trauma centers in the USA. Those recommendations are to avoid 'aggressive' crystalloid volume resuscitation and utilize monitoring techniques rather than blood pressure as endpoints of resuscitation.

Civilian

In addition to the basic science research, civilian clinical research in trauma resuscitation continues in the areas of limited to moderate fluid resuscitation, especially in the patient with chest injury. New solutions which will increase the oxygen-carrying potential for the blood and increase oxygen consumption are being investigated. Hypertonic saline continues to be a focus of research for a limited number of centers. Some civilian centers are focusing on defining time as an independent variable in trauma care and are finding that 'the golden hour' is more a marketing tactic than a scientific reality.

CURRENT RECOMMENDATIONS IN FLUID RESUSCITATION IN PATIENTS WITH CHEST INJURY

Based on the principles discussed above, the following approaches to fluid resuscitation are recommended for patients with thoracic injuries. Intravenous access is preferentially established in the lower extremities whenever possible. The placement of a subclavian line on a side with potential vascular injury is avoided.

In assessing the need for volume replacement, generalized signs of adequate tissue perfusion – such as mentation and urine output – are used, rather than relying on specific blood pressure values. In a patient with adequate perfusion, fluid administration is limited. Mild hypotension (SBP 60–90 mmHg) and hypovolemia are permitted to control hemorrhage in patients who are awaiting definitive repair of their injuries, as long as they exhibit adequate tissue perfusion. Continuous reassessment of perfusion is critical in managing fluid resuscitation in these patients. In patients who are hemodynamically unstable (SBP <60 mmHg) or exhibit other evidence of impaired tissue perfusion, aggressive resuscitation is advocated. Warm crystalloid (lactated Ringer's solution at 40°C) is used initially, followed by warmed blood products as needed.

In the setting of ongoing hemorrhage, autotransfusion devices are used to collect and return shed blood to the patient. In patients with penetrating trauma, a large prospective randomized trial has demonstrated the advantage of limited fluid resuscitation in the patient with penetrating trauma in the urban environment. In patients with blunt trauma, whilst the data relating to penetrating truncal trauma do not specifically relate to blunt trauma, fluid restriction in the patient with isolated chest trauma has a great deal of support.[47] Furthermore, it may be postulated that even for multisystem injured patients, the same mechanisms of prevention of clot disruption, hemodilution, or coagulopathy may be an advantageous effect of fluid restriction. In addition, patients with traumatic disruption of the thoracic aorta would also benefit from prevention of hyper-resuscitation.

Scientifically, a randomized, prospective study similar to the penetrating trauma study is badly needed. In patients with concomitant head injury, maintaining an adequate cerebral perfusion pressure is considered mandatory by neurosurgeons. Whether or not this should be accomplished by aggressive fluid administration, vasoactive drugs, hypertonic solutions or other means is still under investigation. The addition of significant head injury complicates the treatment algorithm. Whilst fluid restriction has advantages, it is in direct conflict with the current thinking of maintaining aggressive oxygen delivery to the brain. It may be that an appropriate middle ground must be developed, as opposed to responding to data applicable to isolated head injury. Until large prospective trials occur, timing and mode of resuscitation should be an individualized, surgeon-directed procedure.[61]

REFERENCES

1. LoCicero J, III, Mattox KL. Epidemiology of chest trauma. *Surg Clin North Am* 1989; **69**:15–19.

2. Mattox KL. Indications for thoracotomy: deciding to operate. *Surg Clin North Am* 1989; **69**: 47–58.

3. Mattox KL. Approaches to trauma involving the major vessels of the thorax. *Surg Clin North Am* 1989; **69**: 77–91.

4. Border JR, Lewis FR, Aprahamian C, *et al.* Prehospital trauma care – stabilization or scoop and run. *J Trauma* 1983; **23**: 708–11.

5. Kaweski SM, Sise MJ, Virgilio RW. The effect of prehospital fluids on survival in trauma patients. *J Trauma* 1990; **30**: 1215–19.

6. Lee WC. Field intravenous lines – Are they worth it? (abstract) *J Trauma* 1986; **26**: 678.

7. Lewis FL. Prehospital intravenous fluid therapy: physiologic computer modeling. *J Trauma* 1986; **26**: 804–11.

8. Smith JP, Bodai BI, Hill AS, *et al.* Prehospital stabilization of critically injured patients: a failed concept. *J Trauma* 1985; **25**: 65–70.

9. Trunkey DD. Is ALS necessary for prehospital trauma care? *J Trauma* 1984; **24**: 86–7.

10. Barnes RW, Merendino KA. Post-traumatic pulmonary insufficiency syndrome. *Surg Clin North Am* 1972; **52(3)**: 625–33.

11. Bass TL, Miller PK, Campbell DB, Russell GB. Traumatic adult respiratory distress syndrome. *Chest Surg Clin North Am* 1997; **7(2)**: 429–42.

12. Bickell WH, Bruttig SP, Millnamoro GA, *et al.* The detrimental effects of intravenous crystalloid after aortotomy in swine. *Surgery* 1991; **110**: 529–36.

13. Boyd AD, Glassman LR. Trauma to the lung. *Chest Surg Clin North Am* 1997; **7(2)**: 263–84.

14. Pepe PE. Acute post-traumatic respiratory physiology and insufficiency. *Surg Clin North Am* 1989; **69**: 157–73.

15. Bickell W, Pepe PE, Mattox KL. Complications of resuscitation. In: Mattox KL (ed.). *Complications of Trauma.* New York: Churchill Livingstone, 1994; 126–31.

16. Behrman SW, Fabian TC, Kudsk KA, Proctor KG. Microcirculatory flow changes after initial resuscitation of hemorrhagic shock with 7.5% hypertonic saline/6% dextran 70. *J Trauma* 1991; **31**: 589–600.

17. Kien ND; Kramer GC, White DA. Acute hypotension caused by rapid hypertonic saline infusion in anesthetized dogs. *Anesth Analg* 1991; **73**: 597–602.

18. Ducey JP, Mozingo DW, Lamiell JM, Okerburg C, Gueller GE. A comparison of the cerebral and cardiovascular effects of complete resuscitation with isotonic and hypertonic saline, Hetastarch, and whole blood for hemorrhage. *J Trauma* 1989; **29**: 1510–18.

19. Gala GJ, Lilly MP, Thomas SE, Gann DS. Interaction of sodium and volume in fluid resuscitation after hemorrhage. *J Trauma* 1991; **31**: 545–56.

20. Gross D, Landau EH, Assalia A, *et al.* Is hypertonic saline resuscitation safe in 'uncontrolled' hemorrhagic shock. *J Trauma* 1988; **28**: 751–6.

21. Gross D, Landau EH, Klin B, *et al.* Quantitative measurement of bleeding following hypertonic saline

therapy in 'uncontrolled' hemorrhagic shock. *J Trauma* 1989; **29**: 79–83.

22. Gross D, Landau EH, Klin B, Krausz MM. Treatment of uncontrolled hemorrhagic shock with hypertonic saline solution. *Surg Gynecol Obstet* 1990; **170**: 106–12.

23. Mattox KL, Maningas PA, Moore EE *et al.* Prehospital hypertonic saline/dextran for post-traumatic hypotension. *Ann Surg* 1991; **213**: 482–91.

24. Reed RL, Johnston TD, Chen Y, Fischer RP. Hypertonic saline alters plasma clotting times and platelet aggregation. *J Trauma* 1991; **31**: 8–14.

25. Hamilton SM. The use of blood in resuscitation of the trauma patient. *Can J Surg* 1993; **36**: 21–7.

26. Klein HG. Allogenic transfusion risks in the surgical patient. *Am J Surg* 1995; **170 (suppl 6A)**: 21S–6S.

27. Edna TH, Bjerkeset T. Association between blood transfusion and infection in injured patients. *J Trauma* 1992; **33**: 659–61.

28. Moore FA, Moore EE, Sauaia A. Blood transfusion: an independent risk factor for postinjury multiple organ failure. *Arch Surg* 1997; **132**: 620–5.

29. Patrick DA, Moore EE, Barnett CC, Silliman CC. Human polymerized hemoglobin as a blood substitute avoids transfusion-induced neutrophil priming. *Surg Forum* 1996; **47**: 36–8.

30. Greenburg AG. New transfusion strategies. *Am J Surg* 1997; **173**: 49–52.

31. Harrigan C, Lucas CE, Ledgerwood AM. The effect of hemorrhagic shock on the clotting cascade in injured patients. *J Trauma* 1989; **29**: 1416–22.

32. Stern SA, Dronen SC, Megoron AJ, *et al.* Effective supplemental perfluorocarbon administration on hypotensive resuscitation of severe uncontrolled hemorrhage. *Am J Emerg Med* 1995; **13**: 269–75.

33. Schultz SC, Hamilton IN Jr, Malcolm DS. Use of base deficit to compare resuscitation with lactated Ringer's solution, haemacoel, whole blood, and diaspirin cross-linked hemoglobin following hemorrhage. *J Trauma* 1993; **35**: 619–26.

34. Xu L, Sun L, Rollwagen FM, *et al.* Cellular responses to surgical trauma, hemorrhage, and resuscitation with diaspirin cross-linked hemoglobin in rats. *J Trauma* 1997; **42**: 32–41.

35. Rabinocivi S, Rudolph AS, Vernick J, Feuerstein G. A new salutary resuscitative fluid: liposome encapsulated hemoglobin/hypertonic saline solution. *J Trauma* 1993; **35**: 121–7.

36. Mattox KL, Walker LE, Beall AC Jr, Jordan GL Jr. Blood availability for the trauma patient – autotransfusion. *J Trauma* 1975; **15**: 663–9.

37. Greenberg AG. New transfusion strategies. *Am J Surg* 1997; **173**: 49–52.

38. Bickell WH, Shaftan GW, Mattox KL. Intravenous fluid administration and uncontrolled hemorrhage. *J Trauma* 1989; **29**: 409.

39. Cannon WB, Faser J, Cowell EM. The preventive treatment of wound shock. *JAMA* 1918; **47**: 618.

40. Harris BH, Shaftan GW, Chiu CJ, Limson A. The treatment of massive venous hemorrhage: an experimental re-appraisal. *Surgery* 1967; **61(6):** 891–5.

41. Harris BH, Shaftan GW, Herbsman H. Maintenance of cardiac output despite deliberate hypotension. *Surg Forum* 1969; **20:** 31.

42. Mattox KL, Bickell W, Pepe P, *et al.* Prospective MAST study in 911 patients. *J Trauma* 1989; **29:** 1104–12.

43. Mattox KL, Feliciano DV. Role of external cardiac compression in truncal trauma. *J Trauma* 1982; **209:** 698–705.

44. *The Medical Department of the US Army in the World War.* Vol. 8, *Field Operations.* US Government Printing Office, 1926; 109–10.

45. *Surgery in World War II, General Surgery.* Washington, DC: Office of the Surgeon General, Department of the Army, US Government Printing Office, 1952; 6–17.

46. Demetriades D, Chan L, Cornwell E, *et al.* Paramedic vs private transportation of trauma patients. *Arch Surg* 1996; **131:** 133–8.

47. Bickell WH, Wall MJ, Pepe PE, *et al.* Immediate versus delayed fluid resuscitation for hypotensive patients with penetrating torso injuries. *N Engl J Med* 1994; **331:** 1105–9.

48. Assalia A, Schein M. Resuscitation for haemorrhagic shock. *Br J Surg* 1993; **80(2):** 213.

49. Kowalenko T, Stern S, Wang X, Dronen S. Improved outcome with 'hypotensive' resuscitation of uncontrolled hemorrhagic shock in a swine model. *J Trauma* 1991; **31:** 1032.

50. Martin RR, Bickell W, Mattox KL, Burch JM, Pepe PE. Prospective evaluation of preoperative fluid resuscitation in hypotensive patients with penetrating truncal injury: a preliminary report. *J Trauma* 1992; **33:** 354–62.

51. Bickell WH, Bruttig SP, Wade CE. Hemodynamic response to abdominal aortotomy in the anesthetized swine. *Circ Shock* 1989; **28:** 321–32.

52. Dronen SC, Stern SA, Wang X, Stanley M. A comparison of the response of near-fatal acute hemorrhage mode with and without a vascular injury to rapid volume expansion. *Am J Emerg Med* 1993; **11:** 331–5.

53. Calhoon JH, Trinkle JK. Pathophysiology of chest trauma. *Chest Surg Clin North Am* 1997; **7(2):** 199–211.

54. Asensio JA, Demetriades D, Berne TV, Shoemaker WC. Invasive and noninvasive monitoring for early recognition and treatment of shock in high-risk trauma and surgical patients. *Surg Clin North Am* 1996; **76:** 985–97.

55. Mattox KL, Beall AC Jr, Jordan GL Jr, *et al.* Cardiorrhaphy in the emergency center. *J Thorac Cardiovasc Surg* 1974; **68:** 886–95.

56. Durham LA, Richardson RJ, Wall MJ, *et al.* Emergency center thoracotomy: impact of prehospital resuscitation. *J Trauma* 1992; **32:** 775–9.

57. Lisagor P, Cohen D, McDonnell B, Lawlor D, Moore C. Irreversible shock revisited: mechanical support of the cardiovascular system: a case report and review. *J Trauma* 1997; **42:** 1182–6.

58. Perchinsky MJ, Long WB, Hill JG, Parsons JA, Bennett JB. Extracorporeal cardiopulmonary life support with heparin-bonded circuitry in the resuscitation of massively injured trauma patients. *Am J Surg* 1995; **169:** 488–91.

59. Flint L. Judgment driven resuscitation – new acquaintance or old friend? *Shock* 1996; **6:** 317–18.

60. Butler FK, Hagmann J, Butler EG. Tactical combat casualty care in special operations. *Milit Med* 1996; **161(suppl):** 3–16.

61. Battistella FD, Wisner DH. Combined hemorrhagic shock and head injury: effects of hypertonic saline (7.5%) resuscitation. *J Trauma* 1991; **31:** 182–8.

5

Blood conservation and blood substitutes in the management of thoracic trauma

GREGORY A NUTTALL AND MICHAEL J JOYNER

INTRODUCTION

Patients receiving surgical treatment for thoracic trauma frequently receive blood products either during surgery or during the immediate postoperative period.[1–5] Transfusion practices during and after such procedures are governed by principles similar to those associated with cardiac and thoracic surgery, other types of surgery, and trauma in general.[1–9] However, there are several unique things about thoracic trauma. First, thoracic trauma can require the use of extra-corporeal circulation and gas exchange. This procedure usually requires systemic anticoagulation and causes marked hemodilution. In this setting, mechanical interactions between the cardiopulmonary bypass pump and oxygenator can damage blood cells and other blood components. Second, while patients undergoing cardiovascular surgery frequently have coexisting vascular disease, and the blood flow to and function of a variety of organ systems are frequently compromised, trauma victims are frequently younger and healthier. However, in thoracic trauma there can be multiple insults to key organs involved in gas exchange and O_2 delivery as a result of conditions such as pneumothorax, cardiac tamponade, and aortic rupture or dissection. In both thoracic trauma and 'routine' cardiac or thoracic surgery the key challenges relate to maintenance of O_2 delivery to tissues, management of intentional or unintentional hypothermia, and recognition and successful treatment of surgical bleeding and coagulopathies.

With this information as a background, the purpose of this chapter is to discuss issues related to blood transfusion and blood substitutes in the treatment of thoracic trauma and compare these concepts to what is known about transfusions in general and transfusions during 'routine' cardiac and thoracic surgery. This is necessary since transfusion practices in trauma are primarily empirical.[2–5] In general, the focus will be on red blood cells and oxygen-carrying capacity. Issues related to coagulation and clotting factors will be discussed in the context of how bleeding might alter oxygen-carrying capacity. Finally, most of the statistical data on transfusion practices that might be germane to thoracic trauma after stabilization of the patient comes from the experience accumulated during cardiac surgery. In the United States coronary artery bypass surgery was performed 485 000 times in 1993, and the transfusion related experience of various centers has been surveyed and reported.[6–8,10–12]

BLOOD USE IN THE USA

Currently, 12–13 million units of red blood cells are transfused to patients each year in the USA.[13–16] About 60–70% of this blood is given to surgical patients in the perioperative period.[13,15,16] Additionally, of all the patients who received red blood cell transfusions, roughly half are 65 years of age or older.[13,15,16] This means that the 'average' patient receiving red blood cell transfusions is an older patient who is either undergoing surgery or has recently undergone surgery. The fraction of the red cells transfused to trauma victims is unknown, but since trauma is a 'disease' of the young it is likely that these patients are much younger and healthier than the 'average' transfusion recipient. Additionally, experience from battlefield situations indicates that the number of 'units' of red cells given to the average combat trauma victim is highly variable and frequently difficult to predict on the basis of the initial events.[1]

About 13–14 million units of red blood cells are collected each year in the USA.[13] When appropriate inventory control and planning is used, very little of this blood becomes 'outdated' and is wasted. About 2% of eligible American citizens donate blood and, whilst the guidelines are changing, blood donation by patients more than 65 years of age is not yet routine.[15,17] If per capita use of red blood cells by various age groups does not change, and the distribution of various surgical procedures and the amount of blood used in each surgical procedure does not change, there will be marked shortages of red blood cells in the reasonably near future.[15,16,18] By the year 2030, this shortage is projected to be 5 million units per year.[15,16,18] This demographic pressure on the blood supply is a primary reason why efforts at blood conservation and development of blood substitutes are essential to sustain medical and surgical practices into the future.

Blood conservation and use of blood substitutes is also attractive in the context of concerns about the 'safety' of the current blood supply. At many centers, use of autologous blood expanded dramatically in the 1980s with concerns over transmission of HIV via the blood supply.[19–24] However, this problem has largely been resolved by the use of advanced screening procedures, and the risk of HIV transmission in blood products is now very low (1 in 300 000–400 000 or less).[18,25,26] Additionally, blood is now screened routinely for several types of hepatitis, and the transmission of hepatitis, which was previously an under-appreciated but serious consequence of transfusions, has now also been reduced dramatically.[27] Taken together, this means that when blood from adequately screened volunteer donors is subject to the appropriate testing, the risk of transmission of infectious diseases is probably far lower than it has ever been.[18]

BLOOD USE DURING THORACIC TRAUMA

Thoracic trauma can cause compromise of one or more organs that are central for gas exchange. In the case of conditions such as pulmonary contusion or cardiac tamponade, transfusion per se might be of limited or no benefit. However, during problems associated with bleeding that are primarily related to damage to the great pulmonary or aortic vessels, the principles of transfusion practices are straightforward. The major goal is to provide the patient with adequate intervascular volume and oxygen carrying capacity so that O_2 delivery to vital organs can be sustained until surgical control of bleeding

is obtained. This means that large-bore intravenous (central or peripheral) access will be required and prompt transfusion of a combination of saline and packed red blood cells may be needed. The timing of transfusion in these patients has recently been questioned, as has value of 'fluid resuscitation' in the field.[2–5]

As a result of safety concerns and demographic pressure on the blood supply mentioned previously, transfusion algorithms and other thoughtful approaches to blood use are now being used routinely during many surgical procedures and for many medical conditions. By contrast, in unstable trauma it may be justified to 'transfuse first and ask questions later'. Under these circumstances little attention is paid to the patient's hemoglobin, since the primary goal is support of blood pressure and treatment of rapid ongoing or anticipated blood loss. Again, the optimal timing of such transfusions remains to be determined.[2–5]

While type specific blood might seem preferable, experience by the US military in Vietnam shows that type O blood (positive or negative in the case of males, negative in the case of females) can be given and may in fact be safer than type-specific blood.[1] Use of type O blood in these circumstances may in fact increase safety since clerical errors associated with the normal confusion in a busy emergency department might be avoided. However, it should be noted that the use of type O positive blood in young males from certain inner-city populations might be problematic, since individuals from particularly violent environments might have been sensitized by previous O positive transfusions. It should also be noted that the key issue is prompt surgical control of bleeding. Use of calcium, platelets, or other adjuvants is probably not necessary on a routine basis until one or more of the patients' blood volumes have been transfused.

A major challenge associated with massive transfusion is temperature regulation in a 'cold' patient. Reductions in body temperature can have a devastating impact on platelet and coagulation factor function. There is also ongoing controversy about the optimal timing of blood transfusions in trauma. Some advocate early transfusion; others advocate a wait-and-see approach if the patient is not obviously unstable.[2,5] Finally, in many instances transfusions are initiated in the emergency department and then a clear cut need for further transfusion is not identified.[1] All of these factors make data collection, analysis and development of evidence based transfusion practices difficult in trauma patients. What can be said with certainty is that (1) patients who are unstable probably warrant blood transfusion; (2) type O blood is acceptable under these circumstances (there is controversy about when it is permissible to switch to type specific units; the usual rule of thumb is to continue with type O blood after 6-8 units have been given); (3) surgical control of bleeding is essential; (4) with massive transfusions, unless one or more of the patients' blood volumes has been transfused, routine use of coagulation factors and platelets is probably not warranted; (5) a fall in body temperature is likely to be a continuing challenge.

While this approach to transfusion for thoracic trauma may not be 'intellectually satisfying' it shares some of the same challenges associated with routine cardiac surgery, where data is now emerging and beginning to allow 'evidence-based' transfusion practices. In this context, the review of blood use during cardiac surgery is especially useful.

BLOOD USE DURING CARDIAC SURGERY

Practice variability

It is interesting to note that there is tremendous practice variability in the use of red blood cells during cardiac surgery.[7] In some centers, many patients successfully undergo coronary artery bypass grafting without the transfusion of allogeneic (donor) blood cells. These patients receive either no red blood cell products or limited amounts of autologous predonated blood or 'cell-saver' blood. By contrast, at some centers, allogeneic red cells are transfused routinely to patients who undergo coronary artery bypass surgery and other forms of cardiac surgery. Additionally, there is probably also large practice variability within institutions where patients cared for by some surgical, anesthesia, and critical care teams receive almost no red blood cell products, whereas other patients at the same institution cared for by other teams frequently receive red blood cell products.

The factors responsible for this practice variability are unknown. There are several possible explanations for this variability which include:

- Patient differences, including perioperative coagulation status, preoperative hemoglobin, and the type of operation required (i.e. a 'redo').
- Philosophical differences about what constitutes an appropriate 'transfusion trigger'.
- Surgical 'skill'.

All things being equal, it would appear to many who care for operative patients that some surgeon's operations are associated with more blood loss than others.[28] Whether this is the result of differences in technical skills or other factors is currently unknown. Taken together, these data highlight the need for more information concerning the causes of practice variability and also the need for outcome-based studies and quality control efforts to reduce the use of allogeneic blood during cardiac surgery.[21,29–31] Similar efforts at understanding transfusion practices in trauma are also needed in an effort to better understand how best to treat these

patients. In both cases this would represent 'quality assurance' efforts directed at real patient care issues as opposed to bureaucratic futility.

The transfusion trigger

While many transfusion for thoracic trauma are 'emergencies' and are given with little concern for the patient's hemoglobin or hematocrit, the transfusion trigger during and after cardiac surgery is now being addressed. In many centers, hemoglobin concentrations of 10 g/dl (Hct of approximately 30) would be considered ideal or nearly ideal for a patient after cardiac surgery, the concept being that this hematocrit and hemoglobin would maximize oxygen delivery to the heart since the rheological properties of blood are nearly ideal in a hematocrit of 30. However, recent guidelines have emphasized the need to individualize the transfusion trigger.[9] In this context, it is the impression of many that the 10/30 values are probably somewhat higher than those which would be tolerated in many patients without known vascular or pulmonary disease. Along these lines, preliminary evidence from a large series of patients who underwent cardiac artery bypass indicates that hemoglobin values in the 8–9 range may, in fact, be optional. Spiess and colleagues have recently reported on a large ($n = 2375$) number of patients who underwent coronary artery bypass grafting surgery at a variety of institutions.[32] They compared perioperative morbidity and mortality from a variety of causes, and demonstrated that when other factors were controlled for, postoperative hemoglobin values of around 8 were associated with fewer postoperative cardiac events in comparison with those with hemoglobins of 10 or more. The overall mortality was also lower in this group. By contrast, patients with hemoglobin in the 12 g/dl or greater range were subject to the highest rate of early postoperative cardiac events. Whilst these data are preliminary and certainly should not be considered conclusive, they highlight the continued need for more information on transfusion practices and outcome.

On a more general note, there is no universal 'transfusion trigger' or series of guidelines that provide hard and fast rules concerning transfusion of red blood cell products to patients under any circumstances, and most transfusions are 'preemptive'. This is true of trauma in general, and especially true of thoracic trauma where concerns over a variety of problems associated with hemodynamic stability and O_2 transport are paramount. This means that clinicians are attempting to transfuse blood *prior* to the onset of problems and not as a result of the problems.[33] Since most clinicians who deal with either trauma patients and/or those undergoing cardiac surgery have seen the dire consequences of exsanguination, most are anxious to not see them again. This means that many transfusions are given in an effort to 'prevent a disaster' as opposed to

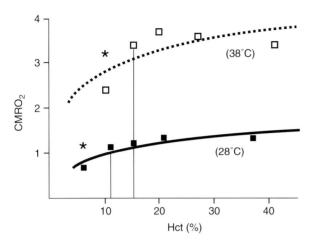

Figure 5.1 *Cerebral metabolic rate (ml/100 g/min) vs hematocrit (Hct) with progressive hemodilution during CPB at 38°C or 28°C (8 dogs per group). As hematocrit is lowered, CMRO$_2$ is constant until Hct reaches 15% at 38°C or 11% at 28°C. CMRO$_2$ is maintained as Hct is lowered by compensatory increases in blood flow. Note the threefold reduction in CMRO$_2$ as temperature is lowered from 38°C to 28°C. *P <0.05 vs previous CMRO$_2$ values at the same temperature. (Adapted from reference 39).*

on the basis of sound outcome-based data. In this context, while improved data on outcomes and transfusion practices would be helpful in determining when to transfuse various patients, it is unlikely that a simple formula will ever be developed that will supplant the individual judgment of the individual clinician dealing with the individual patient. A great deal about transfusion under any conditions is likely to remain subjective.

During cardiopulmonary bypass the anesthesia and surgical team have a high degree of control over what is happening, and sufficient numbers of cases are done to permit well designed trials to be conducted, and relevant animal experiments can be performed. A good example of such information concerns recent attempts to better understand the effects of reduced temperature on the balance between O$_2$ deficiency and uptake by the central nervous system. For example, over the range of clinically relevant cardiopulmonary bypass temperatures (28°–37°C), systemic and cerebral oxygen demand may vary (fall) by more than 300% (Fig 5.1). This allows adequate   tissue oxygen delivery with significantly reduced hematocrits. However, there is no consensus as to what is an appropriate hematocrit when body temperature is reduced. During congenital heart surgery with profound hypothermia, different institutions may hemodilute during CPB to anywhere from a hematocrit of 5%[34] to 30%.[35] Only recently are data characterizing the critical hematocrit[36] as determined by CPB temperature becoming available.[37–39] Figure 5.1 also demonstrates that cerebral metabolic rate is constant over a broad range of hematocrits. In these circumstances, oxygen delivery is maintained when

hematocrit is lowered by reciprocal rises in cerebral blood flow. It also demonstrates the leftward shift of critical hematocrit from 15% at 38°C to 11% at 28°C, and again it is unlikely that transfusion practices during trauma can ever be based on such physiologically elegant concepts, but colder patients may not require normal hematocrit and hemoglobin values to sustain vital organ functions, and if 'trauma' moves to bypass, application of such principles would seem warranted.

STRATEGIES TO CONSERVE BLOOD DURING CARDIAC SURGERY: UTILITY IN TRAUMA

Two basic strategies to conserve allogeneic (donor) blood during cardiac surgery are available. The first centers around the use of autologous donation via predonation of red blood cells for a planned elective operation, and the second centers on the use of procedures that recycle blood obtained from the patient during or after surgery.[18,20–24,40–44] Only the second approach would be available in trauma patients.

'Recycling' of blood from the patient

Cell salvage (cell saver, i.e. intraoperative autotransfusion) is the process of 'recycling' blood from the surgical field (Fig 5.2), concentrating the hemoglobin and hematocrit, and returning the blood to the patient via either intravenous transfusion or, in the case of cardiac surgery, via the CPB bypass pump. This technique can reduce dramatically the amount of allogeneic red blood cells transfused during cardiac surgery.[21,45] This procedure has a long and interesting history, and primitive attempts at cell salvage were made as early as the United States Civil War in the 1860s.[24] Absolute contraindications to cell salvage include malignancy, infection and microfibrillary collagen (e.g. Avitene); relative contraindications include positive viral markers.[22,24]

Reinfusion of shed mediastinal blood is another technique of 'recycling' blood. The blood collected from the mediastinal chest tubes does not clot secondary to defibrinogenation and has a hematocrit between 20 and 35.[44] Several studies have shown reinfusion of shed mediastinal blood without further processing can reduce allogeneic red blood cell transfusions.[42,48] This procedure is not associated with hematological microaggregates which might cause embolic phenomena. However, there is an elevation of serum cardiac enzymes (creatine phosphokinase, glutamic-oxaloacetic transaminase, lactate dehydrogenase, troponin T myoglobin, and 2-hydroxybutyrate dehydrogenase) in patients receiving reinfusion of shed mediastinal blood, which can make diagnosis of myocardial ischemia problematic in these patients.[46]

Cardiopulmonary bypass (CPB) management and coagulation: Lessons for thoracic trauma

Evolving concepts concerning the management of coagulation and coagulopathies during cardiopulmonary bypass are likely to have great utility in the management of coagulation disorders during and after surgery in thoracic trauma patients. This is likely to be true regardless of whether the patient undergoes partial or complete cardiopulmonary bypass. Continued coagulation problems during surgical treatment of thoracic trauma after the major cause(s) of bleeding have been controlled are likely to occur in circumstances where the patient has (a) become cold, (b) undergone massive transfusions, or (c) is experiencing continued microvascular bleeding. In this context, the patient is likely to be hemodynamically 'stable' and the treatment of the coagulopathy can proceed in a more thoughtful fashion. Therefore, a review of current concepts related to management of coagulation during and after standard cardiopulmonary bypass is especially warranted.

Use of transfusion algorithms has been very successful in reducing both red blood cell and coagulation blood product transfusions. A treatment algorithm for transfusion based on routine coagulation tests has reduced the number of transfusions in patients clinically diagnosed as having microvascular (non-surgical) bleeding following cardiac surgery.[29] Goodnough et al. has suggested a transfusion algorithm using routine coagulation tests to guide transfusion therapy in patients undergoing coronary artery bypass grafting surgery.[6] A retrospective study by Spiess et al. found that, after institution of thromboelastograph-guided coagulation studies in the perioperative period, there was a significant reduction in the number of blood transfusions and mediastinal re-exploration for hemorrhage in cardiac surgery patients.[47] A similar approach for the management of the thoracic trauma patient during surgery after hemodynamic stabilization and also during the postoperative period is likely to be helpful.

Multiple drugs have been used in an attempt to decrease the bleeding associated with the use of CPB.[48,49] The most effective of these drug therapies has been the use of antifibrinolytic drugs. Aprotinin, a 58-residue polypeptide isolated from bovine lung, has antifibrinolytic, anti-inflammatory, and possibly platelet-sparing effects. A significant reduction in blood loss and transfusion requirements has been shown with prophylactic aprotinin administration to patients having multiple types of cardiac surgery.[50,51] Unfortunately, the drug is very expensive, can induce allergic reactions, and may induce renal failure in patients with renal dysfunction. Finally, aprotinin, when combined

with heparin, produces a grossly prolonged celate-activated clotting time which makes heparin management of CPB more difficult. For these reasons, aprotinin is usually only given to patients at high risk for blood transfusion following surgery. The synthetic lysine analogues, epsilon-aminocaproic acid (Amicar) and tranexamic acid, are effective antifibrinolytics and have been shown to significantly reduce blood loss and transfusion requirements.[52–54] The effectiveness of this regimen in reducing blood loss in comparison to aprotinin has not been studied thoroughly, and the optimal amount of these drugs to administer is also currently under investigation.[51,53] Desmopressin acetate administration following CPB has been shown to reduce bleeding and transfusion requirements in patients who have platelet dysfunction documented by thromboelastogram.[55]

Multiple drugs have been used in an attempt to decrease the bleeding associated with the use of cardiopulmonary bypass.[48,49] The most effective of these drug therapies has been the use of anti-fibrinolytic drugs. Aprotinin, a 58-residue polypeptide isolated from bovine lung, has anti-fibrinolytic, anti-inflammatory, and possibly platelet-sparing effects. A significant reduction in blood loss and transfusion requirements has been shown with prophylactic aprotinin administration to patients having multiple types of cardiac surgery.[50,51] Unfortunately, the drug is very expensive, can induce allergic reactions, and may induce renal failure in patients with renal dysfunction. Finally, aprotinin, when combined with heparin, produces a grossly prolonged celate-activated clotting time which makes heparin management of cardiopulmonary bypass more difficult. For these reasons, aprotinin is usually only given to patients at high risk for blood transfusion following surgery. The synthetic lysine analogues, epsilon-aminocaproic acid (amicar) and tranexamic acid, are effective anti-fibrinolytics and have been shown to significantly reduce blood loss and transfusion requirements.[52–54] The effectiveness of these regimens in reducing blood loss in comparison to aprotinin has not been studied thoroughly, and the optimal amount of these drugs to administer is also currently under investigation.[51,53] What if any role these drugs have in thoracic trauma in the absence of cardiopulmonary bypass is unknown. Desmopressin acetate administration following cardiopulmonary bypass has been shown to reduce bleeding and transfusion requirements in patients who have platelet dysfunction documented by thromboelastogram.[55]

Excessive bleeding following cardiopulmonary bypass continues to be an important cause of morbidity and mortality and subsequent transfusion. Bleeding following cardiac surgery may result from multiple etiologic factors including hemodilution, massive transfusion, and decreased temperature. These factors are also common in thoracic trauma cases.

In summary, if and when hemodynamic stability has been restored to the patient undergoing surgical treatment of thoracic trauma, a variety of coagulopathies may be encountered. The causes of these coagulopathies include falls in body temperature, massive transfusion, and microvascular bleeding along with (in some cases) extracorporeal circulation. Under these circumstances it is likely that a well-designed transfusion algorithm and the use of 'in the OR' coagulation testing devices could have an important role in guiding transfusion therapy. The role of anti-fibrinollin-like drugs under such circumstances is unclear, particularly if the patient is not undergoing cardiopulmonary bypass as part of the surgical intervention. Finally, use of partial or complete cardiopulmonary bypass can introduce a host of other factors that have the potential to significantly contribute to the development of coagulopathy. Technology and advances in the design of cardiopulmonary bypass equipment is likely to reduce the incidence of equipment-associated coagulopathy in the reasonably near future. Finally, other maneuvers to reduce the bleeding associated with cardiopulmonary bypass such as platelet-rich plasmaphoresis, blood pooling, and hemofiltration have been proposed and had mixed success.[43,56–59] Interpretation of these studies is complicated by the difficulties with blinding of the participating investigations and variations in the techniques performed. When well-designed and blinded studies are performed in a prospective fashion, results are generally negative with these procedures and the use of these procedures in thoracic trauma can not be advocated on the basis of experimental evidence.

POTENTIAL ROLE OF BLOOD SUBSTITUTES IN CARDIAC SURGERY

Thoracic trauma, with its high potential for hemodynamic instability and high risk for death due to exsanguination, is a potential ideal candidate for the use of 'blood substitutes' as a temporizing maneuver to support the circulation and O_2 transport to tissues until definitive surgical treatment can be rendered. Use of blood substitutes is especially attractive in situations such as the battle field, emergency department, helicopter, or when red blood cells are not readily available. The general concept is to 'buy time' and support the circulation. Additionally, extra-corporeal circulation and gas exchange, and the use of a blood substitute as part of the 'prime' in the cardiopulmonary bypass pump, has attracted considerable attention.[18,60,61] This means that a safe and effective blood substitute is attractive for use in thoracic trauma, and also attractive for all types of cases which require cardiopulmonary bypass.

Types of blood substitutes

Currently, three forms of blood substitutes are under development. These include hemoglobin-based solutions, perfluorocarbons, and liposome-encapsulated hemoglobins.[18,60,61] There are also several other promising technologies in the early stages of development.[18]

Hemoglobin-based blood substitutes usually consist of modified hemoglobin in saline solutions.[62–72] Sources of hemoglobin include human red blood cells, animal red blood cells, and biotechnology-related techniques to produce human hemoglobin by microorganisms.[18,60,61] In each case, hemoglobin must be liberated either from the red blood cell (human or animal) or the microorganism. When human or animal red blood cells are used, the hemoglobin tetramers with a molecular weight of approximately 64 kDa can dissociate into dimers and monomers of hemoglobin.[18,60,61] This shifts their P_{50} to the left so that it is more difficult to unload oxygen at tissues and makes it easy for the molecules to leak out of the circulation. It also makes them subject to filtration by the kidney. If the hemoglobin is not adequately purified and the red cell stroma and debris removed from the solution, these 'impurities' can activate the complement cascade and evoke a whole-body inflammatory response.[18] In the case of microorganism-derived hemoglobin, it is also important to remove any bacterial debris, including endotoxin, from the formulation. Additionally, the hemoglobin from microorganisms has been genetically engineered so that several chains are linked together during the synthesis process to limit concerns about dissociation into monomers and dimers and subsequent effects on circulatory half-life, P_{50} and renal filtration.[69]

After obtaining hemoglobin (from whatever source), the smaller units (monomers and dimers) must be chemically modified either to reform tetramers, to be conjugated to other more stable chemical carriers like polyethylene glycol, or to be chemically polymerized.[75–81,83] These maneuvers return the P_{50} of the hemoglobin toward the physiological range [P_{O_2} 25–30 mmHg (3.3–4.0 kPa)] and also limit (to some extent) the leakage of the molecule out of the circulation and limit renal infiltration since in most patients the kidney does not filter molecules with a molecular weight of more than 50 kDa.[18]

Using these procedures, a variety of hemoglobin-based oxygen-carrying solutions have been developed. A number of these have been shown to sustain life in the near absence of red blood cells and have also been shown to be useful in the resuscitation of animals undergoing experimental hemorrhage protocols.[18,62–64,67,68,70,73,74] However, all have several problems. First, the plasma half-life of these solutions is quite low, in the order of hours to days.[62–65,68,73] This contrasts with the half-life of red blood cells which is similar to that of native red blood cells (i.e. 60–120 days). Second, they

Table 5.1 *Success of strategies to conserve blood during cardiac surgery*

Demonstrated	Likely	Developmental
Autologous blood	Pharmacological	Improved biomaterials?
Predonation	DDAVP	Pump
Cell salvage	Erythropoietin	Oxygenator
		Cardiotomy suction
Coagulation monitoring	Improved heparin management	Decreased circuit volume?
Transfusion algorithms	Heparin-bonded circuits	Blood substitutes?
Antifibrinolytic drugs	Platelet-rich plasma? (selected patients)	
Aprotinin		
Tranexamic acid		
Epsilon-aminocaproic acid		
	Hemofiltration	

have limited oxygen-carrying capability. Issues related to osmotic pressure make it difficult to formulate solutions with more than 7–10 g/dl of hemoglobin.[18,60,61,66,75] Third, the solutions cause systemic and pulmonary hypertension when transfused, probably as a result of their binding to the vasodilating substance nitric oxide and other vasoconstricting properties in the hemoglobin.[18,60,61,66,75] Fourth, some of the products undergo rapid transition to methemoglobin which makes the hemoglobin unavailable for oxygen exchange.[73]

While these products appear to have transient and modest effects on renal physiology in various experimental models using young, healthy animals, how will they affect renal function in an older patient with mild elevations in creatinine who is undergoing surgery?[18] It is also not known how these molecules will interact mechanically with the equipment, pumps and oxygenators required for successful CPB and extracorporeal gas exchange. Will their short half-life prevent or limit the use of allogeneic blood, or merely delay transfusion until later in the postoperative course? Finally, is giving a potent nitric oxide scavenger to patients with cardiovascular disease a wise idea? In summary, although a variety of hemoglobin-based oxygen-carrying solutions have been shown to sustain life in the absence of red blood cells, much more needs to be known about them prior to their widespread use in trauma or surgery of any types.

Perfluorocarbons

Perfluorocarbons are organic molecules with high oxygen solubilities.[76,77] These molecules can be put in physical solution with the appropriate addition of various emulsifying agents and surfactants.[18] They can also transport oxygen and, in the late 1970s, Fluasol-DA was approved as the original 'blood substitute'.[78–80] However, this product was not used routinely since only a small amount of it could be given, and even modest systemic oxygen transport required very high P_{O_2}s.[8,60,61]

Newer generations of perfluorocarbons under development have improved the oxygen-carrying capacity. It is now possible for perfluorocarbon-containing solutions to transport significant oxygen at arterial P_{O_2}s of 200–300 mmHg (26.6–39.9 kPa); however, only very small amounts of these solutions (50–100 ml) have been given to patients, and it is unclear if sufficient amounts of perfluorocarbons can be administered to make a difference in red blood cell requirements in cardiac surgery.[18,60,61] In the limited clinical trials to date in humans, many patients report 'flu-like' symptoms, including muscle aches and fever, following transfusion of small amounts of these products.[18] For these reasons, it is unclear if any perfluorocarbon-based blood substitute is likely to be available for use in cardiac surgery in the near future.[81]

Perfluorocarbons are emerging as potentially useful in various liquid ventilation trials and may be helpful to individuals that develop ARDS after thoracic trauma.

Other forms of blood substitutes

In addition to hemoglobin solutions and perfluorocarbons, attempts have been made to make 'artificial erythrocytes' via the use of liposome-encapsulated hemoglobin.[82,83] The concept is that it should be possible to make small liposomes similar in composition to cells and imbed hemoglobin in these liposomes. If this works, it is hypothesized that the half-life of these artificial red blood cells would be in the order of days to weeks and eliminate a variety of concerns related to the short plasma half-lives of hemoglobin-based solutions. Whilst these properties are attractive, liposomes, in fact, are rapidly taken up by the reticuloendothelial system (spleen) and can activate the complement system and evoke whole-body inflammatory responses.[18,60,61,83] There are a variety of other issues that represent barriers to their use. Again, how these compounds might interact with the CPB pump and extracorporeal oxygenator remains to be determined.

Of note in the efforts to generate 'artificial cells' is the recent development of hemoglobin 'microbubbles'. This technology uses the process known as ultrasonic cavitation to generate small (approximately 1 µm) bubbles of hemoglobin.[84] The oxygen-carrying characteristics of these bubbles appear to be good, but whether they can serve as an adequate blood substitute remains to be known. The development of hemoglobin microbubbles demonstrates that new technologies for the creation of blood substitutes are being developed. Although these approaches are conceptually attractive, their utility remains to be determined.

There are several major limitations of the current blood substitutes. First, it is unclear whether sufficient amounts of any blood substitute could be given to make a difference in transfusion required during or after a complex cardiac surgical procedure.[18,60,61] Second, the plasma half-life of these compounds is quite short, and the impact of these limited half-lives and their use in cardiac surgery is now known.[18,60,61] Third, little is known about the interactions of all types of blood substitutes with the CPB pump and extracorporeal oxygenator. Fourth, while these products have been shown to have biological activity in a variety of preparations, it is not known if they can be given in a way that will be of benefit to patients.[18,85,86] The design of a 'clinical trial' in trauma, cardiac, or other forms of surgery that will permit the safety and utility of such compounds to be thoroughly evaluated will be daunting.

SUMMARY

In summary, transfusion practices during the acute stabilization of thoracic trauma victims are likely to remain empirical for some time (Table 5.1). The fundamental issues in the acute phase remain (a) adequate intravascular access, (b) support of intravascular volume and blood pressure, (c) the utility of type O blood, and (d) prompt surgical control of bleeding. After stabilization, use of cell salvage procedures and transfusion algorithms are likely to reduce the use of blood products. Additionally, outcome-based studies designed to understand more about the variability of transfusion practices during all types of surgery and relevant issues related to an appropriate transfusion trigger(s) are clearly needed to better understand the use of allogeneic red blood cells. With these approaches, refining current transfusion practices is probably the surest way to conserve allogeneic blood use during surgery for thoracic trauma. In addition to these simple steps outlined above, better management of perioperative coagulopathies and bleeding disorders might also reduce the use of red blood cells in these patients.[30] Additionally, transfusion management in thoracic trauma patients that require complete or partial cardiopulmonary bypass is likely to be improved as a result of technological improvements including design of lower dead space circuits and oxygenators that require little or no systemic heparinization. These technological innovations, along with the generalized refinement of current transfusion practices, and more data on the appropriate transfusion trigger and outcomes, would appear to be good bets to limit use of allogeneic blood during surgery for thoracic trauma or any other type of surgery. In view of the likely success of the measures outlined above, the safety of type O blood and the uncertainties related to the current generation of blood substitutes, it is unlikely that blood substitutes will result in significant improvement in the current practices. Better management of existing resources, along with improved hardware in those cases requiring bypass, would appear to be the best bet to optimize transfusion practices during the surgical treatment of thoracic trauma. Such efforts would also represent 'quality assurance' initiatives directed at improved patient care.

REFERENCES

1. Bowersox JC, Hess JR. Combat casualties, blood and red blood cell substitutes: a military perspective. In: Winslow RM, Vandegriff KD, Intaglietta M, ed. *Blood Substitutes: Physiological Basis of Efficacy*. Boston, MA: Birkhauser, 1995; 42–52.

2. Craig RL, Poole GV. Resuscitation in uncontrolled hemorrhage. *Am Surg* 1994; **60:** 59–62.

3. Phillips GR, Kauder DR, Schwab CW. Massive blood loss in trauma patients. The benefits and dangers of transfusion therapy. *Postgrad Med* 1994; **95:** 61–72.

4. Bickell WH, Wall MJ, Pepe PE, Martin RR, Ginger VF, Allen MK, Mattox KL. Immediate versus delayed fluid resuscitation for hypotensive patients with penetrating torso injuries. *N Engl J Med* 1994; **331:** 1105–1109.

5. Jacobs LM. Timing of fluid resuscitation in trauma. *N Engl J Med* 1994; **331:** 1153–1154.

6. Goodnough LT, Johnston MFM, Ramsey G, *et al.* Guidelines for transfusion support in patients undergoing coronary artery bypass grafting. *Ann Thorac Surg* 1990; **50:** 675–83.

7. Goodnough LT, Johnston MFM, Toy PTCY. The variability of transfusion practice in coronary artery bypass surgery. *JAMA* 1991; **265:** 86–90.

8. Surgenor DM, Churchill WH, Wallace EL, *et al.* Determinants of red cell, platelet, plasma, and cryoprecipitate transfusions during coronary artery bypass graft surgery: the Collaborative Hospital Transfusion Study. *Transfusion* 1996; **36:** 521–32.

9. American Society of Anesthesiologists Task Force on Blood Component Therapy. Practice guidelines for blood component therapy. *Anesthesiology* 1996; **84:** 732–47.

10. Goodnough LT, Soegiarso RW, Birkmeyer JD, Welch HG. Economic impact of inappropriate blood transfusions in coronary artery bypass graft surgery. *Am J Med* 1993; **94:** 509–14.

11. Ferraris VA, Gildengorin V. Predictors of excessive blood use after coronary artery bypass grafting. A multivariate analysis. *J Thorac Cardiovasc Surg* 1989; **98:** 492–7.

12. Despotis GJ, Filos KS, Zoys TN, Hogue Jr CW, Spitznagel E, Lappas DG. Factors associated with excessive postoperative blood loss and hemostatic transfusion requirements: a multivariate analysis in cardiac surgical patients. *Anesth Analg* 1996; **82:** 13–21.

13. Cook SS, Epps J. Transfusion practice in Central Virginia. *Transfusion* 1991; **31:** 355–60.

14. Surgenor DM, Wallace EL, Hao SHS, Chapman RH. Collection and transfusion of blood in the United States, 1982–1988. *N Engl J Med* 1990; **322:** 1646–51.

15. Vamvakas EC, Taswell HF. Epidemiology of blood transfusion. *Transfusion* 1994; **34:** 464–70.

16. Wallace EL, Surgenor DM, Hao HS, An J, Chapman RH, Churchill WH. Collection and transfusion of blood and blood components in the United States, 1989. *Transfusion* 1993; **33:** 139–44.

17. Pindyck J, Avorn J, Kuriyan M, Reed M, Iqbal MJ, Levine SJ. Blood donation by the elderly. Clinical and policy considerations. *JAMA* 1987; **257:** 1186–8.

18. Dietz NM, Joyner MJ, Warner MA. Blood substitutes: fluids, drugs, or miracle solutions? *Anesth Analg* 1996; **82:** 390–405.

19. American College of Physicians. Practice strategies for elective red blood cell transfusion. *Ann Intern Med* 1992; **116:** 403–6.

20. Birkmeyer JD, AuBuchon JP, Littenberg B, *et al.* Cost-effectiveness of preoperative autologous donation in coronary artery bypass grafting. *Ann Thorac Surg* 1994; **57:** 161–9.

21. McCarthy PM, Popovsky MA, Schaff HV, *et al.* Effect of blood conservation efforts in cardiac operations at the Mayo Clinic. *Mayo Clin Proc* 1988; **63:** 225–9.

22. Tawes RL Jr. Intraoperative autotransfusion: advantages, disadvantages, and contraindications. *Semin Vasc Surg* 1994; **7:** 95–7.

23. Testa LD, Tobias JD. Techniques of blood conservation. Part II. Autologous transfusion, intraoperative blood salvage, pharmacologic agents, and cost issues. *Am J Anesthesiol* 1996; **23:** 63–72.

24. Williamson KR, Taswell HF. Intraoperative blood salvage: a review. *Transfusion* 1991; **31:** 662–75.

25. Dodd RY. The risk of transfusion-transmitted infection. *N Engl J Med* 1992; **327:** 419–20.

26. Selik RM, Ward JW, Buehler JW. Demographic differences in cumulative incidence rates of transfusion-associated acquired immunodeficiency syndrome. *Am J Epidemiol* 1994; **140:** 105–12.

27. Donahue JG, Munoz A, Ness PM, *et al.* The declining risk of post-transfusion hepatitis C virus infection. *N Engl J Med* 1992; **327:** 369–73.

28. Geary V, Sheikh F, Trubiano P, Strickler R, McCloskey D, Lumb P. A review of blood usage in 3215 patients undergoing coronary bypass surgery over a 3-year period at Albany Medical Center. (Abstract) *Anesthesiology* 1996; **85:** A1016.

29. Despotis GJ, Grishaber JE, Goodnough LT. The effect of an intraoperative treatment algorithm on physicians' transfusion practice in cardiac surgery. *Transfusion* 1994; **34:** 290–6.

30. Despotis GJ, Joist JH, Hogue CW Jr, *et al.* The impact of heparin concentration and activated clotting time monitoring on blood conservation. A prospective, randomized evaluation in patients undergoing cardiac operation. *J Thorac Cardiovasc Surg* 1995; **110:** 46–54.

31. Despotis GJ, Santoro SA, Spitznagel E, *et al.* Prospective evaluation and clinical utility of on-site monitoring of coagulation in patients undergoing cardiac operation. *J Thorac Cardiovasc Surg* 1994; **107:** 271–9.

32. Spiess BD, Kapitan S, Body S, *et al.* ICU entry hematocrit does influence the risk for perioperative myocardial infarction (MI) in coronary artery bypass graft surgery. *Anesth Analg* 1995; **80:** SCA1–SCA141.

33. Joyner MJ, Faust RJ. Blood substitutes: what is the target? In: Winslow RM, Vandegriff KD, Intaglietta M (eds) *Blood Substitutes: New Challenges.* Boston, MA: Birkhauser, 1996; 15–33.

34. Eke CC, Gundry SR, Baum MF, Chinnock RE, Razzouk AJ, Bailey LL. Neurologic sequelae of deep hypothermic circulatory arrest in cardiac transplant infants. *Ann Thorac Surg* 1996; **61:** 783–8.

35. Jonas RA. Deep hypothermic circulatory arrest: a need for caution. *Ann Thorac Surg* 1996; **61:** 779–80.

36. van Woerkens EC, Trouwborst A, van Lanschot JJ. Profound hemodilution: what is the critical level of hemodilution at which oxygen delivery-dependent oxygen consumption starts in an anesthetized human? *Anesth Analg* 1992; **75:** 818–21.

37. Cook DJ, MacVeigh I, Orszulak TA, Daly RC. Minimum hematocrit for normothermic cardiopulmonary bypass in dogs. (Abstract) *Circulation* 1996; **94:** I-536.

38. Cook DJ, McGlinch BP, Orszulak TA, Daly RC, Mullany CJ. Cerebral oxygen balance during clinical cardiopulmonary bypass with hemoglobin of 5 g/dL. (Abstract) *Perfusion* 1997; **12:** 40.

39. Cook DJ, MacVeigh I, Orszulak TA, Daly RC, Ayanoglu HO. Critical hematocrit for 28°C cardiopulmonary bypass in dogs. (Abstract) *Perfusion* 1997; **12:** 41.

40. Morris JJ, Tan YS. Autotransfusion: is there a benefit in a current practice of aggressive blood conservation? *Ann Thorac Surg* 1994; **58:** 502–7.

41. National Heart, Lung, and Blood Institute Autologous Transfusion Symposium Working Group. Autologous transfusion: current trends and research issues. Conference Report. *Transfusion* 1995; **35:** 525–31.

42. Owings DV, Kruskall MS, Thurer RL, Donovan LM. Autologous blood donations prior to elective cardiac surgery. *JAMA* 1989; **262:** 1963–8.

43. Petry AF, Jost T, Sievers H. Reduction of homologous blood requirements by blood-pooling at the onset of cardiopulmonary bypass. *J Thorac Cardiovasc Surg* 1994; **107:** 1210–14.

44. Schaff HV, Hauer JM, Bell WR, *et al.* Autotransfusion of shed mediastinal blood after cardiac surgery. A prospective study. *J Thorac Cardiovasc Surg* 1978; **75:** 632–41.

45. Axford TC, Dearani JA, Ragno G, *et al.* Safety and therapeutic effectiveness of reinfused shed blood after open heart surgery. *Ann Thorac Surg* 1994; **57:** 615–22.

46. Hannes W, Keilich M, Koster W, Seitelberger R, Fasol R. Shed blood autotransfusion influences ischemia-sensitive laboratory parameters after coronary operations. *Ann Thorac Surg* 1994; **57:** 1289–94.

47. Spiess BD, Gillies BSA, Chandler W, Verrier E. Changes in transfusion therapy and reexploration rate after institution of a blood management program in cardiac surgical patients. *J Cardiothorac Vasc Anesth* 1995; **9:** 168–73.

48. Fremes SE, Wong BI, Lee E, *et al.* Metaanalysis of prophylactic drug treatment in the prevention of postoperative bleeding. *Ann Thorac Surg* 1994; **58:** 1580–8.

49. Harmon DE. Cost/benefit analysis of pharmacologic hemostasis. *Ann Thorac Surg* 1996; **61:** S21–5.

50. Lemmer JH Jr, Stanford W, Bonney SL, *et al.* Aprotinin for coronary bypass operations: efficacy, safety, and influence on early saphenous vein graft patency. A multicenter, randomized, double-blind, placebo-controlled study. *J Thorac Cardiovasc Surg* 1994; **107:** 543–53.

51. Tabuchi N, De Haan J, Boonstra PW, Gallandat Huet RCG, van Oeveren W. Aprotinin effect on platelet function and clotting during cardiopulmonary bypass. *Eur J Cardiothorac Surg* 1994; **8:** 87–90.

52. DelRossi AJ, Cernaianu AC, Botros S, Lemole GM, Moore R. Prophylactic treatment of postperfusion bleeding using EACA. *Chest* 1989; **96:** 27–30.

53. Pugh SC, Wielogorski AK. A comparison of the effects of tranexamic acid and low-dose aprotinin on blood loss and homologous blood usage in patients undergoing cardiac surgery. *J Cardiothorac Vasc Anesth* 1995; **9:** 240–4.

54. Shore-Lesserson L, Reich DL, Vela-Cantos F, Ammar T, Ergin MA. Tranexamic acid reduces transfusions and mediastinal drainage in repeat cardiac surgery. *Anesth Analg* 1996; **83:** 18–26.

55. Mongan PD, Hosking MP. The role of desmopressin acetate in patients undergoing coronary artery bypass surgery. *Anesthesiology* 1992; **77:** 38–46.

56. Boldt J. Acute platelet-rich plasmapheresis for cardiac surgery. *J Cardiothorac Vasc Anesth* 1995; **9:** 79–88.

57. Walpoth BH, Amport T, Schmid R, Kipfer B, Lanz M, Spaeth P, Kurt G, Althaus U. Hemofiltration during cardiopulmonary bypass: quality assessment of hemoconcentrated blood. *Thorac Cardiovasc Surgeon* 1994; **42:** 162–69.

58. Ereth MH, Oliver WC Jr, Beynen FMK, Mullany CJ, Orszulak TA, Santrach PJ, Ilstrup DM, Weaver AL, Williamson KR. Autologous platelet-rich plasma does not reduce transfusion of homologous blood products in patients undergoing repeat valvular surgery. *Anesthesiology* 1993; **79:** 540–47.

59. Mohr R, Martinowitz U, Lavee J, Amroch D, Ramot B, Goor DA. The hemostatic effect of transfusing fresh whole blood versus platelet concentrates after cardiac operations. *J Thorac Cardiovasc Surg* 1988; **96:** 530–34.

60. Winslow RM. Blood substitutes – minireview. *Prog Clin Biol Res* 1989; **319:** 305–23.

61. Winslow RM. Red cell substitutes: current status, 1992. In: Nance SJ (ed.) *Blood Safety: Current Challenges.* Bethesda, MD: American Association of Blood Banks, 1992; 151–67.

62. Amberson WR, Flexner J, Steggerda FR, Mulder AG, Tendler MJ, Pankratz DS. On the use of Ringer–Locke solutions containing haemoglobin as a substitute for normal blood in mammals. *J Cell Comp Physiol* 1934; **5:** 359–82.

63. Amberson WR, Jennings JJ, Rhode CM. Clinical experience with hemoglobin-saline solutions. *J Appl Physiol* 1949; **1:** 469–89.

64. Amberson WR, Mulder AG, Steggerda FR, Flexner J, Pankratz DS. Mammalian life without red blood corpuscles. *Science* 1933; **78:** 106–7.

65. Hess JR, Fadare SO, Tolentino LS, Bangal NR, Winslow RM. The intravascular persistence of crosslinked human hemoglobin. *Prog Clin Biol Res* 1989; **319:** 351–7.

66. Hess JR, MacDonald VW, Brinkley WW. Systemic and pulmonary hypertension after resuscitation with cell-free hemoglobin. *J Appl Physiol* 1993; **74:** 1769–78.

67. Hess JR, MacDonald VW, Winslow RM. Dehydration and shock: an animal model of hemorrhage and resuscitation of battlefield injury. *Biomater Artif Cells Immobil Biotechnol* 1992; **20:** 499–502.

68. Hess JR, Wade CE, Winslow RM. Filtration-assisted exchange transfusion using $\alpha\alpha$Hb, an erythrocyte substitute. *J Appl Physiol* 1991; **70:** 1639–44.

69. Hoffman SJ, Looker DL, Roehrich JM, *et al.* Expression of fully functional tetrameric human hemoglobin in *Escherichia coli. Proc Natl Acad Sci USA* 1990; **87:** 8521–5.

70. Nho K, Glower D, Bredehoeft S, Shankar H, Shorr R, Abuchowski A. PEG-bovine hemoglobin: safety in a canine dehydrated hypovolemic-hemorrhagic shock model. *Biomater Artif Cells Immobil Biotechnol* 1992; **20:** 511–24.

71. Sehgal LR, Gould SA, Rosen AL, Sehgal HL, Moss GS. Polymerized pyridoxylated hemoglobin: a red cell substitute with normal oxygen capacity. *Surgery* 1984; **95:** 433–8.

72. Snyder SR, Welty EV, Walder RY, Williams LA, Walder JA. HbXL99α: a hemoglobin derivative that is cross-linked between the α subunits is useful as a blood substitute. *Proc Natl Acad Sci USA* 1987; **84:** 7280–4.

73. Lee R, Neya K, Svizzero TA, Vlahakes GJ. Limitations of the efficacy of hemoglobin-based oxygen-carrying solutions. *J Appl Physiol* 1995; **79**: 236–42.

74. Rosen AL, Gould S, Sehgal LR, *et al.* Cardiac output response to extreme hemodilution with hemoglobin solutions of various P50 values. *Crit Care Med* 1979; **7**: 380–4.

75. Jia L, Bonaventura J, Stamler JS. S-nitrosohaemoglobin: a dynamic activity of blood involved in vascular control. *Nature* 1996; **380**: 221–6.

76. Biro GP, Blais P, Rosen AL. Perfluorocarbon blood substitutes. *Crit Rev Oncol Hematol* 1987; **6**: 311–74.

77. Clark LC Jr, Gollan F. Survival of mammals breathing organic liquids equilibrated with oxygen at atmospheric pressure. *Science* 1966; **152**: 1755–6.

78. Kerins DM. Role of the perfluorocarbon Fluosol-DA in coronary angioplasty. *Am J Med Sci* 1994; **307**: 218–21.

79. Spence RK, McCoy S, Costabile J, *et al.* Fluosol DA-20 in the treatment of severe anemia: randomized, controlled study of 46 patients. *Crit Care Med* 1990; **18**: 1227–30.

80. Tremper KK, Friedman AE, Levine EM, Lapin R, Camarillo D. The preoperative treatment of severely anemic patients with a perfluorochemical oxygen-transport fluid, Fluosol-DA. *N Engl J Med* 1982; **307**: 277–83.

81. Stone JJ, Piccione W Jr, Berrizbeitia LD, *et al.* Hemodynamic, metabolic, and morphological effects of cardiopulmonary bypass with a fluorocarbon priming solution. *Ann Thorac Surg* 1986; **41**: 419–24.

82. Chang TMS. Semipermeable microcapsules. *Science* 1964; **146**: 524–5.

83. Rudolph AS. Encapsulated hemoglobin: current issues and future goals. *Artif Cells Blood Substit Immobil Biotechnol* 1994; **22**: 347–60.

84. Wong M, Suslick KS. Sonochemically produced hemoglobin microbubbles. *Proceedings of the Materials Research Society National Meeting*, Symposium W2, Boston, MA, Fall 1994.

85. Fratantoni JC. Points to consider in the safety evaluation of hemoglobin-based oxygen carriers. *Transfusion* 1991; **31**: 369–71.

86. Fratantoni JC. Point to consider on efficacy evaluation of hemoglobin- and perfluorocarbon-based oxygen carriers. *Transfusion* 1994; **34**: 712–13.

FURTHER READING

Dietz NM, Joyner MJ, Warner MA. Blood substitutes: fluids, drugs, or miracle solutions? *Anesth Analg* 1996; **82**: 390–405.

Goodnough LT, Johnston MFM, Toy PTCY. The variability of transfusion practice in coronary artery bypass surgery. *JAMA* 1991; **265**: 86–90.

Goodnough LT, Soegiarso RW, Birkmeyer JD, Welch HG. Economic impact of inappropriate blood transfusions in coronary artery bypass graft surgery. *Am J Med* 1993; **94**: 509–14.

Hess JR, MacDonald VW, Brinkley WW. Systemic and pulmonary hypertension after resuscitation with cell-free hemoglobin. *J Appl Physiol* 1993; **74**: 1769–78.

Williamson KR, Taswell HF. Intraoperative blood salvage: a review. *Transfusion* 1991; **31**: 662–75.

6

Echocardiography in chest trauma

DEAN G KARALIS, JOHN J ROSS JR AND FAROOQ A CHAUDHRY

Cardiac injury is common following blunt or penetrating chest trauma. Most blunt chest trauma is related to motor vehicle accidents and cardiac injury occurs when there is a deceleration impact causing the heart to strike the bony structures of the anterior chest wall. This can lead to traumatic injury of the pericardium, myocardium, valvular structures or great vessels. Penetrating chest trauma can also cause injury to the heart or aorta. Because these cardiac injuries can lead to potentially life-threatening complications and death, early recognition is important.

The clinician caring for the trauma patient has available a number of tools to diagnose cardiac and aortic injury. Electrocardiography, cardiac enzyme determinations, the screening chest radiograph, as well as echocardiographic and radionuclide studies, are commonly used to diagnose cardiac injury in the trauma patient. Electrocardiographic findings and cardiac enzyme determinations are neither sensitive nor specific indicators of myocardial contusion and do not reliably predict cardiac events or mortality. Similarly, the chest radiograph is not accurate enough to reliably diagnose traumatic aortic injury. This is because these tests provide only indirect evidence of cardiac and aortic injury. Echocardiography, however, provides direct visualization of the cardiac structures and can accurately diagnose myocardial, valvular and pericardial injury as well as provide hemodynamic information on cardiac function. Because it uses higher frequency transducers and because of the close proximity of the esophagus to the thoracic aorta, transesophageal echocardiography provides superior imaging of the thoracic aorta as compared with transthoracic echocardiography.

Echocardiography is an ideal diagnostic tool when evaluating the trauma patient for cardiac or aortic injury because it can be performed safely at the patient's bedside and provides rapid and accurate information on cardiac structure and function. This discussion reviews the role of both transthoracic and transesophageal echocardiography in evaluating and risk stratifying the trauma patient for cardiac and aortic injury.

BLUNT CHEST TRAUMA AND CARDIAC INJURY

Cardiac injuries associated with blunt chest trauma

Pericardium

- Laceration
- Hematoma or hemopericardium
- Late pericarditis

Myocardium

- Rupture
- Contusion

Valvular

- Rupture (leaflets, chordae or papillary muscles)

Coronary arteries

- Laceration
- Thrombosis

Great vessels

- Aortic disruption
- Intimal tear
- Aortic aneurysm

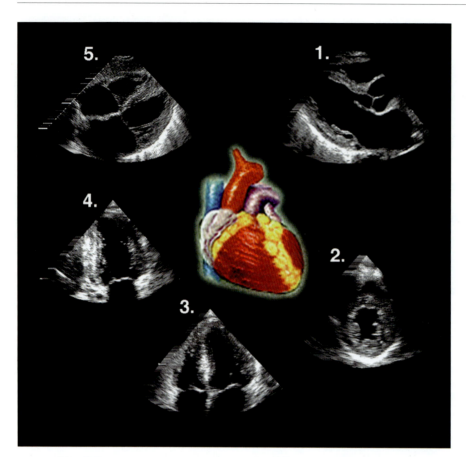

Figure 6.1 *Routine two-dimensional transthoracic echocardiographic views that can be obtained from various positions of the echo-cardiographic transducer on the chest wall: 1, parasternal long-axis view; 2, parasternal short-axis view; 3, apical four-chamber view; 4, apical two-chamber view; and 5, subcostal view.*

The most common cardiac injury following blunt chest trauma is myocardial contusion or rupture. Injury to the pericardium occurs less commonly and damage to the coronary arteries or valvular structures are rare. In an autopsy study of 546 cases of non-penetrating injury to the heart, myocardial rupture was found in 65% of cases, myocardial contusion in 24%, pericardial injury in 11%, whereas the incidence of coronary artery or valvular injury was less than 0.5%.[1] Myocardial rupture is the most common cause of cardiac death following blunt chest trauma and death usually occurs in the field within the first hour following the chest injury.[2] The spectrum of cardiac injury in patients who survive long enough to be brought to the hospital is very different from the spectrum of cardiac injury seen in necropsy studies. Myocardial contusion is the most common cardiac injury among patients who survive to hospitalization, occurring in up to one-third of these patients.[3–6] Less commonly, pericardial injury occurs. Pericardial injury can take the form of a localized hematoma without clinical significance or hemopericardium which can lead to cardiac tamponade and hemodynamic compromise.[7] Isolated case reports have also described injury to the semilunar or atrioventricular valves.[8–10] Injury to the valve leaflets, chordal structures or papillary muscles can lead to significant valvular regurgitation. Patients may remain asymptomatic with the only evidence for valvular injury being a heart murmur on physical examination or, at the other end of the spectrum, patients may develop frank congestive heart failure if severe mitral or aortic regurgitation develops.

THE VALUE OF ECHOCARDIOGRAPHY IN DIAGNOSING CARDIAC INJURY

Echocardiography is an ideal tool to diagnose cardiac injury. Echocardiography uses ultrasound to provide images of the heart and great vessels. Two-dimensional echocardiography provides excellent spatial resolution, thus allowing visualization of cardiac structures in motion in real time. Doppler echocardiography is used to detect blood flow velocity and direction and color-flow Doppler imaging has proven very sensitive in detecting valvular regurgitation and in identifying intracardiac shunts. Several transthoracic echocardiographic views can be obtained by placing the ultrasound transducer at various sites on the chest wall. Common views include the parasternal long- and short-axis views, the apical two- and four-chamber views and the subcostal view (Fig 6.1).

Transthoracic echocardiography is commonly used to image the heart in patients with blunt chest trauma.[11–17] At times the parasternal and apical views are limited due to chest wall bandages, chest tubes or associated chest wall or pulmonary injuries. In these cases the subcostal view can be used to provide satisfactory echocardiographic images. When transthoracic echocardiographic images are technically limited, transesophageal echocardiography overcomes many of these limitations. Transesophageal echocardiography can better visualize the heart due to the close proximity of the esophagus to the cardiac structures, the use of higher frequency transducers and the lack of interfering structures between the transesophageal echocardiographic probe and the heart. Transthoracic and transesophageal echocardiography provide direct anatomical and hemodynamic information regarding cardiac structure and function and can detect myocardial contusion, pericardial effusion and valvular injury.

The diagnosis of myocardial contusion is made echocardiographically by detecting a regional wall motion abnormality of either the left or right ventricle.[17] Furthermore, the contused myocardium appears brighter than areas of normal myocardium. Although the end-diastolic wall thickness is maintained, the systolic thickening of the contused myocardium is decreased.[18]

Echocardiographic characteristics of myocardial contusion

- Regional wall motion abnormality
- Myocardium is more echogenic
- End-diastolic wall thickness is preserved
- Usually involves the right as well as the left ventricle

These characteristics may also be seen with acute myocardial infarction, however; the location of the wall motion abnormality is helpful in differentiating myocardial contusion from myocardial infarction. Following a high speed collision that results in severe blunt chest trauma, the heart is injured as it strikes the anterior chest wall. Since the right ventricle is the most anterior cardiac structure, it bears the brunt of the injury and in almost all cases of myocardial contusion the right ventricle is involved (Fig 6.2).

In a study conducted in our institution, 105 consecutive patients with blunt chest trauma underwent echocardiographic evaluation to detect myocardial contusion.[17] Myocardial contusion was diagnosed echocardiographically in 31 patients (30%). Right and left ventricular contusion was found in 17 of 31 patients (55%), right ventricular contusion alone was found in 12 of 31 patients (39%) and isolated left ventricular contusion was detected in only two patients (6%) (Fig 6.3). Furthermore, when the left ventricle was injured, the contusion was limited to only a small area of the distal anterior septum and apex. At the point of impact during blunt chest trauma this is the region of the left ventricle that will come into contact with the lower pole

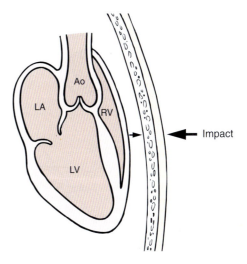

Figure 6.2 *Diagram illustrating the location of the heart to the anterior chest wall. During blunt chest trauma the heart strikes the anterior chest wall and the right ventricle (RV) suffers the greatest injury due to its anterior location. Ao, aorta; LA, left atrium; LV, left ventricle.*

of the sternum and the left rib cage as the heart strikes the anterior chest wall. The degree of right ventricular injury varied. In 72% of right ventricular contusions the degree of injury was small, involving the distal anteroapical right ventricular wall, and the right ventricular function was preserved. In the remaining 28% the myocardial contusion was extensive, involving most of the anterior right ventricular wall and apex, resulting in significant right ventricular dysfunction (Fig 6.4). The right ventricle usually dilates when such extensive injury is present and the finding of a dilated right ventricle with severe global hypokinesis by

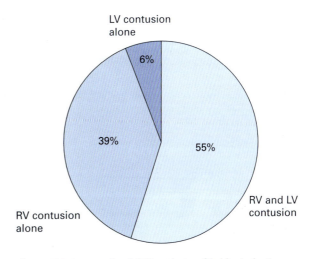

Figure 6.3 *In a study of 105 patients with blunt chest trauma myocardial contusion most commonly involved the right ventricle (RV) and left ventricle (LV); 55% of patients. Isolated RV contusion occurred in 39% of patients while isolated LV contusion was uncommon, occurring in only 6% of the trauma patients.*

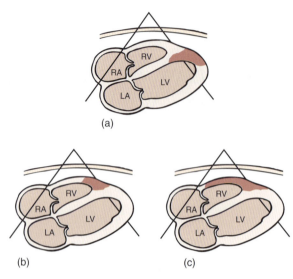

Figure 6.4 *Spectrum of myocardial injury detected by echocardiography following blunt chest trauma. When the left ventricle is injured the myocardial contusion is most often limited to a small area of the left ventricular (LV) septum and apex (a). When the right ventricle (RV) is injured the myocardial contusion may be limited to a small area of the RV anteroapical wall (b) or may be more extensive involving most of the anterior RV wall and apex (c). In patients with extensive RV injury, RV dysfunction can lead to hypotension and hemodynamic compromise. RA, right atrium; LA, left atrium. (From Karalis et al.[17] by permission of the Journal of Trauma)*

echocardiography is also indicative of a right ventricular contusion. It is imperative to image the right ventricle carefully for it is the most common site of

traumatic contusion. The finding of an inferobasal or anterolateral wall motion abnormality of the left ventricle without right ventricular involvement favors the diagnosis of myocardial infarction over myocardial contusion, especially if the patient is older and has a history of coronary artery disease and prior myocardial infarction.

In our experience, the echocardiographic findings correlate poorly with the admission electrocardiogram and serial cardiac enzyme determinations. Understanding which region of the myocardium is most likely to be injured following blunt chest trauma helps explain the limitations of electrocardiography and serial cardiac enzyme determinations in diagnosing myocardial contusion. The right ventricle and left ventricular apex tend to be electrically silent and injury to these areas may not be evident on the 12-lead electrocardiogram. In our experience, the electrocardiogram is very specific for myocardial contusion but not sensitive. There appears to be a critical mass of myocardium that must be injured before electrocardiographic changes appear. Since most myocardial contusions are small it is not surprising that the electrocardiogram is less accurate in diagnosing myocardial injury than is echocardiography. Similarly, a small area of injured myocardium is likely to produce little if any elevations in the MB isoenzyme of creatinine kinase (CK). Furthermore, any minor elevations of the CK-MB could be easily overshadowed by the very high elevations of creatinine kinase that commonly occur following severe chest trauma due to concomitant skeletal muscle injury.

The main limitation of transthoracic echocardiography in detecting myocardial contusion is that the image quality of the echocardiographic study may be poor in

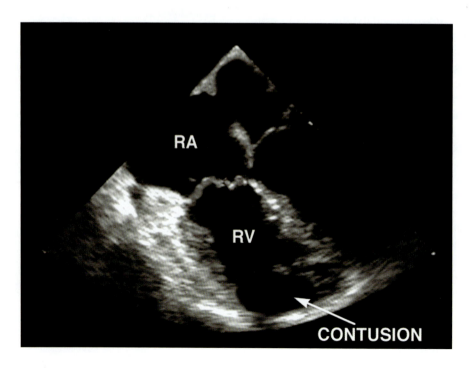

Figure 6.5 *Transesophageal echocardiographic four-chamber view demonstrating a right ventricular (RV) contusion. The RV is dilated and in real-time the anteroapical region (arrow) was severely hypokinetic. No pericardial effusion was present. RA, right atrium.*

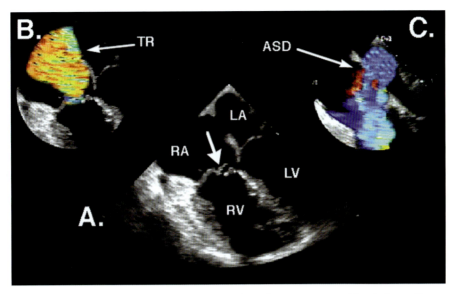

Figure 6.6 *Transesophageal echocardiographic view of a young man with a holosystolic murmur on physical examination following blunt chest trauma from an automobile accident. (A) A flail tricuspid valve leaflet (arrow) is seen in the four-chamber transesophageal echocardiographic view. The right atrium (RA) and right ventricle (RV) are dilated and a RV contusion was present. LA, left atrium; LV, left ventricle. (B) Magnified view of the right atrium. Color-flow Doppler imaging demonstrates severe tricuspid regurgitation (TR). (C) In addition, a traumatic atrial septal defect (ASD) was detected. Color-flow Doppler imaging demonstrates left-to-right flow across a large defect in the atrial septum.*

patients due to chest wall bandages and dressings, chest tubes and associated chest wall and pulmonary injuries. In previous studies[13,16,17] evaluating transthoracic echocardiography in blunt chest trauma, the heart could not be satisfactorily imaged from the transthoracic approach in 13–28% of patients. In these patients, echocardiographic imaging of the heart from the esophagus overcomes many of the limitations of transthoracic imaging.[20-22] This is especially true of those patients with the most severe chest injuries who are most likely to have a myocardial contusion and most likely to have a suboptimal and non-diagnostic transthoracic echocardiogram. We reported a case of a patient who developed clinical and hemodynamic evidence for cardiac tamponade following blunt chest trauma.[19] The transesophageal echocardiographic images were so poor that the cardiac structures could not be adequately visualized. However, transesophageal echocardiography detected a right ventricular contusion with severe right ventricular dysfunction. No pericardial effusion was present (Fig 6.5). It is important to note that severe right ventricular dysfunction may mimic the clinical findings of cardiac tamponade. The transesophageal echocardiographic findings aided the trauma surgeon caring for the patient by directing appropriate therapy and avoiding unnecessary and potentially dangerous pericardiocentesis. This case illustrates the value of echocardiography in the patient following blunt chest

trauma. Transesophageal echocardiography is also of value if traumatic valvular regurgitation or a traumatic shunt such as an atrial septal or ventricular septal defect is present because it provides greater anatomical detail of the cardiac structures (Fig 6.6).

The most accurate method to diagnose myocardial contusion is by performing transthoracic echocardiography, then proceeding to transesophageal imaging if the transthoracic echocardiographic images are suboptimal. It is important to remember, however, that there is no advantage of transesophageal echocardiography over transthoracic echocardiography in diagnosing cardiac injury when the transthoracic echocardiogram provides adequate images of the cardiac structures.

The important question, however, is should all patients with blunt chest trauma undergo transthoracic or transesophageal echocardiography to screen for myocardial contusion? For a test to be of clinical value it must not only be accurate but it must favorably impact upon patient care. This is especially important in today's environment of cost-containment and managed care. To answer the question of which patients following blunt chest trauma would benefit from echocardiographic evaluation one must review the overall prognosis of patients with myocardial contusion with regard to early and late cardiac complications.

Asymptomatic patients with myocardial contusion are thought to be at risk for late cardiac complications.

Myocardial contusion may lead to aneurysm formation which can result in ventricular arrhythmias and sudden death, congestive heart failure or late cardiac rupture. Recent evidence suggests, however, that patients who suffer a myocardial contusion have a favorable prognosis and that late cardiac complications are rare.[23-26] In our experience, patients with myocardial contusion are often asymptomatic, but when symptoms do occur they usually present on admission or develop early in the patient's hospital course. In a study conducted in our institution a cardiac event occurred in 10 of 105 consecutive patients with severe blunt chest trauma.[17] In our study we performed transesophageal echocardiography if the transthoracic approach was not adequate so that all patients had complete echocardiographic assessment of cardiac structure and function. Echocardiography was highly predictive of a cardiac event. Electrocardiography and cardiac enzyme determinations were not predictive of a cardiac event. In only four of these ten patients, representing less than 4% of the entire study population, did the cardiac event lead to symptoms. Furthermore, among the 22 patients with a myocardial contusion who survived to discharge, no late cardiac events occurred for more than a 2-year follow-up period.[27]

Although echocardiography is useful in identifying patients at risk for cardiac complications, the incidence of symptomatic cardiac events is so low that routine echocardiography in patients with blunt chest trauma cannot be recommended. Echocardiography is, however, useful in patients who are hemodynamically unstable or whose cardiac examination is suspicious for cardiac injury. In such patients if the transthoracic echocardiogram is not satisfactory then transesophageal echocardiography should be performed to assess the degree of myocardial or valvular injury and the presence of a pericardial effusion.

> **Recommendations for performing echocardiography in patients with blunt chest trauma**
>
> - Screening echocardiography is not of value in blunt chest trauma since the majority of patients with myocardial contusion remain asymptomatic and have favorable outcomes.
> - Transthoracic echocardiography is indicated in any patient who develops symptoms or whose physical examination suggests underlying cardiac injury.
> - If the transthoracic approach is suboptimal then transesophageal echocardiography is of value.
> - Transesophageal echocardiography is also of value in assessing the thoracic aorta for injury.

THE VALUE OF TRANSESOPHAGEAL ECHOCARDIOGRAPHY IN EVALUATING THE AORTA FOR INJURY

> Any patient with suspected aortic injury should undergo transesophageal echocardiography to evaluate for
> - aortic disruption
> - intimal tear
> - mediastinal hematoma.

Unlike myocardial contusion which often resolves and has a favorable prognosis, rupture of the aorta requires emergency treatment because up to 40% of patients die within the first 24 hours if surgery is not performed.[28] Aortic rupture has been estimated to be responsible for up to 18% of the deaths caused by blunt chest trauma from motor vehicle accidents.[29] The clinician caring for the trauma patient must have a high index of suspicion for traumatic aortic injury, for up to 20% of patients with traumatic aortic injury survive to reach a trauma center and undergo diagnostic evaluation.[1]

The thoracic aorta has several points of attachment to the mediastinal structures. It is attached at the Sinus of Valsalva, at the isthmus by the remnant of the ligamentum arteriosum and again at the diaphragm. The aorta is partially coiled as it traverses from the aortic valve leftward and posteriorly into the lower thoracic cavity. At the point of impact during blunt chest trauma, the aorta at these sites of attachment is subject to extreme torque and compression. The severe stress can lead to tears and rupture of the aortic wall (Fig 6.7). In over 90% of cases of traumatic aortic

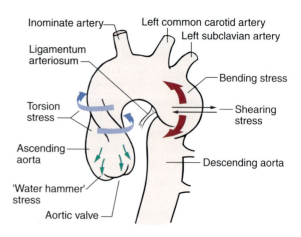

Figure 6.7 *Diagrammatic illustration of the stresses that occur on the thoracic aorta during blunt chest trauma. Shearing and bending stresses are greatest at the aortic isthmus, the most common site of traumatic aortic injury. (From Symbas PN. Cardiothoracic Trauma. Philadelphia: WB Saunders Co., 1989)*

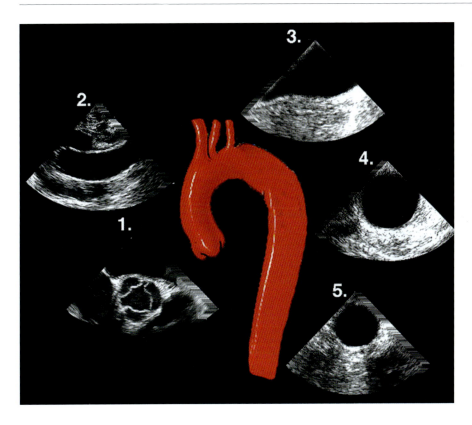

Figure 6.8 *Routine transesophageal echocardiographic views of the thoracic aorta: 1, short-axis view of the aortic valve; 2, long-axis view of the ascending aorta; 3, long-axis view of the aortic arch; 4, short-axis view of the descending thoracic aorta at the level of the aortic isthmus; 5, short-axis view of the descending thoracic aorta at the level of the diaphragm.*

disruption, the isthmus is the involved site of aortic injury, followed less frequently by the ascending aorta and then the thoracic aorta at the level of the diaphragm.

Because of the high mortality associated with traumatic aortic disruption, rapid and accurate diagnosis is essential. The gold standard for diagnosing traumatic aortic injury has been aortic angiography, although accurate aortography is limited by several factors. It is invasive, uses contrast dye and requires transferring the patient to the angiography suite, which can lead to a significant time delay before any suspected aortic injury can be confirmed and surgically corrected. Transesophageal echocardiography has been shown to be ideal for evaluating aortic pathology such as aortic dissection and aortic atherosclerosis and recently has been used to evaluate the trauma patient for aortic injury. This is because of the close proximity of the thoracic aorta to the esophagus. Transesophageal echocardiography can provide high resolution images of the thoracic aorta from the level of the aortic valve to the diaphragmatic aorta (Fig 6.8). There is a blind spot when imaging the aorta by transesophageal echocardiography due to the right bronchus as it courses between the distal ascending thoracic aorta and the esophagus. This is less of a problem in evaluating the trauma patient since aortic injury most commonly involves the aortic isthmus, an area well visualized from the transesophageal approach.

There is a spectrum of injury that can occur to the aorta following blunt chest trauma (Fig 6.9). The

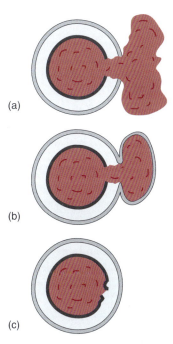

(a)

(b)

(c)

Figure 6.9 *Schematic representing the spectrum of traumatic aortic injury. (a) Complete rupture of all three layers (intima, media and adventitia) of the aortic wall. Death is immediate due to massive exsanguination. (b) Rupture of the intima and media. Blood is contained within a pseudoaneurysm formed by the thin outer adventitial wall. Patients often survive to hospitalization but are at high risk of rupture and death within hours or days of the injury. (c) A tear in the intimal surface. The media and adventitia are intact and the risk of rupture is low. These injuries often resolve without surgical intervention.*

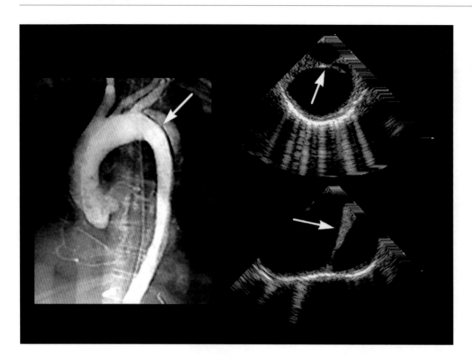

Figure 6.10 *A young man with traumatic aortic disruption following blunt chest trauma from an automobile accident. Left: aortography demonstrates the site of aortic injury (arrow). Right top: transesophageal echocardiographic image of the descending thoracic aorta at the level of the aortic isthmus showing a traumatic aortic disruption with an intraluminal flap (arrow). Right bottom: the true aortic lumen is to the left of the intraluminal flap, the pseudoaneurysm to the right.*

extreme stress on the aortic wall following blunt chest trauma may lead to complete aortic rupture of all three layers of the aorta, the intima, media and the adventitia. These patients usually die at the accident scene from sudden and massive exsanguination. Rupture may involve only the intimal and medial layers of the aortic wall with the adventitial layer remaining intact. This subadventitial disruption will lead to the formation of a pseudoaneurysm. These patients usually survive to reach a trauma center but are at high risk of death from rupture of the thin adventitial layer. The clinician needs a high index of suspicion to diagnose such aortic injury because these patients need prompt surgical repair to prevent rupture and death. Finally, injury may involve only the intimal surface. Such tears do not lead to the formation of a pseudoaneurysm and the relatively stable media and adventitia provide adequate support to the aortic wall such that late rupture does not occur. These lesions are more stable and often resolve without intervention. It is felt that these patients can be managed conservatively with close clinical follow-up.[30]

Echocardiographic criteria for traumatic aortic disruption

- Mobile and thick intraluminal flap
- Asymmetric aortic contour due to the formation of a localized pseudoaneurysm
- Most often localized to the aortic isthmus
- Similar blood flow by color-flow Doppler on either side of the intraluminal flap
- Presence of a mediastinal hematoma suggests aortic injury

The diagnosis of traumatic aortic disruption is made by detecting a disrupted aortic wall with blood flow on either side of the disruption. Echocardiographically this is seen as a thick mobile intraluminal flap which consists of both the intima and media (Fig 6.10). It is important to remember that traumatic aortic disruption is different pathologically from aortic dissection and it is a misnomer to label traumatic aortic disruption as traumatic aortic dissection. Echocardiographically there are differences between traumatic aortic disruption and aortic dissection.[31] In aortic dissection the intraluminal flap tends to be thinner since it is composed of only the intimal layer of the aortic wall and the aortic contour is symmetric. In traumatic aortic disruption the intraluminal flap is thicker since it is composed of both the intima and media and the contour is asymmetric to the formation of a pseudoaneurysm. Furthermore, in traumatic aortic disruption blood flow by color-flow Doppler is equal on both sides of the intraluminal flap whereas in aortic dissection the more sluggish blood flow in the false lumen leads to different blood flow velocities between the true and false lumens.

The finding by transesophageal echocardiography of a mediastinal hematoma (Fig 6.11) is non-specific and may be related to various non-cardiac injuries. It may also indicate injury to the aorta or to aortic branch vessels. When mediastinal hematoma is detected by transesophageal echocardiography, aortography is needed to further evaluate the aortic branch vessels for injury. Le Bret and colleagues[32] used three echocardiographic criteria to diagnose traumatic mediastinal hematoma. The transesophageal echocardiographic signs included:

1. an increased distance between the echocardiographic probe and the aortic wall;

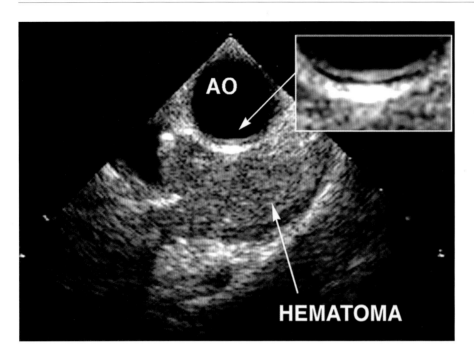

Figure 6.11 *Transesophageal echocardiogram of a mediastinal hematoma. A large hematoma is seen separating the aorta (AO) from the visceral pleura below. The magnified view in the top right corner clearly demonstrates that the intimal surface of the aorta is intact.*

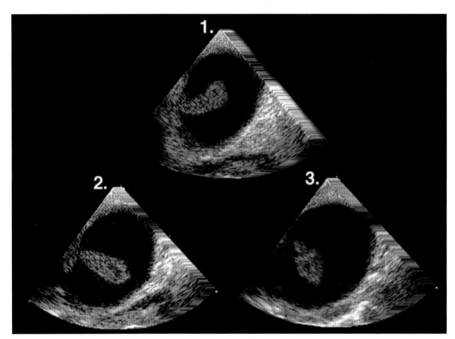

Figure 6.12 *Transesophageal echocardiography in a patient with blunt chest trauma. Serial short-axis echocardiographic views of the descending thoracic aorta at the level of the aortic isthmus obtained at different times of the cardiac cycle show a highly mobile intimal tear. Aortography in this patient was normal and the patient was managed conservatively. Repeat transesophageal echocardiographic imaging one week later was normal.*

2. a double contour of the aortic wall; and
3. the visualization of the ultrasound signal between the aortic wall and visceral pleura.

These authors found that the echocardiographic sign of an increased distance between the transesophageal probe and the aortic wall was the most accurate in diagnosing mediastinal hematoma.

Several recent studies have demonstrated the high sensitivity and specificity of transesophageal echocardiography in diagnosing traumatic aortic injury.[33–37] Transesophageal echocardiography is as specific as, but more sensitive than, aortography in assessing the aorta

for injury. In our experience,[38] and in others,[31] transesophageal echocardiography can detect small intimal tears that are not seen by angiography (Fig 6.12). However, such patients have a favorable prognosis and can be treated conservatively. Furthermore, the finding of a normal angiogram in these patients gives the clinician confidence that they can be treated medically without surgical intervention. Transesophageal echocardiography has several advantages over aortography. It is non-invasive, portable and can more rapidly provide the needed information in the emergency department or operating room without having to transfer the patient to the angiography suite. In a study by Kearny

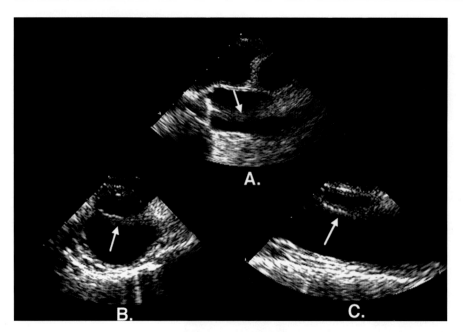

Figure 6.13 *Transesophageal echocardiographic examples of artifact that can mimic traumatic aortic injury. In each case the arrow points to reverberation artifact from the aortic wall that can mimic an intraluminal flap and lead to a mistaken diagnosis of traumatic aortic injury. Operator skill and experience is mandatory when evaluating the aorta in the trauma patient.*

et al.,[33] the average diagnostic time for transesophageal echocardiography was 27 minutes compared with 76 minutes for aortography.

There is, however, a substantial learning curve for the operator and one must be aware of certain pitfalls in imaging the aorta for injury and not misinterpreting other aortic pathology or normal aortic structures as traumatic aortic injury. Transesophageal echocardiographic findings of a total or subtotal traumatic disruption of the aorta tend not to be subtle findings. To diagnose small aortic disruptions or injury limited to the aortic intima, a more skilled and experienced operator is needed. The echocardiographer must be able to distinguish traumatic aortic disruption from other forms of aortic pathology such as aortic dissection and aortic atherosclerotic debris. Difficulty may arise in differentiating a localized intimal tear from focal atherosclerotic debris. Atherosclerotic aortic debris tends to occur in older patients, is diffuse and is associated with calcifications of the intimal surface with overlying thrombus.[39] A localized traumatic intimal tear will lack the intimal thickening and calcifications present in atherosclerotic aortic debris, although overlying thrombus has been described adherent to a traumatic intimal tear. Care should also be taken not to misinterpret the subclavian vein, azygos vein, transverse sinus or reverberation artifact in the ascending aorta as traumatic aortic injury (Fig 6.13). Any equivocal transesophageal echocardiographic findings need to be confirmed or disproved by aortography.

In our opinion, transesophageal echocardiography should be the imaging technique of choice in evaluating the thoracic aorta for injury. However, experience and a skilled operator are essential to make an accurate diagnosis since there are numerous imaging artifacts that can mimic aortic pathology. Transesophageal echocardiography is limited in evaluating aortic branch vessels, specifically the innominate, left carotid and left subclavian arteries and cannot visualize the abdominal aorta. Although traumatic injury to these vessels is unusual, when it is suspected, aortography is necessary. Transesophageal echocardiography cannot safely be performed in combative patients and unless the patient can be adequately sedated transesophageal echocardiography should not be performed. Furthermore, in patients with suspected unstable neck or spine injuries or in patients with oropharyngeal injury, transesophageal echocardiography must be performed with extreme care. If transesophageal echocardiography cannot be performed safely, then aortography should be performed.

Skill and operator experience is mandatory when transesophageal echocardiography is used to evaluate the aorta for injury because numerous imaging artifacts can mimic aortic pathology.

Transesophageal echocardiography and aortic injury

Advantages
- More accurate that aortography
- Can be performed more rapidly than aortography
- Portable, can be performed in the emergency department, the intensive care unit or the operating room
- Requires no contrast agent
- Non-invasive
- Supplies added information on myocardial, valvular or pericardial injury

Disadvantages
- Requires a highly skilled operator
- Cannot adequately visualize branch vessels

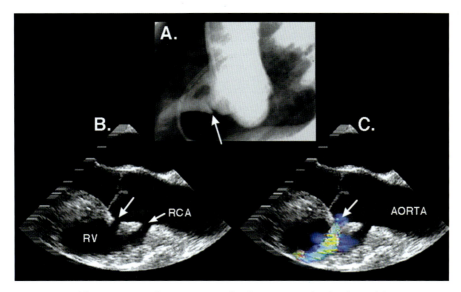

Figure 6.14 *(A) Aortography demonstrates a fistulous communication (arrow) between the aorta and right ventricle (RV) in a young man with a continuous murmur on physical examination following a stab wound to the chest. (B) Transesophageal echocardiographic view of the ascending aorta. The fistula between the aorta and RV (arrow) is clearly seen. The right coronary artery (RCA) is uninvolved. (C) Color-flow Doppler demonstrates continuous flow (arrow) from the aorta into the right ventricle.*

PENETRATING CHEST TRAUMA AND CARDIAC INJURY

Penetrating thoracic injury may lead to laceration of the pericardium, laceration of the myocardium, perforation of the interventricular or interatrial septa, or may damage or disrupt any of the cardiac valves.[40–42] Often the wound involves the pericardium as well as the underlying cardiac structures. The overall mortality increases with more extensive cardiac injury and when definitive surgical repair is delayed, most often due to misdiagnosis. The challenge for the clinician is to accurately and rapidly define the location and extent of cardiac injury.

When a patient develops the classic findings of cardiac tamponade, hypotension, neck vein distension and a pulsus paradox following a penetrating wound to the chest, there is little doubt that injury to the heart has occurred. However, the clinical manifestations of associated injury to the lungs or other organs may overshadow more subtle signs of cardiac injury. The failure of the clinician to recognize underlying cardiac injury may lead to devastating complications. Therefore a thorough investigation for injury to the heart following penetrating thoracic injury is mandatory. A number of algorithms have been put forth to manage patients with penetrating thoracic injury that aim to rapidly diagnose cardiac injury so that definitive treatment can occur. Echocardiography has been shown to be extremely valuable in diagnosing penetrating cardiac injury.[43–47] Echocardiography can detect pericardial

effusion, foreign bodies in the heart and intracardiac shunts. As with blunt chest trauma, if the clinical suspicion for cardiac injury is high and the transthoracic echocardiogram is suboptimal, then transesophageal echocardiography is of value (Fig 6.14).

Echocardiography can aid the surgeon caring for the patient with penetrating chest trauma by directing surgical care. The finding of a significant pericardial effusion by echocardiography would lead to prompt surgical intervention, while the finding of a normal echocardiogram would avoid unnecessary surgery in a patient whose clinical presentation or physical examination may have misled the surgeon in suspecting cardiac injury. However, in a patient who is hemodynamically unstable, therapeutic intervention should not be postponed if the echocardiographic study cannot be performed quickly or if a physician skilled in echocardiography is not readily available.

CONCLUSIONS

Echocardiography is an important tool for the physician caring for the patient following blunt or penetrating chest trauma. Echocardiography provides direct visualization of cardiac structure and function and can rapidly and accurately diagnose cardiac and aortic injury at the bedside. Transesophageal echocardiography offers the advantage of providing superior imaging of the heart when the transthoracic approach is limited and can assess traumatic aortic injury as accurately as, and more rapidly than, aortography. Skill in interpreting the echocardiographic findings is essential to avoid misdiagnosis and maintain accuracy. By understanding the advantages and disadvantages of echocardiography in diagnosing cardiac injury the physician caring for the trauma patient will be able to utilize echocardiography in the trauma patient more effectively. Echocardiography can then lead to earlier diagnosis of cardiac injury and direct appropriate treatment, thereby improving survival in patients who suffer traumatic injury to the heart or great vessels.

REFERENCES

1. Parmley LF, Manion WC, Mattingly TW. Nonpenetrating traumatic injury to the heart. *Circulation* 1958; **18:** 371–96.

2. Mayfield W, Hurley EJ. Blunt chest trauma. *Am J Surg* 1984; **148:** 162–6.

3. Jones JW, Hewitt RL, Drapanas T. Cardiac contusion: a capricious syndrome. *Ann Surg* 1975; **181:** 567–73.

4. Tenzer ML. The spectrum of myocardial contusion: a review. *J Trauma* 1985; **25:** 620–7.

5. Hossack KF, Moreno CA, Vanway CW, Burdick DC. Frequency of cardiac contusion in nonpenetrating chest injury. *Am J Cardiol* 1988; **61:** 391–4.

6. Fabian TC, Mangiante EC, Patterson R, Payne LW, Isaacson ML. Myocardial contusion in blunt chest trauma: clinical characteristics, means of diagnosis, and implications for patient management. *J Trauma* 1988; **28:** 50–6.

7. Leidtke JA, DeMuth WE. Nonpenetrating cardiac injuries: a collective review. *Am Heart J* 1973; **86:** 687–94.

8. Gay JA, Gottdiener JS, Gomes MN, Patterson RH, Fletcher RD. Echocardiographic features of traumatic disruption of the aortic valve. *Chest* 1983; **83:** 150–1.

9. Kleikamp G, Schnepper U, Kortke H, Breymann T, Korfer R. Tricuspid valve regurgitation following blunt chest trauma. *Chest* 1992; **102:** 1294–6.

10. Cuadros CL, Hutchinson JE, Mogtader AH. Laceration of a mitral papillary muscle and the aortic root as a result of blunt trauma to the chest. Case report and review of the literature. *J Thorac Cardiovasc Surg* 1984; **88:** 134–40.

11. Miller FA, Seward JB, Gersh BJ, Tajik AJ, Mucha P. Two-dimensional echocardiographic findings in cardiac trauma. *Am J Cardiol* 1982; **50:** 1022–7.

12. King MR, Mucha P, Seward JB, Gersh BJ, Farnell MB. Cardiac contusion: a new diagnostic approach utilizing two-dimensional echocardiography. *J Trauma* 1983; **23:** 610–14.

13. Reid CL, Kawanishi DT, Rahimtoola SH, Chandraratna PAN. Chest trauma: evaluation by two-dimensional echocardiography. *Am Heart J* 1987; **113:** 971–6.

14. Beggs CW, Helling TS, Evans LL, Hays LV, Kennedy FR, Crouse LJ. Early evaluation of cardiac injury by two-dimensional echocardiography in patients suffering blunt chest trauma. *Ann Emerg Med* 1987; **16:** 542–5.

15. Hiatt JR, Yeatman LA, Child JS. The value of echocardiography in blunt chest trauma. *J Trauma* 1988; **28:** 914–21.

16. Helling TS, Duke P, Beggs CW, Crouse LJ. A prospective evaluation of 68 patients suffering blunt chest trauma for evidence of cardiac injury. *J Trauma* 1989; **29:** 961–5.

17. Karalis DG, Victor MF, Davis GA, *et al*. The role of echocardiography in blunt chest trauma: a transthoracic and transesophageal echocardiographic study. *J Trauma* 1994; **36:** 53–8.

18. Pandian NG, Skorton DJ, Doty DB, Kerber RE. Immediate diagnosis of acute myocardial contusion by two-dimensional echocardiography: studies in a canine model of blunt chest trauma. *J Am Coll Cardiol* 1983; **2:** 488–96.

19. Goldberg SP, Karalis DG, Ross JJ, Chandrasekaran K. Severe right ventricular contusion mimicking cardiac tamponade: the value of transesophageal echocardiography in blunt chest trauma. *Ann Emerg Med* 1993; **22:** 745–7.

20. Shapiro MJ, Yanofsky SD, Trapp J, *et al*. Cardiovascular evaluation in blunt thoracic trauma using transesophageal echocardiography (TEE). *J Trauma* 1991; **31:** 835–9.

21. Brooks SW, Young JC, Cmolik B, *et al*. The use of transesophageal echocardiography in the evaluation of chest trauma. *J Trauma* 1992; **32:** 761–5.

22. Weiss RL, Brier JA, O'Connor W, Ross S, Brathwaite CM. The usefulness of transesophageal echocardiography in diagnosing cardiac contusions. *Chest* 1996; **109:** 73–7.

23. Sturaitis M, McCallum D, Sutherland G, Cheung J, Driedger AA, Sibbald WJ. Lack of significant long-term sequelae following traumatic myocardial contusion. *Arch Intern Med* 1986; **146:** 1765–9.

24. Beresky R, Klingler R, Peake J. Myocardial contusion: when does it have clinical significance? *J Trauma* 1988; **28:** 64–8.

25. McLean RF, Devitt JH, McLellan BA, Dubbin J, Ehrlich LE, Dirkson D. Significance of myocardial contusion following blunt chest trauma. *J Trauma* 1992; **33:** 240–3.

26. Malangoni MA, McHenry CR, Jacobs DG. Outcome of serious blunt cardiac injury. *Surgery* 1994; **116:** 628–33.

27. Karalis DG, Davis GA, McAllister MPJ, *et al*. Are patients with myocardial contusion at risk for late cardiac complications? *J Am Soc Echocardiogr* 1994; **7:** S60.

28. Feczko JD, Lynch L, Pless JE, Clark MA, McClain J, Hawley DA. An autopsy case review of 142 non-penetrating (blunt) injuries to the aorta. *J Trauma* 1992; **33:** 846–9.

29. Greendyke RM. Traumatic rupture of the aorta: special reference to automobile accidents. *JAMA* 1966; **195:** 119–22.

30. Fisher RG, Oria RA, Mattox, KL, Whigham CJ, Pickard LR. Conservative management of aortic lacerations due to blunt trauma. *J Trauma* 1990; **30**: 1562–6.

31. Vignon P, Gueret P, Vedrinne JM, *et al.* Role of transesophageal echocardiography in the diagnosis and management of traumatic aortic disruption. *Circulation* 1995; **92**: 2959–68.

32. Le Bret F, Ruel P, Rosier H, Goarin JP, Riou B, Viars P. Diagnosis of traumatic mediastinal hematoma with transesophageal echocardiography. *Chest* 1994; **105**: 373–6.

33. Kearney PA, Smith W, Johnson SB, Barker DE, Smith MD, Sapin PM. Use of transesophageal echocardiography in the evaluation of traumatic aortic injury. *J Trauma* 1993; **34**: 696–701.

34. Fernandez LG, Lain KY, Messersmith RN, *et al.* Transesophageal echocardiography for diagnosing aortic injury: a case report and summary of current imaging techniques. *J Trauma* 1994; **36**: 877–80.

35. Buckmaster MJ, Kearney PA, Johnson SB, Smith MD, Sapin PM. Further experience with transesophageal echocardiography in the evaluation of thoracic aortic injury. *J Trauma* 1994; **37**: 989–95.

36. Smith MD, Cassidy JM, Souther S, *et al.* Transesophageal echocardiography in the diagnosis of traumatic rupture of the aorta. *N Engl J Med* 1995; **332**: 356–62.

37. Saletta S, Lederman E, Fein S, Singh A, Kuehler D, Fortune JB. Transesophageal echocardiography for the initial evaluation of the widened mediastinum in trauma patients. *J Trauma* 1995; **39**: 137–41.

38. Davis GA, Saverisen S, Chandrasekaran K, Karalis DG, Ross JJ, Mintz GS. Subclinical traumatic aortic injury diagnosed by transesophageal echocardiography. *Am Heart J* 1992; **123**: 534–6.

39. Karalis DG, Chandrasekaran K, Victor MF, Ross JJ, Mintz GS. The recognition and embolic potential of intraaortic atherosclerotic debris. *J Am Coll Cardiol* 1991; **17**: 73–8.

40. Rayner AVS, Fulton RL, Hess PJ, Daicoff GR. Post-traumatic intracardiac shunts. Report of two cases and review of the literature. *J Thorac Cardiovasc Surg* 1977; **73**: 728–32.

41. Thandroyen FT, Matisonn RE. Penetrating thoracic trauma producing cardiac shunts. *J Thorac Cardiovasc Surg* 1981; **81**: 569–73.

42. Cha EK, Mittal V, Allaben R. Delayed sequelae of penetrating cardiac injury. *Arch Surg* 1993; **128**: 836–9.

43. Goldfarb MS, Walpole HT, Landolt CC, McIntyre AB, Felner JM. Two-dimensional Doppler echocardiographic diagnosis of a traumatic intracardiac shunt. *Am J Cardiol* 1986; **57**: 494–5.

44. Freshman SP, Wisner DH, Weber CJ. 2-D echocardiography: emergent use in the evaluation of penetrating precordial trauma. *J Trauma* 1991; **31**: 902–5.

45. Plummer D, Brunette D, Asinger R, Ruiz E. Emergency department echocardiography improves outcome in penetrating cardiac injury. *Ann Emerg Med* 1992; **21**: 709–12.

46. Skoularigis J, Essop MR, Sareli P. Usefulness of transesophageal echocardiography in the early diagnosis of penetrating stab wounds to the heart. *Am J Cardiol* 1994; **73**: 407–9.

47. Aaland MO, Bryna FC, Sherman R. Two-dimensional echocardiogram in hemodynamically stable victims of penetrating precordial trauma. *Am Surg* 1994; **60**: 412–15.

7

Thoracoscopy and chest trauma: its role

GEOFFREY M GRAEBER

Thoracoscopy/video-assisted thoracic surgery (VATS) has a distinct role in the diagnosis and management of chest trauma. The use of video-assisted surgery in treating chest injuries requires mature judgment since the patient must not be unstable and must meet specific criteria before thoracoscopy/VATS is used in diagnosis and/or treatment. Our knowledge of thoracoscopy/VATS and how it may be employed in the evaluation and treatment of trauma patients has expanded since previous reviews.[1,2]

This chapter confirms the role of VATS in treating patients with limited, continued, intrapleural hemorrhage and retained hemothoraces. It also examines the place of thoracoscopy and VATS in treating early fibrothoraces and empyemas resulting from retained hemothoraces. The contribution of thoracoscopy/VATS in evaluating and treating acute diaphragmatic injuries is presented. What part video-assisted thoracoscopy may play in the treatment of pericardial, cardiac and mediastinal injuries is considered. The emerging treatment of spontaneous pneumothorax due to ruptured blebs using minimally invasive techniques is evaluated in light of published experience. Finally, the technical aspects of performing thoracoscopy/VATS are reviewed. In the text that follows, VATS will be used as the term to cover all different modes of video-assisted surgery and various other diagnostic and therapeutic modalities in which video-assisted technology is used in conjunction with minimally invasive techniques to perform surgery.

CONTRAINDICATIONS TO VATS IN TRAUMA PATIENTS

Before exploring those indications for the use of video-assisted thoracic surgery in the evaluation of patients with chest trauma, one needs to understand the absolute contraindications for VATS in trauma patients. The proper use of VATS in trauma patients requires the best judgment of a mature surgeon since miscalculation can be followed by the patient's demise. VATS has a limited but clearly defined role in the diagnosis and treatment of specific chest injuries.

Inappropriate patient selection can lead to a desperate situation which will most likely result in the patient's death (Table 7.1). Obviously, if the patient is hemodynamically unstable, any VATS procedure is contraindicated. No patient with a systolic arterial pressure less than 90 mmHg is a candidate for a VATS procedure. Suspected injuries to the heart or great vessels caused by penetrating trauma also precludes a VATS procedure since immediate catastrophic hemorrhage could occur at any time. These patients are best evaluated and treated using standard incisions.

If the treating surgeon also has any reason to suspect a blunt injury to the same vital structures, VATS procedures should be abandoned in favor of an open approach. A widened mediastinum on standard radiographic examinations could suggest a dangerous injury to the heart or great vessels. Such findings should

Table 7.1 *Contraindications to video-assisted thoracic surgery in thoracic trauma*

Hemodynamic instability
  Signs of hypovolemic shock, particularly arterial systolic blood pressure of 90 mmHg or less
  Cardiac arrhythmia
Suspected injuries to the heart or great vessels
Blunt trauma which is suspected to have caused contusion or other injury to the heart or great vessels
Widened mediastinum
  On PA or AP radiograph
  Loss of architecture on mediastinal pleural reflections
Suspicion of major injuries to the trachea or bronchus
Substantial hemorrhage
  Bleeding of more than 500 ml/h
  Initial drainage by tube thoracostomy of 1500 ml pleural blood and clots
Inability to tolerate one-lung ventilation
  Previous injury or surgery
  Severe pulmonary contusion
  Intercurrent lung disease
Other emergency conditions requiring major operative procedures to stabilize the patient
  Celiotomy
  Craniotomy

Table 7.2 *Indications for VATS in thoracic trauma*

Persistent hemorrhage
  Moderate in nature
  Stable patient
Retained hemothorax
  Evacuation of retained clot, old blood, or other fluids (serum)
  Re-expansion of the lung
Treatment of early fibrothorax
  Early intervention
  Decortication
  Culture
Empyema
  Early intervention
  Evacuation of the pleural space
  Drainage
  Re-expansion of the lung
  Culture
Diaphragmatic injuries
  Diagnosis
  Treatment
Chylothorax
  Diagnosis
  Treatment
Removal of foreign bodies
  Proper instrumentation
  Care to avoid major hemorrhage
Evaluation of pericardium, heart and great vessels
  Questionable diagnostic role
  Therapy requires open procedure for safety
Treatment of persistent air leak
  Identify cause
  Correct source
    Staple
    Coagulate
    Suture
  Re-expand the lung

dictate that the patient be explored through an open approach since catastrophic hemorrhage is possible. Similarly, suspected injuries to the trachea or a major bronchus require repair through an open approach since endoscopic techniques at the present time are inadequate to repair a major tracheobronchial injury. Substantial hemorrhage suggests injury to the heart or an arterial vessel. The immediate loss of 1500 ml of blood on initial tube thoracostomy drainage or blood loss greater than 500 ml/h and persisting over several hours usually heralds an injury to the heart or great vessels sufficient to warrant immediate open exploration. VATS is not indicated if the patient is unable to tolerate collapse of one lung due to previous pleural disease, previous injury, surgical procedures or intercurrent pulmonary disease.

If the patient is suffering from major life-threatening injury to other organs, this condition must be addressed first. Conditions requiring a celiotomy or a craniotomy must be addressed and the patient stabilized before any VATS procedure is considered. Realistically, VATS should only be used in a stabilized patient who can tolerate the procedure to achieve limited diagnostic and therapeutic goals.

EVALUATION AND TREATMENT OF PERSISTENT INTRATHORACIC HEMORRHAGE

Patients who have persistent hemorrhage after trauma may be selected for VATS evaluation and treatment if specific criteria are met (Table 7.2). The patient must be hemodynamically stable; those who are not should be taken to the operating room immediately for open correction through an incision appropriate for the injury.[1-3] If a patient experiences continued moderate hemorrhage (200–500 ml/h) through tube thoracostomies which have re-expanded the lung, then VATS evaluation and treatment are appropriate. In one of the larger studies performed using rigid thoracoscopic evaluation, Jones *et al.* found that moderate continuing hemorrhage could be evaluated and treated in most patients using local anesthesia.[3] In 33 of 36 patients evaluated by this group, local anesthesia was appropriate; only three patients required general endotracheal anesthesia via a double lumen tube.[3] A standard rigid thoracoscope introduced through the sites where chest tubes had been placed in the emergency department and withdrawn in the operating suite was sufficient to evaluate and treat persistent hemorrhage (Fig 7.1). In one of the 36 patients, adhesions prevented successful

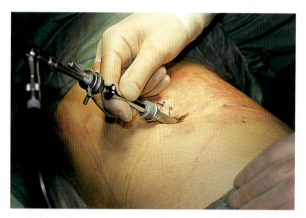

Figure 7.1 *Introduction of the thoracoscope to confirm diaphragmatic rupture after blunt injury to the right chest. (SWTC.)*

thoracoscopic evaluation and treatment. A rigid ventilating bronchoscope replaced the thoracoscope if copious clots were present and a larger orifice was necessary to evacuate the pleural space effectively. In most instances, continuing hemorrhage was due to injured intercostal vessels which were controlled with clipping and/or electrocautery. In patients who had more diffuse hemorrhage, evacuation of retained clot and re-expansion of the lung by means of replaced large (no. 40 French) chest tubes usually stopped continued hemorrhage. The use of a flexible fiberoptic bronchoscope, employed as a thoracoscope, has also been reported to control continuing intrapleural hemorrhage, remove clots and re-expand the lung.[4,5]

Smith *et al.* conducted a prospective trial of videothoracoscopy at an urban trauma center between February 1992 and February 1993, to evaluate the efficacy of this modality in evaluating and treating patients with thoracic injuries.[6] Of the 24 patients (22 penetrating, two blunt injuries), five were taken to surgery for persistent hemorrhage (more than 1500 ml of blood loss in a 24-hour period). In all five, intercostal artery injury was confirmed. The use of diathermy achieved hemostasis in three without the use of thoracotomy.

RETAINED HEMOTHORAX AFTER THORACIC TRAUMA

A logical extension of the use of VATS for control of continued hemorrhage is its use in the drainage of retained hemothoraces and residual pleural clot. Continued retention of liquid and/or clotted blood in the thorax may result in fibrothorax and entrapment of the lung.[1,2,7] In one retrospective review at an urban trauma center, Coselli and his colleagues found that retained hemothoraces after tube thoracostomy placement occurred in less than 4% of 4766 patients presenting with traumatic hemothorax or hemopneumothorax.[7] Although this uncommon complication may be innocuous, it may result in a trapped lung, decreased pulmonary compliance, prolonged time on a ventilator and increased length of hospital stay with a concomitant increase in hospital costs.

Several recent papers have focused on the use of VATS rather than the standard thoracotomy to evacuate retained blood and clot from the traumatized pleural space. Smith and associates found that nine of the 24 chest trauma patients they studied prospectively had clotted hemothoraces that would have required thoracotomies for evacuation.[6] In eight of their nine patients with clotted hemothoraces, videothoracoscopy was used successfully to evacuate the clot and restore normal respiratory dynamics.[6] Success in evacuation of the retained blood and clot is temporally related, as has been shown by Mancini and associates.[8] They showed that retained hemothoraces are more easily removed the sooner they are addressed.[8] Ideally, the clots and old blood should be removed within the first 24 hours of recognition. The longer retained blood and clot remain in the pleural space, the more dense the resolving fibrosis becomes, making complete removal more difficult and time-consuming.

Heniford and his associates at University of Louisville School of Medicine reviewed 25 patients who had retained thoracic collections after trauma.[9] These patients underwent 26 different thoracoscopic procedures to evacuate retained blood in the pleural cavity. In 19 patients, thoracoscopic evacuation was successful. In four patients, thoracoscopy had to be abandoned and an open thoracotomy had to be conducted to evacuate the clot successfully and re-expand the lung. In another two patients, subsequent procedures were required to achieve successful drainage of the retained collections. In their review they found that the failure of thoracoscopy was directly proportional to the time between the injury and the surgical procedure to remove the clot and re-expand the lung. Failure of thoracoscopy could also be correlated with the type of collection present in the chest but not with the mechanism of injury. In their review they found that when thoracoscopy was conducted within 7 days of admission, there were no patients who had an empyema. These authors concluded that videothoracoscopy is an accurate, safe and reliable operative procedure to achieve successful removal of retained thoracic collections after trauma. Ninety percent of the patients in whom the procedure was conducted successfully had good postoperative results. Early evacuation of retained blood and fluid from the pleural space resulted in reduced hospital stay and a concomitant decrease in complications. They suggest that videothoracoscopy should be the initial treatment for the removal of retained thoracic collections in trauma patients and that this modality should be used earlier and more frequently to shorten hospital stay and decrease hospital costs.

A recent paper discussed the role of videothoracoscopy in patients with clotted hemothoraces following chest trauma.[10] The 12 patients evaluated had an average of 1200 ml (range 500–2600 ml) in their thoracic cavities. Evacuation of the hemothorax was much more easily conducted if fewer than 10 days had transpired between the time of injury and the video-assisted thoracic exploration. In all but one patient, videothoracoscopy was successful in removing clots and re-expanding the lung.[10] The sole patient who required thoracotomy was operated on 31 days after a stab wound to the left chest.[10] The adhesions were so dense and the blood clots so organized that the surgeons had to open the chest in order to evacuate the maturing fibrothorax and re-expand the lung.

VATS TREATMENT OF EARLY FIBROTHORAX

Fibrothorax frequently follows a resolving hemothorax. It is differentiated from empyema by a lack of bacterial contamination. Both fibrothorax and empyema may trap the lung as the processes matures. The extent of fibrosis following a hemothorax may be as dense as an empyema. The goal of VATS is directed at eradication of the fibrothorax by evacuating the pleural space and re-expanding the lung against the chest wall. Early intervention is required since successful resolution is inversely dependent on the density of the fibrous adhesions. The earlier decortication is performed, the more easily adhesions will be stripped from the lung and chest wall. If done later, denser adhesions will be encountered and air leaks may result during attempted dissection.

EVALUATION AND TREATMENT OF EMPYEMA

If bacterial contamination complicates a retained intrathoracic collection, empyema thoracis ensues. In most series of patients treated for chest injuries, post-traumatic empyema occurs in only 2–10% of all cases of thoracic trauma.[12] When VATS is used, in a collective series from four hospitals,[10] only one of 42 patients had post-traumatic empyema. The mainstay of therapy to prevent post-traumatic empyema is early evacuation of infected material with complete re-expansion of the lung.[11,12] Initial efforts to evacuate the contaminated blood, clot and serum may include multiple tube thoracostomies.[12] Some authors have suggested that guided percutaneous drainage for post-traumatic empyema thoracis may be as effective as formal open decortication.[13] Chest tubes may, in fact, have detrimental effects

and can facilitate the route though which bacteria can infect residual pleural clot.[14,15] Prolonged emplacement of chest tubes may be correlated with the development of empyema.[14]

The largest number of video-assisted treated patients with empyema thoracis is the 76 reported by Landreneau and associates in 1996.[16] Eight of the empyemas followed retained intrathoracic hematomas, the consequence of chest trauma.[16] O'Brien and associates reported eight cases of empyema thoracis following penetrating chest injury that were treated successfully by thoracoscopy.[17] Two patients required subsequent thoracotomy to release trapped lung and control persistent air leaks.[17]

DIAGNOSIS AND MANAGEMENT OF DIAPHRAGMATIC INJURIES

One of the more perplexing problems of thoracic trauma is the diagnosis of diaphragmatic injuries. According to some sources, approximately 30% of all diaphragmatic injuries are missed even when chest radiography, computed tomography and diagnostic peritoneal lavage are appropriately employed.[18–20] In an attempt to improve diagnostic acumen, some authors have recommended the use of videolaparoscopy to diagnose diaphragmatic injury.[21] Despite some favorable reports, laparoscopy may be inadequate in diagnosing all diaphragmatic injuries and may be potentially dangerous since the air insufflation required for laparoscopy may cause tension pneumothorax by entering the chest through a diaphragmatic defect.[21] Thoracoscopy (VATS), on the other hand, does not require air insufflation, yet gives an excellent view of the diaphragm. For these reasons, some authors are advocating the regular use of VATS to assess the diaphragm and determine whether or not diaphragmatic injury has occurred.[22–24]

The treating surgeon must appreciate that injury to intra-abdominal viscera frequently accompanies diaphragmatic injury and, if left unrecognized and untreated, may lead to critical complications.

The chronicled experience using thoracoscopy (VATS) in evaluating diaphragmatic injuries has increased. Uribe and associates evaluated 28 patients with penetrating thoracoabdominal trauma over a period of 6 months and who underwent thoracoscopy.[24] Patients were hemodynamically stable and had no indication for immediate celiotomy. All patients demonstrated sufficient findings of thoracic injury on chest radiography and physical examination to justify surgical exploration. Twenty-four patients had stab wounds and four had gunshot wounds. The authors were able to identify diaphragmatic injury at thoracoscopy in nine patients (32%). All patients with diaphragmatic injuries underwent celiotomy for confirmation of the injury and appropriate repair. Eight of the nine patients (89%) undergoing celiotomy were found to have significant injuries to intra-abdominal viscera which required direct repair. The authors felt that thoracoscopy was safe in diagnosing diaphragmatic injury; however, their experience underlines the fact that associated intra-abdominal injuries require direct surgical attention.

Nel and Warren assessed prospectively the role of thoracoscopy in evaluating the status of the diaphragm in 55 patients with penetrating knife wounds to the left lower chest.[25] In those with positive thoracoscopic findings laparotomy was performed and those with an uninjured diaphragm were observed. Twenty-two patients went to laparotomy and 32 were observed; one patient had inconclusive findings at thoracoscopy. Two patients were lost to follow-up over the 30-month period of evaluation. With evaluation of the 52 patients (one with an inconclusive thoracoscopy and two lost to follow-up), thoracoscopy was 100% sensitive, 90% specific and 94% accurate in assessing the diaphragm for injury. The authors felt if they had conducted the mandatory laparotomy (celiotomy) for supposed diaphragmatic injuries, there would have been a 63% negativity rate. They deemed thoracoscopy particularly effective since their actual negative rate was only 6% They, therefore, concluded that thorascopy was a safe and reliable method for evaluating the diaphragm in patients with left lower thoracic stab wounds.

Spann and associates conducted a prospective study to evaluate the accuracy of video-assisted thorascopic surgery (VATS) compared with exploratory celiotomy in the assessment of diaphragmatic and thoracoabdominal injuries.[26] They evaluated hemodynamically stable patients who were admitted to a level I trauma center with either blunt or penetrating injury to the lower chest and abdomen. Patients underwent both VATS and subsequent celiotomy under the same general anesthetic. The intraoperative thoracoscopic findings were not presented to the abdominal surgeons who conducted the celiotomies. During their enrollment period of 12 months, 26 patients were entered into the study. Diaphragmatic injuries were identified in eight patients (31%). In their hands, VATS identified all eight injuries in these patients. Six of the eight patients (75%) with diaphragmatic injuries sustained associated injury to intrathoracic or intra-abdominal organs. The authors found that there was no mortality and no procedural morbidity associated with VATS. More importantly, they found that there were no injuries missed by VATS in patients who underwent surgery. They felt that their findings supported the position that VATS was a safe, expeditious and accurate method of evaluating the diaphragm in injured patients. They felt it was at least comparable in diagnostic accuracy to exploratory celiotomy.

Lang-Lazdunski and associates in the French study had 14 patients suspected of having diaphragmatic injuries.[10] In seven of the 14 patients, VATS showed no perceptible injury to the diaphragm. These patients were, therefore, not explored but were observed. In all instances VATS proved to be correct in evaluating the status of diaphragmatic injuries.[10] Four patients had major diaphragmatic injuries and were converted to open thoracotomy. Two additional patients had diaphragmatic injuries of a lesser nature and underwent minithoracotomy (consisting of a 5 cm incision) to repair the diaphragm. One individual had a small diaphragmatic injury closed using endoscopic suture repair techniques.

MANAGEMENT OF CHYLOTHORAX

Chylothorax is a relatively rare, but treatable condition, which may be attributed to trauma. The most extensive experience using VATS has been that of the University of Virginia reported by Graham and associates.[27] In their series conducted between 1987 and 1993, ten patients were treated for chylothorax using video-assisted thoracic surgery. A total of 12 thoracoscopic procedures were performed. The patients ranged from 7 months to 82 years, and causes included iatrogenic (two), congenital (two), caval thrombosis (two), amyloid disease (two), blunt trauma (one) and metastatic carcinoid tumor (one). In these ten cases, video-assisted thoracic surgery was used as the principal mode of therapy. In eight patients, talc pleurodesis alone was used to resolve the chylothorax. One patient had the use of talc pleurodesis in association with clipping of the thoracic duct and application of fibrin glue. The final patient required clipping of a pleural defect with application of fibrin glue. In two patients, video-assisted operation was used in conjunction with pleuroperitoneal shunting. In all cases the effusion resolved after treatment by the video-assisted thoracic operations described and no subsequent surgical intervention was necessary. The authors concluded that video-assisted thoracic surgery offered an effective means of treating chylothorax regardless of its cause, since access could be gained to the thoracic duct and the pleural space without performing a major thoracotomy.

Lang-Lazdunski and associates encountered one patient who had a post-traumatic chylothorax in their experience.[10] They approached the chylothorax with a more direct procedure. Once the injury to the thoracic duct was recognized, a small thoracotomy (5 cm long) was performed and the open end of the thoracic duct was clipped. No pleurodesis was performed.

Complete discussions of chylothorax and the anatomy of the thoracic duct are available. Several different successful surgical techniques besides thoracoscopy have been described. These should be consulted for a more through discussion of the thoracic duct anatomy and the problems of its repair.

MANAGEMENT OF RETAINED FOREIGN BODIES

The most extensive experience reported using VATS to remove symptomatic foreign bodies within the chest is from France.[10] Lang-Lazdunski and colleagues treated four patients in their collected series.[10] One patient had painful metal shrapnel imbedded in the lingula of the left lung which was removed by VATS resection. One patient had a Kirschner wire removed from the right pleural space after it migrated from a scapular repair. Two patients had bullets removed from the chest using VATS. These authors cautioned, however, that assessment of possible cardiac and great vessel injuries could be dangerous since catastrophic hemorrhage or serious arrhythmias could ensue.[10] In one of their patients who had a bullet removed, lethal cardiac arrhythmias claimed the patient's life approximately 36 hours after the projectile had been removed successfully. In another paper, Bartek and colleagues removed glass fragments from a chest using VATS. Had the fragments not been removed thoracoscopically, the patient would have required a thoracotomy for their removal.

EVALUATION OF HEART, PERICARDIUM AND GREAT VESSELS

VATS procedures should not be used to treat injuries to the heart, great vessels and pericardium; only open techniques should be used.[10] Life-threatening hemorrhage is a possibility and VATS techniques are usually inadequate for controlling such hemorrhage and would prove inadequate to achieve successful repair.

Some authors have proposed using VATS for exploring the heart, great vessels and pericardium when a negative evaluation is anticipated (i.e. the chance of finding injury, although its presence has been entertained, is low). Hermansson and his colleagues reported their success in diagnosing pleuropericardial rupture secondary to blunt trauma using VATS. Fortunately, no injury to the heart had occurred. Exploration of the pleural and pericardial spaces using laparoscopic techniques has been described, but it is potentially dangerous on two counts. The patient may suffer tension pneumothorax or tension pneumopericardium with disastrous cardiovascular results. Serious, uncontrollable hemorrhage could ensue secondary to dislodging clot over a major injury. Hence, such approaches are mentioned only to discourage their use.

MANAGEMENT OF PERSISTENT AIR LEAK

Lang-Lazdunski and associates treated five patients for persistent pneumothorax and air leaks in their series of 42 trauma patients treated by VATS.[10] VATS was particularly effective in treating direct lung injuries and in assuring that chest tubes were placed properly. In the five patients the mean period of persistent air leak was 11 days. In one patient with an air leak persisting for 7 days despite tube thoracostomy, CT scan revealed a large rib fragment lacerating the underlying pulmonary parenchyma. The fragment was removed by VATS, the remaining hematoma was evacuated and the lung fully re-expanded. The second and third patients required positive pressure ventilation for multiple trauma. A pneumothorax developed in both patients and persisted despite tube thoracostomies. One patient had ruptured apical blebs which were successfully stapled. The other had a pulmonary contusion and a poorly compliant lung. Both patients had successful VATS pleural abrasions. A fourth patient suffered a large left-sided hemopneumothorax secondary to a stab wound. Tube thoracostomies evacuated the hemothorax but the air leak persisted. VATS was employed and a large pulmonary laceration was identified. VATS stapling techniques were used to control the air leak successfully. The last patient, with a thoracic stab wound, had a persistent pneumothorax despite tube thoracostomy. A VATS procedure was undertaken and demonstrated an extrapleural tube and a small pulmonary parenchymal laceration. Two properly placed tubes were secured in the pleural space using VATS guidance and visualization.

TECHNICAL ASPECTS: ANESTHETIC CONSIDERATIONS

Careful preparation for appropriate anesthesia is mandatory for VATS procedures in treating trauma patients (Table 7.3). Since conditions may arise which dictate a full exploration of the chest, the patient should be prepared for a full thoracotomy. The patient should be prepared and draped widely in case a major incision has to be made. The patient should have a double-lumen endotracheal tube in place. Proper monitoring, including ECG, arterial line and Foley catheter, is necessary in anticipation of a possible major thoracic exploration.

Intravenous access is important since hemorrhage can be substantial.

Although arterial blood gases are frequently

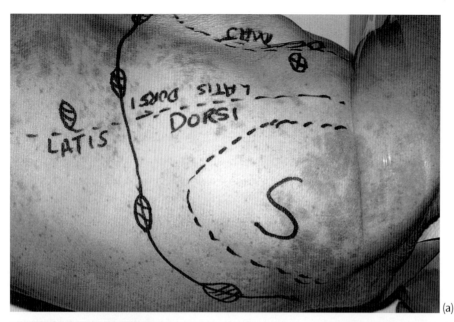

(a)

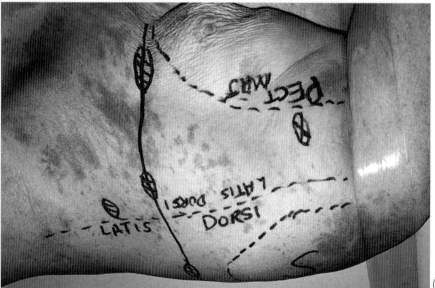

(b)

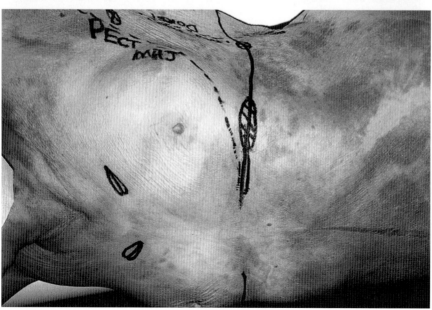

(c)

Figure 7.2 The anticipated left thoracotomy incision relative to the port sites is shown. (a) The posterior aspect is shown with the three potential port sites noted along the longitudinal line describing the thoracotomy. The scapula (S) is outlined with a dotted line. Note that the port sites are placed so as to avoid the anterior border of the latissimus dorsi muscle. (b) This shows the more anterior left aspect of a cadaver used in a teaching session where the port sites are marked as ovals on the chest wall. Note that three of the potential port sites are anterior to the anterior border of the latissimus dorsi muscle. The viewing port is in the middle of the proposed thoracotomy incision. The anterior site is below the left breast and is in the inframammary crease. Note that the port sites avoid the pectoralis major muscle and the latissimus dorsi muscle so that no chest wall hemorrhage is encountered during port placement. (c) This shows the left anterior aspect of the chest wall with the largest and potential utility incision in the crease below the breast. It may be noted also that other anterior port sites which avoid the pectoralis major muscle and the breast as much as possible have been drawn on the anterior chest wall.

Table 7.3 *Anesthetic considerations*

Prepare for full thoracotomy
Double lumen endotracheal tube
Monitoring
   Electrocardiogram
   Arterial line
      Arterial trace
      Blood gases
   Urine output – Foley catheter
Intravenous access
   Large bore lines for blood replacement
   Central line access (introducer)
      Blood replacement
      Placement of Swan–Ganz catheter if it becomes
      necessary
   Lines for medications
      Cardiotropic drugs
      Vasoactive agents
      Antibiotics
Oximeter

Table 7.4 *Surgical considerations*

Placement of patient
   Appropriate thoracotomy position
   Appliances on table to stabilize the patient
      Supports
      Bean bag
      Straps and tapes
Wide preparation
   Prepare for full thoracotomy
   Drape widely
Transfusion requirements
   At least type and screen
   Blood usually should be available
   Universal donor blood
Electrocautery
   At least one, preferably two available
   Bipolar also helpful
Suction
   Best to have two available
   Types available
      Standard Yankauer
      Poole (sump)
      Endoscopy suction
Integrate port sites into thoracotomy incision
   Use existing chest tube sites
   Establish new sites after exploration

monitored, it may be helpful to have an oximeter in place. This allows for a comparison between the oximeter and the actual measured arterial blood gases. Since prolonged ventilation is a possibility, the use of the oximeter and its correlation with the arterial blood gases is most helpful in the prolonged recovery period and in weaning the patient from the respirator.

TECHNICAL ASPECTS: SURGICAL CONSIDERATIONS

The patient must be placed on the operating table so that a full thoracotomy may be performed if it becomes necessary. Appliances which should be placed on the table to stabilize the patient include supports, a bean bag, straps and tapes. The patient is fully secured to the table such that the table may be fully rotated as needed if a thoracotomy becomes necessary (Table 7.4). Preparation of the patient and draping should be wide to prepare for a full thoracotomy and/or any necessary incision to correct any major hemorrhage in the lungs, heart, or in the great vessels.

Transfusion requirements may be substantial if a particularly serious injury to the heart or major vessels is encountered. The patient should at least be typed and screened for blood transfusion. Blood usually should be available since major hemorrhage can ensue. If hemorrhage occurs without proper preparation, universal donor blood may be necessary for immediate transfusion to save the patient's life.

Several other pieces of equipment are necessary in the preparation of a VATS procedure. At least one, preferably two, electrocautery units should be available.

A bipolar unit may also be very helpful in cauterizing intrathoracic bleeders. Suction must also be available since evacuation of large amounts of blood and clot from the chest may be necessary. It is often best to have two suction units available since the hemorrhage can be relatively large. Several different types of suction tips should be available: the standard Yankauer, the Poole (sump), and the endoscopic suction tip.

Every effort should be made to integrate the port sites into the possible thoracotomy incision. One should use the existing chest tube sites, if possible (Fig 7.2). New tube port sites should be used as required by the thoracic exploration. Figure 7.2 shows the placement of these sites relative to the possible thoracotomy incision and final chest tube placement.

REFERENCES

1. Graeber GM, Jones DR. The role of thoracoscopy in thoracic trauma. *Ann Thorac Surg* 1993; **56**: 646–8.
2. Graeber GM. Thoracic trauma. In: Daniels TA, Kizer U (eds). *Thoracoscopic Surgery*. Boston, MA: Little, Brown, 1993; 221–33.
3. Jones JW, Kitahama A, Webb WR, McSwain N. Emergency thoracoscopy: a logical approach to chest trauma management. *J Trauma* 1981; **21**: 280–4.
4. Senno A, Moallem S, Quijano ER, Adeyemo A, Clauss RH. Thoracoscopy with the fiberoptic bronchoscope. A

simple method in diagnosing pleurpulmonary disease. *J Thorac Cardiovasc Surg* 1974; **67:** 606–11.

5. Senno A, Moallem S, Quijano ER, Tan BY, Clauss RH. Fiberoptic thoracoscopy. *N Y State J Med* 1975; **75:** 51–6.

6. Smith RS, Fry WR, Tsoi EKM, *et al.* Preliminary report on videothoracoscopy in the evaluation and treatment of thoracic injury. *Am J Surg* 1993; **166:** 690–4.

7. Coselli JS, Mattox KL, Beall AC. Reevaluation of early evacuation of clotted hemothorax. *Am J Surg* 1984; **148:** 786–90.

8. Mancini M, Smith LM, Nein A, Buechter KJ. Early evacuation of clotted blood in hemothorax using thoracoscopy: case reports. *J Trauma* 1993; **34:** 144–7.

9. Heniford BT, Carrillo EH, Spain DA, *et al.* The role of thoracoscopy in the management of retained thoracic collections after trauma. *Ann Thorac Surg* 1997; **63:** 940–3.

10. Lang-Lazdunski L, Mouroux J, Pons F, *et al.* Role of videothoracoscopy in chest trauma. *Ann Thorac Surg* 1997; **63:** 327–33.

11. Fallon WF Jr. Post-traumatic empyema. *J Am Coll Surg* 1994; **179:** 483–92.

12. Aram KV, Grover FL, Richardson JD, Trinkle JK. Post-traumatic empyema. *Ann Thorac Surg* 1977; **23:** 254–8.

13. Block EFJ, Kinton OC, Windsor J, Vestner M. Guided percutaneous drainage for post-traumatic empyema thoracis. *Surgery* 1995; **117:** 282–7.

14. Eddy AC, Luna GK, Copass M. Empyema thoracis in patients undergoing emergent closed tube thoracostomy for thoracic trauma. *Am J Surg* 1989; **157:** 494–7.

15. Helling TS, Gyles NR, Eisenstein CH, Soracco CA. Complications following blunt and penetrating injuries in 216 victims of chest trauma requiring tube thoracostomy. *J Trauma* 1989; **29:** 1367–70.

16. Landreneau RJ, Keenan RJ, Hazelrigg SR, *et al.* Thoracoscopy for empyema and hemothorax. *Chest* 1995; **109:** 18–24.

17. O'Brien J, Cohen M, Solit R, *et al.* Thoracoscopic drainage and decortication as definitive treatment for empyema thoracis following penetrating chest injury. *J Trauma* 1994; **36:** 536–40.

18. Madden MR, Paul DE, Finkelstein JL, *et al.* Occult diaphragmatic injury from stab wounds to the lower chest and abdomen. *J Trauma* 1989; **29:** 292–8.

19. Feliciano DV, Cruse PA, Mattox KL, *et al.* Delayed diagnosis of injuries to the diaphragm after penetrating wounds. *J Trauma* 1989; **28:** 1135–44.

20. Chen JC, Wilson SE, Diaphragmatic injuries: recognition and management in sixty-two patients. *Ann Surg* 1991; **57:** 810–15.

21. Ivatury RR, Sunign RJ, Weksler B, *et al.* Laparoscopy in the evaluation of the intrathoracic abdomen after penetrating injury. *J Trauma* 1992; **33:** 101–9.

22. Smith RS, Fry WR, Tsoi EKM, *et al.* Preliminary report on videothoracoscopy in the evaluation and treatment of thoracic injury. *Am J Surg* 1993; **166:** 690–5.

23. Kern JA, Tribble CG, Spotnitz WD, *et al.* Thoracoscopy in the subacute management of patients with thoracoabdominal trauma. *Chest* 1993; **104:** 942–5.

24. Uribe RA, Pachon CE, Frame SB, *et al.* A prospective evaluation of thoracoscopy for the diagnosis of penetrating thoracoabdominal trauma. *J Trauma* 1994; **37:** 650–4.

25. Nel JM, Warren BL. Thoracoscopic evaluation of the diaphragm in patients with knife wounds of the left lower chest. *Br J Surg* 1994; **81:** 713–14.

26. Spann JC, Nwariaku FE, Wait M. Evaluation of video-assisted thoracoscopic surgery in the diagnosis of diaphragmatic injuries. *Am J Surg* 1995; **170:** 620–30.

27. Graham DD, McGahren ED, Tribble CG, Daniel TM, Rodgers BM. Use of video-assisted thoracic surgery in the treatment of chylothorax. *Ann Thorac Surg* 1994; **57:** 1507–11.

8

Thoracic drainage

JOHN A ODELL

The insertion of a chest drain is the most frequently performed procedure in chest trauma: it is the only procedure required in the management of most chest injuries (Fig 8.1). Because of its relatively benign risk and frequent need, the procedure is often delegated to junior staff members. There is also a tendency to insert a chest drain prior to the initial chest radiograph. Whilst undertaking chest drainage blindly is usually safe in populations in developed countries where the pleural space is free, in patients where the pleural space is obliterated insertion of the drain may cause considerable morbidity and occasionally mortality.

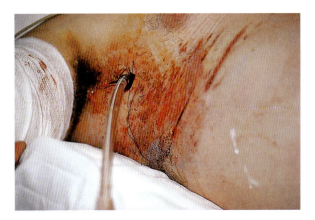

Figure 8.1 *Patient with direct blunt injury to the right hemithorax. A plain chest radiograph (not included) showed a right hemothorax and apparently raised right hemidiaphragm. Diaphragmatic rupture was suspected so the chest drain was inserted at the base of the axilla in the mid-axillary line in order to avoid injury to the prolapsed liver. There is no contraindication to inserting a drain directly through an injured area of chest wall.*

Indications for chest drainage

Pneumothorax

- Tension pneumothorax
- Large pneumothorax
- Bilateral pneumothorax. Larger side first then reassess
- Respiratory distress even if pneumothorax small

Fluid collections

- Hemothorax: where continued blood loss needs to be measured and may be an indication for thoracotomy; when large; when associated with shock
- Chylothorax
- Empyema
- Effusion

As part of the procedure of thoracotomy

PNEUMOTHORAX

The most common blunt injury to the chest is fracture of one or more ribs. Fractured and dislocated rib ends may tear the parietal pleura and lacerate the lung, resulting in alveolar air leak and pneumothorax. Other causes of pneumothorax after blunt trauma include:

- compressive tear of the lung parenchyma;
- rupture of a pre-existing bulla;
- rupture of a pneumatocele following barotrauma or mechanical ventilation; and
- leakage of air from the peritoneal cavity in a patient with a ruptured diaphragm and viscus injury.

In penetrating trauma, a pneumothorax may result from direct underlying lung damage or from ingress of air through the open wound (a sucking pneumothorax).

The size of the pneumothorax and the rate at which it develops is dependent on the rate of air leakage into the pleural cavity and whether a flap-like valve exists at the site of the leak.

Tension pneumothorax

> **Tension pneumothorax**
> - Dyspnea, cyanosis
> - Tachycardia, hypotension
> - Tracheal displacement
> - Hyper-resonance
> - Diminished air entry

A pneumothorax in the vast majority of patients is well tolerated but if a flap-like valve exists, a tension pneumothorax can rapidly develop. In this situation the patient may display tachycardia, hypotension, dyspnea and even cyanosis. The trachea will be displaced, air entry will be markedly diminished on the affected side which will also be hyper-resonant. Fortunately, a tension pneumothorax is relatively uncommon and rarely is seen to develop except during the use of positive pressure ventilation during resuscitative or anesthetic maneuvers.

A tension pneumothorax is a life-threatening condition and any delay can be fatal. If the clinical findings are present and rapid radiographic facilities are not available, then under these circumstances intrapleural drainage should be instituted immediately. It is wise under these circumstances to insert first a large bore needle – air will rapidly egress, confirming the diagnosis and the patient should rapidly improve. An intercostal drain can then be inserted. Occasionally, the clinical diagnosis of tension pneumothorax may be made at the roadside without any medical equipment being available and in these circumstances ingenious techniques of chest drainage may need to be practiced – for example, a hollow pen may be inserted into the

pleural space. The sucking pneumothorax may be more easily tolerated than a tension pneumothorax. To prevent air entering the chest, a condom with the teat cut off, or a cut-off glove finger may be attached to the hollow pen to function like a flutter valve. If rapid radiographic facilities are available, the diagnosis of tension pneumothorax should preferably be confirmed radiographically before intercostal drainage.

Standard pneumothorax

In the vast majority of patients, the size of the pneumothorax does not increase from its initial extent while being observed and to some extent this fact influences further management. Radiological diagnosis of a pneumothorax in the injured patient may be difficult, either because of coexisting surgical emphysema or the inability because of other injuries to take an erect chest radiograph. Intrapleural air can collect in the anterior hemithorax (the highest point in the supine position) without a rim of air being visible around the lung.[1] In these circumstances, one can be reasonably confident, if doubt exists, that the pneumothorax is probably not large and, if the patient is not distressed, an expectant attitude, as will be explained further, is practiced. It may be wise to obtain another opinion about the interpretation of the chest radiograph if doubt exists.

MANAGEMENT OF THE PNEUMOTHORAX

> **The first decision**
> Is a chest drain necessary?

Not every pneumothorax requires the insertion of an intercostal chest drain. In the vast majority of patients, the size of the pneumothorax does not increase from its initial extent while being observed and to some extent this influences further management. The first decision that needs to be made, therefore, is whether a chest drain is, in fact, necessary. A tension pneumothorax is a life-threatening situation and management has already been discussed. A patient who has a large pneumothorax obviously needs chest intubation, but how do we define large? A large pneumothorax is any pneumothorax greater than 2 cm as measured between the visceral and parietal pleura. Smaller pneumothoraces can be observed as discussed further; but, in the patient with limited respiratory reserve, a pneumothorax smaller than 2 cm may cause distress and should be intubated. A patient with a bilateral pneumothorax should have the larger side intubated no matter how small the pneumothoraces are – any increase in either side can be life-threatening. The patient should then be observed and the other side treated on its merits.

The patient with a small pneumothorax whom we have elected to observe should have a repeat chest radiograph immediately if symptoms develop and the chest intubated if the pneumothorax has enlarged; if his/her symptoms have not changed the chest radiograph should be repeated in 6 and 24 hours to document any change.[2] If the pneumothorax has not changed within this time period it is safe, in the vast majority of cases, to discharge the patient with a follow-up appointment in 1 week's time when the chest radiograph is repeated. It should be made clear to the patient that he/she should return immediately if he/she becomes dyspneic.

MANAGEMENT OF CONTINUED AIR LEAK

An important and continuous leakage of air, particularly if the lung remains collapsed, may indicate a major rupture of the trachea or of a bronchus, necessitating tracheobronchial endoscopy. If air leakage persists, bronchoscopy for bronchial toilet should be performed if there is any suspicion of lobar collapse. Occasionally the expansion of a collapsed lobe, even if not responsible for the air leak, may cause the air leak to diminish. Occasionally two chest drains may need to be inserted to 'beat the fistula'. High volume, low pressure suction drainage may also be used.

We are uncertain whether suction, in fact, keeps the 'fistula' open or whether air leakage diminishes quicker without suction being applied to the drain. A recent randomized study suggests that suction compared to water-seal drainage alone significantly decreased both chest tube duration and the time taken for chest tube removal.[3] If air leakage persists after 5 days it is our practice to institute suction if it has not been tried before or to stop it if it has been used. Often this simple change of management seems to result in the air leak decreasing within a short period of time.

If, despite these measures, air leakage remains vigorous, then surgical closure of the leak should be considered. In our practice we generally wait 7–10 days before considering this option. As the usual hospital stay after thoracotomy is 4–5 days, it may be preferable if air leakage is diminishing to persist with a conservative attitude. It is possible that, with increasing enthusiasm and experience with thoracoscopic surgery, these guidelines may change and that thoracoscopic closure of the leak and/or pleurectomy may be instituted earlier. Air leakage is more likely in patients with underlying lung disease and if this type of patient has sustained chest trauma earlier intervention to close an air leak may be necessary.[4]

In ventilated patients, a significant amount of tidal volume can escape through the chest tube (calculated by subtracting the expired minute volume from the inspired minute volume). Management of the air leak in these patients is to prevent or slow the flow of the tidal volume through the fistula tract. Suction should be stopped or decreased if possible. Spontaneous breathing also decreases the tract flow. Avoidance of techniques such as positive end-expiratory pressure, large tidal volumes, high airway pressures and reversed inspiratory:expiratory ratio ventilation may be of assistance. Other more elaborate measures may include high frequency ventilation, mechanical synchronized occlusion of the chest tube during inspiration, or the insertion of a double lumen tube and separate lung ventilation.

If air leakage increases out of proportion to that expected or surgical emphysema develops after the insertion of chest drains, then careful consideration of the possibility of having iatrogenically intubated the lung at the procedure of chest drainage should be considered.

FLUID COLLECTIONS

Interpretation of the chest radiograph

The chest radiograph taken after chest trauma should ideally be taken in the erect position. If taken in the supine position and the pleural space is free, fluid is distributed throughout the pleural cavity; a slight cloudiness may signify an accumulation of several hundred milliliters of fluid; if associated with a pneumothorax the sandwich of air, lung and fluid may even approximate the density of the unaffected opposite side, lulling the inexperienced into a false sense of security. An erect chest radiograph may in these circumstances show a typical fluid level of a hydro-pneumothorax.

'Pleural' opacity after trauma

Early
- Hemothorax
- Rupture of the hemidiaphragm
- Atelectasis
- Extrapleural hematoma

Late (48 hours)
- Chylothorax
- Clotted hemothorax
- Pleural effusion
- Empyema

Occasionally the erect chest radiograph may appear relatively normal because the fluid may be hidden in the recesses of the hemidiaphragm or may be subpulmonic. The only clue in these circumstances may be blunting of the costophrenic angle or a raised hemidiaphragm. The radiographic appearance of a subpulmonic collection typically has its highest point more medial than normal. To differentiate a subpulmonic collection from a normal hemidiaphagm, a ruptured hemidiaphragm or atelectasis, a lateral decubitus chest radiograph should be taken. If fluid is present this will shift to the most dependent point. Others have used computed tomography (CT) scanning but this is expensive and not always readily available.[1,5]

The chest radiographic may show complete opacification of the hemithorax (so-called 'white out'). In these circumstances it is important to observe the position of the mediastinum before proceeding immediately to drainage as the differential diagnosis includes complete collapse of the lung for which intercostal drainage would be inappropriate. Other causes of opacification include, in addition to fluid collections such as hemothorax, rupture of the hemidiaphragm, atelectasis or extrapleural hematoma. If the radiographic appearance is the result of a hemothorax, then there will be marked distress and shift of the mediastinum to the opposite side. In these circumstances it is important to insert an intercostal drain rapidly to relieve the 'tension effect'.

HEMOTHORAX

A hemothorax is the most common complication of thoracic injury, whether blunt or penetrating. It may after blunt trauma be the result of rib fractures, vertebral fractures or laceration of the lung. Occasionally its occurrence may be delayed a few days after injury.[6,7] If the hemorrhage is large and acute, hypovolemic shock requiring rapid fluid replacement may be present; the hemothorax may additionally compress lung, causing atelectasis.

The first decision
Is a chest drain necessary?

Chest drainage in the management of hemothorax

Every patient with a suspected hemothorax should be observed in hospital for at least 24 hours.

Resuscitative treatment by volume replacement occurs simultaneously with local treatment of the hemothorax. Significant blood loss may require rapid transfusion and, if continuing, thoracotomy to control bleeding. If this situation can be anticipated by the patient's clinical condition, then efforts to conserve the blood lost within the chest for autotransfusion should be pursued as often blood banks may not be able to supply sufficient blood rapidly. In some publications it is stated that the presence of a massive hemothorax is a contraindication to chest tube insertion, arguing that the accumulated blood in the pleural space may tamponade the source of bleeding.[8,9] They state that the operating room is more appropriate to manage the patient by open thoracotomy. We disagree for three reasons:

1. There appears to be no scientific basis for such a statement which appears to be based on folklore repeated in the literature.
2. In our large experience we have never seen such a situation.
3. By the nature of the injury the patient needs to be relieved urgently of mediastinal shift and pulmonary compression – the insertion of a chest drain is far more expeditious than transport to an operating room and, in fact, the patient may not ever require a thoracotomy.

Every patient with a suspected hemothorax should be observed in hospital for at least 24 hours. Not every hemothorax requires the insertion of an intercostal chest drain. A significant hemothorax is one which is causing distress to the patient, is larger than 2 cm alongside the parietal pleura as shown on an erect or lateral decubitus chest radiograph, or occupies at least one-third of the expected thoracic cavity. Smaller hemothoraces may be observed if the patient is not distressed. If the patient has multiple injuries, it is wise to insert an intercostal drain, even if small, if only to exclude bleeding from the chest as a cause for any change in the patient's condition. Others practice a policy of 'aggressive resuscitation', arguing that the morbidity of an intercostal chest drain in all patients with suspected hemothorax is justified by the advantages of ensuring rapid emptying of the pleural space of accumulated blood. Clearly this has advantages in communities where the pleural space is likely to be free, but where tuberculosis and trauma are common, the pleural space is likely to be adherent and the potential pleural space nonexistent. To insert intercostal drains in these circumstances can be dangerous. Our policy in South Africa was to treat every patient on his/her merits – small hemothoraces are observed and intervention only undertaken if necessary.

The patient in whom a conservative approach is pursued should be carefully observed with chest radiographs repeated at 6 and 12 hours. If there is any increase in the size of the pleural opacity, then an intercostal drain is inserted. If no change has occurred after 12 hours it is usually safe to discharge the patient with a proviso to return if he/she develops any symptoms.[6,10]

At follow-up in one week the chest radiograph is repeated. In the vast majority the pleural opacity will have decreased or disappeared. In only a small proportion of patients will symptoms develop or the pleural opacity increase, requiring intervention.[6,7] In some groups delayed drainage is more likely – those with a combined hemo- and pneumothorax and those with multiple stab wounds.[6]

In those patients in whom intercostal drainage has been deemed necessary, this should be done at the appropriate site as determined by chest radiographs and the aspiration of blood beforehand. Frequently, a large quantity of blood may initially drain through the chest drain but this may have accumulated within the chest cavity over time and is not necessarily an indication for thoracotomy (Fig 8.2). In the vast majority of cases, where the bleeding is from the low pressure pulmonary circulation, bleeding soon ceases and the chest drain can be withdrawn within a day or two.

Frequent radiographs and observation of the patient are necessary even if the amount of chest drainage

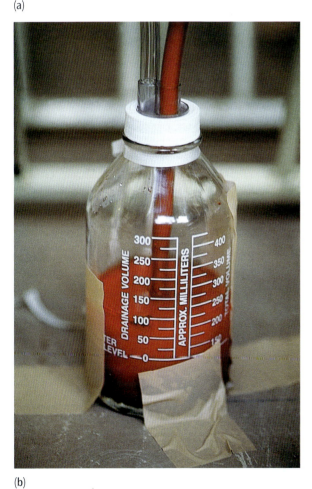

(a)

(b)

Figure 8.2 *(a) Young female patient with a right parasternal stab wound which probably transected the right thoracic artery, causing a substantial hemothorax. Suction on the intercostal drain (–20 cmH$_2$O) produced 800 ml of blood after which drainage stopped. (b) The hemothorax on the chest radiograph was cleared and thoracotomy avoided. (SWTC.)*

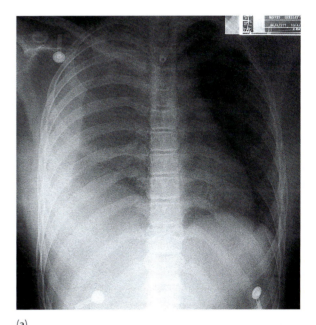

(a)

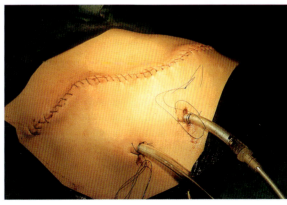

(b)

Figure 8.3 *(a) Clotted right hemothorax after a stab wound to the right chest. A percutaneous intercostal drain did not evacuate the hemothorax so right thoracotomy was performed and apical and basal drains (b) inserted. (SWTC.)*

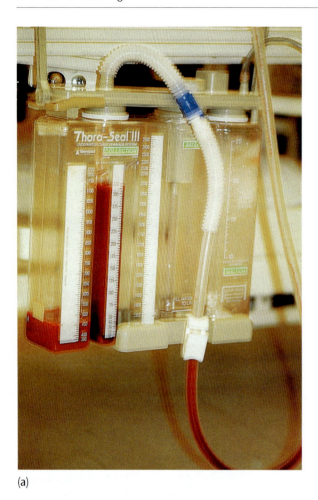

(a)

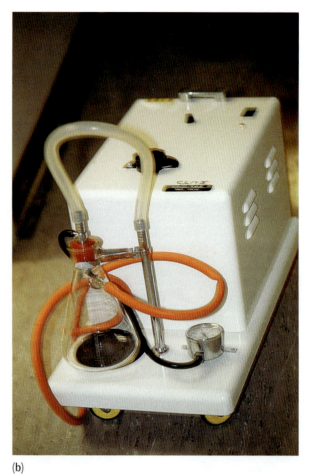

(b)

Figure 8.4 *(a) Multichamber underwater seal drainage system used routinely in cardiac surgery to measure blood loss. A detachable container is used for autotransfusion. (b) Tubbs Barratt high pressure negative suction pump used to evacuate the hemopneumothorax. This pump copes with high volume air leaks whereas the low volume Roberts pump proves obstructive. (SWTC.)*

diminishes. Blood clot may obstruct the chest drainage system and lead to an erroneous impression that bleeding is slowing when, in fact, it may be continuing. A good rule of thumb is to aim for a relatively normal chest radiograph within 48 hours. If not achieved, a different tack in management, for example evacuation of a clotted hemothorax (Fig 8.3),[11] bronchoscopy for atelectatic lung, investigation for concomitant diaphragmatic injury, should be considered.

Before thoracotomy is considered, two basic conditions need to coexist: that is *continuous* and *massive* bleeding. High volume negative pressure (-20 cmH$_2$O) suction should be used to assist complete evacuation of blood, which in certain circumstances may be returned to the patient by autotransfusion (Fig 8.4). No binding rules exist and recommendations vary. A continuous bleed of, say, 50 ml/h even for 12–24 hours is not an indication for thoracotomy as this volume can be easily replaced and the bleeding invariably stops. Drainage of 1000 ml within the first hour after intercostal drainage is an indication for thoracotomy if the injury took place a half hour beforehand but if there was delay in seeing the patient after the injury (say 4 hours), this is not an indication for thoracotomy as blood drained may have collected in the intervening period. If blood loss is greater than 200 ml/h after 3 hours, then thoracotomy is invariably necessary. Bleeding is invariably from a systemic vessel such as an intercostal artery or internal thoracic artery.

LATE MANAGEMENT OF HEMOTHORAX

> When seen late after injury and a pleural opacity exists, concern regarding active bleeding no longer exists.

Occasionally the patient may be seen some time after the injury with a pleural opacity. The patient is usually stable and the concern regarding active bleeding no longer exists.

Management should be aspiration at the appropriate site to determine the nature of the fluid. If the fluid aspirated is serous and bloodstained, then the chest should be aspirated to dryness – there is no need to insert an intercostal drain. If pus or chylothorax are found, then the chest is drained. If only a small quantity of thick/clotted blood can be aspirated, further management will depend upon the condition of the patient, the quantity of blood within the chest cavity and the length of time since the injury. The patient who is apyrexial with a small amount of blood can be observed; the patient with a larger amount of blood, or who is pyrexial, should have the clotted hemothorax evacuated formally through either a small thoracotomy (if the injury occurred more than 10 days earlier then decortication is likely) or by thoracoscopy.[12] Occasionally the chest radiograph after chest trauma may appear quite disorganized with multiple opacities and fluid levels – the so-called disorganized pleural space. In these patients there is no point in attempting multiple drainage procedures – one should proceed directly to thoracotomy.

CHYLOTHORAX

Classically, chylothorax appears late, 2–10 days after injury. The fluid aspirated may be milky-white, suggestive of the diagnosis. Patients with chylothorax who are not being fed enterally have a relatively clear fluid collection. Fluid should be sent for fat and chylomicron analysis to confirm the diagnosis.

Most cases of chylothorax are caused by intraoperative damage to the thoracic duct. In blunt trauma the thoracic duct may be injured because of hyperextension of the back, by a fall from a height, or in association with severe thoracic spinal compression. In 20% of closed injuries of the thoracic duct, spinal fractures or fractures of the posterior ribs exist.[13] Isolated thoracic duct injuries due to penetrating wounds are rare, probably because of its anatomical position, closely applied to major structures. Injury to these major structures are likely to be dominant or fatal, masking the thoracic duct injury.

The chylothorax usually develops on either the left or the right side or on both sides of the chest if the injury occurs in the area where the thoracic duct crosses from the right to the left side (fourth thoracic vertebra) or if a mediastinal chyloma breaks through on both sides.

Chest drainage in the management of chylothorax

> Any sudden decrease in the volume of drainage should be regarded with suspicion as chyle notoriously blocks intercostal drains.

The chest should be drained with a large diameter intercostal drain. Any sudden decrease in the volume of drainage should be regarded with suspicion as chyle notoriously blocks intercostal drains. Vigilance and repeated chest radiographs are necessary to recognize and avoid this complication.

The volume of chyle production should be decreased by intravenous hyperalimentation, or by using an elemental diet if the enteral route for nutrition is used. The nutritional state of the patient should be carefully observed as these patients very rapidly become fluid and nutritionally depleted.

The conservative management of chylothorax as described results in closure of the duct in approximately 50% of patients within 1 week. In those in whom the chyle drainage continues, operative ligation of the duct should be considered before one loses too much ground nutritionally. There is not much point in persisting with conservative management after this period. Most ligate the duct above the diaphragm using a low right-sided thoracotomy. Preoperative feeding with cream or the injection of dye into the wall of the distal esophagus or into the stomach may help to identify the duct. Recently, in patients with left-sided chylothoraces, we have found the leak to be invariably in Poirier's triangle (the triangle formed by the subclavian artery anteriorly, the thoracic vertebra posteriorly and the thoracic inlet superiorly) where the position of the duct is constant and where it can easily be ligated using a small thoracotomy or using thoracoscopic techniques.

After surgical ligation of the thoracic duct, chyle drainage diminishes rapidly. The lymphatic collaterals are extensive and ligation of the duct is well tolerated.

PLEURAL EFFUSION

> **Pleural effusion and chest trauma**
> * Infection – lung, mediastinum
> * Cardiac – chronic tamponade; myocardial contusion; myocardial infarction
> * Hypoalbuminemia

Pleural effusions should not normally develop after chest trauma. If an effusion is found, then one should consider: an effusion associated with infection within the lung or mediastinum (pneumonia or ruptured esophagus); an effusion associated with cardiac pathology (chronic tamponade, myocardial contusion or myocardial infarct secondary to traumatic coronary artery damage); or an effusion associated with hypoalbuminemia.

Management is aspiration to dryness if it is causing respiratory distress and, more importantly, investigation and management of the underlying cause.

EMPYEMA

The development of an empyema after blunt chest trauma is not uncommon. The common associations are listed. It appears that prophylactic antibiotics lessens the risk of the development of empyema, but this is controversial. The frequent finding of resistant organisms suggests that the infection is often hospital acquired. The empyema may be associated with pneumonia which has been acquired either because of bronchial aspiration at the time of injury or the inability to cough adequately because of poor pain relief.

Empyema after trauma: common associations
- Hemopneumothorax
- Delay in evacuating a clotted hemothorax
- Concomitant diaphragmatic or subdiaphragmatic injury
- Chest drains left in too long
- Injudicious attempts at chest drainage

The pus of an empyema typically collects posteriorly in about 90% of cases. Radiographically this will demonstrate on the lateral chest radiograph a typical posterior 'D' with the straight part of the 'D' formed by the vertebral body. The caudal extent of the 'D' is almost always the hemidiaphragm. Occasionally one may suspect a pleural empyema but be unable to localize it on the chest radiograph. In this instance CT scanning may be necessary to locate or exclude the possibility of an empyema.

MANAGEMENT OF EMPYEMA FOLLOWING CHEST TRAUMA

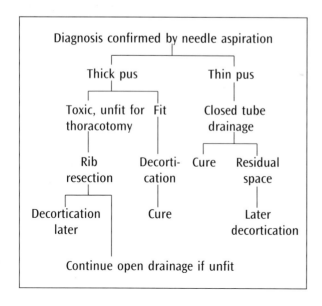

Empyema is a late occurrence after chest trauma and is diagnosed when pus is found at aspiration. If food particles, oral fluids or saliva are aspirated the possibility of esophageal or gastric disruption should be considered. Further management of the empyema depends on the consistency of the pus which can be either thin or thick. If the pus is thin, a large bore intercostal drain is inserted at the most dependent site. Hopefully the underlying lung will rapidly expand and the pleural space will be obliterated by adherence of the visceral and parietal pleura. If the pus is thick, it is unlikely to drain adequately through an intercostal drain and therefore more adequate drainage is necessary. In the patient who is toxic and ill the smallest procedure to achieve this aim, rib resection, is performed, whereas in the patient who is fit for major surgery, a formal decortication is performed.

If the patient managed by closed intercostal drainage fails to improve as measured by fever or persistent pleural opacification, then either rib resection or decortication is planned, depending on the state of the patient.

If the status of the patient managed by rib resection improves, he should be considered for decortication if the empyema space is large. If the empyema space is small, it may be worthwhile waiting for the space to obliterate. If the patient remains unfit, there is no option but to continue with open drainage through the rib resection site. Eventually the space will obliterate and the open drain can be removed; in adults if the underlying lung is normal this may take up to 3 months or longer; in children it occurs more rapidly, approximately 3 weeks.

Almost all empyemas are managed in this way. One can usually assume after chest trauma that the underlying lung is normal, unlike for example, empyema developing in association with bronchiectasis where pulmonary resection may be necessary. If there is an underlying cause for the empyema such as ruptured esophagus then this should be managed simultaneously with the empyema (see Chapter 18).

TECHNIQUE OF INSERTION

After the site for chest drainage has been cleaned, the skin, subcutaneous tissues, intercostal space and parietal pleura are infiltrated with approximately 20 ml of 1% lidocaine (lignocaine). It is important to wait 5–10 minutes for the local anesthesia to become effective before the chest drain is inserted. The waiting period is often neglected. During infiltration of the local anesthetic the pleural space is entered and suction placed on the syringe to confirm the correctly chosen site. Some have contrary views suggesting that the needle may, in fact, damage the underlying lung, but if

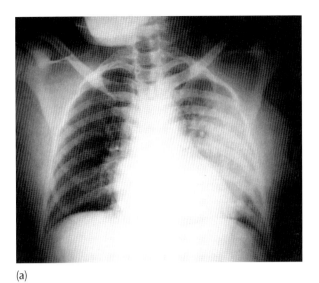

(a)

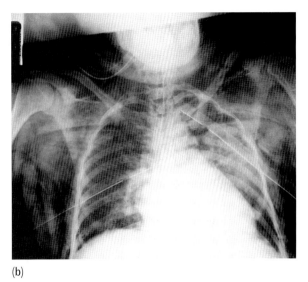

(b)

Figure 8.5 *(a) When a pulmonary opacity after chest trauma does not involve the costophrenic angle, one must be especially careful when considering the insertion of a chest drain. The pleural space is likely to be obliterated from previous pleurisy. The opacity may represent a loculated collection, an intrapulmonary or extrapleural collection. (b) Unfortunately, in this patient a chest drain was inserted into the adherent right lung with the subsequent development of alarming surgical emphysema. Errors were compounded by the insertion of a further chest drain into the left lung (with further subcutaneous emphysema) and the need for ventilation. She was managed by removal of the chest drains and the subcutaneous emphysema slowly resolved.*

there has been correct interpretation of the chest radiograph and the decision made not to drain minor pneumothoraces or fluid collections, then a potential distance of 2–3 cm between the inner surface of the chest wall and the visceral pleura should exist. If perchance the needle enters the lung, the consequences should be minor, because of the small size of the needle and because the chest will be drained in any event.

There are presently two types of drains used. Probably the most common is the plastic drain which may be slid into the chest over a trocar; the other type is a rubber Malecot drain which is stretched over an introducer and then inserted through a metal cannula which is itself inserted with its own trocar.

It is our strong opinion that use of the trocar supplied with the plastic drain should be abandoned as many of the problems associated with chest drainage are associated with its use. The end is extremely sharp (presumably to facilitate penetration of muscle and pleura) and may result in damage to lung, heart, aorta, liver, spleen – in fact, any intrathoracic or intra-abdominal structure. The rigidity imparted to either type of drain, by the trocar for the plastic drain, or the introducer over which the rubber drain is stretched, facilitates injury to these structures because the drain cannot be deflected from a more solid structure.

Probably the best technique is to dissect with sharp or blunt dissection down to the pleural space and then to gently insert the plastic drain without the introducer or with the aid of artery forceps; with the Malecot catheter the trocar and cannulae should be gently

inserted until the ribs are passed (this is easily felt); the trocar is then withdrawn and fluid or air will be seen to escape. Through the open cannula the stretched Malecot drain is gently inserted. Once the drain has passed the end of the cannula, the introducer over which the Malecot drain has been stretched is removed.

A common concern of creating a sucking pneumothorax once one has opened the pleural space, and thus the need to urgently complete the procedure to prevent embarrassing the patient, is probably unjustified. The procedure should be completed in a careful, methodical manner – any air that has entered the pleural space will rapidly drain once the underwater seal is formed.

How does one recognize that the drain has been inappropriately inserted? Most important is when that anticipated to be drained does not drain. The development, after drainage, of massive surgical emphysema invariably means that the lung has been damaged by the drain (Fig 8.5). In these circumstances the pleural space is likely to be obliterated. Management is to remove the offending drain and observe the patient. Surgical emphysema often increases alarmingly, but if the patient is undistressed should not be of concern. Careful interpretation of chest radiographs, often with experts, may be necessary to determine whether an underlying pneumothorax is present and whether it needs to be drained.

If the drain has been inadequately advanced into the pleural space or inadequately fastened to the skin, lateral holes in the drain may lie within the soft tissues or even outside the skin (Figs 8.6 and 8.7). It is essen-

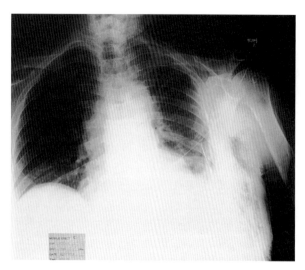

Figure 8.6 *Subcutaneous emphysema in this patient is due to a chest tube drainage hole lying within the subcutaneous tissues. The drain has not been inserted far enough.*

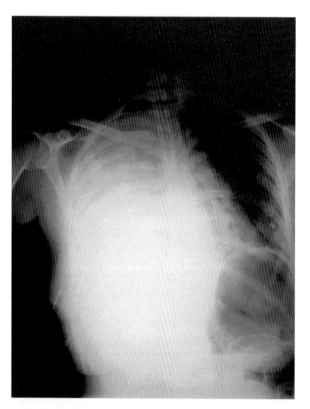

Figure 8.7 *A large traumatic hemothorax causing shift of the mediastinum to the opposite side has not been relieved by the chest drain. The chest radiograph demonstrates that the chest tube is lying within the subcutaneous tissues and has not entered the chest cavity.*

tial after chest intubation to radiographically confirm its correct placement and also to assess the progress of the underlying condition. For example, in severe hemorrhage the drain may be blocked by clot and give the erroneous impression that bleeding has ceased.

COMMON ERRORS IN CHEST INTUBATION

The indications for chest drainage have been previously discussed. Some of the complications seen are more likely when these indications are broadened. For example, the insertion of a chest drain prophylactically in a patient with no pneumothorax or minimal pneumothorax is more likely to result in damage to the underlying lung.

Common errors in chest intubation
- Inserting a drain without a recent chest radiograph
- The wrong interpretation of chest radiographs
- Inserting a drain without obtaining liquid, blood or air freely at needle aspirations prior to drainage
- Drain inappropriately connected, kinks, etc.
- Chest drainage when ventilation or anesthesia is required
- Drains left in for too long a time

Inserting a drain without a recent chest radiograph

A recent chest radiograph should be available and displayed in the room in which the procedure is to be undertaken. It is dangerous to insert a drain on the basis of a radiograph taken a week or a few days earlier. A pneumothorax, hemothorax or pleural effusion that was present previously may have disappeared or even loculated and the need for drainage or the intended site of drainage may have changed.

In some trauma units dealing with the severely injured patient with chest injuries, a spurious sense of urgency is attached to chest intubation and it has become practice to insert chest drains without a chest radiograph. This practice is not recommended as it may expose the patient to unnecessary risk and diminishes the value of subsequent radiographic interpretation because of absent preintubation films (Figs 8.8 and 8.9). The patient is rarely so unwell that he is unfit for a chest radiograph. If proper radiographic facilities are available it takes only a few minutes to position the patient, preferably in the upright position because blood and air can be hidden if taken supine,[14] and to take the radiograph and develop the film. If one considers the time taken from when the injury occurred to when the patient arrived in the trauma unit, these few additional minutes have a negligible influence on the patient's future clinical course. These minutes may, in fact, save him from the sometimes considerable morbidity associated with needless chest intubation (Fig 8.10). Some

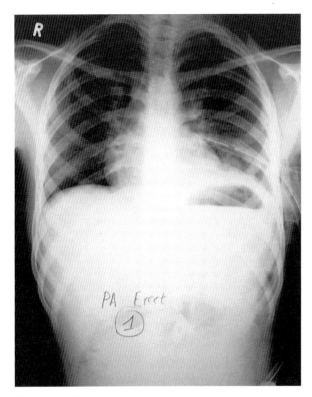

Figure 8.8 *The first chest radiograph in this patient is taken appropriately (erect), but the chest drain has already been inserted. Was an underlying pneumothorax present? Was a chest drain even necessary? The insertion of a chest drain prior to taking a chest radiograph may be unnecessary and may even be dangerous.*

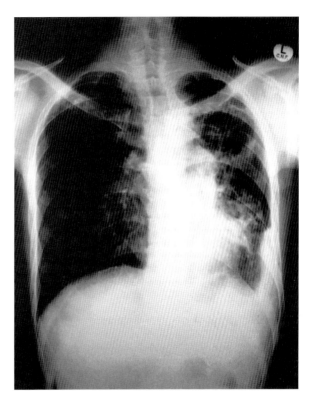

Figure 8.9 *This patient had been stabbed in the left chest and has an apical pneumothorax. The underlying lung is grossly abnormal and the patient was subsequently shown to have pulmonary tuberculosis. The insertion of a chest drain without a chest radiograph would have been unnecessary (the pleural space is invariably obliterated in patients with pleuropulmonary suppuration) and would likely have damaged the underlying lung. The patient was managed without insertion of a chest drain.*

clinicians place reliance on clinical signs, but, with blunt trauma as an example, there is no clinical difference between a pneumothorax and a stomach filled with gas in the left pleural space, or hemothorax and liver in the right pleural space.

The presence of surgical emphysema, especially after trauma, is often interpreted as indicating an underlying pneumothorax. Whilst this assumption is often correct, it is not absolute. The pleural space may have been obliterated by previous inflammation and thus a pneumothorax or hemothorax is an impossibility; the pneumothorax may be small and not, in its own right, require drainage (Fig 8.11). Alternatively, in a partially obliterated pleural space, loculated pneumothoraces under tension may require drainage via special access routes such as the apex (Fig 8.12). There are other causes of surgical emphysema which may be forgotten, for example, damage to the trachea or esophagus. Air is rarely entrained into the tissues from the wound. Extensive surgical emphysema may make radiographic interpretation difficult and consultation with a radiologist may be necessary. A penetrated film made in full expiration or a CT[14,15] may help and serial chest radiographs are far safer than pulmonary intubation across an obliterated pleural space.

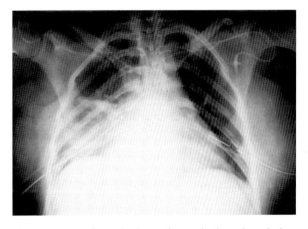

Figure 8.10 *In the enthusiasm of resuscitation, chest drains were inserted into both hemithoraces before the initial chest radiograph and even before careful clinical examination of the patient. The patient had been stabbed only in the right chest and it was unlikely that there was a need for a left-sided chest drain. Why stab the patients ourselves? To act in this manner in this litigious society can result in the physician himself going down the tube.*

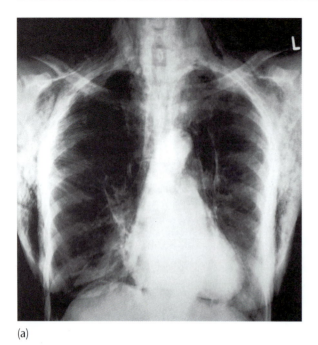

(a)

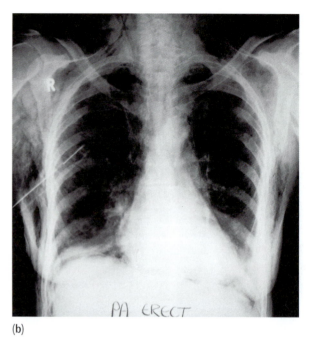

(b)

Figure 8.11 *(a) Subcutaneous emphysema is not synonymous with a pneumothorax. In this patient sustaining penetrating trauma, a chest drain was inserted despite there being no pneumothorax on retrospective careful inspection of the chest radiograph. (b) Unfortunately, an unnecessary chest drain was inserted into the lung and the subcutaneous emphysema worsened.*

The belief by the clinician that he is so experienced in his technique of chest intubation that he will never damage underlying structures and that a chest radiograph is unnecessary, is foolhardy and cannot be supported.

The wrong interpretation of chest radiographs

It is a basic radiographic principle that if the mediastinum is deviated away from an opacity there is space occupation on the opaque side and, where the mediastinum is deviated towards the side of the opacity, there is intrapulmonary shrinkage. Failure to interpret the difference between shrinkage and space occupation may result in inappropriate drainage of atelectatic lung rather than the appropriate investigation – bronchoscopy.

It is often quite difficult to differentiate between pulmonary contusion and hemothorax. To differentiate, lateral and lateral decubitus views should be taken to confirm the movement of fluid. Another common error is the interpretation of a shrunken left upper lobe or shrunken right middle and left lower lobes as pleural (Fig 8.13). The clinician should be aware of their characteristic features – a lateral film, or a decubitis film is often helpful. If, following trauma, an opacity is visible but does not reach the hemidiaphragm, one should be cautious about inserting a chest drain and should be certain, if indicated, of the site of drainage.

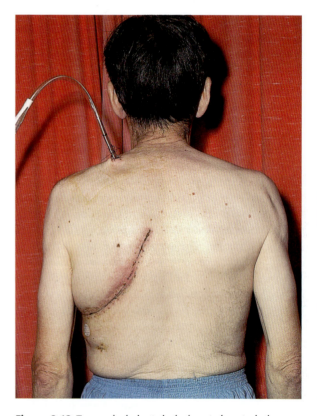

Figure 8.12 *True apical chest drain inserted posteriorly over the scapula between the first and second ribs. This approach is used to drain isolated apical pockets in patients with adhesions or as a more comfortable apical drain in preference to the anterior second intercostal space approach which transfixes the major accessory respiratory muscles. (SWTC.)*

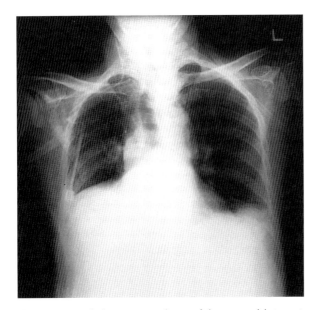

Figure 8.13 *It is important to be careful not to misinterpret the chest radiograph. The opacity at the right base can only be due to shrinkage of the right middle and lower lobe because there is shift of the mediastinum towards the opacity. The correct management is bronchoscopy not chest drainage.*

In these circumstances it is likely that either an intrapulmonary hematoma or loculated hemothorax is present (Fig 8.14).

Bullae are frequently difficult to separate from a pneumothorax. Differentiating features are a relative lack of distress, recent change in symptoms, or change in serial chest radiographs in the patient with bullae. If possible, the views of experts should be obtained before intubating.

The likelihood of stomach herniation may be suspected from the history. The radiographic clues are a dome-shaped upper limit of the 'hemopneumothorax' and the absence of left subphrenic gastric air (Fig 8.15). A useful simple confirmatory procedure that also gives symptomatic relief is the insertion of a nasogastric (NG) tube. This causes the inflated stomach to collapse and the NG tube may, after a repeat chest radiograph, be seen curled up in the stomach within the chest. Occasionally, a congenital[14] or post-traumatic diaphragmatic hernia containing colon may be wrongfully interpreted as a hemopneumothorax or pyopneumothorax (Fig 8.16). Caution in the interpretation of the post-traumatic basal opacity is warranted (Fig 8.17).

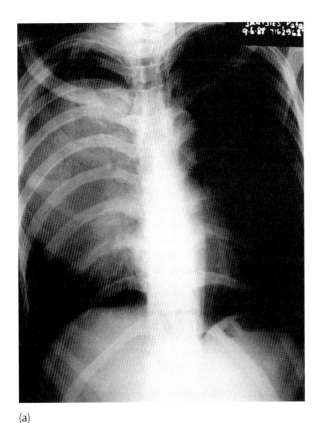

(a)

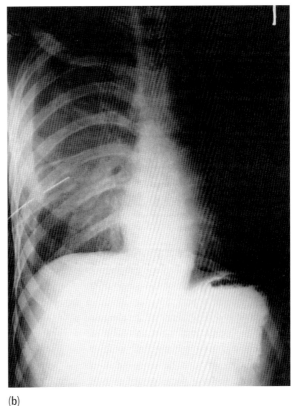

(b)

Figure 8.14 *(a) This patient was stabbed in the right chest. The opacity fails to reach the hemidiaphragm which is a clue that the hemothorax is either loculated or extrapleural. The correct site of drainage needs to be carefully considered (lateral and even a CT may help) and the intended site of drainage should be aspirated to confirm the correct site. (b) The same patient had a chest drain inserted and it is not surprising that the opacity remains in addition to a lateral component. At surgical evacuation the hemothorax was found to be extrapleural.*

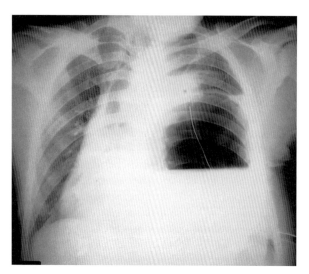

Figure 8.15 *The clue to herniation of stomach through a diaphragmatic defect in this patient is the inferior site of the translucency and the convex upper border. Luckily the inserted chest tube missed the stomach, but it unfortunately entered lung as demonstrated by opacification at the tip of the drain.*

Inserting a drain without obtaining liquid, blood or air freely at needle aspiration prior to drainage

This is probably the most important step in the procedure of chest drainage. Once the intended site of drainage has been selected on the basis of recent chest radiographs, a needle should be inserted into the pleural cavity. If liquid, blood or air does not enter the syringe freely on aspiration, the site selected is incorrect (Figs 8.18–8.20). Small amounts of blood mixed with froth indicates that the needle has entered lung.

If the pus of an empyema is thick and if there is a clotted hemothorax, free flow into the syringe will not occur. Open drainage by rib resection or the procedure of decortication is then required rather than ineffective tube drainage.

A useful hint in the determination of the site of drainage is to determine the relationship of the opacity or translucency to that of the angle of the scapula. This is easily palpable and also easily seen on the chest radiograph and may serve as a reference point. Generally, unless loculation is present, the most appropriate site for chest drainage is the mid-axillary line in the fifth or sixth interspace – here muscle bulk is less, it is comfortable for the patient and it is usually far from mediastinal structures. Air or blood drains equally well from this site. The diaphragm can with expiration rise to the level of the sixth interspace so one should be cautious about inserting a drain below this level (Fig 8.21).[16] Empyemata tend to loculate posteriorly and it is preferable to drain the empyema posteriorly – usually at the angle of the eighth rib.

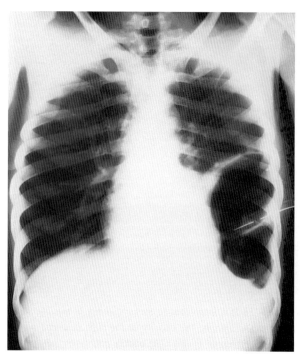

Figure 8.16 *The basal translucency in this patient was wrongly interpreted as a loculated pneumothorax. The correct diagnosis is diaphragmatic herniation through a traumatic diaphragmatic defect which was only made after the splenic flexure of the colon was drained.*

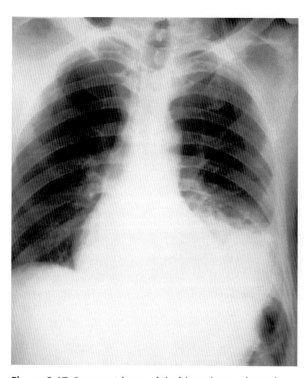

Figure 8.17 *One must be careful of low chest stabs and a basal opacity. This patient had a diaphragmatic herniation of stomach and omentum through a traumatic diaphragmatic defect. Omentum is frequently found in these circumstances as it tends to be sucked into the chest by the normal subatmospheric pleural pressure.*

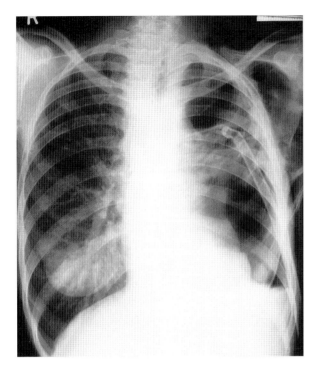

Figure 8.18 *A minor pneumothorax, not requiring chest tube drainage, has been made worse by the insertion of the chest drain. The chest drain has entered lung at the exact spot where the pleura was adherent (it remains against the chest wall). This complication could have been prevented by interpretation of the chest radiograph and careful aspiration to determine the correct site of intended drainage.*

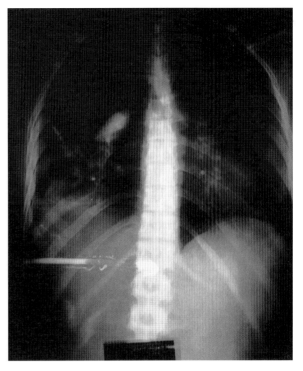

Figure 8.20 *A sinogram in this patient demonstrates that the drain has been inserted directly into the liver. Such a complication could have been prevented by correctly choosing the appropriate site for drainage and confirming the site by aspiration.*

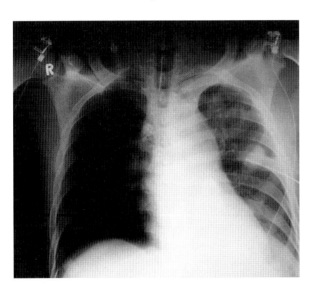

Figure 8.19 *Soon after insertion of the left-sided chest drain this patient developed severe hemoptysis necessitating endotracheal intubation and ventilation. The chest radiograph demonstrates that the chest drain has been inserted into the pulmonary parenchyma; there is a hematoma at the tip of the chest drain and there is opacification of the left lung due to aspirated blood. The chest drain had been inserted without a recent chest radiograph. A pneumothorax or hemothorax was impossible because the pleural space was obliterated.*

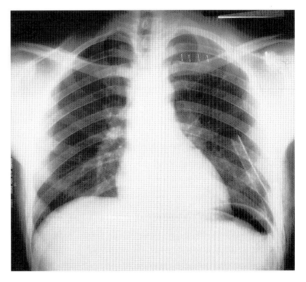

Figure 8.21 *The stapled sole stab wound in this patient is high, thus the cause of subphrenic air on the chest radiograph is likely due to the low insertion of the chest drain.*

There are many examples of considerable morbidity and even mortality attached to the procedure of chest drainage. If the procedure is done carefully with attention to aspiration prior to chest drain insertion (to determine the correct site by aspirating what is to be drained) and the rigid trocar that accompanies many chest drain kits is not used, many of these complications will be eliminated.

Drain inappropriately connected, kinks, etc.

To most this is fairly obvious but on a number of occasions it has been observed, when using the simpler glass bottle container, that the tubing has been connected to the vent port rather than to the rod that is beneath the water seal. With vigorous coughing, bubbles may even be seen. The rod should lie at least 2 cm below the water level – occasionally, especially when transporting the patient, the bottle is lifted up by the tubing, so drawing the rod above the water level and breaking the water seal. With the use of commercial drainage collection containers this is an impossibility. These commercial drainage collection systems are extremely effective and mechanisms exist to alter the amount of suction, if used, and also to retransfuse blood.

Occasionally thrombus or fibrin within the drainage tubes, kinks of the tubing, clamps placed on the drains temporarily during transportation and not later removed, or the plastic occluding device included with commercial systems, may result in inadequate drainage. In a patient with a significant air leak the consequences of an obstructed drain are obvious. The resistance of connectors smaller than the tubing is insignificant when considering air flow, but it is important with fluid/clot drainage as obstruction may occur at the point of greatest restriction, preventing further drainage. Connectors should be appropriately trimmed to provide minimal obstruction.

Chest drainage when ventilation or anesthesia is required

It is frequently believed that if a patient has sustained penetrating trauma to the chest and requires anesthesia or ventilation with high pressures, the likelihood of developing a pneumothorax is high and one should prophylactically insert a chest drain even if a pneumothorax is not present. This presumption is untrue and may lead to needless insertion of chest drains and the likelihood of iatrogenic damage. Although the development of a pneumothorax is possible, it is not inevitable and, in fact, may never occur if the pleural space is obliterated. A pneumothorax may even develop in patients with adult respiratory distress syndrome requiring ventilation and with a chest tube in place.[17] What is advisable is to be aware of the possibility of a pneumothorax and to have a chest drain available. If the clinical status of the patient changes – i.e.

difficulty with ventilation, cyanosis or hypoxemia, a chest radiograph should be taken. In urgent circumstances the chest should be percussed and auscultated – if there is hyper-resonance and decreased air entry a needle should be inserted to confirm the suspicion of a pneumothorax and a chest drain inserted.

OTHER POINTS

Size of the chest tube

The choice depends on the material to be drained. For empyemas this should be large as there is a tendency for fibrin to clog the tubing; with a pneumothorax a smaller diameter tube often suffices.

The post-insertion chest radiograph

It is advisable to view a post-insertion chest radiograph, especially if the anticipated fluid or air does not drain. The drain may have been inserted incorrectly (wrong side, below the diaphragm or in the wrong site, if loculation exists), or drains may be excessively long or may compress or penetrate vital structures (Fig 8.22). Interesting examples of complications due to chest drains include: perforation of the lung and encirclement of the great vessels;[18] vagus stimulation and death due to hemorrhage surrounding the vagus nerve at the apex of the chest cavity;[19] tamponade;[20] a contralateral hemopneumothorax;[21] insertion of a chest drain into the right atrium, repaired successfully 3 days later;[22] phrenic nerve palsy;[23] cardiogenic shock due to compression of the right ventricle[24] and brachial plexus compression[25] or Horner's syndrome.[26] The author is aware of many others, some of which are illustrated.

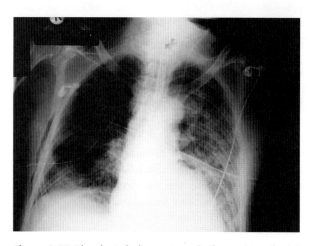

Figure 8.22 *The chest drain must not be inserted too far in! In this patient it traversed the anterior mediastinum into the opposite hemithorax.*

Because of a reluctance to discuss complications, the frequency is probably much higher than suspected.

Removal of the chest drain

When does one remove the chest drain? When the function has been served. There are two ways of assessing the function of intercostal drains – radiographically by observing pulmonary re-expansion and disappearance of pleural contents (air, blood, chyle, or pus) and by observation of the volume and type of drainage. Our rule of thumb is to remove the drain once bubbling has ceased, or if there has been drainage of less than 100 ml per 12-hour period. With a well drained empyema and a residual pleural space, the drain is left in longer, even if minimal drainage occurs. Does suction of drains lead to rapid recovery? Davis and colleagues prospectively randomized patients requiring chest tube drainage after chest trauma to either a suction or water-seal group.[3] The use of suction significantly decreased both chest tube duration and the time taken for chest tube removal. In some circumstances, but only under observation, drains may be removed when the air leak is minimal.[27] Occasionally patients unfit for thoracotomy may be sent home with an open drainage system or with a Heimlich valve.[28]

How does one remove the drain? One removes the drain when the lung remains expanded during the ventilatory cycle. During spontaneous respiration this is during expiration; if on a ventilator, during inspiration. If air enters the pleural space at chest drain removal the volume is frequently small and can often be observed.

A common mistake is to leave drains in too long. The swing in the fluid column within the drain reflects only changes in the intrathoracic pressure with respiration; this may occur even if the lung is fully expanded and the pleural space empty. To always wait until blockage of the tube occurs and swinging ceases will cause needless discomfort to the patient and may result in infection. Chest tube placement rapidly induces significant pleural inflammation and an exudate[29] and by pressure necrosis can cause hemorrhage[30] and perforation of the lung.[31] A residual hemothorax after chest drainage means either loculation or clot formation – if large, a thoracotomy may be required; if small, only observation. Similarly, if after drainage of an empyema the patient remains pyrexial and a pleural collection is still visible on the chest radiograph, formal drainage and/or decortication is required, because the pus is likely to be too thick to drain through a tube.

Antibiotic usage

The frequent finding of multiple resistant organisms with post-traumatic empyema probably reflects hospital-acquired infection rather than infection acquired from the assailant's unsterile weapon and may be the result of inappropriate chest drainage. A number of studies have evaluated the effectiveness of antibiotic usage to prevent infections. In one study, where cefonicid was given intravenously until chest drains were removed, antibiotic usage resulted in a significantly reduced rate of infection compared to a placebo group.[32] In another study, a single dose of ampicillin prophylaxis was as effective as a prolonged course.[33]

Management of the wrongly inserted chest drain

Usually management is fairly obvious. If the intra-abdominal organs are damaged then laparotomy and repair is necessary. Intubation of the lung, particularly if the pleural cavity is obliterated, may result in rapid development of extensive subcutaneous emphysema, which is alarming both to the patient and to the person inserting the drain. The instinctive response by many is to insert another chest drain to drain the excessive air, which compounds the situation. Treatment usually entails no more than removal of the intercostal tube and sedation of the patient (and also assurance of the involved physician that you are not embarking on a dangerous course of action). The surgical emphysema resolves, usually within a week, and blood streaking of the sputum or minor hemoptysis usually abates spontaneously. There are isolated reports of drains placed in the subcutaneous tissues to treat subcutaneous emphysema;[34,35] this is probably unnecessary.

Intubation of the lung may be the cause of a prolonged air leak and may sometimes be difficult to recognize. A CT scan may be helpful. In some instances the diagnosis is only made at thoracotomy or retrospectively after diminitution of the air leak following insertion of a new chest drain and removal of the original. In some instances intubation of the lung is followed by brisk hemoptysis and occasionally death. The author has seen a number of instances of this complication and at post mortem a major pulmonary artery branch was usually damaged. Theoretically, the patient should be managed by immediate thoracotomy and clamping of the hilum with a vascular clamp to prevent spillage and drowning by inhaled blood into the contralateral normal lung. Further repair of the laceration or pulmonary resection is then undertaken. Most patients in these circumstances, however, do not survive.

Chest drainage systems

A single-bottle water-seal drainage system is the simplest and cheapest (Fig 8.23). Emptying of the pleural space depends on gravity and the mechanics of

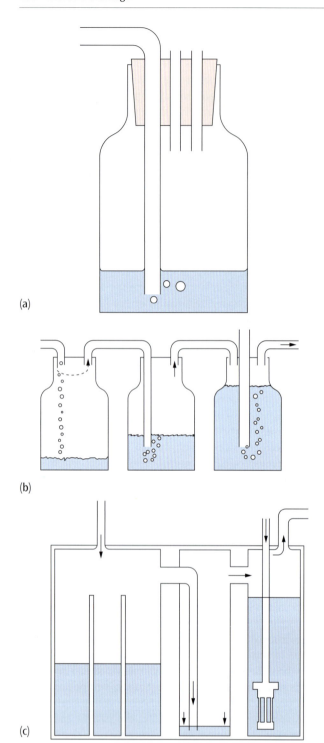

(a)

(b)

(c)

respiration (expiration, coughing and straining). The system is adequate for evacuating air and fluid accumulating at a modest rate. As fluid collects in the trap, increasing resistance to drainage occurs.

Suction can be regulated using either two or three bottles. Some commercial companies provide this system as a plastic integrated system (see Fig 8.23c). The first bottle, or collecting chamber, collects fluid removed from the pleural space and may be a portal for retransfusion (filters will be necessary). The second provides the water seal and is where evidence of an air leak is observed. The third chamber or bottle regulates the vacuum and is commonly controlled by the height of the fluid within the system. Because of convenience and less risk of errors, the commercial system is favored.

Excessive froth

Excessive froth in the collecting bottles in the presence of excessive air leak may be reduced by lowering of the surface tension within the collecting fluid. A few drops of octyl alcohol or Tween in the collecting chamber is effective for this purpose.

REFERENCES

1. Sherck JP, McCort JJ, Oakes DD. Computed tomography in thoracoabdominal trauma. *J Trauma* 1984; **24:** 1015–21.
2. Ordog GJ, Wasserberger J, Balasubramanium S, Shoemaker W. Asymptomatic stab wounds of the chest. *J Trauma* 1994; **36:** 680–4.
3. Davis JW, Mackersie RC, Hoyt DB, Garcia J. Randomized study of algorithms for discontinuing tube thoracostomy drainage. *J Am Coll Surg* 1994; **179:** 553–7.
4. Schoenenberger RA, Haefeli WE, Weiss P, Ritz R. Evaluation of conventional chest tube therapy for iatrogenic pneumothorax. *Chest* 1993; **104:** 1770–2.
5. Toombs BD, Sandler CM, Lester RG. Computed tomography of chest trauma. *Radiology* 1981; **140:** 733–8.
6. Muckart DJJ. Delayed pneumothorax and haemothorax following observation for stab wounds of the chest. *Injury* 1985; **16:** 247–8.
7. Ross RM, Cordoba A. Delayed life-threatening hemothorax associated with rib fractures. *J Trauma* 1986; **26:** 576–8.
8. Kish G, Koxloff L, Joseph WL, Adkins PC. Indications for early thoracotomy in thoracic trauma. *Ann Thorac Surg* 1976; **22:** 23–8.
9. Iberti TJ, Stern PM. Chest tube thoracostomy. [Review]. *Crit Care Clin* 1992; **8:** 879–95.
10. Weigelt JA, Aurbakken CM, Meier DE, Thal ER.

Figure 8.23 *(a) Diagrammatic representation of the simplest chest drainage system. The drainage tubing is connected to a rigid rod which is placed beneath sterile saline. The depth of fluid determines the resistance of the water seal. (b) A three-bottle chest tube drainage system. The first bottle is a collecting bottle; air leakage can be observed at the second bottle and the suction pressure can be regulated in the third bottle by the depth that the open port (center) lies beneath the saline. (c) Diagrammatic representation of the commercial chest tube drainage system. Basically it functions exactly like the three-bottle drainage system in (b).*

Management of asymptomatic patients following stab wounds to the chest. *J Trauma* 1982; **22:** 291–4.

11. Coselli JS, Mattox KL, Beall AC. Reevaluation of early evacuation of clotted hemothorax. *Am J Surg* 1984; **148:** 786–90.

12. Smith RS, Fry WR, Tsoi EK, *et al.* Preliminary report on videothoracoscopy in the evaluation and treatment of thoracic injury. *Am J Surg* 1993; **166:** 690–3.

13. Forster E, Le Maguet A, Cinqualbre J, Piombini JL, Schiltz E. A propos d'un cas de chylothorax consecutif à un traumatisme fermé vertebro-costal. *Chirurgie* 1975; **101:** 605–16.

14. Fein JA, Loiselle J, Eberlein S, Wiley JF, Bell LM. Diaphragmatic hernia masquerading as pneumothorax in two toddlers. *Ann Emerg Med* 1993; **22:** 1221–4.

15. Crabbe MM, Mappin FG, Fontenelle LJ. The use of computed tomography to assess and treat complex pneumothorax. *Milit Med* 1993; **158:** 193–6.

16. Foresti V, Villa A, Casati O, Parisio E, De Filippi G. Abdominal placement of tube thoracostomy due to lack of recognition of paralysis of hemidiaphragm. *Chest* 1992; **102:** 292–3.

17. Ross IB, Fleiszer DM, Brown RA. Localized tension pneumothorax in patients with adult respiratory distress syndrome. *Can J Surg* 1994; **37:** 415–19.

18. Laneri GG, Mitre B, Balsan MJ. Ventilatory management casebook. Lung perforation and encirclement of the great vessels by a malpositioned chest tube. *J Perinatol* 1994; **14:** 150–3.

19. Ward EW, Hughes TE. Sudden death following chest tube insertion: an unusual case of vagus nerve irritation. *J Trauma* 1994; **36:** 258–9.

20. Quak JM, Szatmari A, van den Anker JN. Cardiac tamponade in a preterm neonate secondary to a chest tube. *Acta Paediatr* 1993; **82:** 490–1.

21. Gerard PS, Kaldawi E, Litani V, Lenora RA, Tessler S. Right-sided pneumothorax as a result of a left-sided chest tube. *Chest* 1993; **103:** 1602–3.

22. Shih CT, Chang Y, Lai ST. Successful management of perforating injury of right atrium by chest tube. *Chin Med J* 1992; **50:** 338–40.

23. Odita JC, Khan AS, Dincsoy M, Kayyali M, Masoud A, Ammari A. Neonatal phrenic nerve paralysis resulting from intercostal drainage of pneumothorax. *Pediatr Radiol* 1992; **22:** 379–81.

24. Kollef MH, Dothager DW. Reversible cardiogenic shock due to chest tube compression of the right ventricle. *Chest* 1991; **99:** 976–80.

25. Mangar D, Kelly DL, Holder DO, Camporesi EM. Brachial plexus compression from a malpositioned chest tube after thoracotomy. *Anesthesiology* 1991; **74:** 780–2.

26. Bertino RE, Wesbey GE, Johnson RJ. Horner syndrome occurring as a complication of chest tube placement. *Radiology* 1987; **164:** 745.

27. Kato R, Kobayashi T, Watanabe M, *et al.* Can the chest tube draining the pleural cavity with persistent air leakage be removed? *Thorac Cardiovasc Surg* 1992; **40:** 292–6.

28. Heimlich HJ. Valve drainage of the pleural cavity. *Dis Chest* 1968; **53:** 282–7.

29. Carvalho P, Kirk W, Butler J, Charan NB. Effects of tube thoracostomy on pleural fluid characteristics in sheep. *J Appl Physiol* 1993; **74:** 2782–7.

30. Muthuswamy P, Samuel J, Mizock B, Dunne P. Recurrent massive bleeding from an intercostal artery aneurysm through an empyema chest tube. *Chest* 1993; **104:** 637–9.

31. Resnick DK. Delayed pulmonary perforation. A rare complication of tube thoracostomy. *Chest* 1993; **103:** 311–13.

32. Nichols RL, Smith JW, Muzik AC, *et al.* Preventive antibiotic usage in traumatic thoracic injuries requiring closed tube thoracostomy. *Chest* 1994; **106:** 1493–8.

33. Demetriades D, Breckon V, Breckon C, *et al.* Antibiotic prophylaxis in penetrating injuries of the chest. *Ann R Coll Surg Engl* 1991; **73:** 348–51.

34. Terada Y, Matsunobe S, Nemoto T, Tsuda T, Shimizu Y. Palliation of severe subcutaneous emphysema with use of a trocar-type chest tube as a subcutaneous drain [letter]. *Chest* 1993; **103:** 323.

35. Nair KK, Neville E, Rajesh P, Papaliya H. A simple method of palliation for gross subcutaneous surgical emphysema. *J R Coll Surg Edinb* 1989; **34:** 163–4.

9

Thoracotomy

JOHN A ODELL

Although chest injuries are a contributing cause in 50% of fatal injuries after civilian trauma, only a small percentage, approximately 15%, require thoracotomy as part of their definitive management. In most patients chest injuries can be treated with relatively simple interventions such as tube thoracostomy combined with fluid replacement and observation with serial chest radiography.

Occasionally thoracic trauma may present with dramatic clinical syndromes such as tension pneumothorax, cardiac tamponade and advanced hypovolemic shock, which require rapid and thorough clinical assessment and management. Personnel managing thoracic trauma need to be aware of how to manage these dramatic physiological abnormalities. In this chapter we will discuss the two major factors that characterize thoracotomy and trauma: the timing of the operation and the flexibility of the exposure demanded. For purposes of discussion, immediate thoracotomy is defined as thoracotomy usually performed in the emergency room, in the field at the site of the injury or in the operating room as an integral part of the resuscitative process – often with simultaneous maneuvers directed toward control of the airway and volume restoration. Urgent thoracotomy is defined as that occurring in the operating room soon after resuscitation and soon after the injury has been defined. Elective thoracotomy is defined as the trauma patient who has been fully resuscitated and is stable.

IMMEDIATE THORACOTOMY

This procedure is synonymous with terms such as emergency room thoracotomy, field thoracotomy or resuscitative thoracotomy.

INDICATIONS

There exists considerable debate concerning the value and efficacy of emergency thoracotomy (Fig 9.1). A number of studies have concluded that there is no value in doing the procedure in patients with blunt trauma, those who have no signs of life, those agonal (electromechanical dissociation with no palpable pulse or blood pressure) and those with extrathoracic penetrating injuries.[1-3] The primary indication is penetrating injury to the chest in patients who are on the point of cardiac arrest or have just arrested, or are severely hypovolemic. Patients who have had vital signs within the previous 15 minutes are candidates for resuscitation. Patients having cardiopulmonary resuscitation (CPR) without restoration of their own intrinsic cardiac rhythm within 5 minutes have a dismal prognosis.[4] The immediate objectives of emergency thoracotomy are to relieve pericardial tamponade (Fig 9.2), to control intrathoracic hemorrhage, to provide access for open cardiac massage and cross-clamping of the descending thoracic aorta to redistribute blood flow to the myocardium and brain.[5]

Where should the emergency room thoracotomy be performed?

Most modern busy trauma units are well versed with the equipment and facilities needed for emergency room thoracotomy. There are occasional reports in the literature of successful roadside, or scene resuscitative thoracotomy, but these reports are isolated and probably selective in that only patients with a successful outcome are reported. It is generally accepted that thoracotomy performed at the scene is not rewarding in

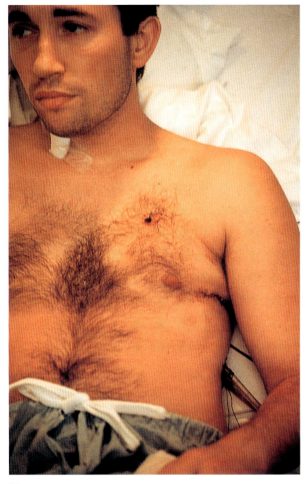

(a)

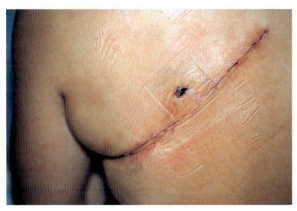

(b)

Figure 9.1 *(a) Young patient saved by emergency room thoracotomy following a low velocity but close range bullet wound to the left chest. The bullet passed directly through the main pulmonary artery in the hilum of the lung and exited posteriorly medial to the scapula (b). He presented moribund with an extensive left hemothorax and no perceptible blood pressure. At thoracotomy the hemothorax was evacuated and a clamp applied across the hilum of the left lung. After fluid resuscitation and stabilization he was transferred to the operating room for direct repair of the left pulmonary artery which required left upper lobectomy. (SWTC.)*

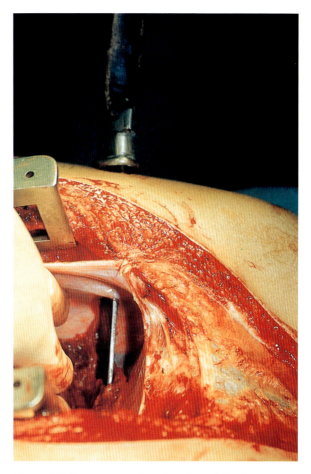

Figure 9.2 *Emergency median sternotomy following a precordial stab wound. The knife appeared to be pulsating and the patient had cardiac tamponade. On opening the pericardium 200 ml of blood were drained. Whilst the knife had lacerated the epicardium no cardiac chamber had been entered and the patient made a rapid recovery. (SWTC.)*

terms of survival and as an aid to resuscitation.[3] The limited efficacy of scene thoracotomy lends support for a 'swoop and scoop' policy; delay caused by performing a scene thoracotomy may be detrimental to overall management. It is more advantageous to do such a procedure with a multidisciplinary team rather than with limited personnel, equipment and facilities. Often a single physician at the scene is unable to coordinate airway and shock management plus the surgical procedure. Occasionally circumstances may advocate a procedure done in such a circumstance, but this is generally not recommended. Besides the low yield in terms of survival following emergency thoracotomy other disadvantages include the high cost (in one series non-survivors received an average of 17 units of blood products[2]) and the risk of trauma team members' exposure to blood-borne infections.[6] Others have advocated a low level of emergency room thoracotomy for resuscitation so that technical expertise can be developed which may provide a more favorable outcome in the occasional patient with amenable injuries.[7]

If emergency thoracotomy is undertaken it is important that a sense of calm prevail in the emergency room. Frequently the patient has multiple injuries and the room is small and crowded with numerous personnel all trying to be as helpful as possible. It is important that somebody take control, get a sense of the priorities and delegate personnel appropriately.

The procedure

The supine position is the most appropriate. Both arms should be positioned at right angles so that venous and arterial access can be obtained. The patient's abdomen, chest and thighs should be draped. Urinary catheterization can occur after resuscitation has been achieved and is not an absolute priority. Although venous and arterial access is ideal, time should not be spent persisting with cannulation of these vessels. The patient may be extremely hypovolemic with a low arterial blood pressure and the vessels may be collapsed. Venous and arterial access can be obtained rapidly after opening the chest and the anesthesiologist should be comfortable that access to venous sites and measurement of arterial blood pressure will be provided by the surgeon. Venous cannulas can be inserted by the surgeon directly into the right atrium, superior cava or innominate vein;[8] others have described inserting a Foley's catheter directly into the cardiac wound – inflation of the balloon controls bleeding and infusion through the port restores blood volume.[9] An arterial cannula can be placed directly into the aorta or left ventricle for pressure measurement. If vascular access is provided via the thoracotomy, certain precautions should be observed. Excessive fluid administration, especially if combined with aortic occlusion, can overdistend the ventricles and compromise cardiac contractility; large volumes of cold solutions or blood may predispose the patient to cardiac arrhythmias because of myocardial cooling and citrate toxicity. There exists the potential for air embolism and, if the catheter is inadvertently dislodged, of excessive bleeding.

The incision decided upon is to some extent determined by the pattern of injury. The initial incision for cardiac resuscitation or relief of cardiac tamponade is a left thoracotomy. The procedure can be rapidly undertaken, and if the incision is extended can give access to the abdomen as a thoracoabdominal incision or to the other chest by extending the incision across the sternum. It requires no specialized instruments apart from a chest wall retractor.

The incision is made along the fifth or sixth interspace, extending from the midpoint on the sternum to the posterior axillary line (Fig 9.3). In women, the inframammary fold is used as an incision guideline. The

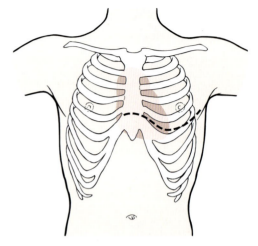

Figure 9.3 *In the patient requiring urgent thoracotomy, particularly for resuscitative purposes, the anterior thoracotomy is ideal. The patient is positioned supine with the side to be operated upon elevated by a pillow to approximately 15°. Arms are positioned at right angles so that vascular access can be obtained simultaneously with thoracotomy. The incision is curved in the inframammary fold following the curve of the fifth rib. The intercostal muscles are opened directly and the pleural space opened. Not infrequently the costochondral junction separates when the spreader is opened. The internal thoracic vessels may need to be controlled. The incision can be extended anteriorly across the sternum using a saw or bone cutters. If required it can be extended posteriorly. Occasionally for higher injuries additional exposure can be obtained by dividing the upper costal cartilages. This, however, results in excessive pain.*

incision should curve and follow the shape of the underlying rib. The incision is extended sharply through the chest wall muscles and will usually come directly upon the underlying rib. The intercostal muscles are incised along its superior edge using either scissors or the knife. Once the pleural space has been entered, the incision is extended anteriorly and posteriorly, taking care to protect the underlying structures. A chest wall retractor is then placed with its handles in the inferior position.

Some surgeons, in order to gain additional room, incise the two superior costal cartilages with a knife blade. This is rarely necessary; and may cause excessive pain in the recovery period. The surgeon should be aware of the internal thoracic arteries anteriorly and these might need to be ligated. The incision can be extended across the sternum, if necessary, using either a Lebsche knife, rib shears, a sternal saw or a Gigli saw. The lung is retracted posteriorly and the phrenic nerve, which is anterior to the hilar vessels is identified. In cardiac tamponade the cardiac pulsations are not visible and the pericardium may be tense. The pericardium is incised parallel to the phrenic nerve (Fig 9.4). After incision of the pericardium, blood and blood clot will

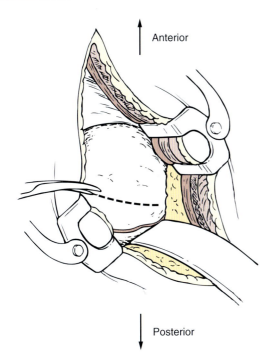

Anterior

Posterior

Figure 9.4 *The pericardium is opened approximately 5 cm in front of the phrenic nerve and extended parallel to the nerve. If tamponade is present, blood and clot should be evacuated and the source of bleeding controlled. If there is asystole or ventricular fibrillation, internal cardiac massage is commenced.*

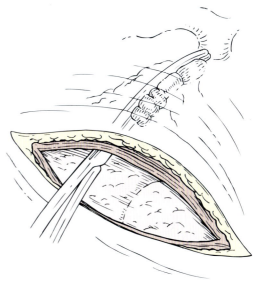

Figure 9.5 *When there is either bleeding from a large laceration of the lung, or, in association with such an injury, air is noted in the coronary arteries, suggesting air embolism, then the hilum of the lung is clamped with a soft vascular clamp to limit further embolism and to control bleeding. The inferior ligament needs to be divided to the inferior pulmonary vein before applying the clamp. This can be accomplished fairly quickly by incising the ligament inferiorly and then sweeping the lung superiorly. In the emergency situation the ligament should not be divided completely with sharp dissection as damage to the inferior pulmonary vein may result.*

rapidly egress from the wound and cardiac action may be observed. In patients who do not have tamponade but who have arrested, internal cardiac massage is initiated. If there is a considerable laceration of the lung, or air bubbles are noted in the coronary arteries, then the hilum of the injured lung should be clamped using a vascular clamp such as a Satinsky clamp (Fig 9.5). Some hypovolemic patients may benefit from clamping of the descending thoracic aorta (Fig 9.6). This may temporarily increase the arterial pressure to the upper extremity and preserve perfusion to the brain and the heart. If survival occurs following such a maneuver, one should be aware of the possible postoperative development of renal failure, necessitating hemodialysis. The exact role of aortic cross-clamping with possible benefit, if any, has not been defined.

Discontinuation of resuscitation

The surgeon involved should have a clear understanding of the passage of time. He should be made aware of the circumstances and time of the injury, the clinical course of the patient and when emergency resuscitation started. Time passes very rapidly under the circumstances of resuscitation. The surgeon should be aware of when further treatment is futile and heroic resusci-

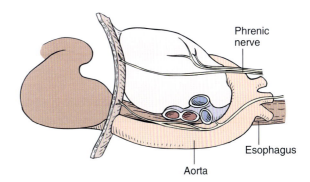

Phrenic nerve

Esophagus

Aorta

Figure 9.6 *Clamping of the descending aorta may be considered to improve perfusion to the upper body. The pleura is incised medial to the aorta and, using one's fingers as a guide, the clamp is positioned. It is not necessary to occlude the aorta completely; attempting to encircle the aorta completely may damage intercostal arteries. When pressure is restored, the clamp should be slowly released while volume is being infused so that a precipitous drop in blood pressure does not occur.*

tation should be discontinued appropriately. Guidelines that suggest that heroic resuscitation should be discontinued include:

- irreparable heart and lung injuries;
- the presence of other lethal injuries, such as massive head injury, spinal cord injury or liver injury;
- if volume resuscitation is not possible within 15 minutes of opening the chest;
- if it is impossible to provide volume and pharmacological resuscitation with self-sustaining rhythm within 15 minutes.

Ideally the patient should maintain a mean blood pressure in excess of 50 mmHg with maximum volume and pharmacological support within 30 minutes. If tamponade is not found, then heroic measures are unlikely to succeed.

URGENT THORACOTOMY

This procedure is usually carried out in the operating room soon after resuscitation has occurred and usually after investigations have delineated the extent of injury. The patient is much more stable than in an emergency room, or immediate thoracotomy situation and usually preparations for the procedure can be undertaken at a more leisurely pace. The usual indications are hemopericardium with tamponade, penetrating cardiac trauma, massive hemothorax or continued intrathoracic bleeding, a ruptured aorta, a rupture of the tracheal bronchial tree, rupture of the diaphragm, rupture of the esophagus and an open chest wound requiring coverage of the wound. An arterial line is usually inserted for continuous arterial blood pressure monitoring and in some patients a Swan–Ganz catheter is used for accessing cardiac performance. A Foley catheter is inserted into the bladder. Double lumen endotracheal tubes may be used in selective cases to provide one-lung anesthesia.

Many patients may be considered relatively stable, yet in some hemodynamics considered stable may be the result of a marked sympathetic drive which may be abolished when the patient is anesthetized. The surgeon and anesthesiologist must be aware of this situation and be prepared to proceed rapidly.

The specific techniques and thoracotomy for these specific procedures are documented under the relevant chapter. The incisions chosen should be appropriate to the site and nature of the expected injury. If there are any preoperative leads to the injury, the patient is positioned and draped accordingly.

TECHNIQUE FOR PERICARDIAL WINDOW

This is a useful technique in patients in whom one suspects the possibility of cardiac injury, but the symptoms and signs are questionable. The procedure

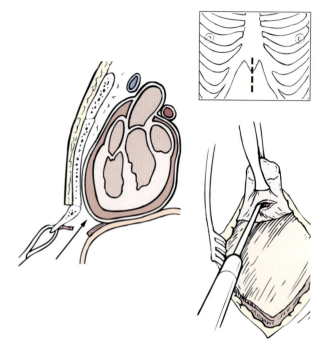

Figure 9.7 *Technique for performance of subxiphoid pericardial window. The xiphoid may be left in place, excised or divided vertically. The muscle slips extending from the xiphoid to the diaphragm are divided and the pericardium exposed and opened.*

may be useful as a definitive procedure in patients who present late after trauma with evidence of pericardial tamponade. In these circumstances the procedure is undertaken to establish drainage as control of ongoing hemorrhage is not a major concern. The procedure is also useful in patients who develop septic pericarditis after trauma and require drainage.

The procedure may be undertaken under either local anesthesia or general anesthesia. The chest and abdomen are cleaned and draped and the patient is placed supine. If necessary, the incision can be extended upwards as a full median sternotomy or downward into the abdomen, if necessary. The incision is made approximately 5–6 cm long, centered over the xiphoid. The incision is extended down to the linea alba and extended over the lower end of the sternum. The xiphoid is dissected free and elevated or excised, if it is large and rigid (Fig 9.7). A small self-retaining catheter is used when spreading the linea alba; a 'third hand,' retracting the sternum upward, may be useful for exposure. The sternal and costal insertions of the diaphragm are incised over approximately 4 cm. The pericardium is then identified in the midline and incised. This allows drainage of pericardial fluid. If blood is found soon after the injury, the incision can be extended upwards as a median sternotomy and the site of intrapericardial trauma controlled. If drainage only

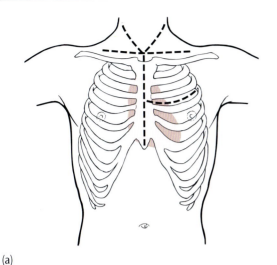

(a)

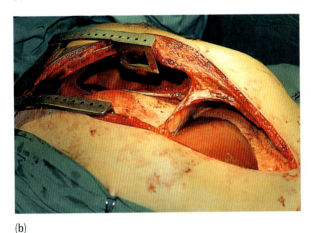

(b)

Figure 9.8 *(a) The median sternotomy is a very versatile incision which can be extended in many directions if necessary. It may be extended either laterally into the pleural space, inferiorly into the abdomen, alongside the anterior border of the sternomastoid muscle if carotid artery or esophageal injuries are suspected, or parallel to the clavicle if the subclavian artery is damaged. (b) Sternolaparotomy used for multiple penetrating injuries to the chest and abdomen wounds which traverse both cavities. This approach is also invaluable to gain control of bleeding in major hepatic trauma, particularly when the hepatic veins are lacerated. (SWTC.)*

is required, drains can be inserted through the incision and brought up through a separate stab wound inferiorly. The linea alba is then approximated with heavy sutures and the skin closed primarily.

MEDIAN STERNOTOMY

The median sternotomy incision is a very versatile incision because it can be extended rapidly to the neck and the abdomen (Fig 9.8). However, specialized instruments to open the sternum are necessary and, if not available and the surgeon is not familiar with these instruments, the procedure can take longer than an anterior thoracotomy. It is the incision of choice whenever there is a suspected injury to the great vessels. In institutions where large volumes of cardiac trauma take place, it is the procedure of choice by many and is used specifically when the injury lies above the third or fourth interspace.

The patient is positioned supine. The neck, anterior chest wall and abdomen are all carefully prepared in case extension of the incision is necessary. The initial incision is made from just below the suprasternal notch to just below the xiphoid process. The incision is deepened, dividing subcutaneous tissues until the anterior aspect of the sternum is visible. The midline at the suprasternal notch, the linea alba and a midline point approximately halfway in between are marked with coagulation and a coagulation line on the periosteum, connecting these midline marks is made. This acts as a guideline for the sternal saw. The sternum can be opened using a sternal saw either from the suprasternal notch toward the xiphoid (Fig 9.9a) or from the xiphoid up toward the suprasternal notch (Fig 9.9b). If extending downward, the surgeon should develop the suprasternal notch using blunt and sharp dissection. The surgeon should keep close to the sternum and not coagulate deeply – the innominate artery lies immediately beneath! Occasionally, in the suprasternal notch there is a strong ligamentous thickening of the interclavicular ligament and the anterior communicating branch of the anterior jugular vein may need to be controlled. If the incision is extended from the xiphoid upwards, then the xiphoid is divided, the diaphragmatic attachments divided, or separated and a finger passed beneath the sternum, separating the pericardium from the sternum. The sternal saw is inserted and moved forward while elevating the saw at the same time. When the manubrium is to be divided, the saw is tilted anteriorly to cut the remaining last centimeters. In some hospitals a right-angled vacillating saw is not available and an oscillating saw (Fig 9.9c) may be used. Occasionally, the sternotomy may be accomplished by the use of Lebsche's knife (Fig 9.9d) or by inserting a Gigli saw in the substernal position.

Depending on the urgency of the situation once the sternum is opened, bleeding from the cancellous surface of the cut sternum may be controlled with bone wax and coagulation may be necessary to control anterior and posterior periosteal bleeding. There is usually excessive bleeding from veins in the suprasternal notch and also where the xiphoid approximates the body of the sternum.

Once the sternal retractor has been inserted and opened, the pericardium and both pleural spaces can be opened, the injury assessed and controlled. The incision may be extended superiorly into the neck on either the right or left side in order to access the distal common

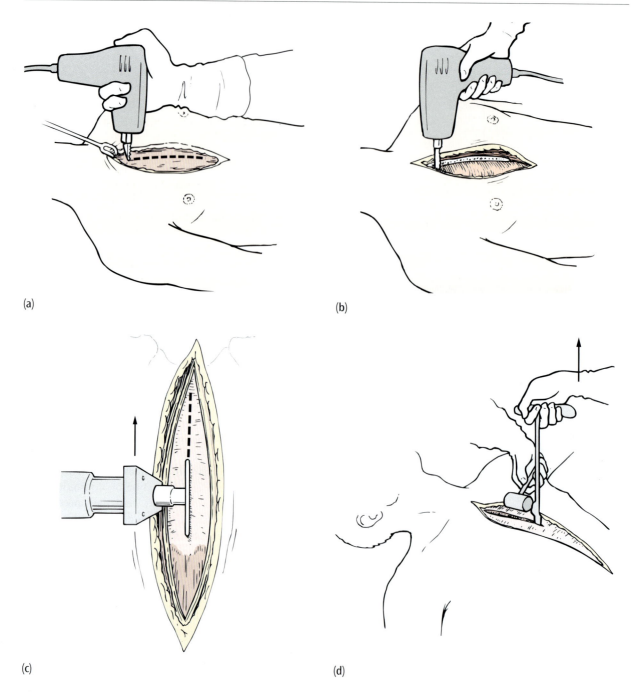

(a)

(b)

(c)

(d)

Figure 9.9 *Specialized instruments are needed to open the sternum. (a, b) The sternum may be opened from either above or below using a vertical cutting saw. The 'toe' of the instrument is positioned beneath the sternum and elevated as the sternum is cut. This lessens inadvertent injury to substernal structures. (c) The oscillating saw is commonly used in orthopedics or in reoperative cardiac surgery. Its advantage is the fact that it does not usually cut soft tissues. It is usually possible to feel when the inner table of the sternum is divided. (d) If no mechanical saw is available, a Lebsche knife or Gigli saw may be used. The Lebsche knife needs to be pulled upwards when striking; it commonly does not follow a straight line.*

carotid and distal subclavian arteries. The head is best turned to the opposite side. When this is undertaken, the skin and platysma are usually divided in a line corresponding to the anterior border of the sternomastoid muscle; if the subclavian vessels require exposure then the incision may be extended laterally parallel and superior to the clavicle. The sternomastoid muscle is

exposed and the sternal head divided from the inner aspect of the manubrium together with the underlying sternohyoid and sternothyroid muscles. On the right side, the junction of the subclavian and common carotid arteries can be readily identified. Further distal control of the right subclavian may require divisional resection of the medial third of the clavicle. The origins

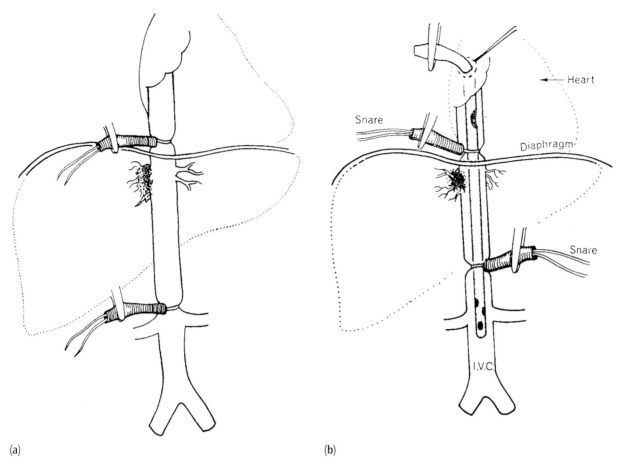

Figure 9.10 *(a, b) Isolation of lacerated hepatic veins through a sternolaparotomy incision. Snares are placed around the inferior vena cava and through the snares to provide continued systemic venous return whilst the ruptured liver and hepatic veins are repaired.*

of the left carotid artery and the left subclavian artery are exposed by dividing the superior limits of the pericardial flexion from the aortic arch, proceeding along the transverse arch of the aorta. The innominate vein may have to be retracted for this purpose. Very rarely does the innominate vein need to be divided but this can be done without serious consequence.

The median sternotomy can also be extended rapidly into the abdomen by continuing the midline incision inferiorly. The midline laparotomy is an excellent incision in the patient who has multiple penetrating injuries to both chest and abdomen. It is also invaluable in the control of bleeding from a severe liver laceration and torn hepatic veins when an intra-vena caval shunt can be employed to all systemic venous return (Fig 9.10).

When the surgical procedure is completed and hemostasis has been achieved, drains are placed. Drains are placed inferiorly, traversing the rectus sheath so that they lie between the peritoneum and the anterior abdominal wall, and positioned within the anterior mediastinum or pericardium; or placed, if the pleura has been opened, laterally directly into the pleural space. The sternum is approximated by using heavy

stainless steel wires swaged on a cutting needle. At least two wires should be placed through the manubrium. The author favors figure-of-eight sutures. After all sutures are placed, the sternum is approximated by twisting the wire suture and inverting the tip. The sheath, skin and subcutaneous tissues are then closed.

THORACOTOMY

The posterior or posterolateral thoracotomy is the standard incision for elective thoracic surgery; by varying the interspace, it is possible to deal with virtually any intrathoracic lesion. Minor variations termed limited anterior thoracotomy or lateral thoracotomy are named according to the extent of the incision – whether more anterior or lateral – and these are chosen depending upon the expected pathology. The trachea and major bronchi, as well as the intrathoracic esophagus, can be dealt with from the right. The left-sided approach provides exposure to the proximal left subclavian artery, the distal aortic arch and descending thoracic aorta and the lower third of the esophagus.

A double lumen endotracheal tube is advantageous but is not necessary in all instances. Intravenous access lines should be placed on the thoracotomy side; the arm, neck and upper chest are more accessible to the anesthesiologist; if a pneumothorax or hemothorax is induced by attempts at subclavian vein or jugular vein puncture, this will be on the same side as the thoracotomy.

The patient is positioned on his side in the center of the operating table. A pad placed under the axilla assists in stabilizing the patient and additionally separates the uppermost ribs. The arms are positioned alongside the head – this extends the scapula forwards and upwards, improving exposure. The dependent leg is placed at a right angle and a pillow placed between the legs. The patient is fixed in position with sandbags placed anteriorly and posteriorly and a broad band of tape over the padded anterosuperior iliac crest (Fig 9.10).

There are a number of important landmarks which guide the skin incision and it is sometimes worthwhile marking these landmarks with a pen. The landmarks are the vertebral spine in the midline; the medial or vertebral border of the scapula; the angle of the scapula; and the inframammary fold. The incision sweeps posteriorly from the mid-axillary line in the inframammary crease, crosses 2–3 cm below the angle of the scapula and ends midway between the vertebral spines and the medial border of the scapula roughly 2–3 cm superior to the angle of the scapula. Coagulation divides the subcutaneous tissues, exposing the chest wall muscles. The muscle immediately exposed is the latissimus dorsi muscle which is divided in the line of the incision. A fatty layer is noted posteriorly and is divided, exposing more readily the posterior border of the serratus anterior muscle. This muscle is conserved as much as possible to preserve function – the digitations are swept off their rib attachments. The appropriate rib is selected by counting from either above or below. The chosen intercostal space is then entered, either in the midline, immediately above the rib or subperiostally. The author resects the posterior end of the rib to prevent fracturing the rib during spreading. Once the intercostal space is entered, the ribs are gently spread with a spreader. If there are pleural adhesions, these need to be freed adequately before spreading the ribs as tearing of the lung can result. In urgent situations where the pleura is fused, the lung may be mobilized in the extrapleural plane.

After adequate hemostasis is achieved, closure is undertaken. Usually two underwater drains are necessary: one anteriorly to evacuate air and another posteriorly to evacuate fluid. The entrance for these drains should be placed anterior to a line extending from the anterior superior iliac spine. This is more comfortable for the patient and drains are less likely to kink. The ribs are approximated with heavy interrupted absorbable sutures. A rib approximater may be necessary when tying the sutures. The muscles, subcutaneous tissues and skin are then closed in layers with running absorbable sutures.

REFERENCES

1. Brown SE, Gomez GA, Jacobson LE, Scherer T, 3rd, McMillan RA. Penetrating chest trauma: should indications for emergency room thoracotomy be limited? *Am Surg* 1996; **62**: 530–3.
2. Lorenz HP, Steinmetz B, Lieberman J, Schecoter WP, Macho JR. Emergency thoracotomy: survival correlates with physiologic status. *J Trauma* 1992; **32**: 780–5.
3. Purkiss SF, Williams M, Cross FW, Graham TR, Wood A. Efficacy of urgent thoracotomy for trauma in patients attended by a helicopter emergency medical service. *J R Coll Surg Edinb* 1994; **39**: 289–91.
4. Bodai BI. Comment on emergency thoracotomy: survival correlates with physiologic status. *J Trauma* 1992; **32**: 780–8.
5. Moore JB, Moore EE, Harken AH. Emergency department thoracotomy. In: Moore EE, Mattox KL, Feliciano DV (eds) *Trauma*. Stanford, CT: Appleton and Lange, 1991; 181–93.
6. Esposito TJ, Jurkovich GJ, Rice CLE. Reappraisal of emergency room thoracotomy in a changing environment. *J Trauma* 1991; **31**: 881–7.
7. Coghill TH, Moore EE, Millikan SE. Rationale for selective application of emergency room thoracotomy in trauma. *J Trauma* 1982; **23**: 453–9.
8. Renz BM, Stout MJ. Rapid right atrial cannulation for fluid infusion during resuscitative emergency department thoracotomy. *Am Surg* 1994; **60**: 946–9.
9. Moulton C, Pennycook A, Crawford R. Intracardiac therapy following emergency thoracotomy in the accident and emergency department: an experimental model. *Arch Emerg Med* 1992; **9**: 190–5.

10

Penetrating trauma: the heart and major vessels

ULRICH O VON OPPELL AND JAMES O FULTON

PENETRATING INJURIES OF THE HEART AND INTRAPERICARDIAL VESSELS

Penetrating injuries of the heart and major mediastinal vessels have become an increasing problem in civilian trauma practice (Fig 10.1). The increasing use of firearms has also resulted in more patients presenting in critical condition with complex cardiac injuries (Fig 10.2). Essential for successful treatment of these injuries is early recognition, immediate transport to hospital by whatever means available,[1] aggressive resuscitation and expeditious surgical intervention, underpinned by a thorough knowledge of the available surgical options.[2–5]

HISTORICAL NOTE

A penetrating wound of the heart was described as early as 950 BC by Homer in *The Iliad*.[6] The second century Greek physician Claudius Galen noted that left ventricular injuries were the most rapidly fatal of all cardiac injuries.[7] Nevertheless, surgery of the heart was thought to be neither possible nor ethically correct by eminent surgeons until the late nineteenth century.[8,9]

The first successful repair of a cardiac injury was done by Ludwig Rehn on 9 September 1896,[10] although first attempted in 1894.[11]

Epidemiology

The incidence of penetrating cardiac injuries varies widely, depending on the levels of civilian violence. In

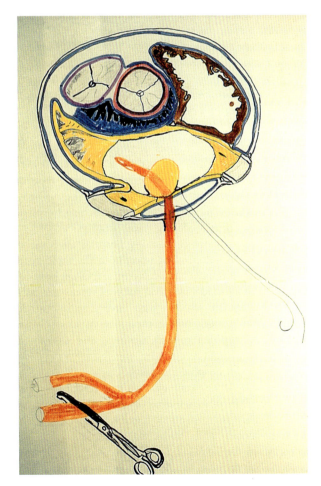

Figure 10.1 *Catheter balloon technique to occlude a laceration in the left atrium pending suture repair.*

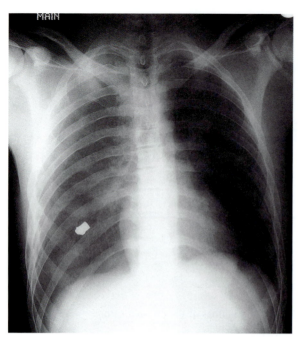

Figure 10.2 *Plain chest radiograph of a young man with a low velocity bullet entry wound in the left parasternal region in the third intercostal space. The bullet passed across the anterior mediastinum, entering the pericardium and the right atrial appendage. The bullet then exited the free wall of the right atrium and pericardium, passing though the right lung. There is a small pneumothorax on the left, a hemothorax on the right and a widened pericardial shadow. Surgical repair was eventually performed 3 hours after the shooting during which time cardiac tamponade and low pressure within the right atrium prevented exsanguination. (SWTC.)*

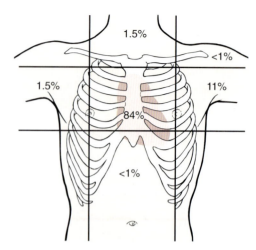

Figure 10.3 *The incidence of the site of the external penetrating wound, associated with confirmed cardiac injuries, in 445 patients treated for penetrating cardiac injuries at Groote Schuur Hospital is shown. The cardiac injury was the result of stab wounds in 98% of patients.*

South Africa, cardiac injuries occur in 6–7% of patients sustaining penetrating chest trauma, accounting for approximately 2000 penetrating cardiac injuries annually – 50 per million population.[12–14] The majority of victims (62–89%) succumb before reaching hospital, either at the scene or during transportation.[2,5,12–14]

Mortality of patients reaching hospital alive varies from 2% to 83% depending upon both the rapidity of transport to hospital,[1,15] as delay in arrival at hospital results in more dead-on-arrival patients versus critically ill but salvageable patients who have a high mortality,[1–3,12,13,16–23] as well as the incidence of more lethal gunshot as opposed to stab wounds, and associated injuries.[1,2,21,24] Right ventricular injuries are associated with the lowest hospital mortality.[12]

In South Africa, stab wounds are responsible for more than 90% of penetrating cardiac injuries, from an array of sharp instruments such as knives, screw drivers, bicycle spokes and traditional weapons.[12–14,25] By contrast, in the USA low velocity gunshot wounds are responsible for up to 70% of penetrating cardiac injuries,[1,3] although stab wounds still predominate in some centers.[4,22] Shotgun wounds and shrapnel injuries are currently rare in civilian practice.

Pathophysiology and clinical presentation

Location of external entrance wound

Patients with penetrating cardiac injuries usually have an external precordial or left chest penetrating wound (Fig 10.3). Nevertheless, cardiac injury can be associated with external penetrating stab wounds located anywhere in the thorax, back, neck or abdomen.[12,13,25–27] Gunshot entry wounds are well known to be poor indicators of associated internal visceral injuries, as bullets pursue unpredictable paths (Fig 10.4).[1,26] A cardiac injury should be considered whenever a projectile may have passed close to or through the mediastinum. In addition, secondary missiles can cause injury remote from the original path, if a bullet strikes bone.

CARDIAC WOUND

The most commonly injured cardiac chamber in clinical series is the right ventricle, followed by the left ventricle, atria and intrapericardial major vessels (Fig 10.5).[4,12,13,15,21,25,28] Coronary artery injuries occur in 2–10% of penetrating cardiac injuries, most commonly the left anterior descending coronary artery.[12,13,25,29,30] Clinically significant intracardiac injuries such as intracardiac fistulae and valvar injuries occur in 5–28% of patients, depending upon postoperative investigation and follow-up,[4,25,30–34] and are more frequently noted in gunshot compared to stab wounds.[27,35]

Penetrating cardiac injuries result in hemorrhage into the pericardial space, and the clinical presentation depends upon whether or not blood accumulates in the pericardial space. If there is free egress of blood into the pleural space or externally through the chest wound, then the patient will manifest hemorrhage and hypo-

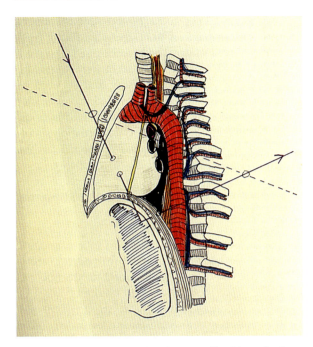

Figure 10.4 *Diagram showing the unpredictable path of a low velocity bullet through the chest. The bullet entered the left parasternal area, passed through the right ventricle with ricochet off the upper aspect of the diaphragm, which altered its path to exit the posterior chest wall. Entry and exit wounds did not predict the path of this missile.*

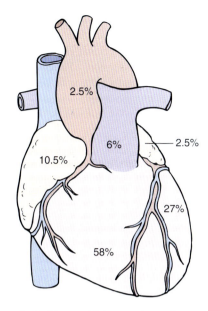

Figure 10.5 *The incidence of injury to the various cardiac chambers in 445 patients treated for penetrating cardiac injuries at Groote Schuur Hospital is shown. The cardiac injury was the result of stab wounds in 98% of patients. Multiple chambers were injured in 5% of patients, and the incidence of coronary artery injuries was also 5%.*

volemia. However, if blood accumulates in the pericardial space, because of sealing of the pericardial wound by clot or surrounding mediastinal tissue, then the presentation will be that of cardiac tamponade (65–80% of patients; Table 10.1).[12,13,25,28]

Pathophysiology of patients presenting with cardiac tamponade

Post-traumatic cardiac tamponade requires 100–200 ml of intrapericardial blood.[24,36] This accumulation of blood raises intrapericardial pressure and compresses the low pressure atria and right ventricle, resulting in

impaired diastolic ventricular filling with consequent reduced cardiac output. Sympathetic augmentation of myocardial contractility combined with this reduced diastolic coronary perfusion (secondary to diminished cardiac output) results in subendocardial ischemia. Raised intrapericardial pressure also independently decreases the diastolic coronary perfusion gradient, causing further myocardial ischemia and diminished myocardial contractility.[37] The rapidity of the development of cardiac tamponade depends upon both the size of the cardiac and pericardial wounds, as well as the contractile pressure of the injured cardiac chamber. Cardiac tamponade is more common with stab wounds as opposed to gunshot wounds.[1]

Cardiac tamponade is a clinical diagnosis. The classic signs of cardiac tamponade are Beck's triad,[38] muffled heart sounds, distended neck veins (raised central venous pressure) and hypotension, which are noted in 10–70% of tamponade patients.[12,39] Useful additional clinical signs include pulsus paradoxus (reduction of pulse pressure more than 15–20 mmHg with inspiration) and Kussmaul's sign (elevation of the central venous pressure with inspiration).[36] Pulsus paradoxus occurs as a result of an accentuated reduction in stroke volume from reduced venous return to the 'preload-dependent' left side of the heart with inspiration.[36] Non-specific signs of shock are usually also present, which include tachycardia, hypotension, cold peripheries, mental obtundation and poor urine output.[12,13,17,27]

Patients with stab wounds presenting with cardiac tamponade have a better prognosis than hypovolemic

Table 10.1 *Incidence and mortality of 445 patients treated for penetrating cardiac injuries at Groote Schuur Hospital, grouped according to their initial clinical presentation on hospital admission*

Clinical presentation	Incidence (%)	Mortality (%)
Moribund	13	63
Hypovolemia	12	22*
Cardiac tamponade		
Unstable	43	6
Stable	51	2

The cardiac injury was the result of stab wounds in 98% of patients.
*P <0.05 compared to either stable or unstable tamponade patients.

patients,[12,14,18] as cardiac tamponade contains the cardiac hemorrhage, and circulation is maintained for a longer period provided critical elevation of pericardial pressure does not develop. Patients with cardiac tamponade, who initially appear to be relatively stable hemodynamically, however, may decompensate suddenly and surgery should not be delayed once the diagnosis is made.

Pathophysiology of patients presenting with hemorrhage and hypovolemia

Patients with cardiac wounds and free egress of blood from the pericardial cavity present with ongoing hemorrhage and hypovolemia. Gunshot cardiac wounds are more frequently associated with hypovolemic shock than stab wounds.[1,23,25] These patients may have similar aforementioned non-specific clinical signs of shock but with a low central venous pressure. There is usually also an associated large hemothorax as a result of a transpleural pericardial defect.

Patients initially presenting with hypovolemia may also have an element of cardiac tamponade, which is not obvious in the hypovolemic patient until after volume resuscitation.

CLINICAL PRESENTATION

Victims with penetrating cardiac injuries can be grouped into three categories as outlined in Table 10.1. Moribund patients should exhibit at least one vital sign of life (respiratory efforts, cardiac activity, reactive pupils) on arrival in the hospital resuscitation area or have been alive immediately prior to hospital arrival whilst being transported.[40,41] Assessment of pupillary reactivity is important in the decision as to whether or not to resuscitate these patients.[40] Patients with cardiac tamponade may present in a clinical spectrum ranging from a relatively stable hemodynamic condition with minimal signs of tamponade to that of severe shock.

Hospital mortality is higher in patients presenting with hypovolemia as opposed to cardiac tamponade (Table 10.1).

Diagnosis and initial management

The diagnosis of a penetrating cardiac injury must be considered in all patients who have a penetrating wound of the chest, neck or upper abdomen, and who manifest cardiovascular instability either as tamponade or hypovolemic shock.

There must be immediate clinical confirmation simultaneous with resuscitation. Advanced life support principles should be applied with securing of airway, breathing and circulation, as well as insertion of wide bore intravenous lines and a central venous catheter. External hemorrhage should be controlled with compression until surgery can be performed. Oxygen is administered by mask to the adequately ventilating patient who can maintain his airway, and the need for endotracheal intubation is determined by associated injuries, level of consciousness and degree of hemodynamic instability. Muscle relaxants and sedation should be avoided in patients with cardiac tamponade, as this can result in precipitous cardiovascular collapse.

The indications for resuscitative emergency room anterolateral thoracotomy include moribund patients, or patients who suddenly decompensate hemodynamically in the resuscitation area.[5,41–45] The objectives of emergency room thoracotomy are to relieve tamponade, control hemorrhage, perform open cardiac massage, occlude the descending aorta for treatment of shock, and rapid intracardiac fluid infusion.[42]

A chest radiograph should be taken in patients not requiring emergency thoracotomy, primarily to confirm the central venous catheter position and to detect any associated hemo- or pneumothorax requiring tube thoracostomy drainage. Chest radiographic features of penetrating cardiac injury (globular heart shadow) are non-diagnostic. Numerous electrocardiogram (ECG) abnormalities are described in patients with penetrating cardiac injuries, but again their non-specific nature does not contribute to making the diagnosis.[21]

Of patients sustaining penetrating cardiac injuries from stab wounds, 18–35% are asymptomatic or hemodynamically stable after initial resuscitation, with few signs of cardiac tamponade, and pose a diagnostic dilemma.[46] Moreover, the clinical signs of cardiac tamponade may be unreliable in the emergency situation.[47] The differential diagnoses that need to be considered and excluded are listed in Table 10.2.

Table 10.2 *The differential diagnosis of an elevated central venous pressure (CVP) following penetrating chest trauma*

Raised central venous pressure after penetrating trauma
True increased central venous pressure
• Cardiac tamponade (signs of shock, pulsus paradoxus, Kussmaul's sign, soft heart sounds)
• Overzealous volume resuscitation (hemodynamic stability, increased urine output, easily palpable apex beat)
• Tension pneumothorax (resonant hemithorax, mediastinal shift to the opposite side)
False increased central venous pressure
• Central venous catheter tip in the right ventricle (rapid oscillation of the CVP water column, position on chest radiograph)
• Combative, straining patient from alcohol intoxication, hypoxia, or acidosis

Useful additional confirmatory clinical signs are shown in parentheses.

THE ROLE OF ECHOCARDIOGRAPHY

Echocardiography can establish the presence of pericardial fluid and suggest cardiac tamponade, as well as detect intracardiac shunts and valve injuries with color-flow Doppler.[35,48,49] However, false-negative echocardiograms have been reported in up to 20% of penetrating cardiac trauma patients,[46] and echocardiograms may therefore be inconclusive.

THE ROLE OF PERICARDIOCENTESIS

Pericardiocentesis was originally suggested by Blalock and Ravitch in 1943.[50] However, early thoracotomy has replaced pericardiocentesis as the primary therapeutic intervention of choice since 1966, with a concomitant decrease in mortality.[24] Therapeutic pericardiocentesis in the deteriorating cardiac tamponade patient is rarely successful because of intrapericardial clotted blood,[12,24,27,28,45] and is thus today only indicated as a temporary therapeutic intervention in patients being transported who cannot undergo an emergency thoracotomy.[42]

Diagnostic pericardial aspiration in penetrating cardiac trauma is also unreliable, with up to 50% false-positive or false-negative results.[28,47] Procedural complications include cardiac laceration, ventricular fibrillation, as well as inadvertent pleural and abdominal penetration with viscus injury.

Technique

The preferred technique for temporary therapeutic pericardiocentesis is to position the patient with the head elevated 30–50° and to insert a long 16–18 gauge intravenous infusion cannula in the angle between the left side of the xiphisternum and adjacent left costal margin with the point directed towards the left shoulder, 45° to the skin (Fig 10.6). If possible, an ECG lead should be connected to the needle hub with continuous ECG monitoring to detect epicardial contact by the needle, which manifests as ST segment elevation. Once blood is obtained, the soft plastic cannula sheath may be advanced over the needle to reduce the likelihood of cardiac injury, and thereafter as much blood as possible is aspirated.

THE ROLE OF DIAGNOSTIC SUBXIPHOID PERICARDIAL WINDOW

The diagnostic procedure of choice in patients suspected of having cardiac injuries who do not manifest all the typical clinical features of cardiac tamponade is a subxiphoid pericardial window.[46,47,51] Subxiphoid pericardiotomy is a safe, expeditious and accurate method of identifying hemopericardium, with no false-positive and few false-negative results, low morbidity, and should be used liberally.[46,47,51] The procedure is carried out under local[4] or light general

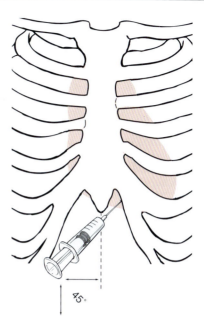

Figure 10.6 *The technique of performing a temporary therapeutic pericardiocentesis is shown. The patient is positioned semi-upright, a 16–18 gauge intravenous cannula is advanced in the angle between the xiphisternum and left costal margin towards the left shoulder, 45° to the skin.*

anesthesia in the operating room. The patient should be cleaned and draped so that, if necessary, immediate extension into a median sternotomy can be done.

Technique

The surgical incision is a 5–6 cm midline incision centered over the xiphoid process, dividing the rectus sheath to expose preperitoneal fat.[46] The xiphisternum can be excised or reflected cephalad once dissected free of its diaphragmatic attachments. The pericardium is now visible and is grasped with hemostats and incised for ± 1 cm with a scalpel, taking care to avoid injury to the underlying myocardium (Fig 10.7).

- If blood is encountered in the pericardial space, a median sternotomy should be done.
- If there is no hemopericardium, then the pericardium is closed, and the wound closed in layers without drains.[46,47]

Currently, the natural history of untreated cardiac injuries is unclear as to whether select patients with cardiac injury and minimal pericardial bleeding require sternotomy and definitive repair as opposed to only pericardial drainage.[46] Nevertheless, non-bleeding epicardial injuries close to the pericardial window do not require further exploration.[4]

SUMMARY

The management of patients suspected of having penetrating cardiac injuries following initial resuscita-

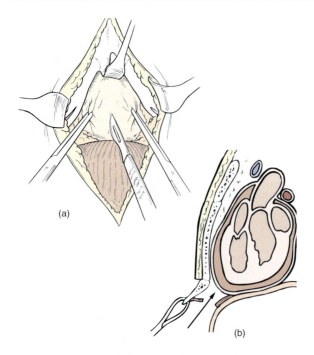

(a)

(b)

Figure 10.7 *(a) The technique of performing a diagnostic subxiphisternal pericardiotomy is shown. The rectus sheath has been divided and the xiphisternum reflected cephalad. The pericardium grasped in hemostats is being incised with a scalpel. (b) The lateral view of procedure.*

tion varies according to the initial clinical presentation, hemodynamic stability and certainty of diagnosis (Fig 10.8).

- Moribund patients with at least one vital sign and who do not immediately respond to volume replacement or deteriorating patients, should undergo emergency room thoracotomy rather than any attempt at temporary therapeutic pericardiocentesis.
- Patients with precordial stab wounds, unexplained

raised central venous pressure or hypotension should be considered to have a cardiac injury until excluded by subxiphoid pericardial window.[47]

Surgical approach and techniques

The surgical approach to a patient with a penetrating cardiac wound should be viewed in distinct phases/decision-making processes. Suture repair of the cardiac wound itself should not be done hastily, but rather with precise and deliberate care (Table 10.3).

SURGICAL INCISION

The optimal surgical incision for exploration of penetrating cardiac injuries depends upon the clinical presentation (tamponade or hemorrhage), likelihood of associated pulmonary injuries (precordial or lateral external wound), and hemodynamic stability (emergency room or operating room thoracotomy).

Anterolateral thoracotomy

An anterolateral thoracotomy on the side of the penetrating injury is indicated in moribund or deteriorating patients suspected of having cardiac tamponade, as well as patients presenting with pleural hemorrhage and lateral chest entry wounds, as the alternative source may be pulmonary hilar injuries which are more easily managed through a thoracotomy.

The chest wall is incised over the left fourth or fifth intercostal space, beginning adjacent to the sternum and extending to the mid-axillary line. The subcutaneous tissue and muscles are divided over the intercostal space. A rib spreader is inserted, exposing the usually tense pericardium. The incision can be extended into the contralateral hemithorax with division of the

Figure 10.8 *Decision-making flow diagram for patients with suspected penetrating cardiac injuries.*

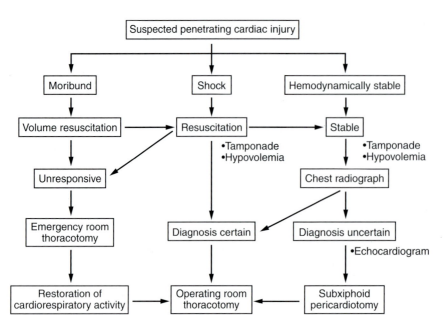

Table 10.3 *Stepwise approach to penetrating cardiac injuries*

Decide on surgical incision
 Median sternotomy
  Cardiac tamponade
  Hemorrhage with hypovolemia in the presence of
  precordial wounds or wounds above the third costal
  cartilage
 Anterolateral thoracotomy
  Emergency room thoracotomy
  Hemorrhage with hypovolemia in the presence of
  lateral chest entry wounds

Relieve cardiac tamponade
 Incise distended pericardium, and extend with scissors
  Adequate suction

Control hemorrhage
 Ventricle: light digital pressure on wound
 Atrium: tangential vascular clamp; traction suture
 Inflow occlusion

Restore calm

Suture cardiac wound
 Polypropylene suture with buttressing pledgets; Dacron,
 Teflon, pericardium
 Avoid occluding proximal coronary arteries
  Horizontal pledgeted under-running sutures
  Suture repair of coronary artery laceration during
  temporary induced ventricular fibrillation
  Saphenous vein coronary artery bypass on the beating
  heart

Prior to closing surgical incision
 Exclude other cardiac and extracardiac injuries

Table 10.4 *Pitfalls of anterolateral thoracotomy*

Thoracotomy incision
 Too high: poor exposure, transection of pectoralis major
 muscle
 Too low: poor exposure, diaphragmatic injury

Pericardial incision
 Phrenic nerve transection
 Iatrogenic cardiac injury from overly aggressive
 pericardial incision

Closure of thoracotomy
 Failure to ligate transected internal mammary artery
 with delayed hemorrhage

---

lower sternum, if necessary, for repair of poorly visualized contralateral cardiac injuries.[3]

Patients undergoing resuscitative thoracotomy in the emergency room should ideally be transferred to the operating room for complete inspection, repair and closure of the thoracotomy after initial stabilization.[43] Pitfalls associated with an anterolateral, especially emergency resuscitative, thoracotomy are listed in Table 10.4.

Median sternotomy

A median sternotomy is the appropriate incision for patients presenting with tamponade, precordial entry wounds as well as wounds superior to the third costal cartilage. A median sternotomy provides excellent exposure of the entire heart, major vessels and right lung hilum.

The midline incision extends from the suprasternal notch to just below the xiphisternum. Significant venous bleeding is usually encountered after skin incision in patients manifesting cardiac tamponade, especially from the anterior communicating jugular vein, and time should not be wasted trying to secure hemostasis. The sternum is divided in the midline with a vertical or circular oscillating saw or Lebsche knife

(hammer and vertical chisel). Deviation from the midline must be avoided in order to prevent transection of the costal cartilages which can cause significant postoperative complications of chondritis, parasternal pain and chest wall instability.

A median sternotomy can be easily extended cephalad into the neck along the anterior border of the sternocleidomastoid muscles or supraclavicularly for further exposure of the major mediastinal and neck vessels.

Prior to closure, the pleura on the side of the penetrating injury should be opened and explored, to exclude an associated injury of the internal mammary artery and other extracardiac structures. The median sternotomy is closed by approximating the sternum with 6–8 interrupted non-absorbable sutures – preferably no. 5 or 6 stainless steel wire or, failing this, no. 5 multifilament polyester suture, passed around or through each sternal half.

RELIEVE CARDIAC TAMPONADE

The tense distended hemopericardium should be initially incised with a scalpel. Released blood obscures the surgical field and the pericardium is opened further with scissors, whilst the fingers of the opposite hand displace the heart posteriorly to avoid iatrogenic cardiac injury. The pericardium is incised in the midline, and inferiorly extended laterally in the form of an inverted T in a median sternotomy approach, and incised anterior to the phrenic nerve in an anterolateral thoracotomy approach. Relief of cardiac tamponade usually produces dramatic improvement in the patient's hemodynamic condition. Remaining intrapericardial blood and clot is then quickly evacuated with strong suction and the source of bleeding located.

IDENTIFY AND CONTROL CARDIAC HEMORRHAGE

Hemorrhage from a wound of the aorta, pulmonary artery or ventricle is usually spurting obviously, and

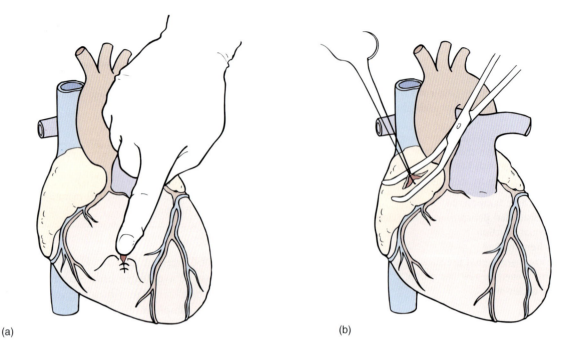

(a)   (b)

Figure 10.9 *(a) Illustration showing digital compression controlling hemorrhage from a penetrating wound of the right ventricle. Suturing of the ventricular wound has been commenced by exposing a small section. (b) Illustration showing a laceration of the right atrium which has been tented up, by a rapidly inserted traction suture, to aid the application of a tangential vascular clamp.*

easily controlled by relatively light digital pressure (Fig 10.9a). The wound is then sutured under the occluding finger. Tangential vascular clamps are useful for the pulmonary artery or aorta but should never be used on the relatively friable ventricular muscle. Standard 6 mm skin staples may be helpful to temporarily rapidly control ventricular wound hemorrhage during emergency room thoracotomy,[52] but should be replaced with secure suture repair in the operating room.

The source of hemorrhage when originating from the atria, vena cavae or pulmonary veins is less obvious as there is a continued 'welling up' of blood in the pericardial cavity. Rapid and careful examination using a strong suction nozzle is necessary. Atrial lacerations can be difficult to control both digitally and with tangential vascular clamps. Application of a vascular clamp is aided by initially grasping the edges of atrial lacerations with forceps or rapidly inserting traction sutures so as to 'tent' the atrial wall (Fig 10.9b). A 30 ml Foley urinary catheter, Fogarty embolectomy catheter or endotracheal tube inserted into the atrial laceration and inflated with subsequent traction is an alternative method to control bleeding, but in our experience is rarely necessary.

If the above methods are not adequate in identifying and controlling ongoing massive hemorrhage, then caval inflow occlusion for up to 3–4 minutes should be used (Fig 10.10).[28] Both vena cavae are occluded with atraumatic vascular clamps or by the surgical assistant pinching the great veins between his index and middle finger. Cardiac output and hemorrhage immediately

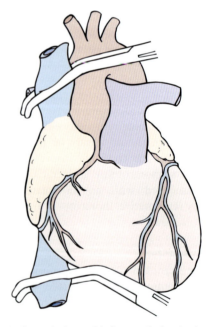

Figure 10.10 *The technique of inflow occlusion is shown. Both the superior and inferior vena cavae have been occluded by a vascular clamp, thus reducing blood flowing into the heart and consequently cardiac output as well. Significantly reduced cardiac output and cerebral perfusion should not be maintained for longer than 3–4 minutes if cerebral ischemic damage is to be prevented.*

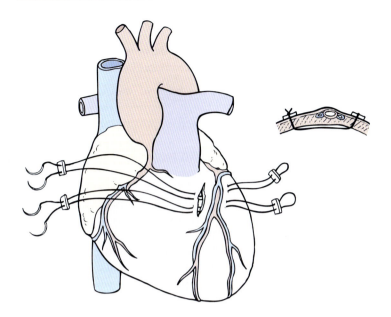

Figure 10.11 *Illustration of a right ventricular stab wound situated close to the left anterior descending coronary artery. Horizontal mattress polypropylene sutures buttressed with Teflon pledgets have been inserted so as to under-run the adjacent coronary artery, and the lateral cross-sectional view shows no obstruction of the coronary artery.*

diminish, allowing identification and control of most cardiac lacerations.

The cardiac wound may already have clotted and no longer be bleeding at surgery in some patients. These wounds should nevertheless be sutured.

SUTURING CARDIAC WOUNDS

A double armed 2/0–4/0 non-absorbable suture, polypropylene or braided polyester, on an atraumatic needle is used to suture the heart or great vessels with simple, figure-of-eight, horizontal mattress or running sutures. Ventricular muscle is surprisingly soft and friable, especially for a tense inexperienced surgeon, and therefore it is advisable to use horizontal mattress sutures with supporting pledgets to prevent sutures cutting through the myocardium (Fig 10.11). Teflon felt pledgets or 0.5 × 1.0 cm pledgets cut from the patient's own pericardium can be used. Widely spaced deep bites are placed approximately 3–5 mm from the edge of the cardiac laceration.

If the cardiac wound is being controlled with digital pressure, the finger is gradually moved to expose small sections which are sutured sequentially (Fig 10.9a); either the assistant ties the sutures down or all sutures are inserted, gently held taut by the assistant, prior to the surgeon tying them individually.

Cardiopulmonary bypass, if immediately available, may very occasionally be necessary to repair inaccessible wounds in the posterior atrioventricular groove.[18,27,53]

Coronary artery injuries

Coronary artery injuries occur in 2–10% of patients sustaining penetrating cardiac trauma,[13,25,29,30,54] and predominantly involve the left anterior descending coronary artery.

Cardiac wounds adjacent to major proximal coronary arteries should be sutured with horizontal

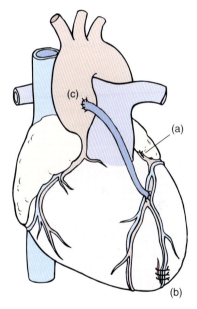

Figure 10.12 *Illustration of three techniques used to repair wounds involving coronaries. (a) A laceration of the proximal left anterior descending coronary artery has been repaired with a single 6/0 polypropylene suture. (b) The left anterior descending coronary artery has been bypassed with a reversed saphenous vein conduit, because of a proximal injury that could not be repaired without occluding the proximal left anterior descending coronary artery. (c) A wound involving the distal left anterior descending coronary artery has been repaired by sutures that have obliterated the coronary artery.*

mattress sutures which under-run the coronary vessel, to avoid occlusion of the coronary artery (Fig 10.11).

Small lacerations of the proximal coronary arteries can be repaired with 6/0 or 7/0 polypropylene sutures on the beating heart with or without inflow occlusion (Fig 10.12).[54] Ventricular fibrillation induced by an electrical fibrillator with leads attached to the epicardium can also improve visualization and allow more accurate fine suture placement for repair of coronary artery injuries, but with a time limitation of 3–4 minutes to avoid cerebral injury. An essential of this technique is the availability of both an electrical fibrillator as well as a defibrillator with internal paddles.

Cardiac wounds with proximal major coronary artery lacerations, although uncommon, usually manifest with low cardiac output, ECG abnormalities and at surgical exploration the relevant myocardium appears cyanotic and akinetic. These proximal major coronary artery injuries may require reversed saphenous vein coronary artery bypass grafting with or without the aid of cardiopulmonary bypass (Fig 10.12).[53–55] Nevertheless, the overall outcome for patients treated with emergency cardiopulmonary bypass is not significantly better than for those treated with coronary artery ligation alone.[29]

Injuries of minor or distal coronary arteries can be safely suture ligated, accepting the inevitable small myocardial infarction (Fig 10.12).[54]

Intracardiac injuries

Intracardiac injuries include ventricular septal defects, valvular injuries, as well as coronary and aortic cameral fistulae, and occur on average in 5–28% of penetrating cardiac trauma victims.[4,25,31–35] Intracardiac injuries may be suggested at surgery by through-and-through wounds or palpable thrills.[32] Nevertheless, immediate exploration and repair with cardiopulmonary bypass is seldom indicated.[33]

Routine postoperative echocardiography reveals abnormalities in up to 31% of patients; however, many of these patients do not require further treatment.[31] Hence, in most units, postoperative heart murmurs or signs of cardiac failure following repair of penetrating cardiac injuries are indications for further investigation. Delayed clinical presentation days or months after the incident of penetrating trauma is also not uncommon,[31] even in the absence of previous emergency cardiorrhaphy,[32] possibly because small initially clinically inapparent fistulae progressively enlarge.[34]

Repair of intracardiac injuries should be undertaken electively after delineating the exact pathology by echocardiography and cardiac catheterization, as multiple lesions are frequent.[33,34] Elective repair is only indicated in symptomatic patients who have significant valvar injuries or intracardiac shunts greater than 40%.[33,34] Spontaneous closure of small traumatic ventricular septal defects has been documented.[56] The majority of significant post-traumatic intracardiac injuries can be repaired 6–12 weeks after injury with low mortalities, at which time the edges of the intracardiac defects are more clearly delineated from fibrosis.[32]

PRIOR TO CLOSING THE SURGICAL INCISION

The following points should be systematically carried out prior to closing the surgical incision.

- Always inspect the back of the heart to exclude through-and-through injuries (the majority of gunshot injuries and approximately 10% of stab wounds).
- Always feel for thrills to detect possible intracardiac injuries.
- Always open the pleural space on the side of the penetrating injury to exclude associated non-cardiac injuries, and specifically to exclude lacerations of the internal mammary or intercostal arteries.
- Always remember to ligate the internal mammary artery after emergency anterolateral thoracotomy.

Two drainage catheters (28–32 gauge) should be inserted, one in the pericardial cavity posteroinferiorly to the heart and one in the anterior mediastinum. The superior two-thirds of the pericardial incision is usually reapproximated.

Conservative management of penetrating cardiac injuries

Conservative non-operative management of penetrating cardiac injuries has been associated with high late mortality from clot lysis, secondary hemorrhage and late tamponade, and is therefore not recommended.[17,26] Nevertheless, select patients with echocardiographic pericardial fluid and minimal clinical manifestations of cardiac tamponade, or pneumopericardium, may be managed conservatively.[50,57,58] However, these patients must be monitored in a high-care setting for a minimum of 3–5 days, as late deterioration may be sudden and surgical intervention is necessary in 14–50% of conservatively treated patients.[13,17] A risk of secondary cardiac tamponade remains for up to 6 weeks after the initial injury in these patients. Hence, we would rather perform at least a subxiphoid pericardiotomy in patients with suspected penetrating cardiac injuries.

Morbidity and mortality of penetrating cardiac injuries

The overall mortality following penetrating cardiac trauma, including prehospital deaths, is approximately 85%.[12] However, hospital mortality varies from 2 to 83%, depending upon admission status, mechanism of injury, site of cardiac injury and other associated injuries (see Table 10.1).[14,20,23] Methods of quantifying both the physiological and anatomical severity of the injury can provide objective methods of evaluating these patients.[20,59]

Table 10.5 *Complications of penetrating cardiac injuries*

Cardiac failure	Cerebral anoxia
Intracardiac injury	Wound infection
Ventricular aneurysm	Mediastinitis
Infective endocarditis	Respiratory infection
Conduction disturbances	ARDS
Pericardial effusion	Pleural effusion
Post-cardiotomy syndrome	Hemorrhagic diathesis
Constrictive pericarditis	

The morbidity in survivors of penetrating cardiac trauma is 27–37% (Table 10.5),[4,22,59] and is primarily related to the duration of poor cerebral perfusion from inadequate cardiac output, specific cardiac chambers involved and associated injuries. Patients surviving emergency room thoracotomy have a 0–58% incidence of neurological deficits on hospital discharge.[41,53] Furthermore, 11–40% of patients undergoing surgery develop wound infections, despite many emergency room thoracotomies having had no prior skin preparation.[12,53] Late pericardial constriction requiring pericardiectomy has been reported in 5% of surviving patients.[53]

Intracardiac missiles

Intracardiac missiles (bullets, pellets, secondary shrapnel) either lodge in the myocardium following direct penetration of the heart, or embolize to the heart after entry into a systemic vein.[21,60,61] Free intracavitary missiles may embolize to the pulmonary or systemic arterial circulation, depending on the chamber in which they are situated. The decision to remove cardiac missiles must be individualized depending on the site and size of the missiles, the presence of associated complications or risk thereof. Complications include infective endocarditis, hemolysis, conduction disturbances, erosion into surrounding vascular structures, embolization of the missile, and secondary thrombus and cardiac neurosis.[60]

MANAGEMENT OF INTRACARDIAC MISSILES

All symptomatic missiles should be removed. The management of asymptomatic missiles should be individualized, as asymptomatic missiles are well tolerated in select patients.[60] If echocardiography or cardiac catheterization suggests a negligible risk of either missile embolization (moving in concert with the heart without tumbling[61]) or thromboembolism (by virtue of encapsulation), then intracavitary missiles partially or completely embedded in myocardium should be left *in situ* unless complications develop.[21,60]

Free intracavitary missiles in the left side of the heart must be removed urgently, because of the potential risk of fatal systemic embolization.[60] Intracavitary right ventricular missiles entrapped in muscular trabeculations can be observed,[61] although embolization to the pulmonary circulation does occasionally occur. However, if the missile traversed a hollow viscus prior to embolization to the right heart, then removal is mandatory, because of the infective risk.[60]

PENETRATING INJURIES OF THE EXTRAPERICARDIAL MAJOR VESSELS

HISTORICAL NOTE

Dshanelidze did the first successful repair of a penetrating thoracic aortic injury in Russia in 1922.[62] Penetrating thoracic vascular injuries were universally fatal in both World Wars as well as during the Korean War,[63–66] and only 15 successfully treated cases of extrapericardial thoracic aortic injuries were reported by 1969.[67] However, increasing civilian injuries to the major arteries at the level of the thoracic inlet are now reported.[26,68–74]

Epidemiology

Approximately 1.2% of patients sustaining sharp penetrating chest trauma have associated injuries to the non-pulmonary great vessels.[26] However, the lethal nature of penetrating non-pulmonary thoracic vascular injuries is evident in that only 1.4% of these patients survive.[26] The majority of victims succumb prior to hospital admission. Victims sustaining penetrating injuries of the aorta and its branches who reach hospital alive, however, have an in-hospital mortality of 5–17%.[73,74] Rapid transport to hospital with immediate resuscitation, which may include resuscitative thoracotomy, rapidity of preparation for operation, and adequacy of surgical exposure, are essential for satisfactory outcome and the reason for decreasing hospital mortalities for these injuries over the last few decades.[75,76]

Injury to the mediastinal vascular structures occurs as a result of gunshot, stab wounds and rarely iatrogenic injuries, and varies according to geographic location. In South Africa, currently approximately 4.8% of patients sustain gunshot wounds, whilst in the USA this proportion is considerably higher at 63.5–79%.[72,76,77] The more lethal nature of gunshot vascular wounds, especially if of high velocity, is well known.

Pathology and clinical presentation

The majority of patients sustaining penetrating mediastinal vascular injuries are young male victims of assault. In stab victims, the external entry wound is in

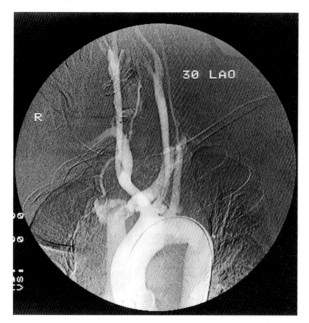

Figure 10.13 *An arch angiogram delineating a complex penetrating injury involving both the innominate vein and artery resulting in an arteriovenous fistula, as well as false aneurysms of the left common carotid and left subclavian arteries. (Reproduced with permission from the Society of Thoracic Surgeons (The Annals of Thorac Surgery 1997; 63, 557–9))*

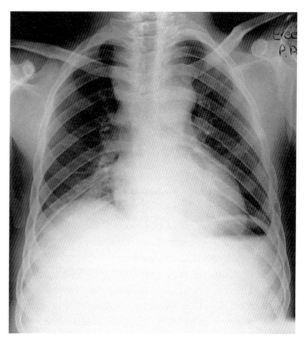

Figure 10.14 *Chest radiograph of a patient with a penetrating mediastinal vascular injury, showing widening of the superior mediastinum from the resultant hematoma.*

the neck in 70% of patients and may appear relatively small and innocuous – injury to the superior mediastinal vessels resulting from the assailant stabbing in a downward direction. Gunshot penetration of the mediastinum should be suspected in any patient in whom the path of the bullet passed through or close to the mediastinum.

The frequency of innominate arterial and venous injuries, or carotid and subclavian artery injuries varies between series,[74,78] and approximately 40% of patients have multiple arterial injuries.[73] Arteriovenous fistulae occur in up to 34% of patients following penetrating injuries,[74] particularly between the innominate artery and vein (Fig 10.13). Isolated venous injuries are rare, accounting for less than 10% of surgically operated major vessel injuries.

Patients with possible mediastinal vascular injury from penetrating injuries to the base of the neck or chest can present with one of the following scenarios:

- Moribund; often requiring resuscitative thoracotomy.
- Active bleeding – shock; exsanguinating hemorrhage, either into the chest or externally through the wound.
- Contained hemorrhage – stable mediastinal hematoma on chest radiography (Fig 10.14), with variable airway or circulatory compromise.

Important clinical signs suggestive of major vascular injuries are pulse deficits, brachial and cerebral

neurological deficits,[74] continuous murmurs over the precordium or neck as well as large cervical hematomas. Signs of cerebral ischemia are present in up to 35% of patients with carotid arterial injuries.[70] Nevertheless, the seriousness of the associated vascular injury may not be recognized unless a high index of suspicion is maintained, as up to 32% of patients with significant vascular injuries have no specific clinical signs.[70]

Diagnosis and initial management

The most critical factor for the survival of patients with significant vascular trauma is the time that elapses from injury to surgical control. Transport to the nearest appropriate facility should be without any delay for 'initial stabilization at the scene', that is, 'scoop and run'.[79]

Initial management includes securing the airway, establishing venous access and appropriately administering intravenous fluid and blood. Moribund patients who fail to respond to resuscitation, or suddenly decompensate, should undergo emergency anterolateral thoracotomy.

In many series, the majority of patients (approximately 60–70% of patients) are hemodynamically unstable with active bleeding and shock and require immediate surgical exploration without angiography.[72,75,77] An emergency method of controlling profuse hemorrhage from subclavian injuries is to

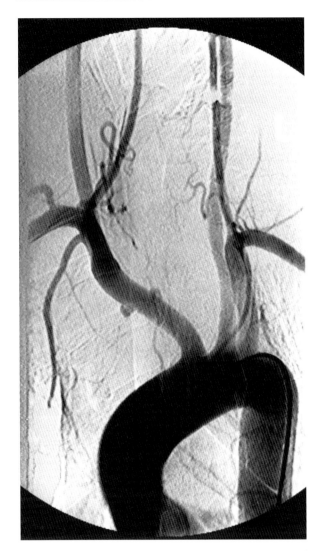

Figure 10.15 *Arch angiogram showing a simple through-and-through laceration of the innominate artery.*

Table 10.6 *Management of penetrating cervicothoracic vascular injuries*

Immediate exploration of wounds entering the mediastinum, manifesting ongoing hemorrhage
    Cervical incision: presumed vascular injury above the cricoid cartilage[82]
    Median sternotomy: presumed injury below the cricoid cartilage
Adequate operative exposure; use of adjunctive incisions without hesitation,[70,76,77] depending on the site of hemorrhage, associated injuries, and need for cardiac resuscitation
    Median sternotomy
    Anterolateral thoracotomy: control of proximal left subclavian artery
    Resection of the medial half of the clavicle; second part of the subclavian artery
Obtain proximal and distal vascular control prior to entering the overlying hematoma

later. Recent studies suggest that careful physical examination combined with color flow Doppler may be a reliable alternative method of evaluating penetrating neck injuries.

Large expanding mediastinal or cervical hematomas cause progressive tracheal compression in up to 15% of patients, and these patients should undergo early nasotracheal intubation.[76] Associated visceral injuries involving the trachea, esophagus, heart or lung occur in up to 66% of patients with major vascular injuries,[76] because of the close proximity of structures in the thoracic inlet, and should be actively excluded either clinically, radiologically or at surgical exploration because of the severe consequences of such missed injuries. Esophageal evaluation should ideally precede aortography.

Surgical management

Acute major penetrating thoracic arterial injuries require surgical repair. However, most venous injuries usually stop bleeding as a result of local compression by surrounding mediastinal tissues and hematoma, and do not generally require surgery unless there is an associated breach of the pleural space with ongoing hemorrhage. Table 10.6 summarizes the more important management considerations of external cervicothoracic wounds with possible mediastinal vascular injuries.

Air embolism - right-sided

Air embolism to the right side of the heart must be considered in any patient with a penetrating injury of the major systemic head and neck veins,[77] who presents with refractory low cardiac output. Air is compressible, and 50–150 ml of air will obstruct right ventricular and pulmonary artery forward flow. Furthermore, 20% of

insert a Foley's catheter through the penetrating entrance wound, blow up the bulb and then apply traction, thereby compressing the vessels against the clavicle and first rib. The initial investigation in stable patients is a chest radiograph to detect mediastinal hematoma, hemothoraces, pneumothoraces and air in the mediastinal tissues, the latter suggesting an associated tracheobronchial or esophageal injury. Thereafter, angiography delineates the vascular abnormality in 90% of cases, and is helpful in planning the operative approach (Figs 10.13 and 10.15),[73] as surgical exploration may require a relatively extensive operative procedure because of the difficulty of exposing the subclavian and innominate arteries. False-negative angiograms occur in up to 23% of patients studied;[78] thus, surgical exploration should still be considered despite a negative angiogram if there is a strong suspicion of significant mediastinal vascular injury.[71,78] Alternatively, progressive false aneurysm formation can be excluded by repeat angiography a few days normal individuals have a patent foramen ovale and thus right-sided air embolism can also result in left-sided systemic arterial air embolism, causing cardiac arrest or cerebrovascular accident. Air embolism might account for the high mortality associated with major venous injuries.[81]

Right-sided air embolism is diagnosed at thoracotomy by palpating crepitus and aspirating air from the pulmonary artery. Left-sided arterial air embolism is discussed in Chapter 11.

Anesthetic

An experienced anesthetist, blood available in the operating room and large bore venous access lines in the lower extremities are important in the successful management of these patients.[77] The airway should be secured with an endotracheal tube and tracheostomy avoided, as hemorrhage may be precipitated by breaching the mediastinal hematoma.[76]

The surgical team should be ready for immediate intervention on induction of anesthesia, as patients with large mediastinal hematomas can decompensate rapidly following the administration of muscle relaxants.

Surgical incision

Extending the neck and bracing the shoulders by means of a bolster placed between the scapulae facilitates exposure of the head and neck vessels. Numerous surgical approaches have been advocated for repair of penetrating thoracic vascular injuries,[69,83] as 73% of patients have injuries to more than one vessel and depending upon the precise location of the injuries.[76]

The incision of choice for cervicomediastinal vascular injuries is a median sternotomy (with or without neck extension), which provides adequate exposure for most injuries of the proximal mediastinal vessels (proximal right subclavian artery, innominate artery, ascending aorta and aortic arch).[69–72,84] Cervical wounds that have a lower suspicion of associated mediastinal vascular injuries should initially be explored by an oblique cervical incision parallel to the anterior border of sternocleidomastoid muscle, with or without lateral supraclavicular extension and resection of the medial half of the clavicle, which is adequate for 97% of common carotid and internal jugular vein injuries.[70] Alternatively, a supraclavicular approach on the respective side is indicated for distal subclavian arterial and venous injuries.[76]

Left subclavian arterial injuries can be managed through a variety of incisions and combinations thereof: a supraclavicular incision (adequate in 20–80% of subclavian injuries[70,76,81]), median sternotomy, anterolateral thoracotomy, or through a posterolateral thoracotomy, depending upon the part of the subclavian artery injured.[71,72,74,76] The sternocleidomastoid, anterior scalenus and strap muscles should be divided close to their sternocleidoclavicular attachments, to expose the distal part of the subclavian artery.[69] Exposure through

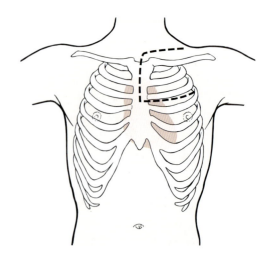

Figure 10.16 *Illustration showing the skin incisions making up the 'trap-door' incision; a left supraclavicular incision, a partial upper median sternotomy and a left anterolateral thoracotomy.*

an initial supraclavicular incision can be improved by either dislocation of the sternoclavicular joint, subperiosteal resection of the medial half of the clavicle, or extended with a median sternotomy.[81] The trapdoor incision (Fig 10.16) does not offer any additional advantage over a median sternotomy with or without dislocation of the sternoclavicular joint.

Descending thoracic aortic injuries are best approached through a left posterolateral thoracotomy.[13]

Temporary vascular shunts in mediastinal vascular injuries

A complete functioning circle of Willis is present in only 20–50% of individuals,[85] and thus carotid or innominate artery clamping may result in inadequate cerebral perfusion. Temporary vascular shunts (e.g. Javid shunt) have thus been advocated during surgical repair of carotid and innominate artery injuries.[67,68,72] Alternatively, innominate and other arterial injuries can be repaired by means of permanent extra-anatomical bypass techniques.[74,75] In our experience, the majority of arterial lacerations following stab wounds are simple lacerations requiring simple arteriorrhaphy following initial digital compression to control hemorrhage (Fig 10.15), and prolonged clamping necessitating temporary vascular shunts is rarely necessary.[86] If it is anticipated that clamping of the innominate or carotid artery will exceed 4 minutes because of more complex vessel transections, then distal carotid stump pressures should be measured and a temporary vascular shunt inserted if the measured pressure is less than 55 mmHg.

Alternatively, cardiopulmonary bypass with deep hypothermic circulatory arrest can be used if clamping of both carotid arteries is anticipated or in complex injuries involving the aortic arch and the origin of the head and neck vessels (Fig 10.13).[73,74,87]

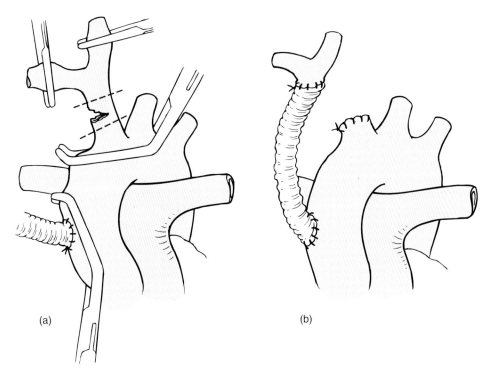

Figure 10.17 *(a) Illustration of a gunshot injury of the innominate artery with vascular clamps in situ. A woven Dacron graft has been anastomosed to the ascending aorta for an extra-anatomical bypass. (b) Completed surgical repair; extra-anatomical bypass of the innominate artery with closure of the proximal stump of the innominate artery.*

SURGICAL TECHNIQUE

Preoperative angiography assists in better surgical planning by delineating the extent of the injury and the possible need for temporary vascular shunts or cardiopulmonary bypass (Figs 10.13 and 10.15). On opening the chest, the surgeon is confronted with variable amounts of hemorrhage and hematoma with obliteration of the usual anatomical planes.

If massive hemorrhage is encountered, digital compression by the assistant can control most bleeding unless extensive injuries are present. The pericardium should be immediately opened in the midline, which provides quick access to the origin of the head and neck vessels, allowing control with encircling tapes or vascular clamps. The adjuncts of caval inflow occlusion, partial aortic cross-clamping, and artificially induced ventricular fibrillation can also be implemented if necessary.[72,88] The innominate vein should be identified, taped and, if necessary, divided. Once proximal control is obtained, hemorrhage lessens and distal control can be secured in a similar fashion. At this juncture the injury can be assessed and a decision regarding the need for a temporary vascular shunt made.

If a large mediastinal hematoma is found, similar maneuvers should be carried out to obtain proximal and distal vascular control but without disturbing the hematoma.

Repair of arterial injury

Simple arterial stab wounds can usually be repaired with monofilament polypropylene sutures (4/0 or 5/0) without difficulty. Transected arteries can usually be reanastomosed, if the vessel edges can be approximated without tension. However, vessel spasm often causes the vessel edges to retract and insertion of an interposition graft may be necessary. Insertion of prosthetic grafts (polytetrafluoroethylene) in a potentially contaminated surgical field, particularly if there is associated hollow viscus injury, is, however, not without risk.

The preferred approach for major proximal innominate arterial transection and gunshot injuries is insertion of a permanent extra-anatomical bypass from the intrapericardial aorta to the carotid and subclavian artery and suture closure of the proximal stump (Fig 10.17).[74,75,77] Extra-anatomical reconstruction of the innominate artery can be done prior to entering the hematoma, and does not require additional temporary vascular shunts or cardiopulmonary bypass.[75,77]

Subclavian artery injuries should be repaired directly or reconstructed, but, if necessary, can be ligated fairly safely.[83]

Carotid arterial injuries associated with neurological signs as a result of hemispherical cerebral hypoperfusion should be repaired as soon as possible, as neurological recovery can occur following restoration of normal cerebral blood flow.[84,85,89] Previous recommendations to ligate the injured carotid artery associated with preoperative neurological injury, because of concern for secondary hemorrhagic cerebral infarction, have not been validated in clinical studies.[85] However, patients admitted in coma have a poor prognosis, regardless as to whether ligation or reconstruction of the carotid arteries is undertaken.[84,85]

Repair of venous injury

The major thoracic veins should always be repaired with 5/0 polypropylene, particularly when the innominate vein has been divided for exposure. However, repair of venous structures can be difficult in the presence of massive hemorrhage from associated arterial lacerations, and obliterated anatomical planes from hematoma, and it thus may be expedient to suture ligate injured great veins. Nevertheless, ligation of the innominate and subclavian veins is associated with transient postoperative upper limb edema and superficial thrombophlebitis, necessitating arm elevation and local therapy,[77] although long-term sequelae are rare.[77,83]

REFERENCES

1. Buckman RF, Badellino MM, Mauro LH, et al. Penetrating cardiac wounds: prospective study of factors influencing initial resuscitation. *J Trauma* 1993; **34:** 717–27.
2. Kulshrestha P, Das B, Iyer KS, et al. Cardiac injuries – a clinical and autopsy profile. *J Trauma* 1990; **30:** 203–7.
3. Mitchell ME, Muakkassa FF, Poole GV, Rhodes RS, Griswold JA. Surgical approach of choice for penetrating cardiac wounds. *J Trauma* 1993; **34:** 17–20.
4. Johnson SB, Nielsen JL, Sako EY, Calhoon JH, Trinkle JK, Miller OL. Penetrating intrapericardial wounds: clinical experience with a surgical protocol. *Ann Thorac Surg* 1995; **60:** 117–21.
5. Mattox KL, Beall AC, Jordan GL, De Bakey ME. Cardiorrhaphy in the emergency center. *J Thorac Cardiovasc Surg* 1974; **68:** 886–95.
6. Homer. *The Iliad.* Book XIII; Vol II. Cambridge, MA: Harvard University Press, 1924.
7. Galen C. *De locis affectis* (translation RE Seigel). Basel: S Karger, 1976; 139.
8. Absolom KB. Theodor Billroth and cardiac surgery. *J Thorac Cardiovasc Surg* 1983; **86:** 451–2.
9. Paget S. *The Surgery of the Chest.* London: John Wright, 1896; 121.
10. Rehn L. Ueber penetrirende herzwunden und herznaht. *Arch Klin Chir* 1897; **55:** 315–29.
11. Cappelen A. Vulnus Cordis: suture of hjertet. *Norsk Magazin Laegevidenskaben* 1896; **6:** 285–8.
12. Demetriades D, Van der Veen BW. Penetrating injuries of the heart: experience over two years in South Africa. *J Trauma* 1983; **23:** 1034–41.
13. Robbs JV, Baker LW. Cardiovascular trauma. *Curr Probl Surg* 1984; **21(4):** 1–87.
14. De Groot M, Von Oppell UO. Management of penetrating injuries of the heart. *Trauma Emerg Med* 1992; **9:** 599–605.
15. Honigman B, Lowenstein SR, Moore EE, Roweder K, Pons P. The role of the pneumatic antishock garment in penetrating cardiac wounds. *JAMA* 1991; **266:** 2398–401.
16. Naughton MJ, Brissie RM, Bessey PQ, McEachern MM, Donald JM, Laws HL. Demography of penetrating cardiac trauma. *Ann Surg* 1989; **209:** 676–83.
17. Blatchford JW, Anderson RW. The evolution of the management of penetrating wounds of the heart. *Ann Surg* 1985; **202:** 615–23.
18. Moreno C, Moore EE, Majure JA, Hopeman AR. Pericardial tamponade: a critical determinant for survival following penetrating cardiac wounds. *J Trauma* 1986; **26:** 821–5.
19. Zakharia AT. Analysis of 285 cardiac penetrating injuries in the Lebanon war. *J Cardiovasc Surg* 1987; **28:** 380–3.
20. Ivatury RR, Nallathambi MN, Stahl WM, Rohman M. Penetrating cardiac trauma: quantifying the severity of anatomic and physiologic injury. *Ann Surg* 1987; **205:** 61–6.
21. Symbas PN. Cardiothoracic trauma. *Curr Probl Surg* 1991; **28(11):** 746–97.
22. Attar S, Suter CM, Hankins JR, Sequeira A, McLaughlin JS. Penetrating cardiac injuries. *Ann Thorac Surg* 1991; **51:** 711–16.
23. Coimbra R, Pinto MCC, Razuk A, Aguiar JR, Rasslan S. Penetrating cardiac wounds: predictive value of trauma indices and the necessity of terminology standardization. *Am Surg* 1995; **61:** 448–52.
24. Sugg WL, Rea WJ, Ecker RR, Webb WR, Rose EF, Shaw RR. Penetrating wounds of the heart: an analysis of 459 cases. *J Thorac Cardiovasc Surg* 1968; **56:** 531–45.
25. Scholtz HJ. Fatal penetrating injuries of the chest. Thesis MMed Path (Forens). Department of Forensic Medicine and Toxicology, University of Cape Town, South Africa, 1996.
26. Lerer LB, Knottenbelt JD. Preventable mortality following sharp penetrating chest trauma. *J Trauma* 1994; **37:** 9–12.
27. Symbas PN, Harlaftis N, Waldo WJ. Penetrating cardiac wounds: a comparison of different therapeutic methods. *Ann Surg* 1976; **183:** 377–81.
28. Trinkle JK, Toon RS, Franz JL, Arom KV, Grover FL. Affairs of the wounded heart: penetrating cardiac wounds. *J Trauma* 1979; **19:** 467–72.
29. Reissman P, Rivkind A, Jurim O, Simon D. Case report: the management of penetrating cardiac trauma with coronary artery injury – is cardiopulmonary bypass essential? *J Trauma* 1992; **33:** 773–5.
30. Fallahnejad M, Kutty ACK, Wallace HW. Secondary lesions of penetrating cardiac injuries: a frequent complication. *Ann Surg* 1980; **191:** 228–33.

31. Demetriades D, Charalambides C, Sareli P, Pantanowitz D. Late sequelae of penetrating cardiac injuries. *Br J Surg* 1990; **77**: 813–14.

32. Antunes MJ, Fernandes LE, Oliveira JM. Ventricular septal defects and arteriovenous fistulas, with and without valvular lesions, resulting from penetrating injury of the heart and aorta. *J Thorac Cardiovasc Surg* 1988; **95**: 902–7.

33. Lindenbaum G, Larrieu AJ, Goldberg SE, *et al.* Diagnosis and management of traumatic ventricular septal defect. *J Trauma* 1987; **27**: 1289–93.

34. Thandroyen FT, Matisonn RE. Penetrating thoracic trauma producing cardiac shunts. *J Thorac Cardiovasc Surg* 1981; **81**: 569–73.

35. Mattox KL, Limacher MC, Feliciano DV, *et al.* Cardiac evaluation following heart injury. *J Trauma* 1985; **25**: 758–65.

36. Shabetai R, Fowler NO, Guntheroth WG. The hemodynamics of cardiac tamponade and constrictive pericarditis. *Am J Cardiol* 1970; **26**: 480–9.

37. Wechsler AS, Auerbach BJ, Graham TC, Sabiston DC. Distribution of intramyocardial blood flow during pericardial tamponade. *J Thorac Cardiovasc Surg* 1974; **68**: 847–56.

38. Beck CS. Wounds of the heart. *Arch Surg* 1926; **13**: 205–27.

39. Jebara VA, Saade B. Penetrating wounds to the heart: a wartime experience. *Ann Thorac Surg* 1989; **47**: 250–3.

40. Vij D, Somoni E, Smith RF, *et al.* Resuscitative thoracotomy for patients with traumatic injury. *Surgery* 1983; **94**: 554–61.

41. Demetriades D, Rabinowitz B, Sofianos C. Emergency room thoracotomy for stab wounds to the chest and neck. *J Trauma* 1987; **27**: 483–5.

42. Knudson MM. Emergency department thoracotomy for trauma: a reappraisal. *Adv Trauma Crit Care* 1992; **7**: 133–57.

43. Ivatury RR, Shah PM, Ito K, Ramirez-Schon G, Suarez F, Rohman M. Emergency room thoracotomy for the resuscitation of patients with 'fatal' penetrating injuries of the heart. *Ann Thorac Surg* 1981; **32**: 377–85.

44. Rohman M, Ivatury RR, Steichen FM, *et al.* Emergency room thoracotomy for penetrating cardiac injuries. *J Trauma* 1983; **23**: 570–6.

45. Siemens R, Polk HC, Gray LA, Fulton RL. Indications for thoracotomy following penetrating thoracic injury. *J Trauma* 1977; **17**: 493–500.

46. Duncan AO, Scalea TM, Sclafani SJA, *et al.* Evaluation of occult cardiac injuries using subxiphoid pericardial window. *J Trauma* 1989; **29**: 955–60.

47. Arom KV, Richardson JD, Webb G, Grover FL, Trinkle JK. Subxiphoid pericardial window in patients with suspected traumatic pericardial tamponade. *Ann Thorac Surg* 1977; **23**: 545–9.

48. Jacoby SS, Gillan LD, Pardian NG, Weyman AE. 2-Dimensional and Doppler echocardiography in the evaluation of penetrating cardiac injury. *Chest* 1985; **88**: 922–4.

49. Plummer D, Bunette D, Asinger R, Ruiz E. Emergency department echocardiography improves outcome in penetrating cardiac injury. *Ann Emerg Med* 1992; **21**: 709–12.

50. Blalock A, Ravitch MM. A consideration of the nonoperative treatment of cardiac tamponade resulting from wounds of the heart. *Surgery* 1943; **14**: 157–62.

51. Andrade-Alegre R, Mon L. Subxiphoid pericardial window in the diagnosis of penetrating cardiac trauma. *Ann Thorac Surg* 1994; **58**: 1139–41.

52. Macho JR, Markison RE, Schecter WP. Cardiac stapling in the management of penetrating injuries of the heart: rapid control of hemorrhage and decreased risk of personal contamination. *J Trauma* 1993; **34**: 711–16.

53. Tavares S, Hankins JR, Moulton AL, *et al.* Management of penetrating cardiac injuries: the role of emergency room thoracotomy. *Ann Thorac Surg* 1984; **38**: 183–7.

54. Espada R, Whisennand HH, Mattox KL, Beall AC. Surgical management of penetrating injuries to the coronary arteries. *Surgery* 1975; **78**: 755–60.

55. Buffolo E, de Andrade JCS, Branco JNR, Teles CA, Aguiar LF, Gomes WJ. Coronary artery bypass grafting without cardiopulmonary bypass. *Ann Thorac Surg* 1996; **61**: 63–6.

56. Walker WJ. Spontaneous closure of traumatic ventricular septal defect. *Am J Cardiol* 1965; **15**: 263–6.

57. Michelow BJ, Bremner CG. Penetrating cardiac injuries: selective conservatism – favorable or foolish. *J Trauma* 1987; **27**: 398–401.

58. De Wet Lubbe JJ, Janson PMC, Barnard PM. Penetrating wounds of the heart and great vessels: experience with 24 cases including 3 with intracardiac defects. *S Afr Med J* 1975; **49**: 512–16.

59. Ivatury RR, Rohman M, Steichen FM, Gunduz Y, Nallathambi M, Stahl WM. Penetrating cardiac injury: twenty year experience. *Am Surg* 1987; **53**: 310–17.

60. Symbas PN, Picone AL, Hatcher CR, Vlasis-Hale SE. Cardiac missiles: a review of the literature and personal experience. *Ann Surg* 1990; **211**: 639–48.

61. Gandhi SK, Marts BC, Mistry BM, Brown JW, Durham RM, Mazuski JE. Selective management of embolized intracardiac missiles. *Ann Thorac Surg* 1996; **62**: 290–2.

62. Dshanelidze IL. Manuscript, Petrograd. Cited by Lilienthal H. *Thoracic Surgery: the Surgical Treatment of Thoracic Diseases*. Philadelphia: WB Saunders, 1926; 489.

63. Makins GH. Gunshot injuries to the blood vessels. Bristol: John Wright & Sons, 1919.

64. De Bakey ME, Simeone FA. Battle injuries of the arteries in World War II: an analysis of 2,471 cases. *Ann Surg* 1946; **123**: 534–79.

65. Jahnke EJ, Seeley SF. Acute vascular injuries in the Korean War: an analysis of 77 consecutive cases. *Ann Surg* 1953; **138**: 158–77.

66. Hughes CW. Arterial repair during the Korean War. *Ann Surg* 1958; **147**: 555–61.

67. Symbas PN, Sehdeva JS. Penetrating wounds of the thoracic aorta. *Ann Surg* 1970; **171**: 441–50.

68. Ecker RR, Dickinson WE, Sugg WL, Rea WJ. Management of the injuries of the innominate and proximal left common carotid arteries. *J Thorac Cardiovasc Surg* 1972; **64:** 618–24.

69. Brawley RK, Murray GF, Crisler C, Cameron JL. Management of wounds of the innominate, subclavian, and axillary blood vessels. *Surg Gynecol Obstet* 1970; **131:** 1130–40.

70. Flint LM, Snyder WH, Perry MO, Shires GT. Management of major vascular injuries in the base of the neck: an 11-year experience with 146 cases. *Arch Surg* 1973; **106:** 407–13.

71. Schaff HV, Brawley RK. Operative management of penetrating vascular injuries of the thoracic outlet. *Surgery* 1977; **82:** 182–91.

72. Pate JW, Cole FH, Walker WA, Fabian TC. Penetrating injuries of the aortic arch and its branches. *Ann Thorac Surg* 1993; **55:** 586–92.

73. Fulton JO, De Groot KM, Buckels NJ, Von Oppell UO. Penetrating injuries involving the intrathoracic great vessels. *S Afr J Surg* 1997; **35(2):** 82–6.

74. Buchan K, Robbs JV. Surgical management of penetrating mediastinal arterial trauma. *Eur J Cardiothorac Surg* 1995; **9:** 90–4.

75. Johnston RH, Wall MJ, Mattox KL. Innominate artery trauma: a thirty-year experience. *J Vasc Surg* 1993; **17:** 134–40.

76. Graham JM, Feliciano DV, Mattox KL, Beall AC, DeBakey ME. Management of subclavian vascular injuries. *J Trauma* 1980; **20:** 537–44.

77. Graham JM, Feliciano DV, Mattox KL, Beall AC. Innominate vascular injury. *J Trauma* 1982; **22:** 647–55.

78. Burnett HF, Parnell CL, Williams GD, Campbell GS. Peripheral arterial injuries: a reassessment. *Ann Surg* 1976; **183:** 701–9.

79. Demetriades D, Chan L, Cornwell E *et al.* Paramedics vs private transportation of trauma patients; effect on outcome. *Arch Surg* 1996; **131:**133–8.

80. Demetriades D, Theodorou D, Cornwell E *et al.* Penetrating injuries of the neck in patients in stable condition: physical examination, angiography, or color flow Doppler imaging. *Arch Surg* 1995; **130:**971–5.

81. Demetriades D, Rabinowitz B, Pezikis A, Franklin J, Palexas G. Subclavian vascular injuries. *Br J Surg* 1987; **74:**1001–3.

82. Blaisdell FW. Discussion: management of major vascular injuries in the base of the neck. *Arch Surg* 1973; **106:** 412–13.

83. Rich NM, Hobson RW, Jarstfer BS, Geer TM. Subclavian artery trauma. *J Trauma* 1973; **13:** 485–96.

84. George SM, Croce MA, Fabian TC, *et al.* Cervicothoracic arterial injuries: recommendations for diagnosis and management. *World J Surg* 1991; **15:** 134–40.

85. Brown MF, Graham JM, Feliciano DV, Mattox KL, Beall AC, DeBakey ME. Carotid artery injuries. *Am J Surg* 1982; **144:** 748–53.

86. Fulton JO, deGroot KM, Von Oppell UO. Stab wounds of the innominate artery. *Ann Thorac Surg* 1996; **61:** 851–3.

87. Fulton JO, Brink JG. Complex thoracic vascular injury repair using deep hypothermia and circulatory arrest. *Ann Thorac Surg* 1997; **63(2):** 557–9.

88. Robicsek R, Matos-Cruz M. Artificially induced ventricular fibrillation in the management of through and through penetrating wounds of the aortic arch: a case report. *Surgery* 1991; **110:** 544–5.

89. Liekwig WG, Greenfield LJ. Penetrating carotid artery injury. *Ann Surg* 1978; **188:** 587–92.

FURTHER READING

Buckman RF, Badellino MM, Mauro LH, *et al.* Penetrating cardiac wounds: prospective study of factors influencing initial resuscitation. *J Trauma* 1993; **34:** 717–27.

Duncan AO, Scalea TM, Sclafani SJA, *et al.* Evaluation of occult cardiac injuries using subxiphoid pericardial window. *J Trauma* 1989; **29:** 955–60.

Johnston RH, Wall MJ, Mattox KL. Innominate artery trauma: a thirty-year experience. *J Vasc Surg* 1993; **17:** 134–40.

Pate JW, Cole FH, Walker WA, Fabian TC. Penetrating injuries of the aortic arch and its branches. *Ann Thorac Surg* 1993; **55:** 586–92.

Symbas PN. Cardiothoracic trauma. *Curr Prob Surg* 1991; **28(11):** 746–96.

Symbas PN, Picone AL, Hatcher CR, Vlasis-Hale SE. Cardiac missiles: a review of the literature and personal experience. *Ann Surg* 1990; **211:** 639–48.

11

Penetrating trauma to the chest wall, lung, esophagus, trachea and thoracic duct

K MARK DE GROOT

Chest wounds are the most lethal of penetrating injuries. In civilian practice stab and small caliber gunshot wounds are the most common penetrating chest injuries. Until recently, high velocity gunshot wounds and shrapnel wounds were exclusive to the military, but the greater availability of handguns in the last three decades has led to a preponderance of gunshot wounds in most urban centers. Proliferation and refinement of legal and illegal armament have caused these types of lethal injuries to be seen more frequently in major trauma centers.

In general terms, the magnitude of the injury depends on the type of weapon, the site of entry and the direction of the missile or stab wound. Amazingly, for patients who present to hospital alive after penetrating injuries of the chest the mortality is low. Most authors agree that the bulk of penetrating chest injuries can be treated non-operatively.[1,2] This policy originated in World War II and continues to the present day.[3]

Mandal[4] observed that only 115 of 1004 patients without cardiac injury required thoracotomy and the overall mortality was 0.8%. In this series the mortality rate for gunshot wounds was three times higher than for stabs. Among the 115 patients who required thoracotomies for bleeding, the sources were lung in 79%, intercostal or internal mammary artery in 65% and internal vascular injury in 29%. In approximately 20% of gunshot wounds to the chest some form of intra-abdominal injury will be present.[5] War injuries require a larger proportion of thoracotomies due to the higher destructive potential of the missiles.[6]

The entrance and exit wounds of missiles may suggest the path and thus the probability of visceral injury but ricochets off bony structures may lead to a false impression. All wounds that penetrate the platysma in the neck should be considered to have a potential visceral injury.

Special consideration should be given to patients with transmediastinal penetration because of vital organs in this region. In the unstable patient who undergoes an emergency operation without preoperative investigations, all viscera, particularly the esophagus and trachea, need to be thoroughly examined in the course of the procedure. For stable patients, a contrast swallow or esophagoscopy, bronchoscopy, and angiography should be performed to rule out injury even if the mediastinal silhouette is normal. Richardson[7] found injuries in 24 of 43 patients investigated under such a protocol. Patients with negative investigation should be closely observed to rule out false-negative studies. The consequences of a missed injury could be fatal.

Transmediastinal injury
- If the patient is unstable, emergency operation – all viscera, particularly the esophagus and trachea, carefully examined.
- If the patient is stable, do contrast swallow or esophagoscopy bronchoscopy and angiography, even if mediastinal silhouette normal.
- Patients should be carefully observed to rule out false-negative studies.

Most survivors of penetrating thoracic trauma recover to near normality[3] and the complication rates are low, with pneumonia, atelectasis and empyema most common.[5] Antibiotic prophylaxis for penetrating chest injuries is not necessary except for esophageal or major bronchial lacerations, deep shock or extensive tissue destruction.[8]

PENETRATING TRAUMA TO THE CHEST WALL AND PLEURA

Pathogenesis

The damage potential of stab wounds depends on the size and shape of the instrument, angle of attack and force behind it. Knife wounds frequently penetrate the chest wall but seldom do severe damage to it. On the other hand, ax or machete wounds can cause extensive superficial damage without a great deal of internal injury. High velocity wounds are often deceptive in that the dissipation of energy causes wider internal damage than the external wounds may suggest. Though these wounds are uncommon in civilian practice, gunshot wounds with hollow-point bullets mimic these closely.

For shotgun wounds tissue damage depends on the distance from the weapon to the victim, pellet size, pattern size and gauge of weapon. An excellent treatise on the subject is given by DeMuth.[9] At close range the entire charge strikes the target as a large missile with the kinetic energy equivalent to a high velocity weapon.[9,10] In patients requiring operative intervention, the injury has a confluent pattern, the destruction is severe and in most cases lethal.[11] The surgeon must always be aware that wadding and plastic casing, as well as skin and clothing, can be forced into the body with close range discharges. This is to be suspected, particularly when wound infection develops and persists despite appropriate treatment.[12] At long ranges the pellets spread out widely before hitting the target, each acting as low kinetic energy projectiles. In the majority of these patients there are no clinical signs of intrathoracic damage.[13] Most of the latter can be treated with simple chest tube drainage if necessary.

Diagnosis

Depending on the site and size of the chest wall wound and damage to underlying viscera, the condition of the patient ranges from asymptomatic to severely distressed. Large defects greater or equal to the diameter of the trachea cause severe respiratory compromise from sucking chest wounds. The inability to develop a sustained negative intrapleural pressure markedly reduces the patient's capacity to ventilate. The open wound also interferes with the ability to raise intratracheal pressure and deliver an effective cough to clear airway secretions. Hemodynamic compromise may result as the loss of intrathoracic negative pressure impedes venous return to the heart. Any shift of the mediastinum tends to kink the venae cavae at the atrio-caval and diaphragmatic junctions.

Management

Most uncontaminated superficial stab wounds of the chest wall can be closed primarily if seen within 6–12 hours. The entrance or exit wounds of gunshot wounds should be debrided if ragged or severely contused. Our policy has been not to attempt primary closure and allow healing by secondary intention.

EMERGENCY CARE OF OPEN WOUNDS OF THE CHEST

> **Emergency care of open wounds of the chest**
> * Occlusive dressing
> * Intercostal drain
> * Intubation and ventilation for massive injury

The diagnosis of open wounds of the chest tends to be obvious with loss of chest wall integrity and wafting in and out of bloody froth with a characteristic to-and-fro sucking sound. The field management differs from the trauma unit care. The optimal primary treatment is covering the wound with an occlusive dressing, thus converting it to a simple pneumothorax. However, this should be accompanied by immediate insertion of an intercostal drain because of risk of creating a tension pneumothorax. In the field a similar result can be attained by an occlusive patch affixed on three sides allowing a 'flap' to vent the pneumothorax while preventing entrainment of air from the outside. Massive wounds in either circumstance are best managed by intubation and ventilation of the patient.

MANAGEMENT OF CHEST WALL TISSUE LOSS

Once the patient's life-threatening injuries are cared for, severe wounds of the chest wall need to be thoroughly debrided prior to attempt at closure. All foreign material, bone fragments and devitalized muscle needs to be removed. Of particular note, in close range shotgun wounds, one must also look for wadding, parts of the shell casing, clothing and other debris. The underlying lung should be thoroughly examined and areas of severe maceration debrided. Careful attention should be made to sealing small bronchi with figure-of-eight absorbable sutures to facilitate complete lung expansion. Two large bore chest drains should be appropriately positioned. All

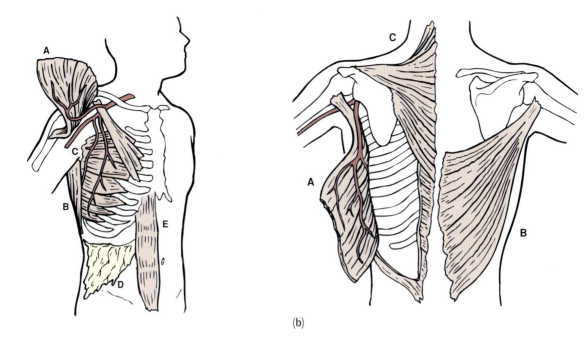

(a)

(b)

Figure 11.1 *(a) Pedicle flaps available for chest wall reconstruction on the anterior chest wall: A, pectoralis major muscle, based on thoracoacromial artery; B, latissimus dorsi muscle, based on thoracodorsal artery; C, serratus anterior muscle, based on thoracodorsal artery; D, greater omentum, based on right or left gastroepiploric artery; E, rectus abdominus muscle, based on superior epigastric artery. (b) Pedicle flaps available for chest wall reconstruction on the posterior chest wall: A, latissimus dorsi muscle, based on thoracodorsal artery; B, latissimus dorsi muscle, based on lumbar and intercostal arteries; C, trapezius muscle, based on transverse cervical artery. (Adapted from Cohen M, ed.* Mastery of Plastic and Reconstructive Surgery. *Volume 2. Boston: Little, Brown, 1994)*

muscle needs to be debrided back to bleeding or twitching elements. A muscle stimulator or low coagulation current is useful for this test. It is advisable to widely debride the wound at first intent irrespective of the size of the resultant defect. The surgeon must resist the temptation to preserve marginally viable tissue in order to attain primary closure. The inevitable result is sepsis, necrosis, wound dehiscence, delay of proper treatment and potential death of the patient. Where the decision is in doubt, re-exploration should be scheduled.

Wounds with a large loss of chest wall integrity may require reconstruction of both the skeletal integrity and superficial coverage. In general, areas of fewer than three ribs and less than 5 cm in length or lying beneath the scapula do not require consideration of chest wall reconstruction. No attempt should be made at the first sitting to use prosthetic material. Local myocutaneous flaps are time consuming and seldom indicated in an unstable patient nor when the complete area to be debrided may not have been demarcated. In the first instance, the wound should be packed and covered with an occlusive dressing. During the first few post-injury days the patient should be returned to the operating room where the wound can be examined and, if necessary, debrided under optimal conditions. This should continue until no further necrotic tissue is found.

Where large sections of chest wall are missing it may be necessary to ventilate the patient with adequate pleural drainage and packing of the wound until a clean granulating wound will allow complete reconstruction. Areas of wide tissue loss should be bridged by rotational muscle flap interposition. Suitable muscles for use are the pectoralis major, the latissimus dorsi or the rectus abdominis (Fig 11.1). Transposition of the diaphragm has also been described for thoracoabdominal wounds.[14] Our preference for structural support is Marlex® mesh reinforced with bone cement though stretched mesh alone or Gore-Tex® sheeting is suitable for this purpose. The choice of reconstruction depends on the size of the defect, the anatomical position, availability of usable surrounding tissue and the necessity for rigidity in the closure. Apical chest wall wounds may occasionally be managed by thoracoplasty where no suitable recourse for reconstruction exists. Rarely, an area involving loss of anterior chest wall can be managed by relocation of the contralateral breast.

PENETRATING TRAUMA TO THE LUNG

Pathogenesis

The lungs so completely fill the chest and surround the intrathoracic viscera that internal penetration usually results in some form of lung injury. Fortunately, the lung is one of the organs of the body most resilient to penetrating trauma. Except for hilar injuries, blood loss usually arrests quickly due to the low pressure of the pulmonary circulation and the presence of high levels of tissue thromboplastins. Air leak is usually of a self-limiting nature, particularly when the pleural surfaces can be brought into apposition using any effective drainage method.

For knife wounds, the length and direction of the blade are the main injury-determining factors. Other modifiers are the presence of the sternum, spine and other bony structure, which cause certain path limitations. Low velocity gunshot wounds tend to cause perforation plus small areas of contusion. Both gunshot and stab wounds primarily manifest by the leaking of blood and air into the pleural space. The clinical presentation tends to reflect the amount of blood or air leak and may be limited in whole or in part by the presence of pleural adhesions. In cases where penetrating injuries present with marked amounts of subcutaneous emphysema, the latter should be suspected.

The amount of damage to the lung sustained with a high velocity bullet wound is less than other viscera because the energy imparted is related to the specific gravity of the tissue, which in this case is low. Notwithstanding, the injury can be extensive with lung maceration, secondary contusion and further damage by vascular thrombosis and supra-infection. Severe lung contusion can even result from the shock wave of a high velocity bullet passing through a contiguous structure without direct injury. The contusion may not manifest clinically or radiologically for the first 24–48 hours. Patients with high velocity gunshot wounds are prone to developing adult respiratory distress syndrome (ARDS) from contusion, blood aspiration, massive fluid resuscitation and sepsis.[15] Traumatic lung cavities produced by high velocity missiles may be persistent and prone to secondary complications. Fortunately, these complications are usually self-limiting.[16]

For shotgun wounds, the extent of damage to the lung varies from massive destruction at short range to relatively minor pellet injuries. The mortality from close range injuries is high.[13] By contrast, the majority of patients with pellet wounds can be managed non-operatively and released after observation.

AIR EMBOLISM

> **Clinical signs of air embolism**
> - Focal or lateralizing neurological deficit
> - Sudden cardiovascular collapse
> - Air or froth noted in arterial blood specimens

Wilson[17] documented six patients with significant penetrating lung injury who had cardiovascular collapse immediately after intubation and positive pressure ventilation. In all cases air was subsequently found in the coronary arteries and the patients could not be resuscitated. Similar experiences have been noted by other authors.[18,19] Air embolism can occur when any bronchial laceration is in proximity to an injury in the pulmonary venous drainage. In patients who are breathing spontaneously, the low pressure differential minimizes the risk but when the patient is intubated and positive pressure ventilation applied, air may be extruded into the venous return. Under experimental trauma, air embolization occurs to some degree in the vast majority of ventilated specimens though generally in amounts not clinically relevant.[20] The amount entrained depends on the intratracheal pressure of inflation;[21,22] therefore care should be taken to minimize this in the clinical setting.

Systemic air embolism must be considered a possibility in any patient who has a neurological deficit and no injury outside the chest. Confirmation can be made by fundoscopic observation of air in the retinal arterioles. If sudden cardiovascular collapse occurs during the course of an operation on a lung injury, air lock or coronary embolism should be considered. Treatment is clamping of the hilar vessels, venting the left ventricle of residual air and cardiac massage until recovery occurs. Vasopressors should be administered to help maintain arterial pressure and drive the air out of the coronary circulation. Consideration should be given to single lung ventilation where this is considered a risk – for example, the hemoptysizing patient with a pulmonary laceration. Definitive management involves isolation of the lung and oversewing the depth of the laceration or resection of the involved area.

Diagnosis

The typical presentation of lung laceration is a simple pneumothorax or hemopneumothorax. The manifestations depend on the amount of air or blood, the presence of pleural adhesions and the underlying pulmonary reserve of the patient. Tension pneumothorax results where air has accumulated under pressure with compression of the ipsilateral lung and contralateral shift of the mediastinum. These are more common in the coughing or struggling patient since with resting ventilation only a modest increase in intrapleural pressure can be attained. Of clinical relevance, a patient with a simple pneumothorax may be converted to a tension pneumothorax by positive pressure ventilation. This is an emergency situation and requires immediate temporization by the venting of the pleural space with a large intravenous cannula, followed by the prompt insertion of an intercostal drain.

Where pleural symphysis is present, a penetrating wound may result in the development of varying degrees of subcutaneous emphysema without a concomitant pneumothorax. Despite the horrendous appearance, this seldom causes respiratory compromise unless a concomitant pneumothorax is present and is not an indication for blind intercostal intubation. Furthermore, the presence of subcutaneous emphysema may make viewing of the chest radiograph difficult and often misinterpretation results. To identify a potential pneumothorax, the clinician must carefully trace the pulmonary bronchovascular markings to the surface of the lung fields.

Intrapulmonary hematomas may follow a penetrating wound to the lung. Usually these are self-limiting but on occasion can become infected and both clinically and radiologically resemble acute or subacute lung abscesses. Bullet tracts through the lung take on a variety of appearances due to the ballistics and path through the lung. The maximal manifestations may not appear for a few days.[23] In most civilian practice the incidence of observable pulmonary contusion with penetrating wounds is low.[5] Occasionally a lung laceration with a bronchial component will develop into a traumatic lung cyst. These rarely become infected and usually resolve in 3–4 months. Occasionally, with damage to more central airways, an enlarging cyst may develop, necessitating exploration and closure of the airway.

Management

In most cases of uncomplicated lung laceration the insertion of a simple intercostal drain is the definitive management. In stable patients, to ensure the diagnosis and avoid pleural adhesions, a good quality upright chest radiograph should be obtained prior to insertion. In patients found to have loculations, the drain should be sited in order to drain the collection and be clinically manageable. Under routine circumstances the drain can

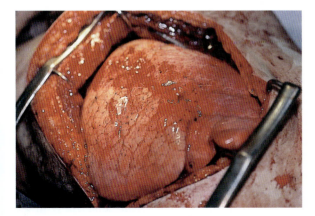

Figure 11.2 *Thoracotomy for bleeding in a patient with penetrating wounds of the right lung. Bleeding was arrested by deep mattress sutures into the lung parenchyma. (SWTC.)*

be inserted in the fifth or sixth intercostal space in the mid-axillary line. Caution needs to be extended where pleural adhesions are present in order not to compound the insult by the insertion of the drain into the lung parenchyma.

Graham[21] found chest drain insertion to be the only required treatment in 76% of 373 patients with penetrating lung injury. Only 45 (12%) required thoracotomies with some form of lung repair (Fig 11.2) and in only eight (2%) was some form of segmental or lobar resection required. Robison[24] compared stab to gunshot wounds of the lung. The incidence of simple pneumonorrhaphy for stabs was 2% compared with 6.3% for gunshot wounds, lung resection 1.1% compared with 2.3%, and hilar repair 0.1% compared with 2.3%. Overall, 10.7% of gunshot wounds compared with 3.3% of stab wounds required some form of intervention.

INDICATIONS FOR OPERATION

> **Indications for surgery in penetrating lung trauma**
> * Massive hemorrhage
> * Uncontrolled air leak
> * Hemoptysis
> * Unstable foreign bodies
> * Hilar injury

The most common indication for surgical intervention in lung injury is massive initial or continued hemorrhage.[24] Most series report the necessity for operative repair to be in the region of 5–15% and resection 1–2%.[21,24,25] Air leak *per se* is seldom an indication alone for thoracotomy. Demetriades[1] conservatively treated 24 relatively massive air leaks lasting more than 3 days with none requiring operative intervention. However, persistent massive air leak raises the suspicion of a central airway injury and this should be ruled out by bronchoscopy.

Bullet fragments and occasionally broken knife points are found to lie within the lung parenchyma. Symptomatic fragments should be removed as well as any sharp or centrally placed piece that may migrate or cause sepsis. Small fragments or shotgun pellets are seldom of consequence. Removal is difficult and may be more traumatic than the original injury. All objects that are removed should be retained and handled in a proper forensic manner.

Patients with severe pulmonary contusion secondary to high velocity gunshot or close range shotgun wounds should have the damaged area resected to prevent the high mortality associated with respiratory failure and sepsis.[15] Fischer[26] advocated resection for high velocity wounds where hypoxia persists despite optimal support or if at thoracotomy for hemorrhage a whole lobe or lung is found to be contused. General treatment for moderately contused lung involves respiratory support and, if necessary, ventilation. Good pulmonary hygiene should be maintained and antibiotics administered if sepsis becomes evident. Fluid balance should be closely monitored and overtransfusion avoided.

TECHNIQUE OF OPERATION

In patients with isolated injury anticipated to require resection it is advisable to approach the area through a posterolateral thoracotomy. Though resection can be accomplished through a sternotomy or anterolateral thoracotomy, associated injuries may make an anatomical lobectomy or pneumonectomy difficult. The vast majority of lung lacerations can be managed by simple pneumonorrhaphy.[21,27] Deep pulmonary lacerations should never be superficially closed but explored to the base to avoid subsequent air embolization. Once opened, care should be taken to oversew all bronchi and vessels. On occasion, hilar or regional vascular clamping may be required to accomplish this. Damaged pulmonary parenchyma has a remarkable ability for recovery from traumatic injury. When in doubt, areas of questionable viability should be retained and, if necessary, re-examined at a subsequent thoracotomy rather than resected.

For central vascular injuries of the lung, it is advisable to attain proximal hilar control before proceeding with exploration. This may not only prevent massive blood loss but may also reduce the risk of air embolization.[28] This can usually be performed outside the pericardium in most cases but the operator should be prepared to attain control by opening the pericardium if necessary. The technique of clamping involves placing a large vascular Satinsky or similar clamp across all vessels including the bronchus (Fig 11.3). Similarly, a hilar snare can be used.[29] Digital control on the area should be maintained while doing this. Dividing the inferior pulmonary ligament facilitates placement.

Resection may be necessary for uncontrolled bleeding or unrepairable vascular or bronchial lacerations. The decision should not be undertaken lightly as resection carries a high morbidity and mortality under these circumstances. Pneumonectomy should only be considered as a last resort because of the high associated mortality under acute trauma conditions.[25,28]

Outcome

If full expansion of the lung can be attained by proper pleural drainage, the vast majority of simple lacerations close spontaneously. If re-expansion cannot be brought about with properly positioned drains and low pressure, high volume suction, a thoracotomy and direct closure should be considered. If the patient is ventilated for

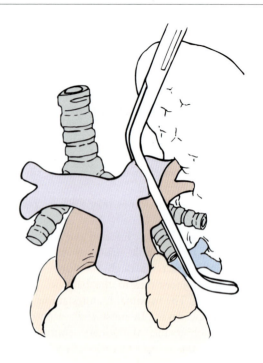

Figure 11.3 *Emergency application of a hilar clamp. Method of clamping the hilum of the lung with a Satinsky clamp to control major hemorrhage. The inferior pulmonary ligament is mobilized and the clamp placed over all hilar structures including the bronchus.*

associated injuries, the probability of persistence of air leak increases. This should only be operatively managed if re-expansion cannot be attained or the leak is interfering with patient care. The resumption of spontaneous ventilation is usually followed by rapid resolution of the air leak. Attempts at operative closure in a patient with active pneumonia or ARDS are unlikely to be gratifying. If a chest drain has been inserted into the lung parenchyma in the presence of pre-existing pleural symphysis, this will result in a persistent air leak until the drain is removed.

Intrapulmonary foreign bodies can migrate into the bronchi or pulmonary vessels, causing hemoptysis or obstructive pneumonia. Hemoptysis followed by chest pain, intermittent cough and recurrent infections are the most common sequelae of retained intrapulmonary foreign bodies.[30] Symptomatic foreign bodies should be removed by pneumonorrhaphy or segmental resection.

Pulmonary arteriovenous fistulae following penetrating trauma are exceptionally rare.[31] The clinical manifestations are similar to those of congenital origin: dyspnea and a low arterial oxygen saturation. Similarly, pulmonary aneurysm occurring after penetrating trauma is very rare[6] and may manifest with hemoptysis, dyspnea, chest pain or a persistent radiodensity in the lung. Despite the high incidence of lung trauma, both these conditions appear only rarely due to the low pressures existing in both the pulmonary arterial and venous systems. Treatment in both cases is resection of the malformation with preservation of as much lung parenchyma as possible.

Through-and-through wounds of the lung and abdominal viscera can lead to late esophageal, gastric, biliary and pancreatic fistulae to the airways. The treatment in all cases is the operative division and viable tissue interposition and treatment of surrounding sepsis. The greater omentum is an ideal interposition in most cases. In rare instances, concomitant lung resection is required due to irreversible damage.

PENETRATING TRAUMA TO THE ESOPHAGUS

Pathogenesis

Traumatic perforations of the esophagus comprise approximately 19% of all types of damage to the esophagus but carry the lowest overall mortality for all causes.[32] Unlike other injuries, the majority of traumatic esophageal wounds are from penetrating wounds rather than blunt trauma. The *in situ* esophagus is an elusive target, being less than the diameter of the index finger in the undistended state. Due to lack of protection from skeletal structures, the cervical esophagus is most at risk. The intrathoracic esophagus is well protected from stab wounds as the depth of penetration required is high and the bony protection good. Accordingly, there are more gunshot wounds of the intrathoracic esophagus compared with stab wounds. In cases where the wounding instrument has managed to traverse the thorax, wounds to the vasculature often determine the immediate fate of the patient.

In our institution the majority of patients with esophageal injury have stab wounds to the neck. This is not the case in most other urban trauma centers where gunshot wounds prevail.[32,33] A common presenting combination is the entrance wound in the mid left neck with a right pneumothorax or empyema indicative of a high transmediastinal injury.[34] One feature of gunshot wounds is the high incidence of injury to adjacent structures.[35] Pass[36] noted 39 associated injuries in 18 patients with esophageal perforation, the most common being pulmonary followed by vascular and tracheal injuries. Most of these injuries can be managed simultaneously.

The clinical presentation depends on the duration, size and anatomical location of the perforation. The perforation may close spontaneously, contaminate the mediastinum, leak into the pleural space or fistulize to the surface. Perforation of the esophagus, if unrecognized, allows air, oral secretions and swallowed food material to contaminate the surrounding space. Except anteriorly, the esophagus lies in a bed of loose areolar tissue bounded by the prevertebral fascia posteriorly

and the pretracheal space anteriorly. Negative intrathoracic pressure draws oral and gastric secretions into the tissue planes outside the esophagus. There are no fascial barriers from the base of the skull to the diaphragm so that any leak and subsequent infection will spread quickly to involve most of the mediastinum. The initial contamination represents the oral flora, including staphylococci, microaerophillic streptococci, fusiform bacilli and spirochetes. These organisms act together to form a symbiotic necrotizing infection resembling aspiration lung abscesses or human bites. Within 1–2 hours, edema, exudate and tissue necrosis ensues. The resulting process may extend through the existing perforation or by spontaneous rupture into the pleural spaces, thereby creating an acute empyema.

Diagnosis

> Diagnosis of esophageal perforations depends primarily on a high index of suspicion.

Esophageal perforations are often difficult to diagnose early because they are asymptomatic initially and often overshadowed by wounds of surrounding viscera. The early diagnosis will be missed unless a high index of suspicion is extended for a penetrating wound whose tract places it in the anatomical vicinity.[33] Morbidity and mortality increase proportionally to the delay in diagnosis.[33,37–39]

Clinical findings vary by time interval, degree of soilage, antibiotic therapy and degree of intervening support of the patient. General signs such as subcutaneous emphysema and cervical hematoma, as well as radiological findings of mediastinal widening or retropharyngeal swelling, have been found to be non-specific.[33,35,40] Pass[36] found cervical or mediastinal air in 14 of 20 patients with esophageal gunshot wounds and noted it was often confused with concomitant lung damage. Large intrathoracic wounds of the esophagus may allow direct pleural fistulization with little or no evidence of subcutaneous emphysema.

When mediastinitis is established, signs of local sepsis and pain on swallowing and with neck movement may be observed. On the plain radiograph this may manifest as mediastinal widening with or without air fluid loculi. This is easily missed in traumatized patients and is usually far advanced when finally detected. Occasionally computed tomography may be helpful to identify loculations of sepsis. With lower perforation of the esophagus, pain and symptoms of upper abdominal rigidity may manifest.

At the time of operation for other injuries, if the wound is in the region of the esophagus and no injury is found, it is prudent to 'air test' the esophagus. With the surgeon's assistance, the anesthetist should insert a nasogastric tube in the esophagus, positioning the holes in the suspected area. With proximal and distal digital occlusion, 50–100 ml of air is then pushed in, using a syringe, while the area is examined under saline. Similarly, a solution of methylene blue can be used. We have found a number of covert injuries using this technique, thus avoiding extensive mobilization of the esophagus.

When a leak is suspected, the radiologist should be advised of this possibility in ordering a contrast swallow. A water-soluble iodinated compound should be administered first to rule out a gross leak. We prefer diatrizoate sodium (Gastrografin®) for this purpose. If a negative study is obtained, a further contrast examination with a thin solution of barium sulfate should follow because extraluminal water-soluble contrast agents may not be seen in up to 50% of cervical perforation and 25% of intrathoracic ones.[40,41] The major disadvantage of barium as the primary agent is its propensity for inciting foreign-body-type reactions if it leaks into the mediastinal tissues. Unfortunately, false-negative studies can be seen in both cervical and intrathoracic perforations despite this methodology.[33,36,40] If a conservative approach to management is being undertaken, the patients should undergo rigid esophagoscopy as well, to rule out injury.[42] Esophagoscopy alone, even in the hands of experienced endoscopists, carries a high chance of missing injury.[33,36] We have performed endoscopy in patients with known leaks diagnosed by contrast studies to plan an operative approach and have been surprised at how innocuous the internal appearance may be. Weigelt[42] showed that both contrast studies and rigid esophagoscopy were reasonably accurate for diagnosis. He observed that only one patient in each group out of nine patients in total with perforations had a false-negative study. Combining both contrast studies and rigid esophagoscopy was diagnostic in 100% of instances. Flexible esophagoscopy was far less accurate, producing false-negative studies in five of eight patients. Despite this, controversy exists on the cost effectiveness, morbidity and appropriateness of aggressive versus conservative treatment approaches. Where there is a clinical indication for exploring the neck for other injuries, the performance of contrast or endoscopy is redundant and the esophagus should be explored directly.

In patients who require immediate exploration for concomitant injuries in other compartments, esophagoscopy should be performed on the table before the end of the procedure. The hole, unfortunately, is often difficult to see and one relies on hematoma, blood clot, air leak and other indirect evidence to suggest the diagnosis. If there is sufficient corroborating evidence, it is better to err on the side of a negative exploration rather than risk an uncontrolled leak.

Occasional late presentation occurs when the patient is noted to have his meals being evacuated by his chest drain. Often there is a history of an early 'traumatic empyema' that went unrecognized as a leak. Easy confirmation is obtained by having the patient ingest a small quantity of methylene blue or food coloring.

Management

Though a non-operative regimen has been advocated in certain types of iatrogenic injuries,[38,43] there is no role for this approach with external trauma. The general philosophy of management is stratified into two groups. On one side are surgeons who advocate exploration of all wounds traversing the platysma in the neck or having an apparent transmediastinal path. This may or may not be preceded by arteriography, contrast studies or endoscopy. Here the bias is one of over-exploration rather than risking missed injury. On the other hand, others advocate a selective approach to exploration, relying on contrast studies, endoscopy and other modalities to exclude esophageal and other injury.

The basic principles of treatment of esophageal perforation are controlling the leak of oral or gastric contents, adequate drainage of involved areas, antibiotics, nutrition and supportive therapy. Isolated injuries to the cervical part of the esophagus should be repaired through an incision anterior to the border of the left or right sternocleidomastoid muscle. This type of incision is particularly useful if unanticipated vascular injuries are encountered. Caution should surround dissection in proximity to the recurrent laryngeal nerves running in the tracheoesophageal groove. Injuries in the upper or middle third should be repaired through a high right posterolateral thoracotomy and those of the lower third through a left. This caveat may be broken if it is found that the perforation has already resulted in pleural soilage in which case it is prudent to operate on the ipsilateral side.

The blood supply of the esophagus enters from the lateral points. Dissection can be extended in the anterior or posterior planes without fear of devascularization. After the wound is identified, the esophagus is rotated to examine the opposite wall to exclude the presence of an exit wound. The repair is achieved in one or two layers with absorbable sutures, the important layer being the mucosa and submucosa. A particular failure of technique is not identifying mucosal tears extending beneath the muscle layers. It is generally prudent to divide this layer longitudinally to ensure that full exposure is attained. Rarely, in complicated wounds or where exposure is limited, the contralateral tear may be repaired from within the lumen. Our preferred technique is to use stay sutures on either side of the wound on the opposing side to rotate the esophagus to allow sutures to be placed from the external aspect.

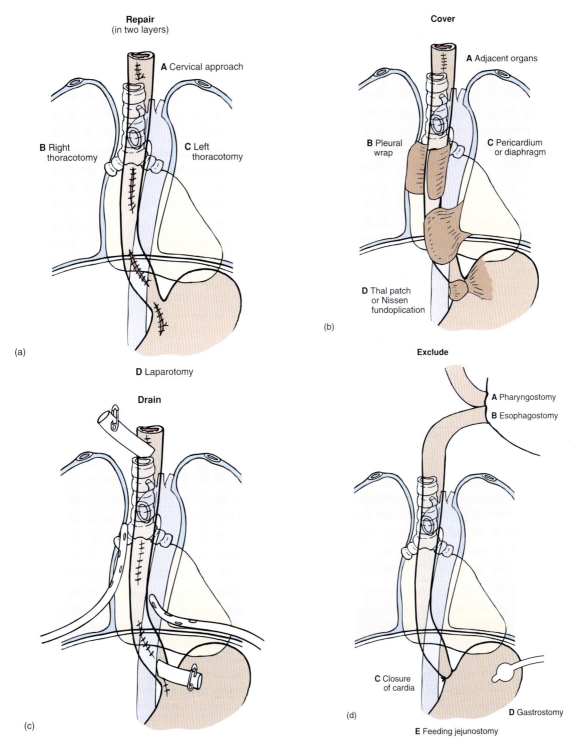

Figure 11.4 *(a) Repair of esophageal perforations. The esophagus is repaired in two layers, an inner mucosal and outer muscular layer, with interrupted absorbable sutures. Cervical perforations can be repaired through a cervical incision, upper and middle third perforations through a right thoracotomy and lower third through a left. The esophagogastric junction is best approached through a laparotomy or thoracoabdominal incision. (b) Reinforcement of esophageal repair. Suture lines should be reinforced with viable tissue in the form of local structures, pedicled wraps of pleura, intercostal muscle, diaphragm or pericardium. Lower esophageal perforations can be buttressed with stomach or omentum. (c) Drainage after repair of the esophagus. All repairs should be drained to surface with soft non-reactive drains. These should be positioned as not to cross major vascular structures or other suture lines. The pleural space should be thoroughly drained prior to closure. (d) Esophageal exclusion for complex injuries. For complex injuries where further soilage is expected exclusion of the esophagus may be a life-saving strategy. Here an end or loop esophagostomy is fashioned in the neck and the esophagogastric junction occluded. A gastrostomy and feeding jejunostomy are fashioned concurrently. (Adapted from Besson A, Saegesser F. A Colour Atlas of Chest Trauma. Volume 2. London: Wolfe Medical, 1983.)*

Bullet wounds are usually low velocity in civilian practice but still may be large with contused edges. Care must be taken to effect the repair without significantly narrowing the residual esophagus. It is important that all involved areas be thoroughly drained.

Buttressing the wound with surrounding tissue or muscle flap is particularly advised in macerated wounds or where the wound is over 12 hours old. Structures to be considered for reinforcement are pleura, diaphragm, pericardium, omentum, intercostal, serratus anterior, sternocleidomastoid and rhomboid muscles.[33,35,37,44–46] If opting for use of an intercostal muscle flap, care must be taken not to include periosteum as late calcification may lead to late esophageal stenosis.[36] Lower esophageal perforations can be adequately reinforced by use of a Thal patch of stomach.[33] Wounds that are macerated or presenting late may be best treated by exclusion methods.[33,35,43,47] Though effective in reducing sepsis the procedure requires further operations to restore intestinal continuity. In uncomplicated high or cervical leaks a nasogastric tube for nutrition usually suffices. In complex repairs we prefer to place both a gastrostomy and feeding jejunostomy.

For late diagnosed perforations, primary repair is often not possible nor indicated. The time frame beyond which repair is likely not to be successful is dependent on numerous variables but is probably not indicated after 12–24 hours.[35,38] Direct surgical repair after 48 hours and even after 24 hours is often impossible due to established sepsis. In these cases the primary intent is debridement and drainage, accepting that a transient fistula will develop. In cases above the thoracic inlet where the process has not involved the pleural space this can usually be managed by a cervical incision. Even where there has been mediastinal extension down to the level of the carina, it usually can be adequately drained through this approach. Where the wound is lower or where pleural soilage has occurred, formal thoracotomy and debridement are required. Here it is important to widely open the mediastinum, thoroughly debride the mediastinum and place drains in proximity to the site of perforation. In this case some authors advocate repair and buttressing with viable tissue as described above, accepting that leak will likely still occur but the course will be more self-limiting.[37] With concomitant vascular injury it is particularly important to interpose pleura or muscle between the suture lines. Dependent pleural drains must be well positioned before closure. Unfortunately, all too often the collections are loculated and recur despite adequate drainage. The surgeon should be prepared for multiple re-explorations.

The timing of reinstitution of oral intake after repair depends on the confidence in the repair. We usually precede feeding with a contrast swallow at day 5 but have observed late leaks despite negative studies also noted by other authors.[36]

Outcome

The importance of early diagnosis on outcome cannot be overemphasized. Defore[33] observed that four of five patients who had a late diagnosis with systemic sepsis died despite apparently adequate drainage procedures. Gunshot wounds of the esophagus carry a mortality of 7–23%.[33,35,36,40] The site of the wound and concomitant injuries often determines outcome.[36] Symbas[47] found that of 48 patients with esophageal gunshot wounds, 38 (79.2%) survived overall but only 11 of 16 (64%) intrathoracic injuries survived. None in whom the injury was identified early and primarily repaired died or developed a suture line disruption.

The major morbidity in most cases occurs from anastomotic leak. In repairs made early, the leak rate is less than 5%.[36] The propensity for prolonged leak appears to be greater with gunshot wounds than stab wounds.[48] Most can be treated successfully by conservative management and long-term complications are uncommon in most series. Where extensive tissue loss has occurred there is an appreciable incidence of late stricture.

PENETRATING TRAUMA TO THE TRACHEA AND CENTRAL AIRWAYS

Pathogenesis

Airway injury should be ruled out in all central penetrating wounds of the chest or neck. Except for the cervical region, most tracheobronchial injuries are due to gunshot wounds. The centrality of the tracheobronchial tree within the chest makes it difficult to penetrate with a knife. The proximity of the central airways to major vascular structures also means that any gunshot wounds involving the central areas will carry a high mortality. Symbas[49] observed that 10 of 20 patients with acute penetrating tracheal injuries had other major associated injuries, the majority being esophageal or vascular injury.

The majority of penetrating airway injuries result in death before medical care can be delivered. In a review by Ecker[50] only one of 15 gunshot wounds to the airways survived to reach hospital whereas 11 of 19 stab wounds did. The intrathoracic trachea was associated with a much higher fatality rate than the cervical. A major factor in the survival rate was the incidence of major associated injuries. Associated stab wounds to the aorta and innominate arteries were uniformly lethal. Age over 30 was also found to be associated with a higher mortality rate.

Diagnosis

Findings that suggest a central airway injury are:
- Transmediastinal injuries
- Rapid progressive subcutaneous emphysema
- Simple or tension pneumothoraces
- Large and persistent air leaks after intercostal drain insertion
- Hemoptysis
- Voice loss

Hemoptysis is very specific to tracheal injuries[51] and in large quantities suggests an associated vascular injury. Notably, death from asphyxiation can occur with a relatively small amount of blood or clot within the airway and should be considered a surgical emergency.

The clinical condition of the patient depends on the site and size of the wound. Wounds in the cervical trachea usually manifest with surgical emphysema of the neck, hemoptysis and dyspnea.[49] Wounds of the intrathoracic central airways have, additionally, the likelihood of simple or tension pneumothoraces with varying degrees of respiratory and circulatory embarrassment. Very rarely the patient presents by expectorating a bullet![49]

The extent of the subcutaneous emphysema is dictated by the amount and pressure of air within the tissues. True subcutaneous emphysema may extend from the eyebrows to the inguinal ligaments. The appearance is usually more distressing than dangerous. On rare occasions deep cervical emphysema may cause severe edema by retarding the venous drainage from the larynx, and may require intubation or a tracheostomy.

Where the pleura is also breached, as is common in deep penetrating knife or gunshot wounds, a simple or tension pneumothorax may be the sole manifestation. A pneumothorax with a massive air leak that does not respond to closed chest drain suggests tracheal or major bronchial injury. If associated vascular injury is suspected, and the victim is stable, angiography is optimal to assist in planning the repair.

The anatomical proximity of the recurrent laryngeal nerves makes damage from the injury or attempted repair a hazard. If possible, the movement of the vocal cords should be documented before surgery, not only as a precaution toward contralateral damage but also for medicolegal considerations.

Chest radiology usually shows mediastinal, cervical or whole body subcutaneous emphysema with or without pneumothoraces. Initially the subcutaneous emphysema is more centered in the neck and upper mediastinum and only at late stages spreads out into the chest wall. If the pleura is breached the process may

vent into the pleural space preferentially and cause minimal external signs apart from a pneumothorax.

Management

Bronchoscopy is indicated where injury is suspected to document the site and extent of injury. Because airway management is critical under such circumstances, we feel this should be carried out exclusively by experienced operative and anesthetic staff, in an appropriately equipped operating room, using a rigid bronchoscope. One must keep in mind that it is not uncommon for even experienced endoscopists to miss or underestimate the extent of injury. Esophagoscopy should be performed at the same time because of the proximity of the structure.

Where the diagnosis is in doubt or a conservative approach is undertaken, the final decision should rest on the findings at bronchoscopy. Isolated injuries of less than 33% of the circumference in a stable patient with no respiratory compromise can be observed expectantly. We feel there is no role for protective intubation; the decision is whether an operation or conservative management is indicated.

EMERGENCY AIRWAY CONTROL

The best form of airway control in complex injuries is a rigid bronchoscope in the hands of an experienced surgeon.

In large complex tears control of the airway is of prime importance. The administration of muscle relaxants before securing the airway is a very dangerous practice. The surest method of airway control is through a rigid bronchoscope in the hands of an experienced operator. The rigid bronchoscope offers the ability to bypass any obstructions and clear secretions while at the same time ascertaining the extent of injury. Anesthesia can be maintained under these circumstances with optimal airway control. With an unstable airway, surgery can continue, using the scope as an endotracheal tube rather than risk reintubation. Blind or nasotracheal intubation should be avoided as it carries the risk of converting a partial tear or transection into a complete one. If all other methods fail, an attempt at emergency tracheostomy is warranted but will be futile for deep intrathoracic injuries. A large external wound communicating with the airway can on occasion be intubated by direct tracheostomy tube insertion rather than by attempting control from above. Immediate suctioning of the airway often restores adequate respiration.

For airway injuries involving the hilum of the lung the situation can be very complex. Injuries may involve the proximal hilar vessels and digital control or proximal cross-clamping may be required to preserve patency of the airway. Only in the rare circumstance of complex injuries is cardiopulmonary bypass necessary.

TECHNIQUE OF REPAIR

Most tracheal injuries can be repaired through a neck incision.[52] In general, the upper three-quarters of the trachea can usually be repaired through a standard cervical approach. In cases where the level is difficult to relate to superficial structures, inserting a sterile needle into the airway from the surface at the time of bronchoscopy may clarify the topical relations. If extreme difficulty is encountered, an upper manubrial split can be performed. Due to difficulties in visualization and for the avoidance of undue traction we prefer to repair low tracheal and carinal injuries or ones compounded with esophageal damage through a right thoracotomy. Isolated left main bronchial injuries beyond 3 cm from the carina should be approached through a left thoracotomy. In rare complex injuries a transpericardial approach may be undertaken through a sternotomy.

Care must be taken not to devascularize the airway during surgery. Material used for repair should be an absorbable suture such as Polyglactin 910 (Vicryl®) but a monofilament non-absorbable material can be used. Recurrent nerve injury is common from the primary insult so care should be taken to avoid creating an iatrogenic contralateral injury. Intrathoracic repairs should be covered with tissue flaps from parietal pleura, pericardium, or other surrounding tissue. Complex injuries of the airway may be best managed by the resection of two to three tracheal rings and end-to-end reanastomosis. This strategy should be reserved for patients who can be extubated postoperatively; otherwise temporary oral or tracheal intubation past the wound should be maintained until definitive repair can be accomplished. For complex repairs with postoperative edema or airway malacia, a silastic T-tube can be used to splint the airway, usually for 3–6 weeks, until stable. We do not routinely insert a tracheotomy tube for simple lacerations as advocated by some authors.[49] Tracheostomy wounds are obligatorily contaminated and thus should be particularly avoided in conjunction with median sternotomies. With combined trachea and major vessel injury, extra-anatomical bypass should be considered rather than putting a tracheostomy in the region of repair. At the termination of repair, careful attention should be directed to bronchial toilet as often blood and oral secretions have been aspirated. Before the termination of anesthetic we prefer to perform flexible bronchoscopy through the endotracheal tube to provide the most optimal airway in the immediate postoperative period. At the end of the procedure the patient should be extubated in the operating room before moving to the recovery unit.

Combined tracheal and esophageal injuries should be synchronously repaired with the interposition of strap or sternocleidomastoid muscle between the suture lines.[41,53,54] In severe injuries with gross contamination of the mediastinum, the trachea should be primarily repaired and consideration given towards an esophageal exclusion procedure.[49] A few weeks post-repair the esophagus can be reconstructed with a higher probability of success.

Outcome

Kelly[53] observed a mortality of 53.8% for intrathoracic tracheal injuries compared with 13.8% for cervical airway injuries. Most of the deaths were attributed to the severity of associated injuries. Concomitant injury to the innominate artery or the thoracic aorta was uniformly lethal in this study. For isolated injuries, primary repair is usually successful and rewarded with early discharge of the patient in most circumstances.

The main late morbid event is stenosis of the airway at the site of repair though this is seldom seen in repair of simple stab wounds. Most cases can be avoided by meticulous repair using absorbable sutures and the avoidance of tension or devascularization. After repair tracheal stenosis is more commonly seen where more than three tracheal rings have been damaged, usually by a gunshot wound.[52] This may not manifest until weeks or months after injury.

PENETRATING TRAUMA TO THE THORACIC DUCT

Pathogenesis

Given a high incidence of penetrating trauma, even the smallest of intrathoracic structures can be damaged. The thoracic duct originates from the cisterna chyli at the level of the second lumbar vertebra and enters the thorax through the aortic hiatus to the right of midline. In the lower thorax it lies between the aorta and azygos vein behind the esophagus. It crosses to the left of midline at the level of the fourth thoracic vertebra, ascending behind the aortic arch on the left side of the esophagus. It then passes behind the left subclavian artery before emptying into the left subclavian vein near the junction with the internal jugular vein. Sixty to seventy percent of the ingested fat is conveyed to the bloodstream by way of the thoracic duct. The normal flow of chyle is up to 2.5 liters in 24 hours.[55]

Chyle is thought to be bacteriostatic as a result of its lecithin and fatty acid content and therefore is usually sterile. Chyle also tends to be non-irritating and does not form any entrapping cortex over the lung. It does tend to form fibrinous clots that regularly block chest drains. The loss of proteins, fats and fat-soluble vitamins in chyle can lead to extreme metabolic deficit in a short time and ultimately to death. The loss of lymphocytes and antibodies can also interfere with the immunological status of the patient. In the past, injury to the duct and a chylous fistula have been associated with mortality in excess of 50%.

Thoracic duct injury is unusual and often overshadowed by accompanying injuries. In a series of eight isolated cases in our department,[56] the vast majority were caused by stab wounds above the sternoclavicular line. The site of injury was most commonly in Poirier's triangle and most frequently resulted in a left-sided chylothorax.

Diagnosis

The accumulation of any pleural fluid including chyle can result in compression of the underlying lung and shift of the mediastinum. In the post-traumatic situation this is often initially considered to be residual traumatic hemothorax and only after a drain is inserted and chyle drained is the diagnosis evident (Fig 11.5). The other common scenario is the patient with a chest drain *in situ* draining serosanguinous effusion for the first 24–48 hours which only becomes chylous after the first meal. Occasionally there may be a long latent period between the injury and the development of a free chylothorax due to initial containment by the mediastinal pleura.[55] Usually diagnosis is obvious but may be confirmed by the finding of free microscopic fat and chylomicrons. Lymphangiography and computed tomography can occasionally be used to demonstrate the site of injury.[57]

Management

Attempts at intravenous replacement are likely to precipitate anaphylaxis and readministration by mouth or rectum is of no benefit. Medium chain triglyceride diets and total parenteral nutrition reduce the amount of chyle formation and may accelerate closure by natural healing. Notably, often the leak under these circumstances does not slow progressively but tends to persist until a time when it stops abruptly. In our series,[56] five of eight patients were initially treated with a medium chain triglyceride diet and two were subsequently converted to total parenteral nutrition. Despite the reduction in volume, none of the leaks ceased at a mean duration of 12 days with a range of 7–29 days. In all cases operative ligation was required. Robinson,[55] however, advocates a period of 2–3 weeks of conservative treatment before resorting to surgery.

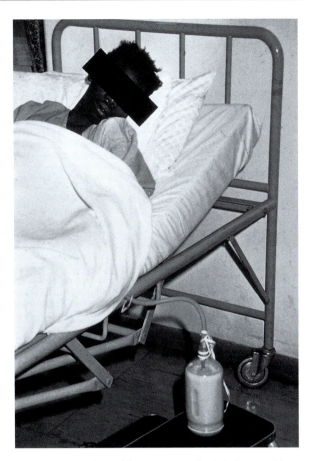

Figure 11.5 *Patient with post-traumatic chylothorax. This young man was stabbed in his left neck with the only identifiable injury being the thoracic duct. Conservative management failed and the thoracic duct was ligated successfully in Poirier's triangle.*

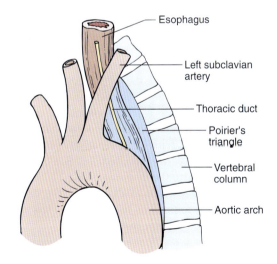

Figure 11.6 *Poirier's triangle. The most likely site of injury and the most convenient for repair lies in Poirier's triangle. This is the area bounded by the vertebral column posteriorly, the aorta inferiorly and the subclavian artery anterosuperiorly. The duct lies in a constant position overlying the esophagus as shown. (Adapted from Worthington et al.[56])*

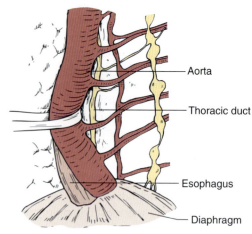

(a)   (b)

Figure 11.7 *(a) Supradiaphragmatic thoracic duct ligation through a right thoracotomy. The inferior pulmonary ligament is incised and the esophagus encircled and retracted. The thoracic duct lies between the azygos vein and the aorta on the vertebral column. Mass ligature is recommended. (b) Supradiaphragmatic thoracic duct ligation through a left thoracotomy. The inferior pulmonary ligament is incised and the aorta carefully dissected along with its intercostal branches. The thoracic duct lies posterior to the aorta and medial to the opposite azygos vein. Mass ligature is recommended. (Adapted from Ross K. Surgery of the thoracic duct and management of chylothorax. In: Rob and Smith's Operative Surgery – Thoracic Surgery. 4th edn. London: Butterworth, 1986)*

Surgical management of chyle leak is ligation of the duct or obliteration of the pleural space. The level of optimal ligation depends on the site of injury as it is of no benefit to ligate the duct downstream from the injury. Anatomically the duct is most easily identified in the chest at the esophageal hiatus or Poirier's triangle (Fig 11.6). Under favorable circumstances a direct attempt at ligature of the leaking site can be attempted. Numerous techniques have been described for operatively identifying the site of leak including the oral administration of cream, olive oil or various vital and lipophilic dyes. We favor the former and recommend that 100 ml should be administered between 2–3 hours before incision. Where a secure closure is in doubt, pleurectomy or pleural abrasion to facilitate pleural symphysis may be advisable. Alternatively or where the site of leak is lower in the chest, ligation should be attempted just above the diaphragm (Fig 11.7). Generally we make no attempt to dissect out the duct but ligate the entire column of tissue with a mass suture ligature of non-absorbable material.

Outcome

In all eight of our patients, complete cessation of chylous leak was present after surgery and a full diet was possible in all patients with 48 hours of surgery. We have seen a case of transient chyloperitoneum after successful duct ligation that was self-limiting. There are no known nutritional complications of the procedure and the chyle is probably absorbed by other pathways.

REFERENCES

1. Demetriades D, Rabinowitz B, Markides N. Indications for thoracotomy in stab injuries of the chest: a prospective study of 543 patients. *Br J Surg* 1986; **73(11)**: 888–90.
2. Borja AR, Ransdell HT. Treatment of penetrating gunshot wounds of the chest. Experience with one hundred forty-five cases. *Am J Surg* 1971; **122(1)**: 81–4.
3. Brewer LA. Wounds of the chest in war and peace, 1943–1968. *Ann Thorac Surg* 1969; **7(5)**: 387–408.
4. Mandal AK, Oparah SS. Unusually low mortality of penetrating wounds of the chest. Twelve years' experience. *J Thorac Cardiovasc Surg* 1989; **97(1)**: 119–25.
5. Oparah SS, Mandal AK. Penetrating gunshot wounds of the chest in civilian practice: experience with 250 consecutive cases. *Br J Surg* 1978; **65(1)**: 45–8.
6. Zakharia AT. Thoracic battle injuries in the Lebanon War: review of the early operative approach in 1,992 patients. *Ann Thorac Surg* 1985; **40(3)**: 209–13.
7. Richardson JD, Flint LM, Snow NJ, Gray LA Jr, Trinkle JK. Management of transmediastinal gunshot wounds. *Surgery* 1981; **90(4)**: 671–6.
8. Mandal AK, Montano J, Thadepalli H. Prophylactic

antibiotics and no antibiotics compared in penetrating chest trauma. *J Trauma* 1985; **25(7):** 639–43.

9. DeMuth WE Jr. The mechanism of shotgun wounds. *J Trauma* 1971; **11(3):** 219–29.

10. Ordog GJ, Wasserberger J, Balasubramaniam S. Shotgun wound ballistics. *J Trauma* 1988; **28(5):** 624–31.

11. Grimes WR, Deitch EA, McDonald JC. A clinical review of shotgun wounds to the chest and abdomen. *Surg Gynecol Obstet* 1985; **160(2):** 148–52.

12. Hoekstra SM, Bender JS, Levison MA. The management of large soft-tissue defects following close-range shotgun injury. *J Trauma* 1990; **30(12):** 1489–93.

13. Flint LM, Cryer HM, Howard DA, Richardson JD. Approaches to the management of shotgun injuries. *J Trauma* 1984; **24(5):** 415–19.

14. Bender JS, Lucas CE. Management of close-range shotgun injuries to the chest by diaphragmatic transposition: case reports. *J Trauma* 1990; **30(12):** 1581–4.

15. Wanebo H, Van Dyke J. The high-velocity pulmonary injury. Relation to traumatic wet lung syndrome. *J Thorac Cardiovasc Surg* 1972; **64(4):** 537–50.

16. Spees EK, Strevey TE, Geiger JP, Aronstam EM. Persistent traumatic lung cavities resulting from medium- and high-velocity missiles. *Ann Thorac Surg* 1967; **4(2):** 133–42.

17. Wilson RF, Soullier GW, Wiencek RG. Hemoptysis in trauma. *J Trauma* 1987; **27(10):** 1123–6.

18. Smith JM III, Richardson JD, Grover FL, Arom KV, Webb GE, Trinkle JK. Fatal air embolism following gunshot wound of the lung. *J Thorac Cardiovasc Surg* 1976; **72(2):** 296–8.

19. Estrera AS, Pass LJ, Platt MR. Systemic arterial air embolism in penetrating lung injury. *Ann Thorac Surg* 1990; **50(2):** 257–61.

20. Ponn RB, Zatarain G, Gerzberg L, Hottinger GF, Haase W, Nelsen TS. Systemic air embolism in experimental penetrating lung injuries. *J Thorac Cardiovasc Surg* 1977; **74(5):** 766–73.

21. Graham JM, Mattox KL, Beall AC Jr. Penetrating trauma of the lung. *J Trauma* 1979; **19(9):** 665–9.

22. Meier GH, Symbas PN. Systemic air embolization: factors involved in its production following penetrating lung injury. *Am Surg* 1978, **44(12):** 765–71.

23. George PY, Goodman P. Radiographic appearance of bullet tracks in the lung. *Am J Roentgenol* 1992; **159(5):** 967–70.

24. Robison PD, Harman PK, Trinkle JK, Grover FL. Management of penetrating lung injuries in civilian practice. *J Thorac Cardiovasc Surg* 1988; **95(2):** 184–90.

25. Thompson DA, Rowlands BJ, Walker WE, Kuykendall RC, Miller PW, Fischer RP. Urgent thoracotomy for pulmonary or tracheobronchial injury. *J Trauma* 1988; **28(3):** 276–80.

26. Fischer RP, Geiger JP, Guernsey JM. Pulmonary resections for severe pulmonary contusions secondary to high-velocity missile wounds. *J Trauma* 1974; **14(4):** 293–302.

27. Millikan JS, Moore EE, Steiner E, Aragon GE, Van Way CW. Complications of tube thoracostomy for acute trauma. *Am J Surg* 1980; **140(6):** 738–41.

28. Wiencek RG Jr, Wilson RF. Central lung injuries: a need for early vascular control. *J Trauma* 1988; **28(10):** 1418–24.

29. Powell RJ, Redan JA, Swan KG. The hilar snare, and improved technique for securing rapid vascular control of the pulmonary hilum. *J Trauma* 1990; **30(2):** 208–10.

30. Vogt-Moykopf I, Krumhaar D. Treatment of intrapulmonary shell fragments. *Surg Gynecol Obstet* 1966; **123(6):** 1233–6.

31. Symbas PN, Goldman M, Erbesfeld MH, Vlasis SE. Pulmonary arteriovenous fistula, pulmonary artery aneurysm, and other vascular changes of the lung from penetrating trauma. *Ann Surg* 1980; **191(3):** 336–40.

32. Jones WG, Ginsberg RJ. Esophageal perforation: a continuing challenge. *Ann Thorac Surg* 1992; **53(3):** 534–43.

33. Defore WW Jr, Mattox KL, Hansen HA, Garcia-Rinaldi R, Beall AC Jr, DeBakey ME. Surgical management of penetrating injuries of the esophagus. *Am J Surg* 1977; **134(6):** 734–8.

34. Shama DM, Odell J. Penetrating neck trauma with tracheal and oesophageal injuries. *Br J Surg* 1984; **71(7):** 534–6.

35. Popovsky J. Perforations of the esophagus from gunshot wounds. *J Trauma* 1984; **24(4):** 337–9.

36. Pass LJ, LeNarz LA, Schreiber JT, Estrera AS. Management of esophageal gunshot wounds. *Ann Thorac Surg* 1987; **44:** 253–6.

37. Cheadle W, Richardson JD. Options in management of trauma to the esophagus. *Surg Gynecol Obstet* 1982; **155(3):** 380–4.

38. Lyons WS, Seremetis MG, deGuzman VC, Peabody JW Jr. Ruptures and perforations of the esophagus: the case for conservative supportive management. *Ann Thorac Surg* 1978; **25(4):** 346–50.

39. Symbas PN, Tyras DH, Hatcher CR Jr, Perry B. Penetrating wounds of the esophagus. *Ann Thorac Surg* 1972; **13(6):** 552–8.

40. Glatterer MS Jr, Toon RS, Ellestad C, *et al.* Management of blunt and penetrating external esophageal trauma. *J Trauma* 1985; **25(8):** 784–92.

41. Feliciano DV, Bitondo CG, Mattox KL, *et al.* Combined tracheoesophageal injuries. *Am J Surg* 1985; **150(6):** 710–15.

42. Weigelt JA, Thal ER, Snyder WH, Fry RE, Meier DE, Kilman WJ. Diagnosis of penetrating cervical esophageal injuries. *Am J Surg* 1987; **154(6):** 619–22.

43. Loop FD, Groves LK. Esophageal perforations. *Ann Thorac Surg* 1970; **10(6):** 571–87.

44. Michel L, Grillo HC, Malt RA. Esophageal perforation. *Ann Thorac Surg* 1982; **33(2):** 203–10.

45. Lucas AE, Snow N, Tobin GR, Flint LM Jr. Use of the rhomboid major muscle flap for esophageal repair. *Ann Thorac Surg* 1982; **33(6):** 619–23.

46. Richardson JD, Tobin GR. Closure of esophageal defects with muscle flaps. *Arch Surg* 1994; **129(5):** 541–7.

47. Symbas PN, Hatcher CR Jr, Vlasis SE. Esophageal gunshot injuries. *Ann Surg* 1980; **191(6):** 703–7.

48. Armstrong WB, Detar TR, Stanley RB. Diagnosis and management of external penetrating cervical esophageal injuries. *Ann Otol Rhinol Laryngol* 1994; **103(11):** 863–71.

49. Symbas PN, Hatcher CR Jr, Boehm GA. Acute penetrating tracheal trauma. *Ann Thorac Surg* 1976; **22(5):** 473–7.

50. Ecker RR, Libertini RV, Rea WJ, Sugg WL, Webb WR. Injuries of the trachea and bronchi. *Ann Thorac Surg* 1971; **11(4):** 289–98.

51. Symbas PN, Hatcher CR Jr, Vlasis SE. Bullet wounds of the trachea. *J Thorac Cardiovasc Surg* 1982; **83(2):** 235–8.

52. Sulek M, Miller RH, Mattox KL. The management of gunshot and stab injuries of the trachea. *Arch Otolaryngol* 1983; **109(1):** 56–9.

53. Kelly JP, Webb WR, Moulder PV, Everson C, Burch BH, Lindsey ES. Management of airway trauma. I: Tracheo-bronchial injuries. *Ann Thorac Surg* 1985; **40(6):** 551–5.

54. Kelly JP, Webb WR, Moulder PV, Moustouakas NM, Lirtzman M. Management of airway trauma. II: Combined injuries of the trachea and esophagus. *Ann Thorac Surg* 1987; **43(2):** 160–3.

55. Robinson CL. The management of chylothorax. *Ann Thorac Surg* 1985; **39(1):** 90–5.

56. Worthington MG, de Groot M, Gunning AJ, von Oppell UO. Isolated thoracic duct injury after penetrating chest trauma. *Ann Thorac Surg* 1995; **60(2):** 272–4.

57. Sachs PB, Zelch MG, Rice TW, Geisinger MA, Risius B, Lammert GK. Diagnosis and localization of laceration of the thoracic duct: usefulness of lymphangiography and CT. *Am J Roentgenol* 1991; **157(4):** 703–5.

FURTHER READING

Besson A, Saegesser F. *A Colour Atlas of Chest Trauma.* London: Wolfe Medical, 1983.

Defore WW Jr, Mattox KL, Hansen HA, Garcia-Rinaldi R, Beall AC Jr, DeBakey ME. Surgical management of penetrating injuries of the esophagus. *Am J Surg* 1977; **134(6):** 734–8.

DeMuth WE Jr. High velocity bullet wounds of the thorax. *Am J Surg* 1968; **115(5):** 616–25.

Feliciano DV, Bitondo CG, Mattox KL, *et al.* Combined tracheoesophageal injuries. *Am J Surg* 1985; **150(6):** 710–15.

Hood RM, Boyd AD, Culliford AT. *Thoracic Trauma.* Philadelphia: WB Saunders, 1989.

Webb WR, Besson A (eds) *Thoracic Surgery: Surgical Management of Chest Injuries.* St Louis: Mosby Year Book, 1991.

12

Penetrating trauma to the inlet and outlet regions of the chest

JOHN V ROBBS

This chapter deals with vascular injuries within the superior mediastinum and penetrating injury to the diaphragm. Penetrating trauma to the aerodigestive tract is dealt with in Chapter 11.

SUPERIOR MEDIASTINAL VASCULAR INJURY

The surgical management of these injuries may present the most challenging in vascular trauma in view of the anatomical confines of the space and hence the difficulty in obtaining adequate control of hemorrhage. In addition, these injuries often occur at times of the night which preclude ready availability of many facilities while immediate therapy is demanded in view of the life-threatening nature of the injury.

In order to provide perspective as to the incidence of these injuries, in the last 18 years the computerized database of the Metropolitan Vascular Service of the University of Natal Hospitals has data on 3500 major vascular injuries treated surgically by the unit. Twenty percent of these involve the cervicomediastinal vessels of which approximately one-third are within the superior mediastinum. The most frequently injured vessels are the proximal subclavian (Fig 12.1) and common carotid, with the brachiocephalic being least frequently involved. This may well reflect on-site mortality due to massive hemorrhage.

The review that follows is based on lessons learnt from this experience.

Pathological considerations

The vast majority (97%) of mediastinal arterial injuries follow penetrating trauma, of which in our experience, more than half are low velocity gunshot wounds.[1-7] High velocity missile injuries (muzzle velocity of more than 600 m/s) in this region are probably incompatible with survival. Close range shotgun wounds warrant special consideration in view of the extensive associated soft tissue and visceral injury, in addition to multiple vessel perforations. An added component is the presence of multiple foreign bodies such as pellets,

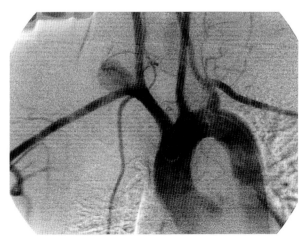

Figure 12.1 *Aneurysm at the root of the right subclavian artery after a fractured clavicle penetrated this vessel. (SWTC.)*

cartridge wadding and clothing fragments. Possibly not unique to the rural areas of South Africa is the use of homemade ammunition, which contains a wide variety of missiles akin to the 'blunderbuss' used in military conflict in days of yore.

Although outwith the scope of the present report, it is interesting to note that the commonest injuries following blunt trauma, mainly crush and acceleration/deceleration injuries of the superior mediastinal vessels, involve the brachiocephalic and left subclavian arteries.[8–10]

In order to treat these injuries rationally, it is essential that there is a good understanding of the pathology. Penetration may result in partial transection of the artery, complete transection, or in the case of missiles, percussion trauma with thrombosis.

Iatrogenic injuries in this region are uncommon and arterial lacerations may follow attempts at subclavian venous cannulation or operative misadventure during neck dissections, usually for malignant disease.

Most frequently associated with laceration of major arteries is significant hemorrhage which when contained gives rise to a false aneurysm. Frequently, however, significant hemorrhage is not a consequence of complete transection because the ends of the artery develop intense spasm with associated thrombosis. Delayed hemorrhage may occur due to lysis of the clot but the precise mechanism of this phenomenon is ill understood as it occurs 5–7 days later, but that may possibly be due to low-grade infection. The consequence of false aneurysm is compression of adjacent nerves and viscera, but in the acute situation the trachea is the most vulnerable and immediately life-threatening. Of particular importance in relation to nerve compression is the vagus and the lower trunks of the brachial plexus. The prognosis for recovery of either in the presence of significant compression is poor.

Concomitant perforation of adjacent artery and vein frequently results in an arteriovenous fistula with or without an associated false aneurysm (Fig 12.2). More than a third of the superior medistinal injuries in our experience presented with this pathology and most frequently involved the left common carotid or brachiocephalic. This may reflect the fact that hemorrhage had not occurred at the time of initial injury as the artery decompressed directly into the vein. In the region of the fistula there is marked dilatation of the vein draining the fistula, which eventually develops degenerative change with aneurysmal dilatation most frequently seen in the internal jugular vein. The extensive hypertrophy and dilatation of collateral veins may compound the difficulties in the technical exercise of repairing the fistula. The shunting of blood away from the distal circulation is a potential cause of cerebral ischemia but even quite significant distal arterial flow does not in practice seem to lead to any cerebral dysfunction *per se*. The major import of reduced distal arterial flow is the

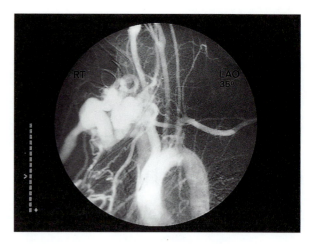

Figure 12.2 *Large arteriovenous fistula following stab wound to the right side of the thoracic inlet. (SWTC.)*

frequent development of partially occluding thrombus in the artery just distal to the fistula. We have frequently encountered this at surgery and on several occasions patients have developed acute cerebral embolization while awaiting operation, presumably from this source. This is illustrated in Fig 12.3. It has also become apparent to us that neurological deficit following repair of fistulae of these vessels may be a consequence of embolization. The systemic hemodynamic effects of the shunt are directly proportional to the extent and duration of the arteriovenous communication.[11,12] The presence of a significant fistula results in a fall in diastolic blood pressure because of the drop in peripheral resistance. There is also a significant increase in pulse rate and a concomitant increase in cardiac output. The blood volume also increases for reasons which are not understood.[13] The ultimate net effect of this hyper-

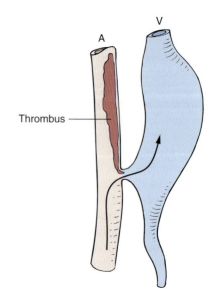

Thrombus

Figure 12.3 *Development of thrombus in relation to traumatic arteriovenous fistula. A, artery; V, vein.*

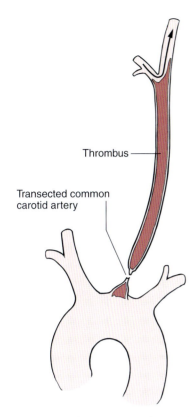

Thrombus

Transected common
carotid artery

Figure 12.4 *Pattern of propagation of thrombus in common carotid artery injuries.*

dynamic state may be cardiac decompensation. In our experience, however, the only patients who do develop significant cardiac decompensation have some other underlying cardiomyopathy.[11] Subacute bacterial endocarditis may also occur at the site of the fistula but is a rare late complication which we have only documented on one occasion.[14]

Thrombosis of an artery in relation to the passage of a missile in close proximity is an interesting phenomenon. It may be postulated that the mechanism of injury is in fact an acute distraction-type force caused by rapid displacement of the artery by the shock wave as the bullet traverses the tissue. The intima is relatively inelastic in relation to the media and adventitia. The application of any type of distraction force would result in the intima tearing before the other layers. The artery therefore tears in layers from the inside out and the degree of disruption of the vessel would depend upon the extent of the force applied. These intimal tears expose thrombogenic media, initiating the coagulation process. There is also the possibility of an intimal flap developing with distal dissection along the media. On observation at surgery, however, it would appear that dissection does not occur in an otherwise normal vessel and it is apparent that the basic pathogenesis is focal thrombosis in the area of intimal damage.

An important associated problem when flow is interrupted in the common carotid artery is that there is propagation of the clot proximally and distally to the point at which there is blood flow, that is, up to the carotid bifurcation. This must be a major consideration when restoring prograde flow after repair of these vessels in the mediastinum and neurological deficit in association with injuries to carotid and brachiocephalic systems may result from embolism from distal propagated thrombus (illustrated in Fig 12.4). Care must be taken to ensure distal patency before releasing clamps after repair. A further compounding issue in relation to neurological deficit is associated hypovolemia and shock.

Clinical considerations

It is extremely important to realize that the actual site of entry of low velocity penetration, particularly gunshot wounds, does not often give an indication of the precise direction of the missile through the tissues. Certainly probing is ill advised and not to be recommended as it may initiate torrential hemorrhage. Massive overt hemorrhage makes the diagnosis of major arterial injury obvious and this occurs in approximately a third of our patients. However, spontaneous hemostasis due to arterial spasm or thrombosis at the site of injury may manifest in a more subtle manner and the clinician must remain alert to the possibility of arterial injury. In the patient presenting with unexplained hypovolemia or anemia associated with a penetrating wound in the lower neck or mediastinal area, a bruit or a palpable thrill may be the only manifestation of an arteriovenous fistula or a partially occlusive thrombus at the site of trauma. This type of injury may be associated with an apparently insignificant cervical puncture wound and, in the case of arteriovenous fistula due to the rapid decompression from a high to a low circulatory pressure system, may have minimal if any associated false aneurysm formation. In our own series, approximately 30% of the patients presented with a bruit and in half of those it was the only physical sign of arterial injury.[6,11] With regard to arteriovenous fistula, we found that almost half of the patients only presented for treatment more than a week after injury, the longest being 12 years after a stab in the lower neck. It is also interesting to note that in those presenting within a week of injury only about a half had a machinery murmur whereas this was a universal finding in those presenting later. Possible explanations are that there is initially thrombotic occlusion of the fistula, which later lyses, or an initially small communication enlarges with time due to the pressure. Congestive cardiac failure and obvious superficial venous dilatation were relatively uncommon findings in our patients and were only noted in those presenting months to years later. In addition, patients with congestive heart failure all had evidence of underlying cardiomyopathy, whether ischemic or nutritional.

False aneurysm occurring in the superior media-stinum frequently causes severe compressive symptoms, most significant of which is compression of the trachea with resultant stridor. This invariably increases as the hematoma expands and is a mandate for prompt action. Under these circumstances tracheostomy or crycothy-roidotomy is of little use in view of the anatomical site of the compression and any ill-considered attempt to improve the airway in this way invariably precipitates torrential hemorrhage. Under these circumstances urgent surgical decompression with control of the bleeding vessel is life-saving.

Compression of the brachial plexus involving mainly the lower trunks has been encountered in a number of patients with stab wounds involving the proximal common carotid and subclavian arteries. This may be an acute phenomenon but in most the patients presented some days or weeks later. Under these circumstances the vascular injury was not diagnosed at the time of clinical presentation and the patient returned 7–21 days later with obvious nerve lesions associated with the development of false aneurysm. This delayed onset is presumably the result of clot lysis as discussed earlier. Prognosis for limb function is variable and at least a year is required before final assessment can be made. In our experience the outlook for intrin-sic hand function recovery is poor although some recovery of upper trunk function, responsible for shoul-der and elbow movement, can be anticipated in most cases.[15] Most patients with subclavian artery trauma have a definite pulse deficit although this may be subtle in view of the rich collateralization, especially if there is partial disruption of the patent vessel. About a quarter of patients with penetrating mediastinal trauma with involvement of brachiocephalic or carotid vessels will present with a neurological deficit ranging from coma to hemiparesis or hemiplegia. It may be extremely diffi-cult to assess the actual contribution made by focal cerebral ischemia as the problem is compounded by the fact that many patients sustaining this type of injury have an associated head or craniofacial injury. The issue is further clouded by alcoholic or drug intoxication and hypovolemic shock. Of increasing importance is the realization that delayed neurological deficits may occur in patients with arteriovenous fistulae involving the carotid or brachiocephalic vessels. This is presumably due to dislodgment of clot either at the fistula site or in the segment of artery distal to the fistula, as described earlier.

Diagnosis and management

The most important facet in diagnosis is to have a high index of clinical suspicion in every patient who sustains a penetrating neck injury. In our own practice we have had to adopt a selective management policy for penetrating neck trauma due to the large patient load on the trauma services. This has proved highly satisfac-tory in dealing with stab wounds.[16] Arch-angiography in selected cases is the gold standard for diagnosis and is also essential for planning the operative approach, particularly to injuries within the superior mediastinum and root of neck (zone 1).[17] It is difficult to trace trajec-tory in stab and in particular low velocity gunshot wounds and digital probing is strongly discouraged. It must be emphasized that the ancillary investigations must only be performed in the hemodynamically stable patient. In addition, stridor is a mandate for immediate exploration and in the absence of obvious false aneurysm in the neck it can be assumed that the lesion is situated in the superior mediastinum and the appro-priate exposure should be obtained. Failure to do so results in a prohibitive mortality in this group of patients. A detailed description of resuscitation is dealt with in Chapter 4.

The initial investigation in the stable patient should be a plain erect chest radiograph and a superior mediastinal shadow (widening) is often found in patients who have superior mediastinal arterial injuries. This may not be the case if an acute arteriovenous fistula has developed. However, emergency room radiographs of this nature must be interpreted with caution as they are often taken in the recumbent position and more often than not one is dealing with an uncooperative and unruly patient, which may give a false picture of mediastinal widening due to positional errors. Arch-angiography must be employed if there is clinical suspicion of superior mediastinal injury. Signs include an upper limb pulse deficit which may be noted with brachiocephalic or subclavian injuries, presence of a false aneurysm or evidence of previous hemorrhage. The latter may be overt or subtle as in the patient who presents with unexplained shock or is found to have a low hematocrit or hemoglobin value with no obvious blood loss. The presence of a bruit is also an important sign. Shotgun injuries mandate routine angiography. There is still some debate, however, about low velocity handgun wounds, although we usually perform angiog-raphy in these injuries. A widened mediastinum on good quality chest radiographs also mandates angiogra-phy. Indications for angiography are summarized in Table 12.1. Angiograms may be difficult to interpret, however, due to the multiplicity of vessels and bony landmarks within the narrow confines of these areas although digital subtraction angiography (DSA) largely eliminates this problem. It is also compounded by technical difficulties in managing inebriated uncooper-ative patients. Arteriovenous fistulae may be difficult to define accurately in view of the rapid circulation time and this applies particularly when multiple fistulae are present. In general this has proved an accurate investi-gation in our hands and, as far as we can ascertain, tends to overdiagnose injuries because approximately

Table 12.1 *Indications and contraindications for angiography*

Indications
Wound
    Stab root of neck/parasternal
    Cervical/upper thoracic gunshot
    Shotgun wounds neck/thorax
Evidence of previous haemorrhage
    History of major bleed
    Low hemoglobin level
    Unexplained hypovolemia
Upper limb pulse deficit
False aneurysm
Bruit
Superior mediastinal widening (chest radiograph)

Contraindications
Stridor
Hemodynamic instability

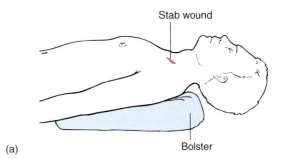

(a)

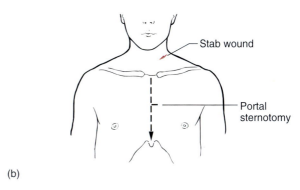

(b)

Figure 12.5 *(a) Patient positioning for superior mediastinal exploration. (b) Optimum incisions for superior mediastinal exploration.*

2% of our patients have had negative explorations for suspected superior mediastinal injury. The complication rate of angiography has proved extremely low and to date there has been only one significant femoral artery laceration which required surgical treatment. On rare occasions unexplained episodes of mental confusion which have resolved completely have followed selective carotid angiography but no patients have had permanent neurological deficit.

Color-flow Doppler has proved accurate in the neck but has been very disappointing in evaluation of superior mediastinal vascular injury.[18] Transesophageal echocardiography also has proved disappointing. CT scanning may prove valuable in accurately defining the exact site of a false aneurysm in the mediastinum and may also prove valuable in patients with neurological deficit in order to exclude some intracerebral pathology such as surgically treatable hematomas. It is of little use in defining cerebral infarction in the acute situation as these take 2–3 days to develop sufficient definition to manifest.[19]

Operative management

In view of the complications due to delayed hemorrhage and false aneurysm formation, we believe that all penetrating arterial injuries should be routinely explored and appropriately managed. As already discussed, it is foolhardy to attempt exploration of superior mediastinal injuries without the benefit of angiography in order to adequately plan the procedure although active life-threatening hemorrhage or stridor precludes investigation and are indications for immediate exploration.[17]

The standard position of the patient should be supine with the arms alongside with a bolster placed between the scapulae and with the neck extended. In addition, the head should be rotated away from the injured side (Fig 12.5). It is advisable to prepare and drape the area from mastoid to xiphisternum so that access can be widened as required. Standard median sternotomy presents the widest exposure to the superior mediastinum and is the optimum utility incision. This provides excellent access to all vessels, including the left subclavian. Access to the latter may be improved by rotating the patient towards the operator standing on the patient's right side. We have never found it necessary to use the variety of trap-door incisions or excision of the clavicle in order to gain access to the proximal subclavian artery. On occasion, however, we have used a limited sternal split with lateral division of the sternum just below the angle. With retraction, this then slides apart as a unit and obviates the postoperative morbidity often associated with mobility of the sternal ends as the intact segment of sternum acts as a splint.[17,20,21]

Anatomically the key to the superior mediastinum is the left brachiocephalic vein. Once detected and isolated with a vessel loop, all tissue on a plane anterior to this may be divided with equanimity as these muscles are devoid of important structures, and this will greatly improve access to the mediastinal vessels.

The arteries lie immediately behind the left brachiocephalic vein and can be located by palpation. In the event of the anatomy of the superior mediastinum

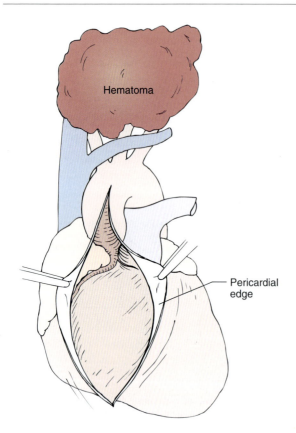

Hematoma

Pericardial edge

Figure 12.6 *Access to major arch branches in the presence of superior mediastinal hematoma (when landmarks obscured).*

being obscured by hematoma or distorted by a large false aneurysm, it is wisest to open the pericardium and to locate these vessels along the aortic arch by palpation through this clean plane (Fig 12.6). It must be emphasized that the superior mediastinal arteries are surprisingly friable and that dissection and various maneuvers such as looping these vessels should be done gently and meticulously. There is no place for blind clamping.

GENERAL PRINCIPLES OF VASCULAR REPAIR

The technical options available are ligation, lateral suture, patch angioplasty, end-to-end anastomosis or placement of an interposition graft.[22] Ligation is reserved for branches of the subclavian vessels such as the vertebral or internal thoracic or may be entertained for the major trunk vessels in the presence of gross sepsis in patients presenting with infected false aneurysms.

Once the site of the laceration has been clearly identified and proximal and distal control obtained, the edges of the vessel wall should be debrided back to healthy tissue and cleaned of adventitia. Simple lateral suture, usually with interrupted vascular sutures, can be used when there is no risk of narrowing the vessel

lumen. Otherwise it is safer to perform a patch angioplasty, using a segment of vein; long saphenous vein is most suitable under these circumstances in view of its relative strength. End-to-end anastomosis is practicable only when there is no tension on the anastomosis. Tension can be judged to be excessive if the initial single tethering stitch fails to hold the ends together without tearing out. Under these circumstances it is preferable to place an interposition graft. In the case of the mediastinal vessels, with adequate mobilization of the vessel one can usually accept approximately 0.5 cm of tissue loss. The circumstances under which end-to-end reconstruction is optimal is in the presence of through-and-through wounds where it is preferable to completely transect the vessel and debride it so that healthy tissue is reanastomosed. If an interposition graft is deemed advisable, it seems acceptable to use prosthetic material in the superior mediastinum as the saphenous vein is frequently of insufficient caliber. The situations under which interposition grafting is necessary are where there is significant tissue loss or there are multiple perforations as would be seen in the presence of shotgun wounds.

A frequently encountered injury is perforation of the vessels close to their origins on the aorta with a very short proximal arterial stump. Under these circumstances attempts at end-to-end anastomosis are fraught with difficulty and are potentially disastrous in view of the tendency for the inner aortic wall layers to retract, creating difficulty in proximal control and also in obtaining good intima-to-intima apposition. In the case of the brachiocephalic trunk or left common carotid it is advisable to oversew the short proximal remnant on the aorta and to restore continuity by the placement of an inline graft taken from the intrapericardiac portion of the aorta.[1,2,21] This can be partially occluded using a side biting clamp and the proximal graft then placed in an end-to-side manner. End-to-end anastomosis is then made distally (Fig 12.7a, b). When the left subclavian is injured close to its origin, after oversewing of its proximal end continuity is best restored by making a separate supraclavicular incision and transposing the subclavian to the side of the common carotid artery. If this proves technically difficult the distal end may be ligated and flow restored by means of an interposition graft placed from the side of the common carotid to the side of the third part of the subclavian artery (Fig 12.7c–e).

The importance of meticulous technique and adherence to the principles of vascular repair must be stressed. This includes, as already mentioned, adequate debridement of the vessel ends, the avoidance of tension and intima-to-intima apposition, ensuring that the anastomoses are not narrowed and free of adventitial incorporation into the lumen. It must also be emphasized that these mediastinal vessels are extremely friable and great care must be taken when performing the anastomoses not to tear the vessel. In addition, excessive force must not be used in ill-considered attempts to approximate the ends. The finer the suture that will be tolerated the better and we have found that on these vessels a 4/0 or 5/0 vascular suture is most appropriate. On completion of the anastomoses where the cerebral circulation is involved, with clamp release meticulous attention must be paid to avoidance of embolization of thrombus or air into the cerebral circulation. Prior to commencing reconstruction, distal thrombus must be extracted by gentle balloon catheter passage and back-

bleeding. Before completing the suture line, back-bleeding as well as forward flushing should be allowed to occur by release of the proximal clamp. The final suture should be tied in the presence of active back-bleeding.[22]

With regard to the use of temporary intraluminal shunting, we have used the stump pressure technique as desribed by Moore *et al.*[23] as an index of the need for temporary shunting. However, in relation to the superior mediastinal vessels, we have never found this to be necessary. The only indication for the use of an

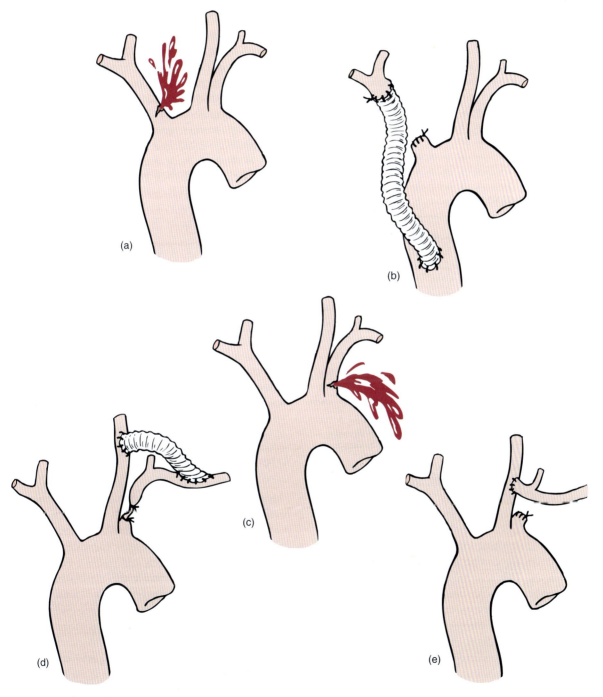

Figure 12.7 *Methods of arch reconstructions for injuries close to vessel origins. (a, b) Brachiocephalic artery. (c, d, e) Left subclavian artery.*

intraluminal shunt has been simultaneous injury of the brachiocephalic and left common carotid arteries. We have only seen this on one occasion following a gunshot wound. Under these circumstances a silastic shunt was placed from the intrapericardiac aorta into the left common carotid while the brachiocephalic was repaired. The shunt was then withdrawn and the left common carotid repaired and the patient made an uneventful recovery.

Arch continuity using interposition grafts as described can easily be performed without the use of cardiopulmonary bypass.[2,6,11] Indications for cardiopulmonary bypass in the event of trauma to these stem vessels would be the presence of late trauma where technical difficulty in defining the injury may be encountered or possibly in the presence of long-standing arteriovenous fistulae. It is also probably wiser to use cardiopulmonary bypass electively if multiple vessels are injured and well defined by preoperative angiography and this would certainly provide for safer surgery.[24-26]

SPECIFIC PROBLEMS

Associated preoperative neurological deficit

The approach to patients with a central neurological deficit associated with carotid or brachiocephalic injury remains a largely unresolved problem. The theoretical risk associated with revascularization is the creation of an hemorrhagic infarct in an area of ischemic cerebral softening. The difficulties of accurate assessment and localization of the patient's neurological lesion is bedevilled by the frequent association of intoxication and associated head injury. In addition, on occasions active hemorrhage precludes detailed preoperative investigations.

In our own practice we have adopted an aggressive policy and revascularized virtually all patients irrespective of their neurological status. This approach evolved by virtue of the fact that most were young adult males, usually manual laborers. The proviso before undertaking vascular reconstruction is the presence of back-bleeding down the carotid system once thrombus has been extracted. This is to prevent the theoretical danger of intracerebral embolization once flow is re-established. Angiography is extremely difficult to interpret, for technical reasons, on the operating table and has proved of little value in our practice. We have found a far more favorable outcome in patients in whom reconstruction has been performed than in those in whom ligation was done. Over the last 10 years we have felt that there is no need to change this approach which has been supported in recent times by others.[27,28] At present

we perform ligation only in patients whose general clinical condition precludes a complex reconstructive procedure or in those patients who have severe compound cerebral injury with a Glasgow coma scale <4. In the latter the prognosis is known to be extremely poor. In general it would appear that reconstruction yields far better results than ligation.

Trauma in the presence of congenital arch anomalies

The surgeon should be aware of the possibility of the existence of these anomalies before embarking upon exploration, particularly in the emergency situation (Fig 12.8). Anomalies range from hypoplasia or absence of vessels, in particular the vertebrals, to the full Lusorian anomaly in which the common carotids arise from a common trunk and the right subclavian arises from the descending aorta and traverses the posterior mediastinum behind the esophagus. It is this latter anomaly that we have encountered most frequently, albeit rarely (six patients). The problem confronting the surgeon under these circumstances should the common trunk be injured is to ensure that cerebral perfusion is maintained while reconstruction is performed. Even with good quality angiography unless this is borne in mind it may be missed in the emergency situation. During an emergency exploration the surgeon should be alerted if what is identified as the brachiocephalic is considered to be shorter than expected. Under these circumstances, if it is necessary to clamp the common trunk it is safer to insert a shunt into one or both branches from the ascending aorta. In Fig 12.9 an arch-angiogram done for suspected mediastinal vascular injuries, which was negative, showed a common origin (arrowed) for the left common carotid and brachiocephalic trunk.

Arteriovenous fistula

These patients are usually stable enough to enable full preoperative investigation and assessment to be performed. Arteriovenous fistulae[11] explored more than a week or so after injury create formidable technical problems due to the fibrosis and massive venous dilatation in the neck, particularly the mediastinum, when massive venous bleeding may present a major problem. The veins lie on a more superficial plane and the fistula usually constitutes a relatively small perforation in the vessels. It is therefore wisest to dissect the venous component out initially and the perforation can be localized transvenously by palpation of the thrill and the defect controlled by direct pressure, if required. Once the fistula is isolated it is much easier to identify and isolate the feeding artery and control this component.

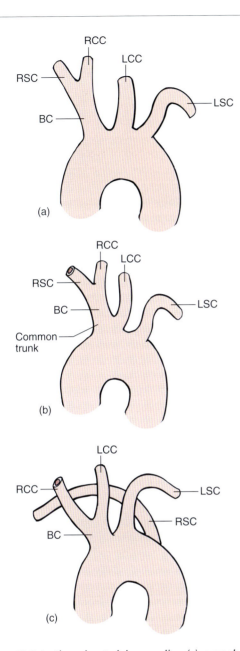

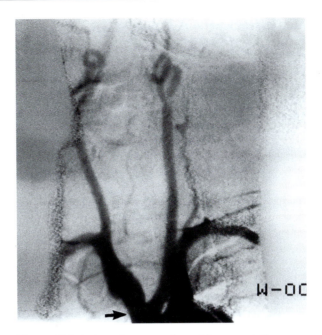

Figure 12.9 *Arch angiogram performed for suspected superior mediastinal arterial injury, but proved negative, showed a common origin (arrowed) for the left common carotid and brachiocephalic arteries.*

Figure 12.8 *Aortic arch arterial anomalies: (a) normal; (b) common trunk; (c) Lusorian anomaly (retroesophageal right subclavian). BC, brachiocephalic; LCC, left common carotid; LSC, left subclavian; RCC, right common carotid; RSC, right subclavian.*

If necessary, particularly in the carotid artery, it may be possible after controlling the feeding vessels to approach the fistula transvenously. As a rule, however, it is better to separate the vessels at the site of the fistula and to repair them on their merits. The artery is repaired as described earlier with the method of reconstruction depending upon the circumstances; usually simple lateral suture or end anastomosis suffices. Simple venous lacerations can be be dealt with in the same way.

Embolism from the clot in the arterial segment just distal to the fistula is a distinct hazard. It is extremely important to be meticulous and gentle in the dissection of the vessels and to ensure that there is no residual thrombus in the artery prior to repair and restoration of prograde flow. This entails back-bleeding and gentle thrombectomy using a small balloon catheter. There is also a theoretical risk of air embolism through the venous component. To avoid this it is important to clamp the veins at an early stage and to fill the venous segment with saline prior to final closure.

Recurrent arteriovenous fistula has not occurred in our experience and in the few patients in whom there was residual evidence of fistula this was found to be due to an additional lesion undetected at the original operation. In no case could this be attributed to repeat fistulation at the site of repair and we have not made a fetish of interposing tissue between the arterial and venous repairs, which has been the classical teaching. It is important to search for evidence of a second fistula at operation by carefully tracing the trajectory of the stab or missile. This applies especially to multiple missiles, as in shotgun injuries, and the surgeon must ensure that all palpable thrills have disappeared once the repair is complete.

It must be emphasized that if a policy of selective management of penetrating wounds is to be followed, particularly in the neck and supraclavicular area, the patients in whom vascular injury is not detected at the time of initial assessment should receive thorough clinical re-evaluation at least 1 week later and thereafter at intervals of at least 1 month for an arbitrary period of 3 months in order to detect undiagnosed arteriovenous fistulae or late-onset false aneuryms.

Mediastinal venous injuries

Guidelines for the management of superior mediastinal venous injuries have not been well defined. It has been empirically stated that repair should always be attempted in this situation. However, this may present formidable technical problems as anatomical location and control of the bleeding site frequently present difficulties in view of the high flow rate and low pressures. Certainly venous repair at whatever site cannot match the excellent results obtained with arterial reconstruction in view of the friability of the vessels, and the patency rates of interposition grafts in major veins are significantly lower than those to be expected from arterial reconstructive procedures. A frequent problem facing the surgeon is that of horrific venous bleeding in the mediastinum that is difficult to localize or control and is eventually found to be the result of a ragged laceration in which simple lateral suture or reanastomosis is not feasible. The dilemma presented is whether or not to attempt repair by some form of interposition graft or to perform simple ligation.

Classical phlebographic studies were performed by Barret in the late 1950s on patients with idiopathic superior mediastinal fibrosis.[29] These studies showed that when a single brachiocephalic vein is obstructed, a ready collateral pathway to the superior vena cava develops through the anterior jugular system and the anterior communicating veins in the neck. With obstruction of the superior vena cava cephalad to the azygos vein the main alternative pathways are the superior intercostal veins which carry blood to the azygos and hemi-azygos systems and to the heart. These collaterals appear adequate under these circumstances so that the superficial veins on the chest wall do not dilate or become prominent. When the azygos vein becomes involved, the superficial veins on the chest wall dilate and, together with the azygos system, drain into the inferior vena cava. Although not visualized on phlebography, it must be postulated that the internal and external vertebral plexuses play a major part in this collateralization. The development of these collateral pathways is largely possible because of the absence of valves in the great veins of the neck and mediastinum. Similarly, ligation of one or both internal jugular veins is well tolerated and is well described. Collateral flow occurs through the visceral plexuses, the vertebral plexuses and the superior intercostal veins.

It has been our policy to perform simple repair to these veins, such as lateral suture or end-to-end anastomosis. If continuity can only be restored by the use of an interposition graft, we have simply ligated these veins if the the injury is situated cephalad to the azygos. Complex venous injury of the superior vena cava caudad to the azygos has not been encountered in our experience and is probably incompatible with survival.

It must be emphasized that if the vein is to be reconstructed, meticulous and gentle technique is essential, using a fine 6/0 gauge vascular suture.

We have not encountered major permanent morbidity as a result of this approach.[30] Temporary facial and upper limb edema occurred in one patient who had ligation of the left braciocephalic vein which resolved completely within a period of 4–5 days. Two additional patients developed upper limb edema after ligation of the distal subclavian vein but this has also not resulted in long-term morbidity. No patients have developed problems related to massive air embolism or pulmonary embolism, although it has been our practice to ensure that the vein contains either saline or is actively bleeding at the time of final closure.

The increasing use of the subclavian vein for venous access for monitoring or drug therapy has resulted in some complications. Venous catheter transection is the most commonly encountered and, unless the catheter is removed, it will certainly migrate into the heart or pulmonary artery. It is folly to attempt surgical removal without preparation for sternotomy. On two occasions an interventional radiologist has successfully removed catheter emboli by means of transluminal interventional techniques.

Interventional catheter techniques

Under certain circumstances embolization of disrupted arteries or restoration of arterial continuity by the use of covered stents seems an attractive alternative.[31] Occlusion of vessels using a spring coil has been reserved for injuries to branches of the subclavian artery, such as the internal thoracic or proximal vertebral. Figure 12.10 shows a false aneurysm arising from a laceration of the thyrocervical trunk. There was also a small fistulous communication with the internal jugular vein. This was successfully occluded by means of a spring coil placed in

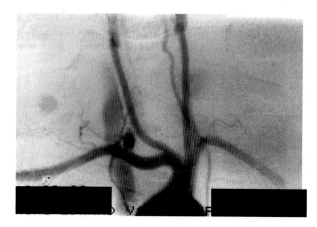

Figure 12.10 *Arteriovenous fistula between thyrocervical trunk and internal jugular vein. This was successfully treated by interventional catheter techniques.*

the artery. Obviously, under these circumstances thrombus in relation to the fistula is of no significance in relation to cerebral embolization. The use of a covered Palmaz-type stent using a polytetrafluoroethylene (PTFE) graft has been used for partial lacerations of the subclavian artery with mixed success. We have not advocated these procedures for carotid lesions or for arteriovenous fistulae involving the cerebral circulation for fear of precipitating embolization either of pre-existing thrombus or of the device itself. It is probably not to be recommended under these circumstances. Although we have not encountered neurological sequelae due to vertebral artery interruption, there is a possibility of this occurring if the posterior communicating vessels on the circle of Willis are deficient.[32,33]

Penetrating diaphragmatic injury

It must be realized that diaphragmatic lacerations may occur as a consequence of any penetrating injury to the chest, although obviously those situated in the lower chest wall are more likely to be associated with diaphragmatic wounds. Small puncture wounds of the right hemidiaphragm are of little consequence in view of the protection afforded by the liver. On the left, however, neglected perforations may result in the development of evisceration into the chest months or even years later. The organs most frequently involved in these hernias are the stomach and colon and occasionally the spleen.[34]

Most busy trauma centers follow a selective conservative management policy for penetrating wounds of the lower chest and upper abdomen and exploration is only entertained if mandated by signs of intra-abdominal injury, including positive peritoneal lavage. In our own practice, if free air is noted under the diaphragm on chest radiography, laparoscopic inspection of the diaphragm is undertaken and repair effected by this technique. The proviso is that there is no other indication for laparotomy such as hemoperitoneum or peritonitis. A three-port[35] technique is used and the diaphragm repaired with 0-gauge braided monofilament suture.

Delayed presentation with post-traumatic diaphragmatic hernia is most frequently associated with acute upper abdominal symptoms. In our practice the majority presented with acute intestinal obstruction. Others had acute upper abdominal pain; in a few patients the diagnosis was made with repeat presentation for trauma and this proved to be an incidental discovery on chest radiography. Gravier and Freeark[36] stated that diaphragmatic hernia should be considered if any one of the following four criteria were present:

- Intestinal obstruction and a history of past trauma
- Intestinal obstruction associated with radiological changes at the left lung base and small bowel obstruction in patients having no abdominal hernias or scars
- Large bowel obstruction in young patients.

Radiographic studies are the most useful diagnostic aids. Plain films may show equivocal signs or signs suggestive only of diaphragmatic hernia. Obvious air fluid levels in the chest make the diagnosis apparent. Barium studies have proved most useful in our practice. Contrast examination should start with a barium enema and if that is negative it should be followed by a barium meal and follow-through. The contrast examination should continue until the entire alimentary tract has been demonstrated. The passage of a nasogastric tube may also be helpful. Thoracocentesis for diagnosis should be avoided because of the risk of fistula formation between the alimentary tract and the pleural space.

Figure 12.11 shows the chest radiograph of a 27-year-old man stabbed in the lower chest 4 years earlier. He presented with acute upper abdominal pain associated with distension. A pleural effusion can clearly be seen on the left with an associated gas shadow (arrowed). Abdominal x-ray (Fig 12.12a) shows distended small and large bowel. Note the loop which appears to be above the diaphragm (arrowed). Barium meal and follow-through showed no small bowel in the chest, but barium enema revealed total obstruction at the level of the splenic flexure (arrowed, Fig 12.12b).

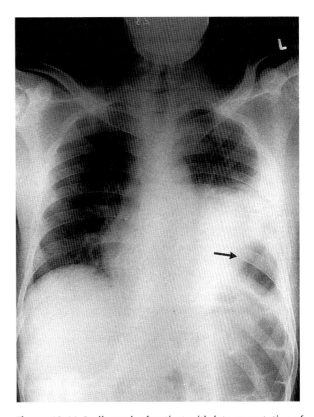

Figure 12.11 *Radiograph of patient with late presentation of a diaphragmatic hernia.*

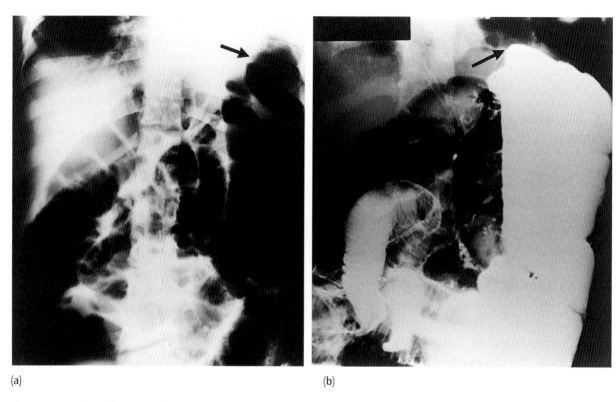

(a)   (b)

Figure 12.12 *(a) Straight abdominal radiograph of same patient as in Figure 12.11. (b) Barium meal and follow-through and enema in the same patient, showing colon obstruction at the splenic flexure.*

Note that the air-filled loop above the diaphragm (arrowed in Fig 12.12a) fails to fill with contrast.

Thoracotomy was performed which revealed that this was a gangrenous loop of transverse colon. The hernia was reduced and the colon resected via a separate laparotomy, and the diaphragm repaired. After a stormy postoperative course complicated by septicemia, the patient eventually recovered.

Increasing use of laparoscopic techniques has also provided a valuable ancillary aid to diagnosis. Once the diagnosis is made and the patient adequately resuscitated, operation is mandatory. Most authors agree that traumatic diaphragmatic hernias with delayed presentation should be approached through the chest since the adhesions within the chest can then be easily freed. Once the organs are freed and reduced, the edges of the defect can be debrided and repaired using a fairly heavy (0-gauge) interrupted braided monofilament absorbable suture. If there is gangrenous bowel or other viscera, these are best approached via a separate laparotomy and dealt with accordingly.[34]

REFERENCES

1. Buchan K, Robbs JV. Surgical management of penetrating mediastinal arterial trauma. *Eur J Cardiothorac Surg* 1995; **9(2):** 90–4.

2. Graham JM, Feliciano DV, Mattox KL, Beall AC Jr. Innominate vascular injury. *J Trauma* 1982; **22(8):** 647–55.

3. Johnston RH, Wall MJ, Mattox KL. Innominate artery trauma; a 30 year experience. *J Vasc Surg* 1993; **17(1):** 134–9.

4. Li MS, Smith BM, Espinosa J, Brown RM, Richardson P, Ford R. Non-penetrating trauma to the carotid artery. Seven cases and a literature review. *J Trauma* 1994; **36(2):** 265–72.

5. Perry MO, Thal ER, Shires GT. Management of arterial injuries. *Ann Surg* 1973; **173:** 403.

6. Robbs JV, Baker LW, Human RR, Vawda IS, Duncan HJ, Rajaruthnam P. Cervicomediastinal arterial injuries. *Arch Surg* 1981; **116(5):** 663–8.

7. Robbs JV, Baker LW. Major arterial trauma: review of experience with 267 injuries. *Br J Surg* 1978; **65(8):** 532–8.

8. Batzdorf U, Bentson J, Machleder H. Blunt trauma to the cervical carotid artery. *Neurosurgery* 1979; **5(2):** 195–201.

9. Costa MC, Robbs JV. Nonpenetrating subclavian artery trauma. *J Vasc Surg* 1988; **8(1):** 71–5.

10. Davis J, Holbrook T, Hoyt D, *et al.* Blunt carotid artery dissection: Incidence, associated injuries, screening, and treatment. *J Trauma* 1990; **30(12):** 1514–17.

11. Robbs JV, Carrim AA, Kadwa AM, Mars M. Traumatic arteriovenous fistula; experience with 202 patients. *Br J Surg* 1994; **81(9):** 1296–9.

12. Sako Y, Varco RL. Arteriovenous fistula: results of management of congenital and acquired forms, blood flow observations and observations on proximal arterial degeneration. *Surgery* 1970; **67(1):** 40–61.

13. Warren JV, Elkin DC, Nickerson JL. The blood volumes in patients with arteriovenous fistulas. *J Clin Invest* 1951; **30:** 220.

14. Hook EW, Wainer HS, McGee TJ, *et al.* Acquired arteriovenous fistula with bacterial endarteritis and endocarditis. *JAMA* 1957; **164:** 1450.

15. Robbs JV, Naidoo KS. Nerve compression injuries due to traumatic false aneurysm. *Ann Surg* 1984; **200(1):** 80–2.

16. Campbell FC, Robbs JV. Penetrating injuries of the neck: a prospective study of 108 patients. *Br J Surg* 1980; **67:** 582–6.

17. Robbs JV, Baker LW. Cardiovascular trauma. *Curr Probl Surg* 1984; **21(4):** 1–87.

18. Fry WR, Dort JA, Smith RS, Sayers DV, Morabito DJ. Duplex scanning replaces arteriography and operative exploration in the diagnosis of potential cervical vascular injury. *Am J Surg* 1994; **168(6):** 693–5.

19. Mohr JP, Biller J, Hilal SK, *et al.* Imaging in acute stroke. *Stroke* 1992; **23:** 142.

20. Robbs JV, Keenan J. Exploration of the neck. In: Champion HR, Robbs JV, Trunkey D, eds. *Rob and Smith's Operative Surgery*, 4th edn. London: Butterworths, 1989.

21. Robbs JV. Injuries to vessels of the neck and superior mediastinum. In: Champion HR, Robbs JV, Trunkey D, eds. *Rob and Smith's Operative Surgery*, 4th edn. London: Butterworths, 1989.

22. Robbs JV. Vascular trauma. General principles of surgical management. In: Champion HR, Robbs JV, Trunkey D, eds. *Rob and Smith's Operative Surgery*, 4th edn. London: Butterworths, 1989.

23. Moore WS, Yee JM, Hall AD. Collateral cerebral blood pressure. An index of tolerance to temporary carotid occlusion. *Arch Surg* 1973; **106:** 520–4.

24. Fulton JO, de Groot KM, Buckels NJ, Van Oppel UO. Penetrating injuries involving the intrathoracic great vessels. *S Afr J Surg* 1997; **35(2):** 82–6.

25. Fulton JO, de Groot KM, Von Oppel UO. Stab wounds of the innominate artery. *Ann Thorac Surg* 1996; **61(3):** 851–3.

26. Fulton JO, Brink JG. Complex thoracic vascular injury repair using deep hypothermia and circulatory arrest. *Ann Thorac Surg* 1997; **63(2):** 557–9.

27. Robbs JV, Human RR, Rajaruthnam P, Duncan H. Vawda I, Baker LW. Neurological deficit and injuries involving the neck arteries. *Br J Surg* 1983; **70(4):** 220–2.

28. Ramadan F, Rutledge R, Oller D, Howell P, Baker C, Keagy B. Carotid artery trauma: a review of contemporary trauma center experiences. *J Vasc Surg* 1995; **21(1):** 46–55.

29. Barret NR. Idiopathic mediastinal fibrosis. *Br J Surg* 1958; **46:** 207.

30. Robbs JV, Reddy E. Management options for penetrating injuries to the great veins of the neck and mediastinum. *Surg Gynecol Obstet* 1987; **165(4):** 323–6.

31. Marin ML, Veith FJ, Panetta TF, *et al.* Transluminally placed endovascular stented graft repair for arterial trauma. *J Vasc Surg* 1994; **20:** 466–72.

32. Thomas GI, Anderson KN, Hain RF, *et al.* The significance of anomalous vertebro-basilar artery communications in operations on the heart and great vessels. *Surgery* 1956; **46:** 747–57.

33. Monson DO, Saletta JD, Freeark RS. Carotid vertebral trauma. *J Trauma* 1969; **9:** 987–99.

34. Hegarty MM, Bryer JV, Angorn IB, Baker LW. Delayed presentation of traumatic diaphragmatic hernia. *Ann Surg* 1978; **188:** 229–33.

35. Marks JM, Ramey RL, Baringer DC, Aszodi A, Ponsky J. Laparoscopic repair of a diaphragmatic laceration. *Surg Laparosc Endosc* 1995; **5:** 415–18.

36. Gravier L, Freeark RJ. Traumatic diaphragmatic hernia. *Arch Surg* 1963; **86:** 363–7.

Transfixion injuries

STEPHEN WESTABY

Transfixion injuries are rare, unpredictable and often spectacular. The transfixing implement may have been withdrawn at the time of presentation, particularly after wounds from swords or spears. Alternatively, after impalement the patient may be brought to the emergency room with the offending object in place (Fig 13.1). The etiology of transfixion injuries may broadly be classified into:

- Aggression: in this group transfixion occurs with low velocity implements including knives (Fig 13.2), swords and spears or high velocity missiles projected from explosive devices. Explosions in confined spaces may result in glass or parts of furniture or machinery being driven through the torso (Fig 13.3).
- Road traffic accidents: these are the commonest source of transfixion injuries in civilian life, commonly when a motor vehicle occupant or motor cyclist leaves the road and collides with a fence post or farm machinery (Fig 13.4).
- Falls from a height may also result in impalement or transfixion injuries usually on fencing (Fig 13.5).

The great majority of transfixion injuries or impalement are low velocity in nature so that the outcome depends on the size of the offending instrument and the anatomical structures involved. Transfixion often involves more than one body cavity, usually chest and abdomen but sometimes neck and chest or chest,

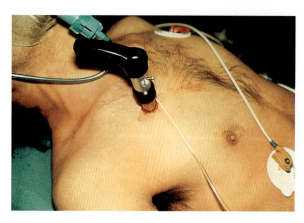

Figure 13.1 *Transfixion of the right upper chest with an electric drill. During the assault the drill bit passed through the anterior chest wall, pleural cavity and into the posterior chest wall. Thoracotomy was required for pleural bleeding which required partial right upper lobectomy.*

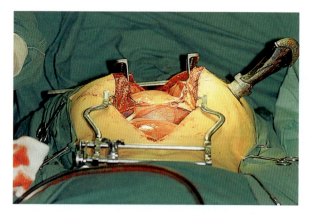

Figure 13.2 *Precordial transfixion with an oriental dagger. The long blade passed through the pericardium, lacerating the epicardium without entering a cardiac chamber. The blade then passed through the central tendon of the diaphragm and into the right lobe of the liver. The knife handle moved with the cardiac cycle and the patient presented with cardiac tamponade. Sternolaparotomy was performed before the knife was removed; no vital structures were damaged and the patient made an uneventful recovery.*

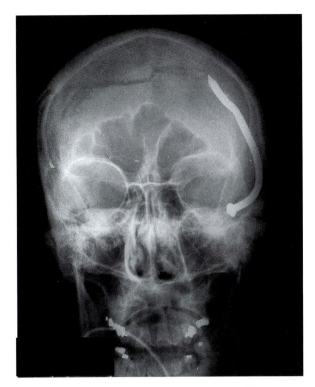

Figure 13.3 *Open injury to the brain after a nail bomb explosion.*

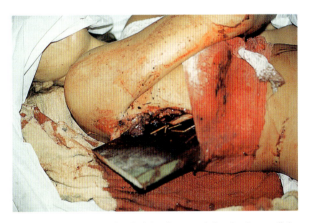

Figure 13.4 *Rapidly fatal right thoracoabdominal transfixion injury with a fence post. The victim lost control of a sports car which careered through a fence and into a field. Death occurred through hemorrhage from the liver and inferior vena cava.*

abdomen and pelvis. Major cardiac or vascular penetration usually results in early mortality whilst parenchymal injury to the lung, liver, guts or spleen is compatible with survival with expert treatment (Fig 13.6).

Transfixion or impalement usually generates both chest wall and visceral injury. Added to this are the risks of contamination by clothes, dirt or debris, together with bacteria such as clostridia, streptococci and staphylococci.

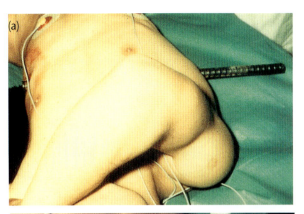
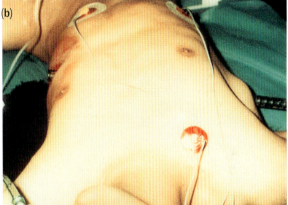
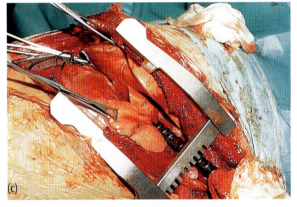
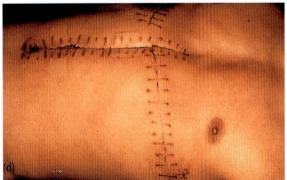

Figure 13.5 *Fall from a height onto metal railings. (a, b) The patient was transfixed from side to side but the metal bar missed all major vascular structures. (c, d) Surgical exploration was via bilateral lower thoracotomies and laparotomy. The implement was removed and, surprisingly, had not damaged any vital structures. (Courtesy of Professor K. Kobayashi.)*

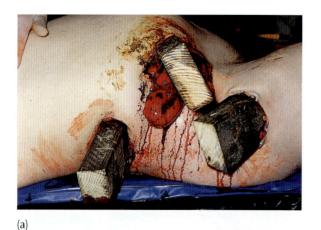

(a)

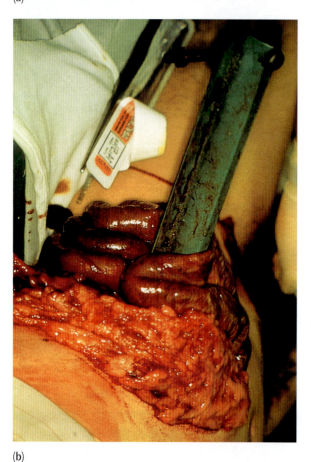

(b)

Figure 13.6 *Transfixion injuries involving the abdomen. (a) Impalement on multiple fence posts after a motor vehicle accident. After major surgery the patient made an uneventful recovery. (b) Extensive evisceration after a fall onto scaffolding. There was laceration of the gut and inferior vena cava which the patient did not survive.*

PREHOSPITAL CARE

Impalement seldom prevents exsanguinating hemorrhage if a major blood vessel is lacerated. However, as a precaution no attempt should be made to remove a transfixing implement at the site of injury. Retrieval

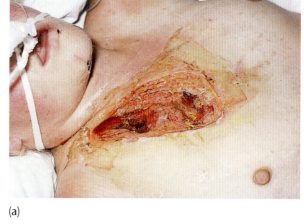

(a)

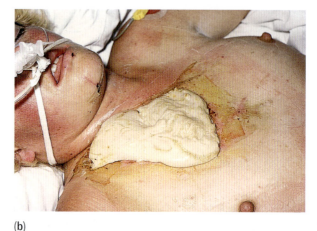

(b)

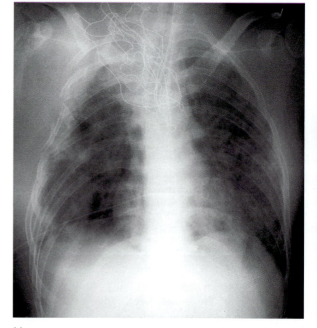

(c)

Figure 13.7 *(a) Transfixion injury with extensive rib fractures, chest wall disruption and bacterial contamination. (b, c) The wound was debrided then covered with a dressing rather than attempt primary closure.*

may be problematic until the arrival of heavy cutting gear to cut through wooden fence posts or metal railings. Pending rescue it may be necessary to begin intravenous fluids, pain relief or supplemental oxygen. On occasions endotracheal intubation and positive pressure ventilation may be established on site before transport. From an early stage it is possible to predict the extent of visceral injury from the site of entry and exit wounds.

If the patient is extricated from the transfixing implement on site, both entry and exit wounds are sealed with clean dressings and the patient brought rapidly to hospital (Fig 13.7).

RESUSCITATION IN HOSPITAL

The transfixing object is left *in situ* until large bore intravenous cannulae are inserted (Fig 13.8), blood is cross-matched and the patient intubated, ventilated and positioned for surgical exploration in the operating room. On removal of the instrument, tamponaded major vascular injury poses the greatest threat and it is important to have a strategy to obtain proximal and distal control of lacerated vessels from the outset. Injury to the major airways may result in massive air leak and loss of tidal volume after removal of a transfixing object (Fig 13.9).

Resuscitation should follow basic principles irrespective of the extent of damage. The airway is cleared or endotracheal intubation undertaken. The mechanics of breathing are restored by stabilization of a flail segment or covering of a chest wall defect. Hemothorax or pneumothorax is managed with an intercostal drain and blood volume replacement is undertaken cautiously. When hemodynamically stable, radiographs or endoscopy techniques are used to ascertain the extent of visceral damage. Emergency surgery may be required to arrest bleeding or control an air leak by partial lung resection. Liver injuries may require urgent laparotomy, particularly in the presence of damage to the inferior vena cava or hepatic veins. For those without immediately life-threatening injuries, early surgery is undertaken to debride devitalized tissues and remove sources of bacterial contamination. Tetanus prophylaxis and broad spectrum antibiotic cover are given before surgery begins.

ASPECTS OF SURGICAL TECHNIQUE

If the transfixing object is still in place, a surgical incision is planned to expose all potentially damaged major blood vessels in the affected body cavities. This may involve bilateral thoracotomies (by the anterior

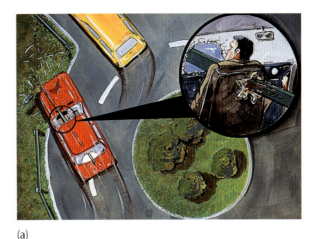

(a)

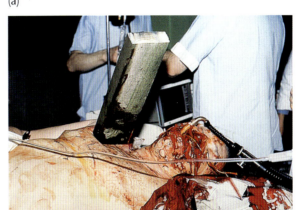

(b)

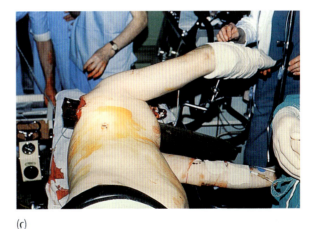

(c)

Figure 13.8 *Transfixion with a roadside fence post. The motor vehicle was involved in a high speed chase. (a) Mechanism of injury. (b) Resuscitation and preparation in the operating theatre. Faciomaxillary injuries caused difficulty in endotracheal intubation. (c) Patient positioned for left thoracotomy and removal of the fence post. At thoracotomy the transfixing implement was found to have removed the pleura from the apex of the chest and right pulmonary artery. There was anterior and posterior chest wall disruption but no vascular injury. After debriding the chest wall and right upper lobe, the pleural cavity was irrigated and primary closure undertaken. The patient made an excellent recovery. (Courtesy of Mr J. Gibbon FRCS.)*

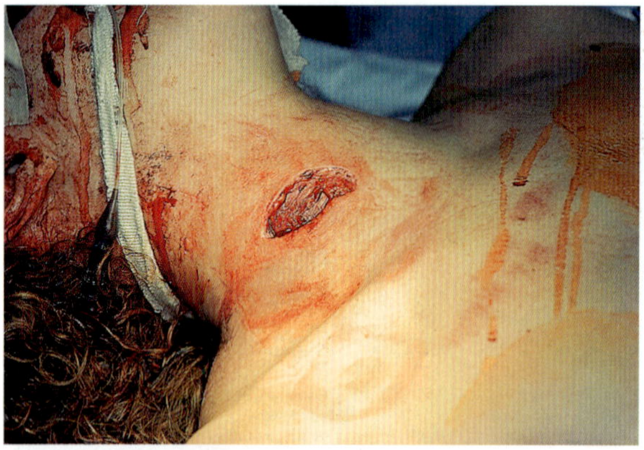

Figure 13.9 *(a) Young female patient with transfixion injury at the neck and thoracic inlet during a car crash. The stake was removed at the site followed by a brisk air leak from the wound. She was also profoundly hypovolemic with a left hemothorax. The airway was procured by rigid bronchoscopy. (b) Emergency left thoracotomy for repair of a lacerated left subclavian artery. (c) Attention was then turned to the neck. Exploration of the thoracic inlet provided access to a hemi-transected trachea. After debridement the trachea was closed directly. (d) The surgical incision closed, but the contaminated neck wound is left open with a corrugated drain to the site of repair. Delayed primary closure of the traumatic wound was performed 5 days later.*

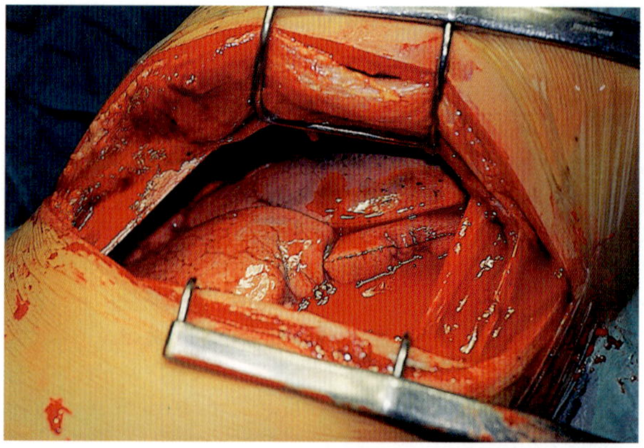

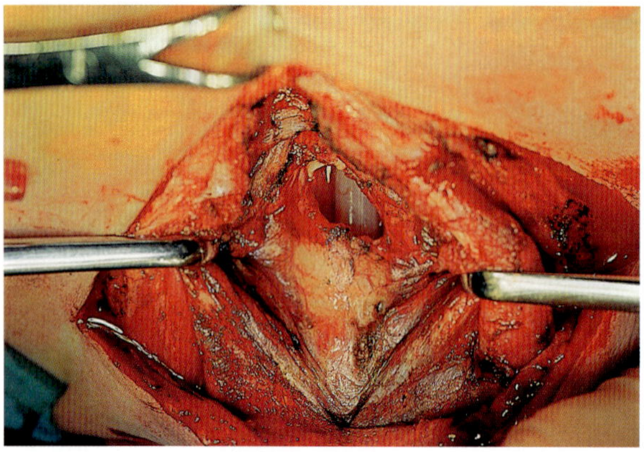

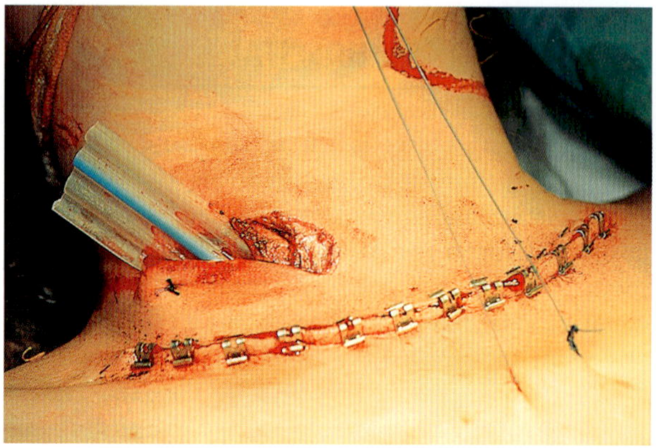

clam shell approach), sternolaparotomy or a thoro-coabdominal incision. The size of incision is of secondary importance to the safety aspects of extensive exposure. If the transfixing object is large (e.g. fence post) with a substantial chest wall defect, a plastic surgeon should be involved at the primary procedure. Infection-resistant material such as antibiotic sterilized homograft aorta, a pericardial patch or tube, or saphenous vein opened longitudinally and rolled into a tube should be available for major vascular replacement (Fig 13.10). It is particularly important to avoid synthetic material such as Dacron grafts in heavily contaminated wounds.

With the damaged structures exposed, the transfixing object is removed. Vascular clamps or a Foley catheter should be readily available to control bleeding from a damaged major vessel. Some vessels may be safely sacrificed by ligation but major arteries or veins should be occluded with a clamp or snare prior to repair with biological material and monofilament sutures. After vascular repair, full wound debridement is undertaken by excising damaged skin edges, subcutaneous tissue, devitalized muscle or bone and injured

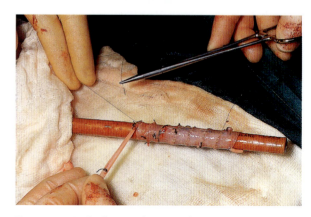

Figure 13.10 *The long saphenous vein rolled into a tube and sutured to provide a replacement for the superior or inferior vena cava.*

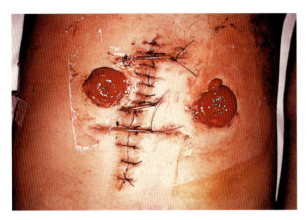

Figure 13.11 *Exteriorization of bowel after laparotomy for transfixion injury with colonic and small bowel lacerations.*

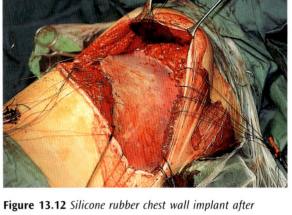

Figure 13.12 *Silicone rubber chest wall implant after extensive debridement of a penetrating injury.*

lung. On occasions when hilar bronchi or pulmonary vessels are damaged, a formal pneumonectomy or lobectomy may be required. Splenectomy or partial hepatic resection may be required for thorocoabdominal injuries. In the presence of esophageal, colonic or small bowel perforation, consideration should be given to the merits of primary repair versus formation of a cutaneous fistula (esophagostomy, colostomy or iliostomy) with delayed reconstruction (Fig 13.11). These decisions are made after assessment of the degree of bacteriological contamination, the integrity of the arterial and venous systems, and the length of gut affected. Foregut defects (esophagus, stomach, ileum) are sterile so that contamination does not preclude primary repair. Direct suture of stomach and ilial defects is feasible whilst esophageal perforation is best covered with a pedicled graft of diaphragmatic muscle. Tracheo-bronchial defects are usually treated by resecting the damaged part and end-to-end anastomosis.

Whilst penetrating injury to the aorta or bracheo-cephalic vessels is usually fatal, bleeding hypotension and local tamponade often stops bleeding from extensive venous defects. In this case the vessel may be reconstituted with biological material. Diaphragmatic defects can usually be closed directly but if there is tension on the repair a patch of pericardium or silicone may prove useful.

Reconstructive surgery may be required for large chest wall defects. Pectoralis or latissimus dorsi muscle flaps can be transposed to fill gaps. In lightly contaminated cases sheets of silicone rubber may be used in the same way (Fig 13.12). Realistic decisions must then be made about primary or delayed closure of the skin and subcutaneous tissues. In the event of primary skin closure over prosthetic material in the chest wall, prolonged antibiotic prophylaxis should be considered. In particular, this must cover potentially fatal organisms such as clostridia or streptococci which may spread unchecked along the tissue plains. Anaerobic conditions and foci of necrotic muscle constitute a life-threatening infection risk and in the event of uncertainty about the effectiveness of debridement delayed closure is preferable.

14

Management of foreign bodies within the chest

JOHN A ODELL

BULLETS AND SHELL FRAGMENTS

Brewer and Burford in an excellent chapter, based on extensive experience, estimated that in the Second World War a retained intrathoracic foreign body could be anticipated in approximately one of every four patients with penetrating chest wounds.[1] Retained bullets and shell fragments are usually innocuous and in the majority of circumstances surgical removal is associated with greater morbidity and mortality than if left alone. If a foreign body is a bullet (Fig 14.1), it is less likely to cause complications than if it were an irregular shell or rib fragment because the jagged edges are more apt to cause lung damage.[1] Those fragments lying adjacent to important structures[2] and larger irreg-

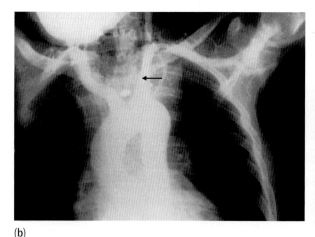

(b)

Figure 14.1 *(a, b) A widened mediastinum in this patient with a bullet wound prompted aortography which revealed intact arterial structures. Bleeding causing the hematoma was presumed venous and the patient was observed without surgical intervention. The mediastinal widening shown radiographically slowly resolved. This illustrates that widening of the mediastinum is not by itself an indication for surgical exploration and that retained bullets can often safely be observed.*

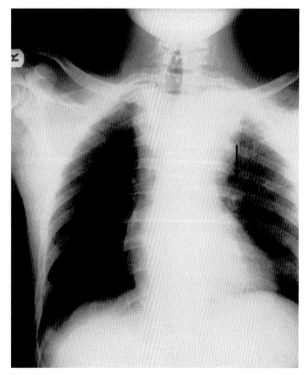

(a)

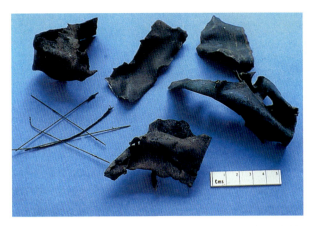

Figure 14.2 *Fragments of bomb casing after explosion which distributes these missiles at high velocity.*

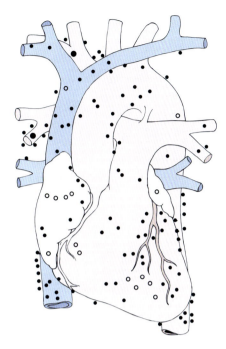

Figure 14.3 *The illustration documenting the site of the retained missile from Dwight Harken's classic paper describing removal of missiles from the mediastinum and heart without cardiopulmonary bypass. The paper, demonstrating the safety of intracardiac surgery, gave impetus for the era of closed cardiac surgery.*

ular fragments (Fig 14.2) should be removed soon after the injury when the patient is stable.[3] Operative removal is recommended for complications such as hemoptysis, lung abscess or gangrene, bronchial obstruction, bronchiectasis, chronic pneumonia and suspicion of scar carcinoma.[4] In those patients with carcinoma related to a bullet or shell fragment, the fragment had been retained for many years (average 24 years) and most had symptoms of hemoptysis and infection.[5] Shell fragments are easily localized radiographically within the lung and at surgery. In most cases removal is possible by simple incision down to the bullet or fragment; where there is permanent lung damage, resection of lung tissue, which should be as conservative as possible, is necessary.[4]

One of the classic papers in cardiac surgery, which stimulated many to attempt closed cardiac surgery, is that of Dwight Harken describing removal of 134 missiles from the mediastinum, including 55 from the pericardium and 13 from chambers of the heart, without mortality (Fig 14.3).[6] The latter were removed using clamps introduced through small incisions and hemostatic sutures. Indications for immediate operative management in patients with metallic fragments involving the heart wall or cardiac chambers are essentially the same as those with cardiac injuries without foreign bodies. Immediate extraction depends on factors such as size, location, potential for embolization and ease of extraction. If the bullet is imbedded within cardiac muscle, multiple sutures can be placed beneath the missile and the muscle incised and the fragment removed. Knowledge by the patient of a retained missile within the heart can contribute to intense psychological unease.

Accurate localization of intracardiac foreign bodies is important in determining acute care and monitoring for late sequelae if a conservative approach is decided upon. Transthoracic and transesophageal echocardiography (TEE) and CT scanning may be useful.[7] There exists uncertainty regarding management of embolized

bullets to the heart. Symbas advocates a selective approach[8] whereas Shannon *et al.*[9] in their review of 102 cases since 1930 found 25% with embolus-related complications and death in 6%. They advocate mandatory removal. Missiles completely imbedded within the myocardium, those in the pericardial space, and intracavitary right-sided missiles lodged within the trabeculae may be managed non-operatively. Surgical intervention is recommended for symptomatic, large (>5 mm) or irregular shaped missiles, those within a left-sided cavity or partially imbedded. The medical guidelines in patients managed expectantly with regard to frequency of follow-up, anticoagulation and antibiotic prophylaxis have not been established.[10] Another difficulty with the conservative approach is that delayed systemic embolization can occur.[11] Some bullets, particularly those that have embolized via the venous system to the heart, may require cardiopulmonary bypass for removal; others have digitally palpated the missile with a finger introduced through a purse-string in the right atrium, positioned the missile against the right ventricle, and then cut down upon it. It is advisable to have a means of determining the exact site of the bullet prior to instituting bypass (chest radiograph or intraoperative TEE) to ensure that further migration to a pulmonary artery has not taken place. In occasional circumstances controlled embolization, under fluoroscopy, to a peripheral vein may facilitate removal.[12]

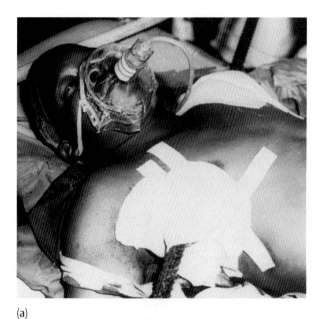

(a)

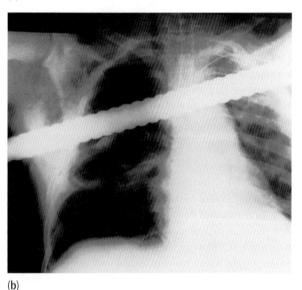

(b)

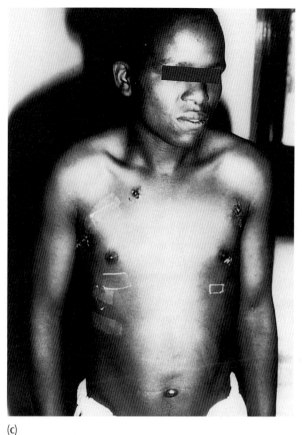

(c)

Figure 14.4 *(a, b, c) This patient, a construction worker, fell and impaled himself on a reinforcing steel rod. We deduced that the anterior mediastinum had been traversed: any other site would have resulted in death. A right pneumothorax and left pulmonary contusion are shown on the chest radiograph. A happy and lucky patient without scars of a thoracotomy at discharge demonstrates that many patients with significant chest trauma can be managed easily by chest drainage.*

Bullets can enter the esophagus and can migrate in the gastrointestinal tract;[13] in some instances the esophageal perforation may close spontaneously and not be demonstrated.[14,15] Bullets may also enter the airway and a single report documents removal via a bronchoscope.[16] Burihan described a case of arterial embolism and reviewed the literature;[17] most had bullet wounds of the heart, but some involved the pulmonary veins and ascending aorta. Factors contributing to embolization and affecting where the bullet lodges are the diameter of the artery, the position of the patient with regard to trajectory and the caliber and velocity of the bullet. Suspicious clinical and radiographic features are the absence of an exit wound and the position of the retained bullet away from the site of injury and variability in the site of the bullet on serial radiographs.

PLASTIC BULLETS

Plastic bullets, primarily designed for wounding and the prevention of injury to innocent bystanders, were introduced in Northern Ireland[18] and have also been used in the Middle East for riot control. The bullet used in Northern Ireland is large (10 cm length, 3.7 cm diameter) whereas the Israeli bullet is smaller (5.62 mm diameter, 1.5 cm long) and is shot by conventional military weapons.[19] Because of the low weight of the plastic bullet the estimated kinetic energy is similar to that of a hand gun. Although designed primarily to wound, the spectrum of injury is very similar to other gunshot wounds; management is no different from other gunshot wounds.

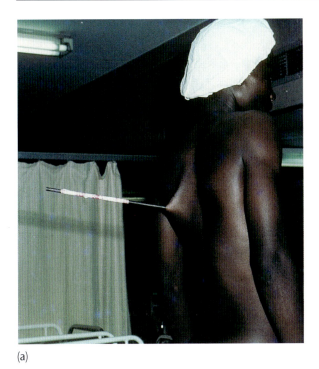
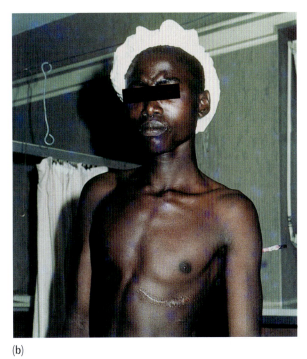

(a)   (b)

Figure 14.5 *(a, b) This patient seems to attract metallic foreign bodies. He was admitted with a metallic rod projecting from his left chest posteriorly. A few years previously he had a left anterior thoracotomy for removal of a needle from his left ventricle (sustained while doing press-ups). It was assumed that intrapleural adhesions, because of his thoracotomy, would obviate the development of a pneumothorax or hemothorax and the rod was removed with local anesthesia and sedation.*

LEAD POISONING

Retained bullet fragments after gunshot wounds with lead bullets generally do not cause lead poisoning, but poisoning can result when the lead comes into contact with body fluids, such as the pleura,[20] which can solubilize lead. Surgical removal of the lead can result in decreased lead levels and improvement in symptoms, which result from severe systemic lead toxicity. Chelation therapy using succimer (DMSA), which can be taken orally, may be used in conjunction with surgical removal.[21]

RADIOLUCENT FOREIGN BODIES

It is important to have a high index of suspicion for a retained foreign body which may be translucent, with any instance of penetrating trauma. The fragment is usually organic such as a piece of wood and can cause considerable morbidity if initially missed.[22]

IMPALEMENT

These dramatic injuries often result in single case reports.[23] Although uncommon in the clinical setting, many more cases with this injury die before reaching a hospital. Most follow motor vehicle or horse riding accidents or a fall from a height onto a fence post or tree; in combat situations, a projectile traveling at speed may hit a stationary victim.[24]

In the field the impaling object should be manipulated as little as possible, but may be shortened to expedite transport. Unnecessary movement or injudicious removal under less than ideal circumstances may cause further damage to nerves and blood vessels. Upon arrival in the hospital and after resuscitation, full assessment is undertaken. During this phase advanced studies such as arteriography and CT scan may be performed. In the operating room the impaled object is removed and the wounds debrided. In a personal patient a reinforced rod was removed without thoracotomy (Fig 14.4) and chest radiographs were taken at repeated intervals in the operating room; pneumothoraces that developed were treated with chest tube insertion only;[25] wooden fence posts, because of the greater likelihood of contamination and retained foreign material should have a thoracotomy to adequately debride the damaged lung as well as the entrance and exit wounds.[26]

TRANSFIXION INJURIES

These, differing only in magnitude and terminology, are similar to impalement injuries. Usually the patient is

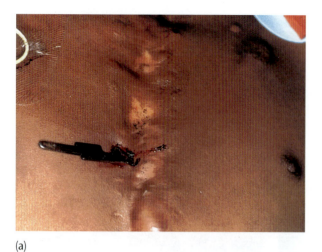

(a)

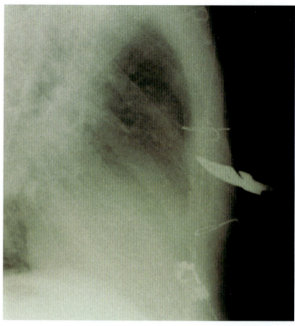

(b)

Figure 14.6 *(a, b) A similar situation as that in Figure 14.5 occurred in this patient who was stabbed through his previous median sternotomy incision, also for a heart stab. The lateral chest radiograph and obliqueness of the blade suggests that cardiac injury is unlikely; if present, tamponade is unlikely because of obliteration of the pericardial space, the result of his previous surgery. In this patient the knife blade was removed without incident under general anesthesia.*

seen with a knife blade, knife or arrow protruding from the chest or abdomen (Fig 14.5). One may be tempted to remove the knife blade, arguing that in the total scheme of thoracic injuries most knife wounds enter and leave the chest and are usually innocuous, yet injury and even death may be produced by removal of the knife blade. The knife blade may be situated within a vessel or acting as a tampon, reducing bleeding (Fig 14.6). This circumstance, for obvious reasons, is not commonly described in the literature. It is recommended that the transfixing object be left *in situ* and then removed, usually in the operating room under controlled circumstances, with preparation for immediate thoracotomy or chest tube insertion, if necessary. In our experience, the object is removed while the patient is anesthetized and carefully monitored. A radiographer is available and chest radiographs are taken immediately after removal of the object and 10 minutes later. If a significant pneumothorax or hemothorax develops, a chest drain is inserted; if the patient is stable he is observed for 24 hours prior to possible discharge; if bleeding is significant, or a hemodynamic change is apparent while being observed, the chest is immediately opened and the cause dealt with appropriately. In some circumstances clinical and preoperative investigations reveal a high likelihood of vascular injury which is managed by immediate thoracotomy and removal of the object with the chest open and the arterial defect managed appropriately (Fig 14.7).[27,28]

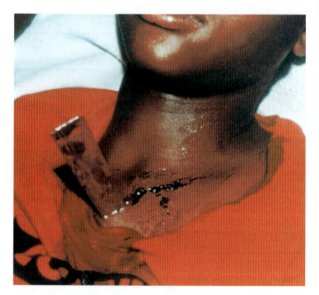

Figure 14.7 *The site of this retained knife blade is strongly suggestive of underlying great vessel injury and the approach was median sternotomy.*

REFERENCES

1. Brewer LA, Burford TH. Management of retained intrathoracic foreign bodies, Mediterranean (Formerly North African) theater of operations. In: *Medical*

Department, US Army. Surgery in World War II. Thoracic Surgery. Washington, DC: US Government Printing Office, 1963; 325–51.

2. Sommer G, McColloch CH. Surgical problems of retained foreign bodies. *Am J Surg* 1949; **77:** 314.

3. Jaffe H, O'Conor J. War wounds of the chest. *Am J Roentgenol* 1947; **58:** 183.

4. Vogt-Moykopf I, Krumhaar D. Treatment of intrapulmonary shell fragments. *Surg Gynecol Obstet* 1966; **123:** 1233–6.

5. Siddons AHM, MacArthur AM. Carcinomata developing at the site of foreign bodies in the lung. *Br J Surg* 1952; **39:** 542–5.

6. Harken DE. Foriegn bodies in, and in relation to the thoracic blood vessels and heart. *Surg Gynecol Obstet* 1946; **169:** 117–25.

7. LiMandri G, Gorenstein LA, Starr JP, Homma S, Auteri J, Gopal AS. Use of transesophageal echocardiography in the detection and consequences of an intracardiac bullet. *Am J Emerg Med* 1994; **12:** 105–6.

8. Symbas PN, Vlasis-Hale SE, Picone AL, Hatcher CR Jr. Missiles in the heart. *Ann Thorac Surg* 1989; **48:** 192–4.

9. Shannon FL, McCroskey BL, Moore EEE. Venous bullet embolism: rationale for mandatory extraction. *J Trauma* 1987; **27:** 1118–22.

10. Gandhi SK, Marts BC, Mistry BM, Brown JW, Durham RM, Mazuski JE. Selective management of embolized intracardiac missiles. *Ann Thorac Surg* 1996; **62:** 290–2.

11. Fisk RL, Addetia A, Gelfand ET, Brooks CH, Dvorkin J. Missile migration from lung to heart with delayed systemic embolization. *Chest* 1977; **72:** 534–5.

12. Pecirep DP, Hopkins HR. Removal of a bullet from the right heart using controlled embolization to a peripheral vein. *Ann Thorac Surg* 1994; **58:** 1748–50.

13. Hughes JJ. Bullet injury to the esophagus detected by intestinal migration. *J Trauma* 1987; **27:** 1362–4.

14. Montano JN, Mandal AK, Lou MAE. A 'wandering' bullet in the thoracic esophagus. *J Natl Med Assoc* 1983; **75:** 835–6.

15. Symbas PN, Hatcher CR, Vlasis SE. Esophageal gunshot injuries. *Ann Surg* 1979; **191:** 703–7.

16. Choh JH, Adler RH. Penetrating bullet wound of chest with bronchoscopic removal of bullet. *J Thorac Cardiovasc Surg* 1981; **82:** 150–3.

17. Burihan E, Pepe EV, Miranda F Jr. Bullet embolism following gunshot wound of the chest. Case report and review of the literature. *J Cardiovasc Surg (Torino)* 1980; **21:** 711–16.

18. Millar R, Rutherford WH, Johnston S, Malhorta VJ. Injuries caused by rubber bullets: a report on 90 patients. *Br J Surg* 1975; **62:** 480–6.

19. Yellin A, Golan M, Klein E, Avigad I, Rosenman J, Lieberman Y. Penetrating thoracic wounds caused by plastic bullets. *J Thorac Cardiovasc Surg* 1992; **103:** 381–5.

20. Aly MH, Kim HC, Renner SWE. Hemolytic anemia associated with lead poisoning from shotgun pellets and the response to Succimer treatment. *Am J Hematol* 1993; **44:** 280–3.

21. Meggs WJ, Gerr F, Aly MH, *et al.* The treatment of lead poisoning from gunshot wounds with succimer (DMSA) [see comments]. *J Toxicol Clin Toxicol* 1994; **32:** 377–85.

22. Chalmers JA, Graham TR, Magee PG. A concealed impalement injury of the chest – an unusual intrathoracic foreign body. *Eur J Cardiothorac Surg* 1989; **3:** 267–9.

23. Hyde MR, Schmidt CA, Jacobson JG, Vyhmeister EE, Laughlin LL. Impalement injuries to the thorax as a result of motor vehicle accidents. *Ann Thorac Surg* 1987; **43:** 189–90.

24. Robicsek F, Daugherty Y. Massive trauma due to impalement. *J Thorac Cardiovasc Surg* 1984; **87:** 634–6.

25. Odell JA, Whitton ID. Impalement of the chest with a reinforced steel rod. *J R Coll Surg Edinb* 1985; **30:** 132.

26. Kron IL, Unger S, Crosby IK. Fence post impalement injury of the chest with air embolus: a case report. *Va Med* 1983; **110:** 666–8.

27. Fradet G, Nelems B, Muller NL. Penetrating injury of the torso with impalement of the thoracic aorta: preoperative value of the computed tomographic scan. *Ann Thorac Surg* 1988; **45:** 680–1.

28. Odell JA, Shama D, Crause L. Retained knife blade and acute superior vena cava obstruction. *J Trauma* 1988; **28:** 416–17.

15

Blunt thoracic vascular trauma

ULRICH O VON OPPELL

TRAUMATIC RUPTURE OF THE THORACIC AORTA

Epidemiology

Blunt traumatic rupture of the thoracic aorta is an injury sustained predominantly from motor vehicle accidents, and is responsible for 12–27% of motor vehicle accident fatalities.[1–3]

Motor vehicle accidents account for 57-80% of aortic ruptures, pedestrian–vehicle accidents for 18–43%, motor cycle accidents for 3–10%, and airplane crashes, direct blows, compression injuries, and falls from heights for 1–10%.[3–5] The majority of traumatic aortic ruptures occur in males in the third and fourth decade, and only rarely in children.[4,6]

Natural history

Less than 5% of patients sustaining traumatic aortic rupture will survive if not treated, and develop chronic false aneurysms.[7] Post-traumatic aneurysms are considered to be chronic if of more than 2 weeks' duration.[8]

The majority of accident victims sustaining aortic rupture die at the scene of the accident and survival for more than 1 hour after injury, enabling patients to reach hospital alive, occurs in only 6–23% of patients.[2,3,9,10] The instantaneous risk of death for these initial survivors, in the absence of specific treatment, then decreases progressively; the probability of survival for 24 hours without treatment, on admission is 73%, at 24 hours 89%, and by day 5 increases to 96%.[8] Nevertheless, a risk of sudden death persists in untreated patients, as 41% of patients with chronic false aneurysms will develop signs or symptoms of aneurysm expansion or die from sudden rupture within 5 years of injury.[11]

Pathophysiology

Aortic rupture is usually caused by either a direct impact on the stationary sternum, rapid deceleration of the cranially or caudally moving body, or a combination of these mechanisms.[12] Traction, inertial, and shearing forces are produced between the relatively immobile descending aorta and relatively mobile aortic arch (Fig 15.1).

Blunt blows on the sternum displace the heart downwards and to the left, causing tensile stretch and rupture of the ascending aorta. Alternatively, sternal impact may cause an 'osseous pinch' mechanism, whereby the descending aorta tears as a result of compression against the spine by the anterior bony complex (manubrium, clavicle, first rib) rotating posteriorly and inferiorly about the posterior articulations.[13] A cranially directed impact on the lower chest may cause a 'shoveling effect', whereby the heart and mediastinum are displaced cranially, which causes tensile stretch and rupture of the proximal descending aorta.

On the other hand, rapid deceleration of the cranially moving body by impact on the head or chest creates inertial forces that displace the aortic arch towards the head, resulting in tensile stretching and rupture of the aortic isthmus. Caudally directed deceleration (falls from a height) also generate inertial forces by caudal displacement of the thoracoabdominal viscera.

Less likely postulated mechanisms of aortic rupture are sudden increased hydrostatic aortic pressure causing

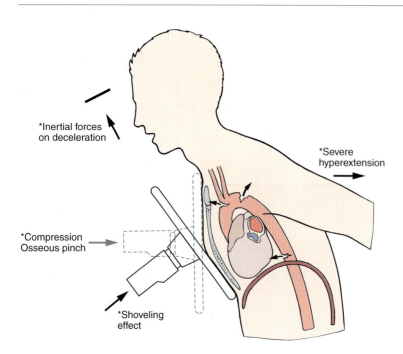

Figure 15.1 *Four pathophysiological mechanisms of blunt traumatic thoracic aortic rupture showing the direction of forces (*) acting during motor vehicle accidents are illustrated. Three different sites of rupture are shown.*

*Inertial forces on deceleration

*Severe hyperextension

*Compression Osseous pinch

*Shoveling effect

the aorta to 'burst', and posteroanterior deceleration inertial forces. More than one mechanism may be operative in any individual patient.

Rupture occurs at the aortic isthmus in 60% of patients; the region between the origin of the left subclavian artery and the ligamentum arteriosum, the ascending aorta or aortic arch in approximately 20%, and in the more distal descending thoracic aorta in a further 20%.[10,14,15] Multiple aortic tears occur in 12–16% of patients.[14,15] Ruptures of the distal descending thoracic aorta are frequently associated with thoracic vertebral fractures and severe hyperextension is the probable pathophysiological mechanism at this site.[16]

The spectrum of traumatic aortic rupture varies from only a tear of the intima to involvement of all three layers – intima, media and adventitia – which is invariably immediately fatal.[15] The resilience and integrity of the adventitia of the aorta surrounding the ruptured tunica intima and media determines the patient's immediate survival at the time of the accident, by containing the expanding hematoma. The intima and media tear is usually transverse and linear, and circumferential in 40–60% of cases in which case the ends of the intima and media retract for up to 3–6 cm.

The mediastinal hematoma contained by the adventitia, in the initial survivors of traumatic aortic ruptures, accounts for the radiographic manifestations suggestive of this injury. Subadventitial dissection of the hematoma for a few centimeters can occasionally cause the torn distal intima and media to fold into the aortic lumen, causing 'pseudo-coarctation' resulting in distal ischemia. The more elastic pediatric aortic tissue may account for the apparent high 40% incidence of pseudo-coarctation in children sustaining aortic rupture.[6]

Clinical presentation and diagnosis

There is no characteristic clinical presentation of blunt aortic rupture and up to 20% of patients will be asymptomatic with respect to the aortic injury. Non-specific symptoms of shock and dyspnea are reported in 20–50% of patients, and retrosternal or interscapular chest pain in 30–50%. Post-traumatic pseudo-coarctation, i.e. diminished blood pressure in the legs compared to the arms, occurs in 7–40% of patients,[5,6,17] and is highly suggestive of acute aortic rupture.

Multisystem trauma is prevalent in the majority of aortic rupture patients and many patients have no external evidence of thoracic trauma, which may distract the emergency room physician from further thoracic investigations. Hence, maintaining a high index of suspicion for acute traumatic aortic rupture in all patients who have sustained violent deceleration impacts is essential (Table 15.1).

Table 15.1 *Blunt traumatic thoracic aortic rupture – diagnosis*

High index of clinical suspicion
All major deceleration accidents
    Increased risk if ejected from a vehicle[1]
    Increased risk if pedestrian-vehicle accident[15]
Pseudo-coarctation syndrome (discrepant arm–leg blood pressure)

Screening investigations for mediastinal hematoma
Chest radiography (erect PA film from 2 m)
Dynamic computerized tomography (CT) of the chest

Diagnostic investigations for traumatic aortic rupture
Multiplane transesophageal echocardiography
Arch-aortography

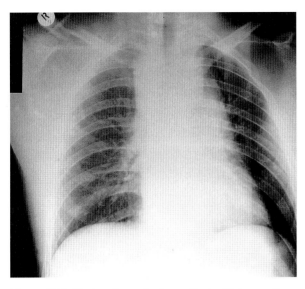

Figure 15.2 *Chest radiograph of a patient with traumatic rupture of the aortic isthmus, illustrating a wide mediastinum, loss of the sharp contour of the aortic knob, loss of the clear angle between the aorta and pulmonary artery, as well as a left apical pleural cap.*

Table 15.2 *Non-specific chest radiographic signs of blunt traumatic thoracic aortic rupture*

- Wide mediastinum; greater than 8 cm at the aortic knob
- Left apical pleural cap; opacification of the supramedial aspect of the left pleural apex
- Blurring of the sharp aortic knob contour
- Obliteration of the clear angle between the aorta and left pulmonary artery
- Tracheal shift to the right
- Esophageal shift to the right at the aortic knob, as evidenced by displacement of a nasogastric tube
- Depression of the left main bronchus greater than 40° below the horizontal
- Abnormal paraspinal stripe
- Left hemothorax
- Fracture of the first rib

Associated thoracic injuries include cardiac contusion in up to 62% of aortic rupture patients,[18] and blunt diaphragmatic rupture in up to 16%.[19]

CHEST RADIOGRAPH

The basic screening investigation for patients sustaining blunt traumatic injuries is an erect chest radiograph. The chest radiographic features suggestive of aortic rupture (Fig 15.2), are non-specific radiographic signs of mediastinal hematoma (Table 15.2).[20] None is diagnostic of aortic rupture. The most consistent sign is a widened mediastinum, greater than 8 cm at the aortic knob, which has a sensitivity of approximately 92% but a specificity of only 10%.[21] The detection of these chest radiographic signs should alert the emergency room physician to proceed with further diagnostic procedures in order to actively exclude an aortic rupture.

A normal chest radiograph, however, does not exclude the diagnosis of an aortic rupture as a normal admission chest radiograph occurs in up to 27% of confirmed aortic rupture patients, especially in patients over the age of 65 years.[22]

COMPUTERIZED TOMOGRAPHIC SCAN

The resolution of dynamic chest computerized tomography (CT) is not satisfactory for detecting specific aortic intimal irregularities, and therefore CT should be viewed as an ancillary screening method for detecting the presence of periaortic mediastinal hematoma and not as a primary method of diagnosing aortic injury.[23] The specificity of an abnormal chest CT for an aortic

tear is only 21–54%,[24–26] and thus patients with chest CT evidence of mediastinal bleeding still require angiography because of this high false-positive rate.

CT as an adjunct to chest radiography in the screening for traumatic aortic tears can decrease the need for angiography by 25–56%, and may be cost-effective in triaging patients.[25,27,28] However, the sensitivity for detecting signs of aortic injury is only 55–88%,[24,29] and the rate of false-negative chest CTs can be as high as 17%.[30] Thus a negative CT may also not reliably exclude aortic injury.[24,26,29] The possible detrimental effect of delay in initiating definitive surgical treatment caused by inappropriate routine use of chest CT, because angiography must still be performed, should also be considered.[31] The value of preliminary chest CT to avoid thoracic aortography in patients with blunt trauma is therefore limited,[27,29,31] and probably only indicated in patients undergoing CT evaluation of other injuries.[28]

Dynamic CT should probably only be used as an additional screening examination for patients with equivocal or normal chest radiographs in the presence of a history of violent blunt trauma.[20,23,30] Chest CT may also, by excluding the presence of a mediastinal hematoma, assist in establishing the correct diagnosis in patients having an equivocal aortogram, e.g. an isolated intimal defect, 'ductal bump' or pre-existing atherosclerotic aneurysm,[29,30,32,33] in whom surgery is not indicated.

TRANSESOPHAGEAL ECHOCARDIOGRAPHY

Transesophageal echocardiography (TEE) is proving to be a rapid, reliable and cost-effective method of accurately diagnosing injuries of the descending thoracic aorta by visualizing an intimal flap or intimal disruption as well as periaortic hematoma. Contraindications to TEE include suspected esophageal trauma, a history of previous esophageal pathology or surgery, severe maxillofacial trauma, unstable cervical spinal

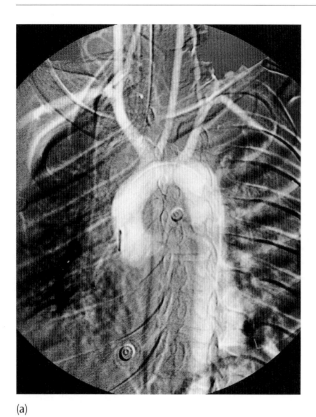

(a)

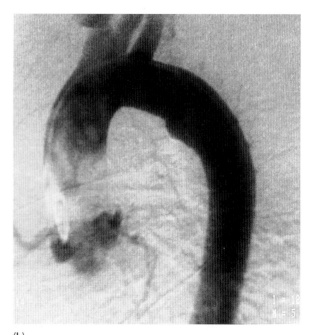

(b)

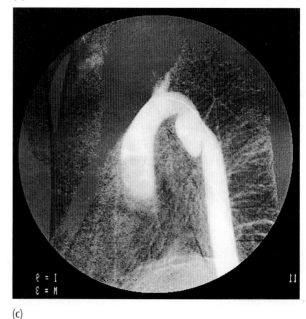

(c)

Figure 15.3 *(a) Angiogram of a traumatic rupture at the isthmus of the descending thoracic aorta, illustrating a relatively indistinct periaortic false aneurysm. (b) Angiogram of a 56-year-old patient with a 'ductal bump'. (c) Angiogram of a traumatic rupture at the aortic isthmus, demonstrating a false aneurysm as well as distal subadventitial dissection causing compression of the distal aortic lumen; pseudo-coarctation narrowing.*

injury, or an uncooperative patient. TEE can be successfully performed in approximately 92% of emergency room patients suspected of having aortic rupture.[34] False-positive and false-negative TEEs have been reported and the sensitivity ranges from 63% to 100% and specificity from 84% to 100%, which is similar to that for aortography.[34–37]

Multiplane TEE is usually performed in the trauma unit by cardiologists,[37] can accurately identify a descending or ascending aortic intimal defect, and can also assess associated cardiac injuries and function. Nevertheless, TEE is operator dependent and is unreliable in assessing injuries of the aortic arch and brachiocephalic vessels. Equivocal TEE findings should be further evaluated with angiography.

AORTOGRAM

Aortography is currently still the diagnostic gold standard for all patients suspected clinically of having blunt aortic rupture. In our experience, the liberal use of angiography yields positive angiograms in approximately 12% of victims of blunt trauma who have abnormal chest radiographs.[17] Intra-arterial digital subtraction aortography is now more frequently used than conventional film angiography.

The angiographic appearance of blunt aortic rupture is based on the detection of a false aneurysm, extravasation of contrast medium outside the normal aortic contour, or an intimal tear. This angiographic appearance can vary from a slight irregularity of the aortic outline which can be confused with a 'ductal bump', a linear defect produced by a flap of intima or media, subadventitial dissection, pseudo-coarctation narrowing or to a large false aneurysm (Fig 15.3).

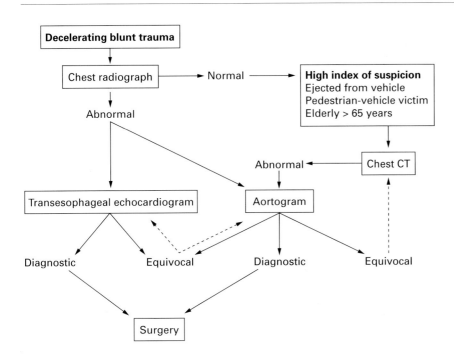

Figure 15.4 *Diagnostic flow diagram for patients suspected of having acute blunt traumatic rupture of the aorta.*

False-positive angiograms occur as a result of diagnostic confusion with a ductal bump (Fig 15.3b) or pre-existing atherosclerotic aneurysm, and can be excluded by the absence of any signs of mediastinal hematoma on CT scan or TEE.[38] False-negative angiograms have also been reported,[36] and in our experience even on review have not shown any abnormality, as the adventitial hematoma maintained luminal continuity without the formation of an expanding false aneurysm.[5] Hence, the sensitivity of aortography is 73–100% and specificity 99%.[24,36]

Summary

The high mortality rate associated with missed aortic rupture necessitates liberal use of diagnostic investigations in victims of blunt trauma, the current gold standard being aortography in all patients having abnormal admission chest radiographs. Chest CT is a non-diagnostic screening investigation for the presence of a mediastinal hematoma. TEE is proving to be as accurate as aortography in diagnosing aortic rupture; however, patients with an equivocal TEE, suspected arch or brachiocephalic vessel injury should preferably or additionally undergo aortography. Furthermore, an additional diagnostic investigation should be performed despite an initial normal chest radiograph if there is a high index of clinical suspicion for blunt aortic rupture (Fig 15.4).

Surgical management

The first successful repair of a traumatic aortic rupture was accomplished in 1923.[8] The current controversial

Table 15.3 *Controversial issues in the surgical management of acute descending thoracic aortic rupture*

- Timing of surgical repair in relation to the treatment of associated injuries
- Operative techniques to minimize the risk of paraplegia complicating the surgical procedure
- Method of repairing the aortic rupture, either direct suture repair or prosthetic graft insertion

issues in treating patients with aortic rupture are outlined in Table 15.3.

The mortality of moribund acute traumatic aortic rupture patients undergoing emergency room thoracotomy on arrival in hospital is 94%.[39] By contrast, potentially salvageable aortic rupture patients reaching hospital alive have a mortality of 32%; 14% of these hospitalized patients die prior to definitive surgery.[39,40] Thus, the most important issue is patient survival and the 'optimal method' might not always be available or appropriate at all times.

The surgical mortality of patients undergoing 'non-resuscitative' surgical intervention is 21%, and in an international meta-analysis mortality was higher in patients treated either by simple aortic cross-clamping or with bypass techniques requiring full systemic heparinization.[39,40] Age greater than 25 years,[41] and associated cardiac contusion,[18] have also been implicated as surgical risk factors.

ISOLATED INTIMAL TEARS

On the one end of the spectrum of traumatic aortic rupture is the 'isolated intimal tear', seen on angiography as a small area of intimal irregularity with no extravasation of contrast material outside the normal contour of the aorta. An additional chest CT is advisable in these patients with suspected isolated intimal tears, to exclude the presence of any periaortic hematoma. These patients can then be treated medically; however, it is essential that repeat aortography be performed after a few days, to confirm that healing is occurring without false aneurysm formation.[32] The final diagnosis of an isolated intimal tear should be 'retrospective' as false-negative angiograms in the presence of circumferential ruptures of both the intima and media have been documented.[5]

PREOPERATIVE MEDICAL MANAGEMENT AND TIMING OF SURGICAL REPAIR

Initial medical management to decrease the risk of precipitous exsanguination

The instantaneous risk of death at the time of hospital admission is approximately 27%, as previously discussed,[8] and nearly half of hospital deaths occur prior to definitive surgery, often as a result of delays in diagnosing the contained aortic rupture.[39,40] Hypertension, which is common after initial resuscitation and replacement of blood losses in these patients, is considered a risk factor for exsanguination from precipitous rupture of the periaortic hematoma. Hence, once an aortic rupture is suspected, even prior to any definitive diagnostic investigations, appropriate pharmacological therapy to diminish aortic wall stresses should be commenced.[42] The drug of choice is a β-blocker such as intravenous esmolol [1–2 mg/kg i.v. infusion (IVI) repeated as necessary; half-life ±10 minutes, or 50 mg IVI bolus and then infused at 0.05–0.3 mg/kg/min] or propranolol hydrochloride (0.5–1 mg IVI repeated as necessary; half-life ±2–3 hours), which decreases the force of ejection of the left ventricle. Blood pressure should be monitored continuously and systolic pressure kept below 100 mmHg (mean arterial pressure less than 80 mmHg), and additional vasodilators such as sodium nitroprusside introduced as second line therapy for resistant hypertension.[43]

Timing of surgical intervention

Historically, surgical repair of acute aortic rupture has taken precedence over the treatment of most other associated injuries. Progressive cerebral signs of intracranial compression or evidence of continued intra-abdominal bleeding possibly warrant prior management.

The risk of dying after hospital admission from exsanguination as a result of rupture of the aortic adventitia as opposed to associated injuries, and therefore the need for immediate surgical repair, can be extrapolated from various studies. The instantaneous risk of death in the absence of treatment decreases with time; within the first 24 hours of injury it is 94%,[3] but within 24 hours of hospital admission decreases to 27% and by day 5 decreases further to 4%.[8] Furthermore, approximately 64% of traumatic aortic rupture patient deaths are due to exsanguination; ±50% of deaths at the scene, ±86% of deaths prior to or within 30 minutes of arrival at hospital, and 14% of hospitalized patients before the diagnosis of aortic transection is made.[9] However, others have found that approximately 67% of all pre- and perioperative hospital deaths are due to exsanguination, often as a result of diagnostic and treatment delays, albeit in the absence of routine pharmacological therapy.[5,44] Nevertheless, the axiom of immediate surgical intervention for all acute aortic ruptures is now being questioned.[42] A policy of pharmacological aortic wall stress reduction with delayed more elective surgical repair of the aortic rupture after stabilization and treatment of associated injuries may be indicated in selected patients.[42,45,46] However, elective delay of definitive surgical treatment, albeit with appropriate medical therapy and monitoring in an intensive care unit, is not without risk, and is associated with a 4.5% risk of death from aortic rupture within 72 hours of admission.[47]

Modern increasingly rapid paramedical transportation of accident victims to hospital facilities increases the number of potentially salvageable patients at high risk of exsanguination,[9] and this should therefore also be taken into account when assessing policies. We would therefore advise a policy of immediate β-blocker therapy in all suspected aortic ruptures, and surgical intervention as soon as the diagnosis has been established. The risk/safety of elective surgical delay when the diagnosis of aortic rupture is made within 24 hours of injury in the presence of β-blocker therapy is not yet firmly established. Elective delay can only be advised for selective patients who have complex associated injuries in whom the risk of immediate surgery is thought to be higher than the risk of elective delay,[45] provided pharmacological aortic wall stress reduction is commenced and facilities exist for careful continuous monitoring. Possible indications for delay include associated severe cerebral trauma, respiratory insufficiency, significant myocardial contusion or infarct, extensive burns or sepsis.[47] Clinical signs indicative of high risk for precipitous exsanguination are left hemothorax, supraclavicular hematoma and pseudocoarctation, and contraindicate elective surgical delay.[48] Renal failure and paraplegia from pseudocoarctation may resolve with prompt surgical treatment.[49]

When the diagnosis is made 24 hours after injury, operation may be undertaken on the next available scheduled surgical list rather than as an emergency as the risk of precipitous exsanguination is lower, provided there is no evidence of active bleeding nor a very large hematoma, and that arterial hypertension is avoided with β-blocker therapy.[8]

Surgical approach – descending thoracic aortic ruptures

ANESTHESIA

Patients 'should receive β-blocker therapy preoperatively, to decrease aortic wall stress and the risk of precipitous exsanguination, as previously discussed. Careful hemodynamic monitoring during the procedure is essential, as perioperative arterial hypotension, hypoxemia and proximal hypertension during aortic clamping have been associated with increased risks of paraplegia, complicating the procedure, and should therefore be avoided.[50] Furthermore, the use of sodium nitroprusside or trinitroglycerine to decrease proximal hypertension during simple aortic cross-clamping is contraindicated because it increases the risk of perioperative paraplegia by decreasing spinal cord perfusion.[51,52]

An arterial line for pressure monitoring should be placed in the right radial artery, as the left subclavian artery might be clamped during the procedure, and an additional arterial line should be inserted into the right pedal artery for distal aortic pressure monitoring during aortic cross-clamping. Double lumen endotracheal intubation with single-lung ventilation is recommended as it improves exposure of the aorta and ameliorates iatrogenic pulmonary injury from surgical retraction, especially if the patient is heparinized.

INCISION AND INITIAL DISSECTION

The patient is positioned in a right-side-down posterolateral position, with the pelvis rotated ±40° posteriorly to the left to allow access to the left groin. The patient is prepped and draped to allow simultaneous exploration of the chest and, if necessary, the left groin and abdomen.[53] The incision is a left posterolateral thoracotomy entering the pleural space through the fourth intercostal space (above the fifth rib).

The mediastinal pleura on either side of the aorta, just distal to the hematoma, is incised and a tape passed around the aorta for later easy placement of the distal aortic cross-clamp. If the hematoma is extensive, this distal clamp can be reapplied closer to the site of rupture after the aneurysm has been opened, so as to limit the possibility of inadvertent occlusion of a critical intercostal artery (Table 15.4, Fig 15.5).

Table 15.4 *Perioperative spinal cord ischemia in surgery for acute descending thoracic aortic rupture*

Etiological factors	Ameliorating factors
Occlusion of the major radicular artery Maximum safe period of total occlusion in the absence of collateral flow is ±15–18 min[56]	

Temporary occlusion within aortic segment isolated by aortic cross-clamps.
  The major radicular artery originates just distal to the isthmic rupture (between T5 and T8) in 12–15% of patients.[54,55]
	Apply/reapply cross-clamps close to the rupture so as to occlude the minimum number of intercostal vessels
	Systemic hypothermia (32°C)
	  Metabolic rate decreases at 5%/°C[57]
	    Cooling blanket
	    Pleural lavage with iced saline

Permanent ligation of critical intercostal artery	
Hypotensive perfusion of major radicular artery Maximum safe period of hypotensive (<40 mmHg) perfusion is 30 min[39,40,58,59]	
Proximal aortic clamping in the absence of collateral circulation or additional distal perfusion Perioperative systemic hypotension[44,50]	**Augment distal perfusion/partial bypass**[39,40] Intrathecal papaverine (3 ml 1% solution[60]) **Systemic hypothermia (32°C)**
Increased cerebrospinal fluid pressure Reduces spinal cord perfusion gradient; minimal safe gradient is 30 mmHg[61]	
Proximal hypertension accompanying simple aortic clamping Paradoxically aggravated by vasodilators which divert blood flow away from spinal cord collaterals[51,52]	**Augment distal perfusion/partial bypass** Exsanguination technique[62] Cerebrospinal fluid drainage[63]
Reperfusion injury	
	Methylprednisolone (30 mg/kg IVI) 10 min before cross-clamping and 4 h later[64] Free radical scavengers – iron chelators (deferoxamine 50 mg/kg)[65] Calcium channel blockers

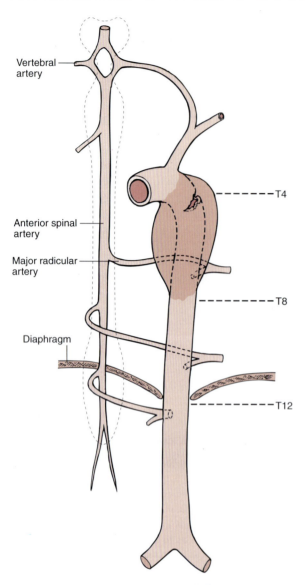

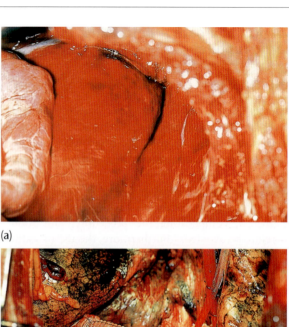

(a)

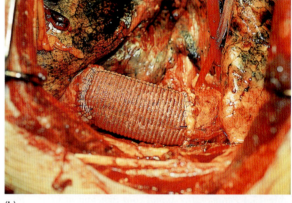

(b)

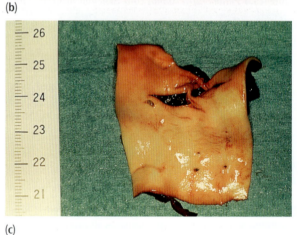

(c)

Figure 15.5 *The possible close relationship of the origin of the major radicular artery, which supplies the anterior spinal artery of the spinal cord, to an isthmic aortic rupture is shown. The major radicular artery arises between T5 and T8 in 12–15% of patients, and may be included in the aortic segment cross-clamped if the distal cross-clamp is not kept close to the aortic tear.*

Figure 15.6 *(a) The appearance of an extensive mediastinal hematoma at left thoracotomy for blunt traumatic aortic injury. No anatomical structures can be defined apart from the lung (left) retracted downwards away from the superior mediastinum. (b) Graft replacement of the injured segment of descending thoracic aorta immediately distal to the left subclavian artery. (c) The resected specimen of aorta showing the traumatic laceration. Sometimes these can be closed by direct suture, thereby avoiding graft interposition. (SWTC.)*

Mediastinal dissection around the proximal aortic arch can result in precipitous hemorrhage if the hematoma is inadvertently entered (Fig 15.6), and therefore at this stage it is prudent to prepare and commence partial heparinless bypass as discussed below.

OPERATIVE TECHNIQUES TO MINIMIZE THE RISK OF PARAPLEGIA COMPLICATING THE SURGICAL PROCEDURE

The incidence of associated spinal cord injuries with paraplegia occurring at or shortly after the traumatic

event in patients sustaining traumatic aortic rupture is 2.6%.[39] This 'preoperative' paraplegia occurs as a result of either direct spinal cord injury with or without associated spinal fractures or dislocations, spinal arter-

Table 15.5 *Traumatic descending thoracic aortic rupture: surgical techniques and risk of new paraplegia*

	Incidence of paraplegia (%)
Simple aortic cross-clamping	19.2
Risk of paraplegia increases if cross-clamp time exceeds 30 min	
Augmenting distal perfusion – passive shunts	11.1
Risk of paraplegia increases if cross-clamp time exceeds ±40 min	
Augmenting distal perfusion – active perfusion	2.3
Partial heparinless bypass (no oxygenator)	
Centrifugal vortex pump (standard or heparin-bonded tubing)	
Femoral veno-arterial bypass (heparin-bonded tubing)	
Partial or complete bypass with systemic heparin (with oxygenator)	
Overall average incidence	9.9

International meta-analysis[39,40]

ial injury or consequent to pseudocoarctation-induced ischemia. Most of the paraplegia associated with acute descending thoracic aortic ruptures, however, occurs as a complication of the surgical procedure undertaken to repair the aortic rupture. The global incidence of new postoperative paraplegia complicating surgical repair of the traumatic aortic rupture is 9.9%.[39]

Patients with acute traumatic aortic rupture have neither collateral circulation to the distal aorta as in coarctation of the aorta, nor spinal cord collaterals that potentially evolve during chronic disease processes such as atherosclerotic aortic aneurysms, and therefore have a greater risk of developing postoperative paraplegia than after operations for more chronic lesions. Paraplegia occurs as a result of inadequate spinal cord perfusion, which is provided by the anterior spinal artery that arises cranially from the vertebral arteries, as well as via

a few radicular arteries originating from intercostal arteries (Fig 15.5).[54,55] Inadequate perfusion of these radicular arteries, and predominantly that of the single major radicular artery (artery of Adamkiewicz) which originates between T5 and T8 in 12–15% of patients, T9 and T12 in 60–75%, and below L1 in 10–25% of individuals,[54,55] is the major cause of perioperative spinal cord ischemia, and therefore paraplegia (Table 15.4).

The incidence of new postoperative paraplegia in relation to the type of surgical technique used to augment perfusion distal to the aortic cross-clamp highlights the importance of this single variable (Table 15.5). The risk of paraplegia increases substantially if the aorta is cross-clamped for longer than 30 minutes and if the surgeon does not augment distal perfusion during the period of cross-clamping (Fig 15.7).

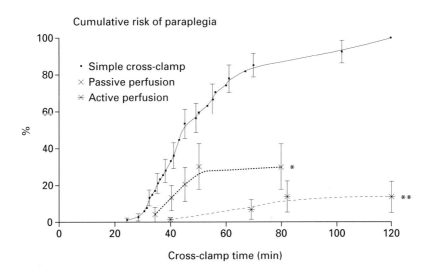

Figure 15.7 *The cumulative risk of new paraplegia complicating surgical repair of acute traumatic descending thoracic aortic rupture (with standard errors) in relation to different surgical techniques as well as the duration of aortic cross-clamping is shown. The shortest cross-clamp time at which the risk of paraplegia in the simple cross-clamp group exceeded that in distally perfused patients was at 31 minutes (P <0.05). *P <0.005 'passive' methods of augmenting distal perfusion versus simple cross-clamping. **P <0.001 'active' methods of augmenting distal perfusion versus 'passive' methods. (Reproduced with permission from Von Oppell et al.)[40]*

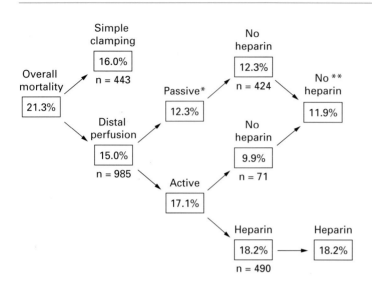

Figure 15.8 *The operative mortality for repair of acute traumatic descending thoracic aortic rupture in relation to different surgical techniques is shown. *P <0.05 'passive' methods of augmenting distal perfusion versus 'active' methods. **P <0.01 all methods of augmenting distal perfusion without using heparin versus methods requiring heparin. (Reproduced with permission from Von Oppell et al.)[40]*

Cognizance should also be given to the fact that in surgical practice we cannot confidently predict whether surgical repair can be accomplished within 30 minutes. Furthermore, complex and multiple tears (12–16% of patients[14,15]) might only be identified after applying the aortic cross-clamps. Individual surgical experience with these injuries is also limited, which affects outcome,[5] as on average only 2.6 patients per year are treated in any single institution and the global average cross-clamp time needed to treat this injury is 41 minutes.[39]

The recommended surgical technique, which minimizes the risk of paraplegia occurring during repair of acute descending thoracic aortic ruptures, is the provision of 'active' distal perfusion during the aortic cross-clamp period. Partial bypass techniques not only ameliorate the risk of paraplegia by preventing hypotensive distal spinal cord perfusion but also prevent proximal hypertension and physiological overload of the left ventricle consequent to aortic clamping, as well as ameliorating hemodynamic and metabolic changes of declamping. Adjunctive mild systemic hypothermia (32°C) can also be easily instituted by topical pleural cooling, which extends neurological ischemic tolerance by approximately 25%.[57]

An additional preventable but rare cause of postoperative paraplegia (0.08% of thoracotomy incisions) is the use of excessive electrocautery or wound packing with oxidized cellulose in the costovertebral angle of the thoracotomy incision,[66] which should be avoided.

Cardiovascular system failure causes 14–49% of pre- and perioperative deaths in acute aortic rupture patients,[44] which may be related to the high 62% incidence of associated cardiac contusion in these patients.[18] The operative mortality following simple aortic cross-clamping in an international meta-analysis was 16% which was higher than that for heparinless partial bypass methods, possibly as a result of the consequent increased left ventricular afterload aggravating associated myocardial contusion or pre-existing cardiac

disease (Fig 15.8).[39,40] Systemic heparinization may, however, also contribute to both surgical mortality and morbidity by aggravating other multisystem injuries, especially cerebral injuries, in these patients.[67] Distal perfusion methods not using heparin are associated with an operative mortality of 11.9%, whilst partial or complete bypass with full systemic heparinization have a higher average mortality of 18.2%.[39,40] Hence, partial heparinless bypass without an oxygenator is the technique of choice, and this is usually done with a centrifugal vortex pump and standard polyvinylchloride tubing.

Heparinless femoral venoarterial partial bypass without an oxygenator using a roller pump, heparin-bonded tubing and cannulae has only been used in a few patients to date.[68] This method is dependent on cannulation of the right atrium via the femoral vein, maintenance of high mixed venous oxygen saturation, as well as high perfusion pressures and flow rates.[69]

PARTIAL HEPARINLESS BYPASS USING A CENTRIFUGAL VORTEX PUMP

Partial heparinless bypass can be instituted without groin dissection, by placing purse-string sutures for the 'arterial' outflow line in the distal descending thoracic aorta (alternatively the left femoral artery), and in the left atrial appendage for the 'venous' inflow line (alternatively the left inferior or superior pulmonary vein) (Fig 15.9). Standard polyvinylchloride tubing can be used for the bypass circuit, although heparin-bonded tubing may be preferable. Flow rates should be maintained at 1.5–3.0 l/min (distal aortic pressure maintained at 50–70 mmHg) with either the Biomedicus (Biomedicus Inc., Minneapolis, MN) or Sarns (Sarns; 3M Health Care, Ann Arbor, MI) centrifugal pumps.[70] Experimental studies suggest that distal aortic pressure needs to be maintained above 60 mmHg to prevent paraplegia.[58] A single low dose (activated clotting time

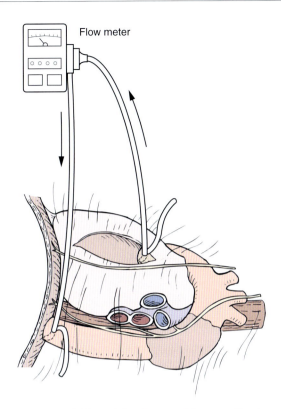

Figure 15.9 *Partial heparinless bypass with a centrifugal pump providing 'active' perfusion of the aorta distal to the cross-clamped segment of aorta is shown. Oxygenated blood is pumped from either the left atrial appendage, superior or inferior pulmonary veins to either the descending thoracic aorta or left femoral artery.*

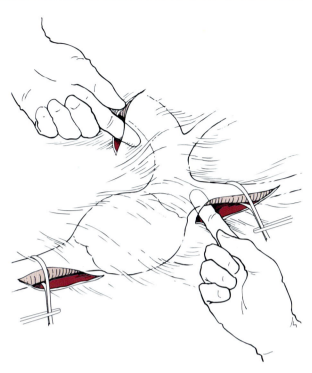

Figure 15.10 *Illustration of a traumatic rupture at the aortic isthmus showing the overlying hematoma. The mediastinal pleura has been incised over the distal aorta, the subclavian artery, and aortic arch. Tapes have been passed around the distal aorta and subclavian artery. A plane is developed posterolaterally behind the aortic arch and above the hematoma by blunt dissection with a finger, commencing behind the left subclavian artery.*

less than 200 seconds) of intravenous heparin (3000–5000 IU) has been used by some surgeons if non-heparin-bonded cannulae are inserted into the left atrium, because of concern for clot formation. [The centrifugal pump is a non-occlusive pump and there-fore, in order to prevent retrograde flow of blood from distal aorta to left atrium and possible embolization of any air contained in the 'left atrial venous line' (after connection of cannulae), pumping at 2000 r.p.m. should be commenced prior to release of line clamps. To avoid stasis-induced clot formation in non-heparin-bonded cannulae, partial heparinless bypass should be commenced immediately after cannulation, prior to dissection and placement of the proximal aortic clamp on the aortic arch, and the patient should be decannu-lated promptly after stopping partial bypass.]

DISSECTION AND PLACEMENT OF PROXIMAL AORTIC CLAMP

The mediastinal pleura over the left subclavian artery is incised and a tape passed twice around the left subcla-vian artery or a Rummel tourniquet applied, to allow for later occlusion. The left phrenic and vagus nerves are identified and taped.

A plane is then developed behind the aortic arch, commencing behind on the right lateral aspect of the left subclavian artery by blunt finger dissection, staying anterosuperior to the mediastinal hematoma and site of rupture (Fig 15.10). The mediastinal pleura over the concavity of the arch is similarly incised and a medial plane developed. The aortic arch, between the left carotid and left subclavian, can now be taped or a cross-clamp applied. If the mediastinal hematoma is extensive, proximal control can also be obtained by extending the pericardial incision cephalad across its reflection on the ascending aorta, to permit finger dissection around the transverse aortic arch.[53] Alternatively, the aorta is dissected intrapericardially; the right lateral pericardial reflection is dissected from the anterior aspect of the ascending aorta, a tape is then passed from the previous dissection below the left subclavian behind the arch anterior to the ascending aorta, the ascending aorta is separated from the pulmonary artery and the tape then brought posterior to the ascending aorta and anterior to the pulmonary artery, thus isolating the aortic arch. A large blunt-tipped curved vascular clamp should be used for proximal aortic clamping of both the subclavian and aortic arch between the left carotid and subclavian arter-ies (Fig 15.11).

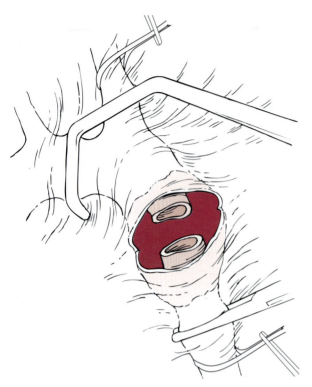

Figure 15.11 *Illustration of a traumatic rupture at the aortic isthmus showing aortic cross-clamps in situ. The adventitial hematoma has been opened transversely and a circumferential rupture of the tunica media and intima is seen. The ends of the intima and media have retracted for 2–3 cm.*

The mediastinal pleura and adventitia overlying the hematoma is then incised transversely; a transverse incision is preferred if direct suture repair of the tear is to be attempted,[71] and with blunt dissection the transected ends of the aorta (tunica intima and media) are identified.

SURGICAL TECHNIQUES; DIRECT SUTURE REPAIR OR INTERPOSITION PROSTHETIC GRAFT

Primary end-to-end suture repair of the ruptured aorta with either 3/0 or 4/0 polypropylene is the ideal. The adventitial hematoma causes partial separation of the adventitia from the aorta, and the ends (tunica intima and media) of circumferentially ruptured aortas usually retract for 2–3 cm. Sutures placed under tension in only the retracted intima and media tend to tear out. However, primary repair may be possible without mobilizing the aorta, especially of incomplete tears, by gentle traction of multiple preplaced sutures and including the more resilient adjacent mediastinal and adventitial tissue in the suture line (Fig 15.12a).[72] Alternatively, if all layers of the aorta including the adventitia are mobilized for 2–4 cm proximally and distally (ligation of intercostal arteries is usually not required) and additional fine straight vascular clamps are applied

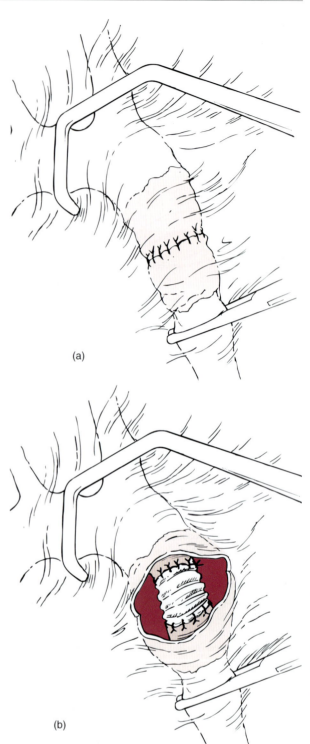

Figure 15.12 *Illustration of completed surgical repair of a traumatic rupture at the aortic isthmus. (a) Direct suture reapproximation of the ruptured tunica intima and media, with inclusion of the overlying adventitia in the suture line. (b) Reapproximation of the ruptured tunica intima and media by insertion of an interposition woven Dacron graft.*

within a centimeter of the edge of the aortic tear to approximate the ends, then primary repair without tension may be possible.[73–75]

The majority of surgeons insert an interposition graft between the retracted ends, in order to avoid suturing under tension (Fig 15.12b). This might be the safer option, especially if surgical experience with this injury is limited.[5] Prosthetic grafts used include polytetra-fluoroethylene (PTFE), although the rigidity of this graft might require additional techniques to facilitate suturing,[76] or the more pliable zero-porosity woven Dacron grafts. 'Sutureless' intraluminal grafts should not be used in these patients because the size of the normal non-aneurysmal ruptured aorta necessitates insertion of intraluminal grafts of extremely small internal diameter, resulting in high postoperative pressure gradients and iatrogenic coarctation.[77]

POSTOPERATIVE MANAGEMENT

These patient are usually ventilated postoperatively, and associated multisystem injuries dictate further management. Intercostal drains can usually be removed within 24–48 hours.

Oral β-blocker therapy is often necessary for the treatment of postoperative hypertension, but can usually be discontinued within a few months. Anti-aggregatory or anticoagulatory agents are not required, regardless of whether prosthetic grafts were inserted.

Surgical approach – ascending aorta or aortic arch ruptures

The less common ascending aorta and aortic arch ruptures are repaired through a median sternotomy on heparinized cardiopulmonary bypass, if necessary with the aid of deep hypothermic circulatory arrest to provide cerebral protection. The hematoma around the ascending aorta should not be disturbed when instituting cardiopulmonary bypass, and therefore a single right atrial venous cannula and femoral arterial cannula are used.

TEARS OF THE ASCENDING AORTA

After commencing moderate hypothermic cardiopulmonary bypass, the pericardial reflection over the distal portion of the ascending aorta is dissected and a cross-clamp placed just proximal to the origin of the innominate artery. Cardioplegic solution can be administered either retrograde via the coronary sinus or antegrade by direct cannulation of the coronary ostia after opening the aorta through the hematoma/transection. In the absence of an obvious anterior rupture, the aorta should be opened to allow inspection of the posterior aortic wall. The aortic tear is repaired either by direct suture reapproximation or by inserting an interposition prosthetic graft.

TEARS OF THE AORTIC ARCH

If the aortic rupture involves the innominate artery or aortic arch, deep hypothermic circulatory arrest (18–20°C) is necessary. Circulatory arrest is commenced once the appropriate nasopharyngeal temperature is reached, the hematoma opened and the aortic tear identified under direct vision in a relatively bloodless field and repaired. The head and neck vessels need not be clamped, provided the patient is placed in a head-down position. The maximum safe period of deep hypothermic circulatory arrest is 45 minutes, which can be extended to approximately 90 minutes if retrograde cerebral perfusion via the internal jugular vein/superior vena cava is used during the period of circulatory arrest.[78]

BLUNT INJURY OF THE EXTRAPERICARDIAL MAJOR VESSELS

Blunt injuries of the extrapericardial major intrathoracic vessels are relatively rare, because of the protective musculoskeletal tunnel of the thoracic inlet. Mechanisms of injury are similar to those of blunt aortic rupture, but with the addition of direct crush injuries as well as acute stretching of the major head and neck vessels from hyperextension of the neck and shoulder joints.[79] Blunt injuries can result in vessel tears with hemorrhage, false aneurysm or arteriovenous fistula formation, as well as arterial dissection and thromboembolism. Blunt injury to the carotid arteries predominantly causes dissection.

Suggestive findings on clinical examination following blunt trauma include unilateral diminished or absent radial pulse, brachial plexus palsy (50% of patients), cerebral deficits, fractured clavicle (up to 50% of patients), supraclavicular hematoma, and a pulsatile cervical mass with a bruit.[80–82] Radiographic features are similar to traumatic aortic rupture, and include a widened mediastinum and more specifically an associated fractured first rib.

The diagnosis is established by aortography, and concomitant aortic tears are found in 4–12% of patients.[79]

Surgical approach

The surgical incision depends upon the side that is injured and the location of the arterial disruption. Direct entry into the hematoma should not be attempted, before proximal and distal vascular control has been achieved.

BLUNT RUPTURE OF THE SUBCLAVIAN ARTERY

Injuries at the origin of the left subclavian artery can be approached through a left thoracotomy. However, disruptions distal to the vertebral artery should be approached initially through a supraclavicular incision, with either dislocation of the sternoclavicular joint or subperiosteal resection of the medial portion of the clavicle if required. If necessary, either a median sternotomy or left anterolateral thoracotomy in the third or fourth intercostal space can be performed to obtain proximal control. The trap-door incision, a partial upper median sternotomy connecting the supraclavicular incision with an anterolateral thoracotomy,[80] is not recommended as it does not offer any advantage over a full median sternotomy with or without sternoclavicular dislocation.

Right-sided subclavian artery disruptions should be approached through a supraclavicular incision, extended if necessary into a median sternotomy. Supraclavicular exposure is facilitated by placing a sandbag beneath the upper spine and rotating the chin to the opposite side, and dividing both the sternocleidomastoid, strap muscles and scalenus anterior muscles near their origins.

Arterial reconstruction either directly with an interposition reversed saphenous vein or with a prosthetic graft is desirable depending upon the operative findings. Collateral circulation surrounding the subclavian artery is generally good; however, this may be altered by associated injuries, making subclavian artery ligation unpredictable in patients who have sustained blunt trauma. Ligation of the proximal subclavian artery should only be used as a last resort in the unstable or complex patient.

BLUNT INJURY OF THE INNOMINATE AND COMMON CAROTID ARTERIES

Conservative non-operative management with anticoagulation may be indicated in blunt carotid arterial injuries presenting with hemiplegia as a result of arterial dissection with thrombosis.[82,83] The neurological deficit can be expected to improve in 60% of patients with blunt carotid dissections.[83]

Surgical repair of innominate and common carotid arterial lacerations should be approached through a median sternotomy (Fig 15.13), if necessary with cervical extension along the medial border of the appropriate sternocleidomastoid muscle.

The primary issue in the surgical management of innominate and carotid arterial injuries is cerebral protection. Curved tangential occlusive clamps may allow control of the origin of the innominate and common carotid artery. However, the need for a temporary vascular shunt for cerebral protection during clamping should be established, although shunting is rarely necessary as 80% of individuals have a normal circle of Willis.[79] 'Stump pressure', pressure distal to the clamp on the innominate or carotid artery, should be measured and should remain above 55 mmHg.[79,84] Heparin should be administered after obtaining vascu-

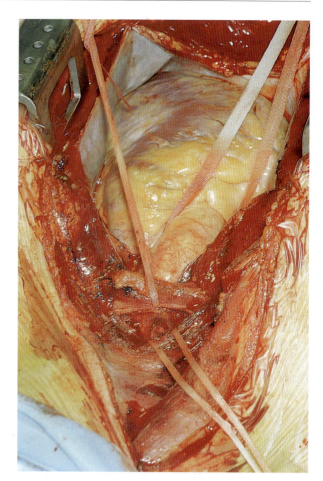

Figure 15.13 *Surgical exposure for blunt traumatic rupture of the innominate artery. Median sternotomy has been performed and the pericardium opened to sling the ascending aorta. The incision is carried up into the neck and a second sling used to retract the innominate vein caudally. A third sling is placed around the root of the innominate artery. (SWTC.)*

lar control to avoid embolic complications. Arterial reconstruction is done either directly or with an interposition prosthetic graft (woven Dacron or polytetrafluoroethylene). Cardiopulmonary bypass with deep hypothermic circulatory arrest (18–20°C) can also be used for injuries of both the innominate and left common carotid arteries, but the disadvantage is the need for systemic heparinization.

Alternatively, extra-anatomical reconstruction of proximal innominate injuries without entering the hematoma,[85,86] is the surgical approach of choice in many units. Oversewing of the ruptured ends can then be performed without cardiopulmonary bypass or shunts.

Mortality and morbidity

The overall mortality for blunt injuries of the innominate and subclavian arteries is approximately 5%, and is related to hemorrhagic complications and associated injuries.[81] Morbidity includes pseudoaneurysm formation, thrombosis, distal ischemia with gangrene, subclavian steal syndrome, and limb loss, in 5–10% of patients. Furthermore, the involved extremity may be rendered functionally useless in a number of patients because of the associated brachial plexus lesions which are usually permanent, as well as from associated major bony and soft tissue injuries.[81]

REFERENCES

1. Greendyke RM. Traumatic rupture of aorta: special reference to automobile accidents. *JAMA* 1966; **195:** 119–22.

2. Smith RS, Chang FC. Traumatic rupture of the aorta: still a lethal injury. *Am J Surg* 1986; **152:** 660–3.

3. Williams JS, Graff JA, Uku JM, Steinig JP. Aortic injury in vehicular trauma. *Ann Thorac Surg* 1994; **57:** 726–30.

4. Eddy AC, Rusch VW, Fligner CL, Reay DT, Rice CL. The epidemiology of traumatic rupture of the thoracic aorta in children: a 13-year review. *J Trauma* 1990; **30:** 989–92.

5. Von Oppell UO, Brink J, Hewitson J, Pinho P, Zilla P. Acute traumatic rupture of the thoracic aorta: a comparison of techniques. *S Afr J Surg* 1996; **34:** 19–24.

6. Trachiotis GD, Sell JE, Pearson GD, Martin GR, Midgley FM. Traumatic thoracic aortic rupture in the pediatric patient. *Ann Thorac Surg* 1996; **62:** 724–32.

7. Akins CW. Major injuries: aortic rupture. In: Grillo HC, Eschapasse H, eds. *International Trends in General Thoracic Surgery.* Vol 2. *Major Challenges.* Philadelphia: WB Saunders, 1987; 268–72.

8. Kirklin JW, Barratt-Boyes BG, eds. *Cardiac Surgery: Morphology, Diagnostic Criteria, Natural History, Techniques, Results, and Indications.* New York: Churchill Livingstone, 1986; 1451–69.

9. Hartford JM, Fayer RL, Shaver TE, *et al.* Transection of the thoracic aorta: assessment of a trauma system. *Am J Surg* 1986; **151:** 224–9.

10. Parmley LF, Mattingly TW, Manion WC, Jahnke EJ. Nonpenetrating traumatic injury of the aorta. *Circulation* 1958; **17:** 1086–101.

11. Finkelmeier BA, Mentzer RM, Kaiser DL, Tegtmeyer CJ, Nolan SP. Chronic traumatic thoracic aneurysm. Influence of operative treatment on natural history: an analysis of reported cases, 1950–1980. *J Thorac Cardiovasc Surg* 1982; **84:** 257–66.

12. Sevitt S. The mechanisms of traumatic rupture of the thoracic aorta. *Br J Surg* 1977; **64:** 166–73.

13. Cohen AM, Crass JR, Thomas HA, Fisher RG, Jacobs DG. CT evidence for the 'osseous pinch' mechanism of traumatic aortic injury. *Am J Roentgenol* 1992; **159:** 271–4.

14. Tribble CG, Crosby IK. Traumatic rupture of the thoracic aorta. *South Med J* 1988; **81:** 963–8.

15. Moar JJ. Traumatic rupture of the thoracic aorta: an autopsy and histopathological study. *S Afr Med J* 1985; **67:** 383–5.

16. Arajärvi E, Santavirta S, Tolonen J. Aortic ruptures in seat belt wearers. *J Thorac Cardiovasc Surg* 1989; **98:** 355–61.

17. Von Oppell UO, Thierfelder CF, Beningfield SJ, Brink JG, Odell JA. Traumatic rupture of the descending thoracic aorta. *S Afr Med J* 1991; **79:** 595–8.

18. Kram HB, Appel PL, Shoemaker WC. Increased incidence of cardiac contusion in patients with traumatic thoracic aortic rupture. *Ann Surg* 1988; **208:** 615–18.

19. Rizoli SB, Brenneman FD, Boulanger BR, Magissano R. Blunt diaphragmatic and thoracic aortic rupture: an emerging injury complex. *Ann Thorac Surg* 1994; **58:** 1404–8.

20. Woodring JH, Dillon ML. Radiographic manifestations of mediastinal hemorrhage from blunt chest trauma. *Ann Thorac Surg* 1984; **37:** 171–8.

21. Kram HB, Appel PL, Wohlmuth DA, Shoemaker WC. Diagnosis of traumatic thoracic aortic rupture: a 10-year retrospective analysis. *Ann Thorac Surg* 1989; **47:** 282–6.

22. Gundry SR, Williams S, Burney RE, Cho KJ, Mackenzie JR. Indications for aortography in blunt thoracic trauma: a reassessment. *J Trauma* 1982; **22:** 664–71.

23. Weiss JP, Feld M, Sclafani SJA, Scalea T, Vieux E, Trooskin SZ. Traumatic rupture of the thoracic aorta. *Emerg Med Clin North Am* 1991; **9:** 789–804.

24. Durham RM, Zuckerman D, Wolverson M, *et al.* Computed tomography as a screening exam in patients with suspected blunt aortic injury. *Ann Surg* 1994; **220:** 699–704.

25. Raptopoulos V, Sheiman RG, Phillips DA, Davidoff A, Silva WE. Traumatic aortic tear: screening with chest CT. *Radiology* 1992; **182:** 667–73.

26. McLean TR, Olinger GN, Thorsen MK. Computed tomography in the evaluation of the aorta in patients sustaining blunt chest trauma. *J Trauma* 1991; **31:** 254–6.

27. Fisher RG, Chasen MH, Lamki N. Diagnosis of injuries of the aorta and brachiocephalic arteries caused by blunt chest trauma: CT vs aortography. *Am J Roentgenol* 1994; **162:** 1047–52.

28. Hunink MGM, Bos JJ. Triage of patients to angiography for detection of aortic rupture after blunt chest trauma: cost-effectiveness analysis of using CT. *Am J Roentgenol* 1995; **165:** 27–36.

29. Miller FB, Richardson JD, Thomas HA, Cryer HM, Willing SJ. Role of CT in diagnosis of major arterial injury after blunt thoracic trauma. *Surgery* 1989; **106:** 596–603.

30. Tomiak MM, Rosenblum JD, Messersmith RN, Zarins CK. Use of CT for diagnosis of traumatic rupture of the thoracic aorta. *Ann Vasc Surg* 1993; **7:** 130–9.

31. Hills MW, Thomas SG, McDougall PA, Hewitt-Falls EA, Graham JC, Deane SA. Traumatic thoracic aortic rupture: investigation determines outcome. *Aust N Z J Surg* 1994; **64:** 312–18.

32. Wigle RL, Moran JM. Spontaneous healing of a traumatic thoracic aortic tear: case report. *J Trauma* 1991; **31**: 280–3.

33. Morse SS, Glickman MG, Greenwood LH, *et al.* Traumatic aortic rupture: false-positive aortographic diagnosis due to atypical ductus diverticulum. *Am J Roentgenol* 1988; **150**: 793–6.

34. Smith MD, Cassidy JM, Souther S, *et al.* Transesophageal echocardiography in the diagnosis of traumatic rupture of the aorta. *N Engl J Med* 1995; **332**: 356–62.

35. Kearney PA, Smith DW, Johnson SB, Barker DE, Smith MD, Sapin PM. Use of transesophageal echocardiography in the evaluation of traumatic aortic injury. *J Trauma* 1993; **34**: 696–701.

36. Buckmaster MJ, Kearney PA, Johnson SB, Smith MD, Sapin PM. Further experience with transesophageal echocardiography in the evaluation of thoracic aortic injury. *J Trauma* 1994; **37**: 989–95.

37. Saletta S, Lederman E, Fein S, Singh A, Kuehler DH, Fortune JB. Transesophageal echocardiography for the initial evaluation of the widened mediastinum in trauma patients. *J Trauma* 1995; **39**: 137–42.

38. Sparks MB, Burchard KW, Marrin CAS, Bean CHG, Nugent WC, Plehn JF. Transesophageal echocardiography: preliminary results in patients with traumatic aortic rupture. *Arch Surg* 1991; **126**: 711–14.

39. Von Oppell UO, Dunne TT, De Groot MK, Zilla P. Traumatic aortic rupture: twenty-year metaanalysis of mortality and risk of paraplegia. *Ann Thorac Surg* 1994; **58**: 585–93.

40. Von Oppell UO, Dunne TT, De Groot KM, Zilla P. Spinal cord protection in the absence of collateral circulation: meta-analysis of mortality and paraplegia. *J Card Surg* 1994; **9**: 685–91.

41. Sturm JT, Billiar TR, Dorsey JS, Luxenberg MG, Perry JF. Risk factors for survival following surgical treatment of traumatic aortic rupture. *Ann Thorac Surg* 1985; **39**: 418–21.

42. Pate JW, Fabian TC, Walker W. Traumatic rupture of the aortic isthmus: an emergency? *World J Surg* 1995; **19**: 119–26.

43. Warren RL, Akins CW, Conn AKT, Hilgenberg AD, McCabe CJ. Acute traumatic disruption of the thoracic aorta: emergency department management. *Ann Emerg Med* 1992; **21**: 391–6.

44. Duhaylongsod FG, Glower DD, Wolfe WG. Acute traumatic aortic aneurysm: the Duke experience from 1970 to 1990. *J Vasc Surg* 1992; **15**: 331–43.

45. Walker WA, Pate JW. Medical management of acute traumatic rupture of the aorta. *Ann Thorac Surg* 1990; **50**: 965–7.

46. Kipfer B, Leupi F, Schuepbach P, Friedli D, Althaus U. Acute traumatic rupture of the thoracic aorta: immediate or delayed surgical repair? *Eur J Cardiothorac Surg* 1994; **8**: 30–3.

47. Maggisano R, Nathens A, Alexandrova NA, *et al.* Traumatic rupture of the thoracic aorta: should one always operate immediately? *Ann Vasc Surg* 1995; **9**: 44–52.

48. Clark DE, Zeiger MA, Wallace KL, Packard AB, Nowicki ER. Blunt aortic trauma: signs of high risk. *J Trauma* 1990; **30**: 701–5.

49. Herendeen TL, King H. Transient anuria and paraplegia following traumatic rupture of the thoracic aorta. *J Thorac Cardiovasc Surg* 1968; **56**: 599–602.

50. Mattox KL, Holzman M, Pickard LR, Beall AC, DeBakey ME. Clamp/repair: a safe technique for treatment of blunt injury to the descending thoracic aorta. *Ann Thorac Surg* 1985; **40**: 456–63.

51. Marini CP, Grubbs PE, Toporoff B, *et al.* Effect of sodium nitroprusside on spinal cord perfusion and paraplegia during aortic cross-clamping. *Ann Thorac Surg* 1989; **47**: 379–83.

52. Gregoretti S, Gelman S, Henderson T, Bradley EL. Hemodynamics and oxygen uptake below and above aortic occlusion during crossclamping of the thoracic aorta and sodium nitroprusside infusion. *J Thorac Cardiovasc Surg* 1990; **100**: 830–6.

53. Grosso MA, Brown JM, Moore EE, Moore FA. Repair of the torn descending thoracic aorta using the centrifugal pump with partial left heart bypass: technical note. *J Trauma* 1991; **31**: 395–400.

54. Svensson LG, Klepp P, Hinder RA. Spinal cord anatomy of the baboon – comparison with man and implications for spinal cord blood flow during thoracic aortic cross-clamping. *S Afr J Surg* 1986; **24**: 32–4.

55. Wadouh F, Lindemann EM, Arndt CF, Hetzer R, Borst HG. The arteria radicularis magna anterior as a decisive factor influencing spinal cord damage during aortic occlusion. *J Thorac Cardiovasc Surg* 1984; **88**: 1–10.

56. Adams HD, van Geertruyden HH. Neurologic complications of aortic surgery. *Ann Surg* 1956; **144**: 574–610.

57. Hägerdal M, Harp J, Nilsson L, Siesjö BK. The effect of induced hypothermia upon oxygen consumption in the rat brain. *J Neurochem* 1975; **24**: 311–16.

58. Laschinger JC, Cunningham JN, Nathan IM, Knopp EA, Cooper MM, Spencer FC. Experimental and clinical assessment of the adequacy of partial bypass in maintenance of spinal cord blood flow during operations on the thoracic aorta. *Ann Thorac Surg* 1983; **36**: 417–26.

59. Katz NM, Blackstone EH, Kirklin JW, Karp RB. Incremental risk factors for spinal cord injury following operation for acute traumatic aortic transection. *J Thorac Cardiovasc Surg* 1981; **81**: 669–74.

60. Svensson LG, Stewart RW, Cosgrove DM, *et al.* Intrathecal papaverine for the prevention of paraplegia after operation on the thoracic or thoracoabdominal aorta. *J Thorac Cardiovasc Surg* 1988; **96**: 823–9.

61. Berendes JN, Bredèe JJ, Schipperheyn JJ, Mashhour YAS. Mechanisms of spinal cord injury after cross-clamping of the descending thoracic aorta. *Circulation* 1982; **66(Suppl I)**: 112–16.

62. Cooley DA, Baldwin RT. Technique of open distal anastomosis for repair of descending thoracic aortic aneurysms. *Ann Thorac Surg* 1992; **54**: 932–6.

63. Woloszyn TT, Marini CP, Coons MS, *et al.* Cerebrospinal fluid drainage and steroids provide better spinal cord protection during aortic cross-clamping than does either treatment alone. *Ann Thorac Surg* 1990; **49**: 78–83.

64. Laschinger JC, Cunningham JN, Cooper MM, Krieger K, Nathan IM, Spencer FC. Prevention of ischemic spinal cord injury following aortic cross-clamping: use of corticosteroids. *Ann Thorac Surg* 1984; **38**: 500–7.

65. Qayumi AK, Janusz MT, Jamieson WRE, Lyster DM. Pharmacologic interventions for prevention of spinal cord injury caused by aortic crossclamping. *J Thorac Cardiovasc Surg* 1992; **104**: 256–61.

66. Attar S, Hankins JR, Turney SZ, Krasna MJ, McLaughlin JS. Paraplegia after thoracotomy: report of five cases and review of the literature. *Ann Thorac Surg* 1995; **59**: 1410–16.

67. Ketonen P, Järvinen A, Luosto R, Ketonen L. Traumatic rupture of the thoracic aorta. *Scand J Thorac Cardiovasc Surg* 1980; **14**: 233–9.

68. Young JN, Stallone RJ, Iverson LIG, Ennix CL, Ecker RR, May IA. Surgical management of traumatic disruption of the descending aorta. *West J Med* 1989; **150**: 662–4.

69. Grossi EA, Krieger KH, Cunningham JN, Culliford AT, Nathan IM, Spencer FC. Venoarterial bypass: a technique for spinal cord protection. *J Thorac Cardiovasc Surg* 1985; **89**: 228–34.

70. Olivier HF, Maher TD, Liebler GA, Park SB, Burkholder JA, Magovern GJ. Use of the BioMedicus centrifugal pump in traumatic tears of the thoracic aorta. *Ann Thorac Surg* 1984; **38**: 586–91.

71. Fernandez G, Fontan F, Deville C, Madonna F, Thibaud D. Long-term evaluation of direct repair of traumatic isthmic aortic transection. *Eur J Cardiothorac Surg* 1989; **3**: 327–34.

72. Schmidt CA, Wood MN, Razzouk AJ, Killeen JD, Gan KA. Primary repair of traumatic aortic rupture: a preferred approach. *J Trauma* 1992; **32**: 588–92.

73. Orringer MB, Kirsh MM. Primary repair of acute traumatic aortic disruption. *Ann Thorac Surg* 1983; **35**: 672–5.

74. McBride LR, Tidik S, Stothert JC, *et al.* Primary repair of traumatic aortic disruption. *Ann Thorac Surg* 1987; **43**: 65–7.

75. McGough EC, Hughes RK. Acute traumatic rupture of the aorta: a reemphasis of repair without a vascular prosthesis. *Ann Thorac Surg* 1973; **16**: 7–10.

76. Antunes MJ. Acute traumatic rupture of the aorta: repair by simple aortic cross-clamping. *Ann Thorac Surg* 1987; **44**: 257–9.

77. McCroskey BL, Moore EE, Moore FA, Abernathy CM. A unified approach to the torn thoracic aorta. *Am J Surg* 1991; **162**: 473–6.

78. Murase M, Maeda M, Koyama T, *et al.* Continuous retrograde cerebral perfusion for protection of the brain during aortic arch surgery. *Eur J Cardiothorac Surg* 1993; **7**: 597–600.

79. Rosenberg JM, Bredenberg CE, Marvasti MA, Bucknam C, Conti C, Parker FB. Blunt injuries to the aortic arch vessels. *Ann Thorac Surg* 1989; **48**: 508–13.

80. Sturm JT, Dorsey JS, Olson FR, Perry JF Jr. The management of subclavian artery injuries following blunt thoracic trauma. *Ann Thorac Surg* 1984; **38**: 188–91.

81. Posner MP, Deitrick J, McGrath P, *et al.*Nonpenetrating vascular injury to the subclavian artery. *J Vasc Surg* 1988; **8**: 611–17.

82. George SM, Croce MA, Fabian TC, *et al.* Cervicothoracic arterial injuries: recommendations for diagnosis and management. *World J Surg* 1991; **15**: 134–40.

83. Fabian TC, George SM, Croce MA, Mangiante EC, Voeller GR, Kudsk KA. Carotid artery trauma: management based on mechanism of injury. *J Trauma* 1990; **30**: 953–63.

84. Ehrenfeld WK, Stoney RJ, Wylie EJ. Relation of carotid stump pressure to safety of carotid artery ligation. *Surgery* 1983; **93**: 299–305.

85. Johnston RH, Wall MJ, Mattox KL. Innominate artery trauma: a thirty-year experience. *J Vasc Surg* 1993; **17**: 134–40.

86. Graham JM, Feliciano DV, Mattox KL, Beall AC. Innominate vascular injury. *J Trauma* 1982; **22**: 647–55.

FURTHER READING

Kirklin JW, Barratt-Boyes BG, eds. *Cardiac Surgery: Morphology, Diagnostic Criteria, Natural History, Techniques, Results, and Indications.* New York: Churchill Livingstone, 1986; 1451–69.

Olivier HF, Maher TD, Liebler GA, Park SB, Burkholder JA, Magovern GJ. Use of the BioMedicus centrifugal pump in traumatic tears of the thoracic aorta. *Ann Thorac Surg* 1984; **38**: 586–91.

Sevitt S. The mechanisms of traumatic rupture of the thoracic aorta. *Br J Surg* 1977; **64**: 166–73.

Sturm JT, Dorsey JS, Olson FR, Perry JF Jr. The management of subclavian artery injuries following blunt thoracic trauma. *Ann Thorac Surg* 1984; **38**: 188–91.

Von Oppell UO, Dunne TT, De Groot KM, Zilla P. Spinal cord protection in the absence of collateral circulation: meta-analysis of mortality and paraplegia. *J Card Surg* 1994; **9**: 685–91.

Blunt cardiac injury

STEPHEN WESTABY

Cardiovascular injury occurs in up to 30% of trauma patients and blunt cardiac injury is almost exclusively related to rapid deceleration motor vehicle collisions.[1] A small percentage of injuries may follow crushing industrial accidents or a severe direct blow to the precordium (Fig 16.1). The mechanisms of injury include compression of the heart between the sternum and spine with deceleration forces directly proportional to the square of the speed of the vehicle and inversely related to the stopping distance (Fig 16.2).[2]

Whereas penetrating injury to the heart is obvious in its manifestations, blunt cardiac trauma is often obscured by associated visceral or skeletal injuries. Diagnosis depends on a high index of suspicion and the assumption can be made that any patient who has sustained high speed deceleration trauma with head, thoracic, abdominal or long bone injuries will also have cardiac contusion. Clinical and autopsy studies report between 15% and 75% incidence of myocardial injury in patients with blunt chest trauma.[3,4] In one series, cardiac contusion was the most common unsuspected visceral injury responsible for trauma deaths and it is apparent that life-threatening cardiac contusion can occur with minimal or absent external signs. If blunt cardiac injury is not excluded by deliberate investigation and then treated appropriately, the first clinical event may be cardiogenic shock, ventricular fibrillation, tachycardia or complete heart block, frequently during an anesthetic for orthopedic injuries.

THE SPECTRUM OF BLUNT CARDIAC INJURY

High speed deceleration impact of the anterior chest wall against the steering wheel and severe crush injuries cause acute depression of the sternum and costal cartilages. These compress the heart against the vertebral column posteriorly. In children and young adults the chest wall may spring back into position with no external evidence of the severity of injury. Older adults may sustain a transverse fracture of the sternum, anterior costochondral dislocation or multiple rib fractures, producing an anterior flail segment. These findings guarantee blunt cardiac injury, though the spectrum of severity is wide. Pulmonary contusion, ruptured diaphragm, liver or spleen, head injury, faciomaxillary trauma, aortic transection and long bone fractures commonly coexist.

In the setting of multiple injuries, cardiac trauma is virtually always overlooked unless accompanied by tamponade dysrhythmia or left ventricular failure. The range of potential cardiac injuries is shown in Table 16.1. In practice, pericardial effusion and partial or full thickness myocardial contusion with conduction disturbances or dysrhythmia are common but well tolerated in patients with major deceleration injury.[5] Valve disruption, cardiac rupture and ventricular septal defect are rare in patients who reach hospital alive. Blunt cardiac rupture into the pericardium is usually

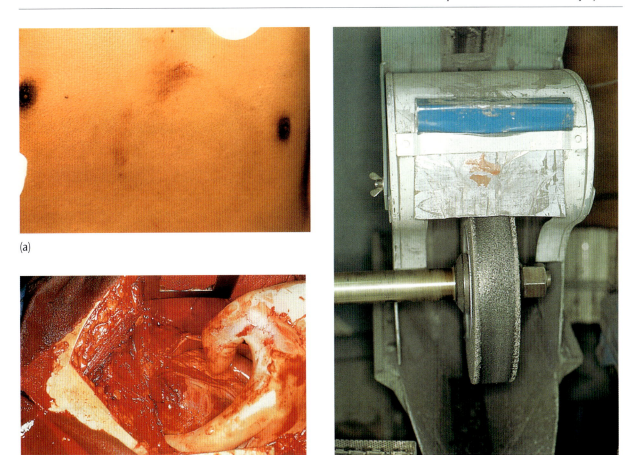

(a)

(b)

(c)

Figure 16.1 *Blunt cardiac rupture following a direct blow. (a) Evidence of impact on the anterior chest wall. (b) The lathe at which the patient had been working. The lathe broke free from its bearings, hitting the patient directly in the precordium. (c) The patient presented moribund with distended neck veins. Emergency room thoracotomy was performed to evacuate blood clot and control hemorrhage from an apical rupture of the left ventricle. (Courtesy of Professor K. Kobayashi.)*

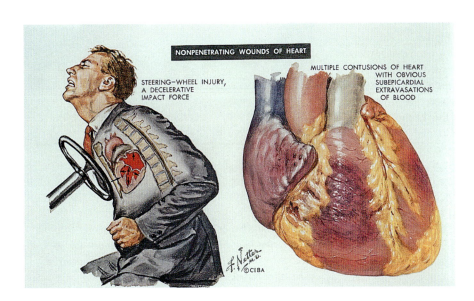

Figure 16.2 *Mechanism of cardiac injury following impact with the steering wheel. The right ventricle lies directly behind the sternum. A violent blow may cause the sternum to impact against the spine.*

Table 16.1 *The spectrum of blunt cardiac injury*

Myocardium
Acute cardiac rupture
Full or partial thickness contusion (= acute MI)
Delayed free wall rupture or ischaemic VSD
Right or left ventricular aneurysm

Valves
Torn aortic cusp
Tricuspid 'blow-out' laceration
Mitral papillary muscle dysfunction
Mitral or tricuspid chordal rupture

Conduction tissue
Partial or complete heart block
Bundle branch block
Ventricular dysrhythmia
Atrial fibrillation

Coronary arteries
Acute thrombosis
Coronary artery fistula
Coronary aneurysm

Pericardium
Rupture with cardiac herniation
Reactive pericardial effusion
Hemorrhage with tamponade
Pneumopericardium

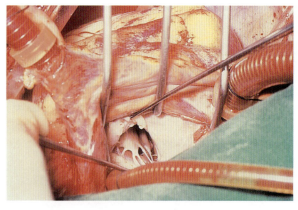

Figure 16.3 *Surgical access in a patient with severe mitral regurgitation following blunt chest injury. The valve leaflets were intact but the anterior papillary muscle was ischemic. Valve repair failed and mitral replacement was necessary.*

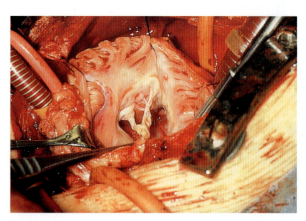

(a)

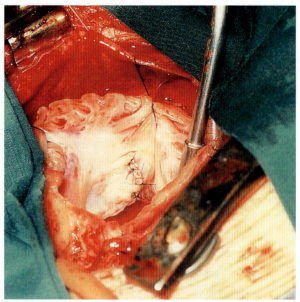

(b)

Figure 16.4 *Blow-out type rupture of the anterior tricuspid valve leaflet following severe deceleration injury. (a) The shredded valve on first appearance. (b) The reconstructed valve after meticulous repair.*

fatal before hospital admission. In order of frequency, traumatic cardiac rupture affects the right ventricle, left ventricle, right atrium and left atrium. Rupture of the interventricular septum may occur acutely from a direct blow or as a delayed event in the follow-up period when the patient develops cardiac failure with a loud systolic murmur. This condition was identified in 5% of Parmley's large but historic series of autopsies, occurring as an isolated defect in less than 1%.[6] Injuries to the tricuspid, mitral and aortic valves are usually detectable at an early stage, though heart failure may not be recognized early and the cardiac murmur may be obscured by ventilation sounds or a pericardial effusion. Papillary muscle ischemia may lead to late tricuspid or mitral regurgitation (Fig 16.3).[7] Rupture of the chordae tendineae and mitral or tricuspid leaflets is extremely rare, though we have successfully repaired 'blow-out' type tricuspid rupture on two occasions (Fig 16.4). Whereas aortic cusp tears are rare in patients, they are intermittently seen in the homograft valve bank when human valves are obtained from trauma patients (Fig 16.5). Acute occlusion of a non-atherosclerotic left anterior descending coronary artery may occur in blunt trauma and produce myocardial infarction or cardiogenic shock. We have also seen false aneurysm formation of the left anterior descending coronary artery and blunt rupture of the right coronary with aorto-right atrial fistula (Fig 16.6).[8] Right ventricular aneurysm has been described after severe right ventricular contusion.[9]

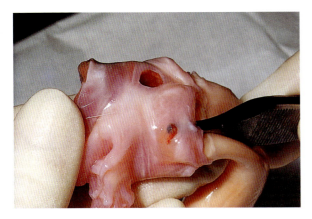

Figure 16.5 *Inverted aortic homograft harvested from a young donor following death from head injury in a motor vehicle accident. There is a laceration at the base of the right coronary cusp.*

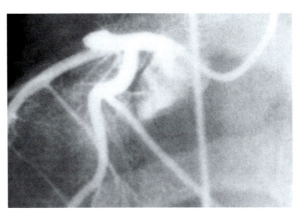

Figure 16.6 *False aneurysm of the proximal left anterior descending coronary artery after blunt impact. The injury caused acute myocardial infarction.*

Although blunt cardiac contusion is considered similar to acute myocardial infarction, there are important morphological and clinical differences.[10] Coronary artery occlusion is rare in cardiac contusion and myocardial blood flow may be normal or increased. Nevertheless, in severe cases, transmural injury is subject to the same sequelae as infarction. Initially there is hemorrhage into the myocardium which varies from scattered petechiae to large transmural hematomas. Small arteries and arterioles are disrupted. Erythrocytes leak into the interstitial space and myocytes are fragmented. Hemorrhage and edema produce a decrease in myocardial compliance. Most patients show patchy areas of necrosis in scattered portions of muscle bundles rather than complete coagulation necrosis and the transition from normal to abnormal myocardium is more abrupt than in acute myocardial infarction. Healing is by patchy scarring rather than fibrosis.

By contrast, acute myocardial infarction may occur if a proximal coronary artery is occluded. A previously normal coronary artery may sustain disruption of the intima, subintimal hemorrhage and obstructive intraluminal thrombus formation on the injured arterial wall. Traumatic thrombosis of a saphenous vein bypass graft has been described as have traumatic occlusion of both left anterior descending and circumflex coronaries, and thrombosis of the left main coronary.[11,12]

DIAGNOSIS OF BLUNT CARDIAC INJURY

Occasionally the presentation is dramatic with circulatory collapse suggesting a major cardiovascular injury. The description of the accident from paramedics is useful since major blunt cardiovascular injuries are virtually restricted to high speed deceleration trauma or severe crushing. Bruising on the anterior chest wall adds

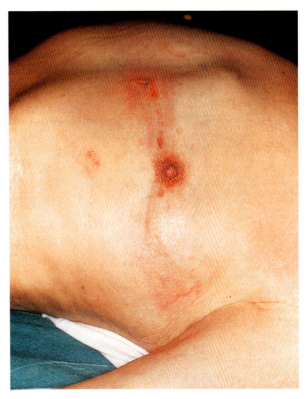

Figure 16.7 *Extensive bruising to the left anterior chest wall with underlying right ventricular contusion.*

to the suspicion (Fig 16.7). If the patient is unconscious, pulseless but has ECG complexes, consideration should be given to diagnosis by emergency room thoracotomy.[13] However, the ECG remains long after irreversible cerebral death, so the pupils should be inspected first. In the presence of fixed dilated pupils no further action should be taken. If the patient is warm with reactive pupils and no cardiac output, left anterolateral thoracotomy may provide the diagnosis and allow cardiac tamponade or cardiac herniation to be corrected. We have salvaged a patient with blunt rupture of the pericardium and cardiac herniation with strangulation of the atrioventricular sulcus. Severe deceleration compression injury pushed the ventricles into the left pleural cavity and when the heart was relocated into the pericardium, resuscitation proved successful. Severe contusion of the right ventricular free wall and ventricular septum were treated by intra-aortic balloon pumping with survival. Limited blunt cardiac rupture may also be salvaged by relieving massive hemopericardium followed by direct suture repair. Blunt pericardial rupture is a hallmark of severe direct precordial impact and may be associated with laceration of the pulmonary veins (Princess Diana's injury).

Conscious patients may complain of midthoracic constrictive pain and severe dyspnea eased by the sitting position. Clinical signs of tamponade include cyanosis of the head, neck and upper chest with dilatation of the jugular veins, sometimes increasing on inspiration. There is usually hypotension and tachycardia. A waxing and waning (paradoxical) pulse has a 10–20 mmHg drop at the end of the inspiratory phase. This classic sign is of little practical value in the general agitation of a patient with severe thoracic injuries. The heart sounds are usually muffled, occasionally with a pericardial rub. These signs are distinct from those of hypovolemic shock, the commonest manifestation of penetrating cardiac injuries. Early invasive monitoring should always be used to guide resuscitation if a cardiac or aortic injury is suspected. In hypovolemic shock, the central venous pressure is less than 5 cmH$_2$O. In cardiac tamponade, central venous pressure rises to above 15 cmH$_2$O (and sometimes as high as 40 cmH$_2$O). Whilst tamponade may occur with less than 500 ml blood loss into the pericardial cavity, the venous pressure may be lowered by simultaneous bleeding from abdominal viscera, pelvis or long bones. An arterial line allows accurate recording of blood pressure, blood gases and acid–base balance during resuscitation. In a suspected cardiac or thoracic injury, controlled hypotension should be used before surgical access to the injury. Elevation of intravascular pressure may precipitate rapid deterioration and death before the bleeding site can be closed.

The electrocardiogram in tamponade shows QRS waves of low voltage, especially in the precordial leads. The standard antroposterior chest radiograph in trauma may offer little clue to the extent of injury apart from an abnormally globular shape to the cardiac shadow. This is because an intact pericardium does not distend and emergency radiography is usually obtained from a short distance in difficult conditions with a recumbent patient with incomplete inspiration. All these factors predispose to pseudo-widening of the mediastinum. In an urgent situation, pericardiocentesis can be used for diagnosis of tamponade, but is rarely effective in a therapeutic sense. In less urgent cases, two-dimensional echocardiography provides accurate diagnosis of an intrapericardial collection and allows the wall motion of right and left ventricles and the integrity of the valves to be assessed.

Diagnosis of tamponade is critically important during initial resuscitative maneuvers since a compromise must be found between transfusion in hemorrhagic shock and restriction of intravenous fluids in the cardiogenic shock of tamponade. Pericardiocentesis on suspicion of hemopericardium is falsely negative in 25–40% of cases, often because the blood has clotted or the attempt is too timid. On the other hand, the tap is falsely positive in about 15% of cases and may damage the right coronary artery. Emergency surgery is indicated and preoperative resuscitation should be as brief as possible. Regardless of the origin of tamponade, surgery alone makes it possible to identify and treat the source of bleeding. Subxiphoid pericardiotomy is effective in relief of tamponade, but will not provide access to the cause and may result in exsanguinating hemorrhage. The median sternotomy provides the best access to mediastinal structures, but the means to perform median sternotomy are rarely present in the emergency room. By contrast, a left anterior fifth space thoracotomy is easy and provides immediate access to the left side of the heart. Exposure to the right atrium can be achieved by transecting the sternum. After cardiac arrest or in the case of exsanguinating hemorrhage, the mortality of urgent thoracotomy is between 60 and 90%.

Delayed thoracotomy performed in the operating theatre in the event of initial resuscitation followed by relapse carries a mortality of about 40%. Survival with ongoing resuscitation only occurs in those with a remediable injury dealt with by an experienced cardiac surgeon. Only very rarely will resuscitation for a blunt cardiac injury proceed to cardiopulmonary bypass and repair of an intracardiac structure. Most valve or coronary injuries have a subacute presentation and rupture of a cardiac chamber can usually be repaired whilst the heart supports the circulation. In the event of a large lateral rupture of the pericardium, there is the potential for further dislocation of the heart if the edges are not approximated. The repair is performed loosely so that a reactive pericardial effusion can drain into the left pleural cavity.

In the subacute phase of blunt cardiac injury, hemopericardium without tamponade is common and only occasionally requires pericardiocentesis. Pneumopericardium (Fig 16.8) is a condition whereby air enters the pericardial sac, either through a limited laceration in the presence of pneumothorax or where severe barotrauma causes air to track around the pulmonary arteries or veins. Pneumopericardium is often a hallmark of bronchial rupture and we have reported tension pneumopericardium with tamponade in this circumstance. Pleural drainage will usually resolve the problem, though a pigtail catheter can be placed in the pericardium itself.

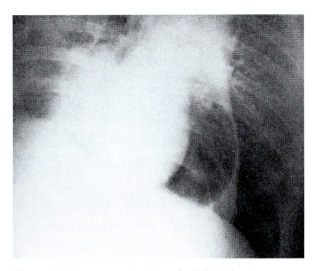

Figure 16.8 *Pneumopericardium after blunt chest trauma. Lateral decubitus chest film.*

Diagnosis of blunt cardiac injury in the stable patient

The possibility of cardiac trauma should be considered in every patient who sustains a high velocity deceleration injury. Precordial bruising, tire or seat belt marks reinforce suspicion of cardiac injury. Petechial hemorrhages over the chest and neck, together with subconjunctival hemorrhage suggest traumatic asphyxia due to severe anteroposterior crush injury (Fig 16.9). Cardiac contusion must be assumed to coexist in patients with aortic transection, blunt tracheobronchial injuries, lacerated diaphragm and ruptured liver or spleen, all of which are an index of the severity of trauma. A pericardial friction rub, cardiac murmur or irregular pulse suggests acute cardiac injury in the absence of a previous history of cardiac disease.

Elevated jugular venous pressure prior to volume replacement is suspicious, especially in the face of blood loss from other injuries. An inappropriately raised venous pressure suggests either cardiac tamponade or severe right ventricular dysfunction due to myocardial contusion or tricuspid regurgitation. It is extremely difficult to assess the severity of myocardial contusion, the spectrum of which ranges from barely perceptible to that sufficient to cause complete myocardial disruption.

The appearance of the heart shadow on the chest radiograph may be entirely normal, but, with radiological evidence of pulmonary contusion or edema, implies an element of cardiac contusion. With more severe cardiac trauma, the chest radiograph may show cardiac enlargement or pulmonary venous congestion. Apparent cardiac dilatation may result from a hemopericardium and true dilatation from an acute valve injury with left ventricular failure. Pneumopericardium can be

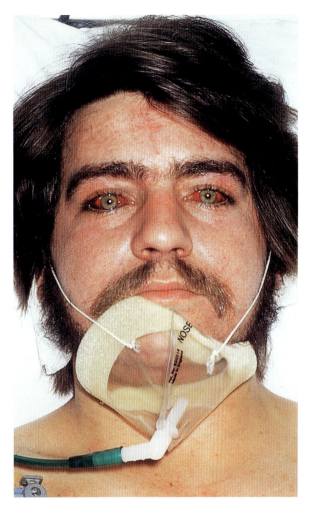

Figure 16.9 *The facial appearance with subconjunctival hemorrhages after traumatic asphyxia.*

distinguished from pneumomediastinum by tipping the patient into the left lateral decubitus position (Fig 16.8).

The electrocardiographic findings are variable. The ECG may show non-specific ST and T wave changes, sinus tachycardia, supraventricular tachycardia and conduction abnormalities such as right bundle branch block. Bundle branch block, left anterior hemiblock, or first or second degree heart block may progress to complete heart block and sudden death with worsening of the edema around the conduction tissue. The most frequent clinical manifestation of cardiac contusion is ventricular tachycardia, the nature of which seems unrelated to the size of contusion or the extent of morphological damage. Electrical instability at the sites of unevenly perfused tissue may initiate re-entry responses conducive to tachyarrhythmia formation. These electrical events often occur in the convalescent period after injury when no chest or cardiac injury has been suspected.

It is virtually impossible to quantify myocardial injury and in practice this is never done in the setting of multiple injuries. In a prospective study to assess the relative contribution to the diagnosis of cardiac trauma made by electrocardiography, serial measurement of creatine kinase (CKMB) isoenzyme and echocardiography, about half the patients with echocardiographic evidence of abnormal wall motion showed no ECG or enzyme abnormalities.[14] Similarly, two-thirds of the patients with raised enzyme levels showed no echocardiographic changes. In practice, the use of echocardiography to define wall motion abnormalities is extremely difficult in trauma patients. Contact of the transducer with the injured chest wall frequently causes pain, and it is virtually impossible to turn the patient with rib fractures into the left lateral decubitus position. Nevertheless, identification of interventricular septal akinesia is sinister since these patients may die suddenly in complete heart block during the recovery period. When septal wall motion abnormalities are identified, the patients should be monitored with a view to antidysrhythmic therapy pacemaker insertion or use of the intra-aortic balloon pump.

In another large series of blunt trauma victims, a rise in CKMB isoenzyme greater than 6% of total serum creatine kinase provided a sensitive and accurate index of important myocardial injury which was not obtained by other investigations.[15] Dysrhythmia, conduction defects, ST segment and T wave changes, and a pathological QT interval were present more often when CKMB exceeded 6%. Chest radiograph appearances of cardiac dilatation, venous congestion, pulmonary edema and, in particular, pulmonary contusion, were seen more frequently when CKMB was raised. More often than not, catastrophic events such as complete heart block and ventricular tachycardia occur 36 hours or more after the initial traumatic event without the possiblity of suspected cardiac injury having been discussed. When the ECG suggests myocardial infarction with classic complexes, either the patient has pre-existing coronary disease and myocardial infarction which caused the accident, or acute coronary thrombosis occurred. Measurement of the cardiac specific factor Troponin C will provide the answer. Whilst early coronary bypass surgery has been undertaken in this situation, this is rarely feasible in practice.

TREATMENT OF BLUNT CARDIAC TRAUMA

Early intervention depends on the extent of associated injuries. Hypoxia and acidosis due to blood loss, hemopneumothorax or airway obstruction will seriously compound a head or cardiac injury and must be corrected at the earliest opportunity. There should be a low threshold for intubation and ventilation, and

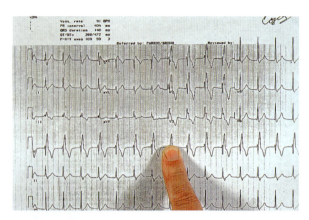

Figure 16.10 *The electrocardiogram with right bundle branch block and ischemic changes over the right ventricle after severe blunt chest trauma.*

care must be taken not to overtransfuse the patient. There is an early and consistent depression of cardiac output following myocardial contusion. The damaged heart has less reserves with which to compensate for abnormal hemodynamic states. Meticulous fluid management is therefore necessary to avoid the dangerous sequelae of hyper- or hypovolemia.

With careful treatment, most patients with myocardial contusion make a complete functional recovery within a relatively short period of time (4–6 weeks) with no residual disability.

Severe cases characterized by altered wall motion abnormalities, raised CKMB and ECG changes (Fig 16.10) are subject to the same delayed events as acute myocardial infarction. These include ventricular septal rupture, left or right ventricular scar formation with dysrhythmia, and ventricular aneurysms. Cardiogenic shock is rarely seen with myocardial contusion alone but occurs in the event of cardiac tamponade, valve disruption, or ventricular septal defect. The thin-walled right ventricle which lies directly behind the sternum may fail acutely. This may contribute to death from chest trauma of apparently moderate severity (particularly when subject to volume overload).

Patients who sustain cardiac injury should be managed along the lines of an acute myocardial infarction, particularly during surgery for associated abdominal trauma or long bone injuries. Although operations for associated injuries are mandatory, it is important that they be undertaken by experienced surgeons and anesthetists who can minirnize the duration of surgery. Dysrhythmia prophylaxis should be discussed beforehand, if necessary with a cardiologist. Bed rest with continuous ECG monitoring, serial CKMB measurement and repeat two-dimensional echocardiography should be employed until the risks of complete heart block, ventricular fibrillation or delayed cardiac rupture are considered extinct.

In patients with cardiogenic shock, it is important to use two-dimensional echocardiography to diagnose or rule out cardiac tamponade, pericardial laceration with cardiac herniation or acute laceration of the tricuspid, mitral or aortic valves. Injury to the cardiac valves can usually be managed conservatively for a period until the patient's condition is stabilized. These then require cardiopulmonary bypass for valve replacement or repair.

In the setting of multiple injuries, it is imperative to optimize cardiac filling pressures and a pulmonary artery catheter is used unless the patient has undergone cardiac surgery with placement of a left atrial line. With severe right ventricular contusion, the right atrial pressure may substantially exceed the left atrial or pulmonary arterial wedge pressure. Tricuspid regurgitation, due to papillary muscle dysfunction, ruptured chordae or laceration of the anterior leaflet will result in a characteristic right atrial pressure trace. In cardiac tamponade, both left and right atrial pressures are elevated and equal.

In established cardiogenic shock, inotropic drugs may be required early. However, inotropic support in isolation increases cardiac work and oxygen consumption and provides an ideal setting for fatal dysrhythmias. Maintenance of adequate perfusion pressure to uninjured areas of cardiac muscle is vital and the intra-aortic balloon pump provides an effective means of increasing coronary perfusion and reducing afterload.

Pericardial effusion may compound the effects of myocardial contusion and lead to late deterioration. Post-traumatic pericardial effusions may be reactive and serous or traumatic and frank blood. Serous effusions can be successfully tapped with a needle and, if necessary, an indwelling catheter. Whole blood in the pericardium may clot, requiring surgical decompression. Blood clot that is not evacuated will eventually liquefy with an increase in volume by osmosis and the risk of increasing cardiac compression with time. Two-dimensional echocardiography should be repeated daily and occasionally more frequently if hemodynamic deterioration occurs.

Delayed hemodynamic deterioration may follow worsening myocardial edema delayed thrombosis of the left anterior descending coronary artery, increasing papillary muscle dysfunction or ventricular septal or free wall rupture following hemorrhage into ischemic myocardium (Fig 16.11). Cardiac catheterization may then be necessary to check the status of the coronary arteries or the significance of a new murmur.

A lacerated aortic valve requires early repair or replacement. The tricuspid valve can be repaired satisfactorily, even with leaflet laceration. Great care should be taken in assessing a severely regurgitant mitral valve since if the leaflets and chordae are intact the valve will appear normal and the problem will lie in an infarcted papillary muscle. Under these circumstances the mitral valve should be replaced.

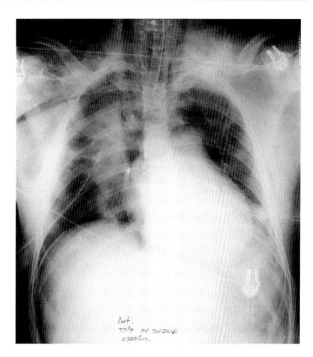

Figure 16.11 *Plain chest radiograph after severe blunt myocardial injury and pulmonary contusion.*

HEMORRHAGIC SHOCK

Those patients who arrive moribund with hemorrhagic shock should undergo immediate thoracotomy on the side of injury. The object is to control hemorrhage from the cardiac laceration and then restore blood volume and acid–base status. Accident department thoracotomy is performed only when the patient arrives warm with reactive pupils but with circulatory arrest, or when acute deterioration, uncontrolled hemorrhage or cardiac arrest occurs in a patient whose injuries suggest cardiac involvement. In this situation, transfer to an operating room is not feasible since a 5–10 minute delay is not compatible with survival. These patients are rapidly intubated before thoracotomy and infused with a crystalloid solution such as Ringer's lactate. Unmatched type-specific or non-specific universal donor blood is given as soon as possible. Arterial pH and blood gas measurements are taken early and sodium bicarbonate administered intravenously if necessary. Anesthesia is not required in the moribund patient and survivors do not recall the surgical events.

Resuscitive emergency thoracotomy for patients with cardiopulmonary arrest was commonly used in the 1940s and 1950s. Introduction of external defibrillating equipment (1956) and techniques for closed chest cardiac massage (1960) caused accident center thoracotomy to fall into disuse. An increasing incidence of penetrating cardiac wounds, together with the development of urban trauma centers in the USA and increased expertise in cardiac and vascular surgery, revived immediate resuscitative thoracotomy for exsanguinating cardiopulmonary wounds in the 1970s. An anterolateral approach through the left fifth intercostal space is used most frequently. The incision can be taken across the sternum for access to the right atrium and venae cavae or through the costal cartilages on the left side superiorly for involvement of the great vessels. The technique is also useful for patients with blunt thoracic trauma with flail or crushed chest who have suffered cardiopulmonary arrest and cannot undergo external cardiac compression safely. Profoundly hypotensive patients with blunt or penetrating abdominal trauma can sometimes be stabilized for transport to the operating room by accident center thoracotomy and cross-clamping of the descending thoracic aorta. This arrests intra-abdominal hemorrhage, facilitates internal cardiac massage and allows resuscitation of the brain and myocardium in preference to other organs. Patients with ruptured abdominal aortic aneurysms can be revived in the same way. Median sternotomy gives better access to all cardiac chambers but sternal saws are not readily available in most accident departments.

The surgical management of cardiac laceration depends on the location. Control of hemorrhage can usually be obtained by digital or manual compression and the wound sutured directly or over felt pledgets. A small number of patients who survive with laceration of a major coronary artery or valvular or septal destruction with cardiac decompensation may require early cardiopulmonary bypass shortly after urgent thoracotomy. Holes in the atria or pulmonary veins may be controlled by inserting a Foley catheter and inflating the balloon which then allows direct suture repair of the defect. Air embolism is a serious risk during exposure of lacerated atria or pulmonary veins. Autotransfusion is a valuable adjunct in the face of major cardiac laceration, though few patients with this problem survive to reach hospital. Frequently, the lacerated heart has already arrested or is fibrillating. Control of the penetrating wound must then be carried out in association with cardiac massage and defibrillation.

All patients who respond to this treatment are transferred to an operating room for formal exploration, more secure surgical repair, and if necessary, management of associated injuries and cleansing and closure of the chest incision. Intravenous antibiotics, such as gentamicin, flucloxacillin and penicillin, are administered postoperatively for periods of 5 days or more. Treatment with steroids, mannitol or hypothermia may be considered for patients exhibiting cerebral hypoxia. Potential complications of the procedure relate to the uncontrolled operative circumstances and the pressure to intervene rapidly. Iatrogenic lacerations of the heart, coronary arteries and lung may contribute to failure of the procedure. Considerable experience in trauma is essential in deciding which patient should be explored

in the accident department. The heart is relatively easy to resuscitate. The outcome depends more frequently on cerebral status.

Young age, a brief period of cerebral hypoxia and lack of major intracardiac structural injury are good prognostic features. Outcome is less satisfactory after blunt versus penetrating injury. Factors associated with high mortality in penetrating cardiac injuries include shotgun wounds (100% mortality), left ventricular injury (47% mortality), unconsciousness at the time of arrival (86% mortality), and the absence of measurable blood pressure on arrival (66% mortality). Usually a lower mortality is associated with knife wounds compared with gunshot wounds.

CARDIAC TAMPONADE

In those patients whose circulatory status remains good and in whom there may be doubts as to whether the heart has been damaged, a plain chest radiograph or two-dimensional echocardiography can be carried out once the venous lines have been inserted (Fig 16.12). On a plain chest radiograph the cardiac shadow is typically of an abnormally globular shape and on two-dimensional echocardiography a pericardial effusion with compression of the cardiac chambers and abnormal ventricular filling will be apparent.

Patients with tamponade who survive prolonged transfer to hospital will usually survive a further short transfer to an operating room. The great majority of centers that receive large numbers of penetrating cardiac wounds have abandoned pericardiocentesis in favour of thoracotomy since the pericardial blood has usually clotted. Some workers advocate a surgical trans-diaphragmatic pericardotomy by small subxiphoid incision with midline opening of the diaphragm and pericardial cavity for diagnosis and relief of suspected tamponade. This may produce temporary clinical improvement until definitive median sternotomy or thoracotomy can be carried out. However, it may also disturb the blood clot in the cardiac wound and precipitate fatal hemorrhage before adequate surgical access is possible.

Median sternotomy is the incision of choice. This provides access to all aspects of the heart and both pleural cavities can be inspected by opening the pleura when necessary. When the sternum is opened a bulging, dark blue pericardium is encountered. When this is opened, blood clot is evacuated rapidly and is usually followed by fresh bleeding from the site of injury. Control of the wound can then be obtained with a finger, followed by suture. It is important to inspect the rest of the heart carefully for other wounds. Only rarely is cardiopulmonary bypass required at this stage.

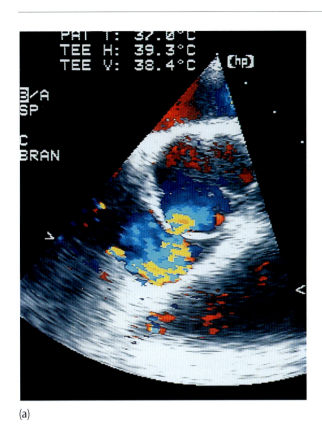

(a)

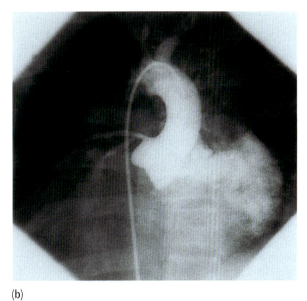

(b)

Figure 16.12 *(a) Two-dimensional echocardiography and (b) aortography in a patient with blunt fistula formation between the aortic root and the right atrium. (Courtesy of Dr Chris Knott-Craig.)*

THE CARDIAC CONSEQUENCES OF MAJOR BURNS

Extensive (>30%) dermal burns lead to a substantial reduction in cardiac output which is only partly dependent upon plasma volume changes. Heart rate and arterial blood pressure often remain normal or somewhat elevated. This low stroke volume, high peripheral vascular resistance form of circulatory shock develops within the first hour of injury, persists for over 24 hours and contributes to early mortality, even in aggressively treated patients.

The mechanism of these cardiac effects remains poorly understood, particularly in relation to whether inotropic failure might play a role. Adams and colleagues studied contraction/relaxation properties of isovolumic left ventricular preparations isolated from guinea pigs 24 hours after full thickness burn to approximately 47% total body surface area. Compared with controls, hearts from burned subjects consistently generated significantly lower values for left ventricular systolic pressure and maximal rates of left ventricular pressure rise and fall. The left ventricular contractile deficit of burn hearts could not be correlated with changes in tissue water content and was not surmountable by excess glucose and insulin, increased coronary flow or maximal preload elevation.

In addition, end-diastolic pressure/volume relationships in burn hearts were shifted upwards and to the left of controls in the direction of decreased compliance.

Thus, left ventricular sequelae of thermal trauma manifested in isolated hearts as decreased contractility, slowed isovolumic relaxation and decreased diastolic compliance. In the intact animal, this combination would reduce ejection and impede filling of the ventricle, with diastolic pressures reflecting changes in compliance as well as contractile function.

This study has important clinical implications for the treatment of patients with burns. The triad of reduced contractility, impaired relaxation during early diastole and increased chamber stiffness during late diastole would impede filling and reduce ejection of the ventricle. The resulting decrement in stroke volume would further reduce cardiac output and exacerbate the poor tissue perfusion already present in the burned patient. Moreover, if the observed end-diastolic pressure/volume relationship occurs in humans, then diastolic pressure indices in burn patients may yield spuriously high predictions of ventricular filling volumes owing to changes in compliance. This possibility should be considered when pulmonary wedge pressures are used to determine cardiac status in burn patients.

CASE STUDIES IN BLUNT CARDIAC TRAUMA

Case 1

A 23-year-old male motorcyclist sustained rapid deceleration and severe blunt anterior chest compression in collision with another vehicle. He suffered a fractured right femur and a blow to the head without unconsciousness. On admission to hospital, there was bruising over the precordium but no rib fractures. The electrocardiogram showed right bundle branch block and there was a soft pansystolic murmur over the sternum. On closer inspection during preoperative assessment for fracture fixation, the jugular venous pressure was seen to be raised with a suspicion of cardiac tamponade (Fig 16.10). Two-dimensional echocardiography then showed only a narrow rim of fluid in the pericardium but torrential tricuspid regurgitation and an akinetic right ventricle. The anterior leaflet of the tricuspid valve was flail, with the appearance of complete disruption. Consequently, a decision was made to explore the tricuspid valve with a view to repair. A CT scan of the brain was carried out first to exclude intracranial hemorrhage which may worsen with systemic heparinization. On cardiopulmonary bypass the right atrium was opened when total disruption of the tricuspid anterior leaflet was readily apparent (see Fig 16.4). This proved amenable to direct repair which restored competence. Cardiopulmonary bypass was discontinued uneventfully though the right ventricle appeared diskinetic. The cardiac output was sufficient to allow fixation of the femoral fracture after reversal of heparin with protamine. Postoperative recovery was uneventful.

Case 2

A 35-year-old motor vehicle driver who was not wearing a seat belt sustained a severe high velocity impact of the chest against the steering wheel. The chest wall remained intact without sternal or rib fractures. No cardiac abnormality was noted on admission to hospital, but 5 days later he was noticeably dyspneic at rest. On auscultation of the heart sounds there was a pansystolic murmur in the mitral area and a gallop rhythm suggesting heart failure. Two-dimensional echocardiography showed akinesia of the interventricular septum with severe mitral regurgitation. The right ventricle was dilated whilst the left ventricular free wall was normal. The findings suggested severe blunt injury to the interventricular septum and septal papillary muscle of the mitral valve. With continued observation and diuretic therapy there was little symptomatic improvement. It was therefore decided to explore the mitral valve with a view to surgical repair (see Fig 16.3). At operation, the mitral leaflets appeared normal and repair was attempted by commissural plication and insertion of an annuloplasty ring. There was no symptomatic improvement, and with the onset of pulmonary edema, mitral valve replacement was undertaken. After this, recovery was uneventful. Histological examination of the septal papillary muscle showed necrosis with areas of new fibrosis.

Case 3

A 64-year-old male was working at a lathe when the movable part detached, striking him directly in the precordial area. The severe blow left a circular mark over the left pectoral region and the victim became acutely dyspneic (see Fig 16.1). On arrival at the emergency room, he was clinically shocked with raised jugular venous pressure and sinus tachycardia. The chest radiograph showed a globular pericardial outline. The radial pulse was barely perceptible. Two-dimensional echocardiography demonstrated cardiac tamponade with a 2 cm rim of blood around the ventricles. Urgent thoracotomy was performed and an apical tear in the left ventricle identified and sutured (Fig 16.1). Postoperative recovery was uneventful.

Case 4

A 19-year-old motor vehicle driver sustained a high speed deceleration injury with impact of the left chest against the steering wheel. He was not restrained by a seat belt and was unconscious when retrieved from the vehicle. Twenty-four hours later, when awake, he complained of chest pain and was noted to have a sinus tachycardia and blood pressure of 90/60 mmHg. Two-dimensional echocardiography showed akinesia of the anterolateral wall of the left ventricle and the electrocardiogram showed the classical picture of an anterior acute myocardial infarction. Five days after the accident, coronary angiography was performed. This demonstrated an aneurysm at the origin of the left anterior descending coronary artery (LAD) (Fig 16.6). Distal flow down the artery was sluggish, with the appearance of a recanalized vessel. When chest pain and ischemic ECG signs persisted, he was referred for surgery.

Median stenotomy was performed and the left internal mammary artery harvested. Inspection of the heart confirmed an akinetic anterolateral wall with scattered petechiae and contusion of the right ventricle. A subepicardial hematoma marked the site of the aneurysm. On cardiopulmonary bypass the proximal left anterior descending coronary was explored and the aneurysm plicated to maintain continuity of the native vessel. The left internal mammary artery was anastomosed to the distal LAD. Postoperative recovery was uneventful with no further chest pain.

Case 5

A 3-year-old girl was kicked directly in the precordium by a horse. Despite the severity of the blow, the injury was thought to be restricted to bruising on the left anterior chest wall. Six days later she was listless and clearly disabled by breathlessness. On examination the venous pressure was raised with a sinus tachycardia. There was a harsh systolic murmur at the apex and over the precordium. Two-dimensional echocardiography confirmed the suspicion of traumatic ventricular septal rupture with a small pericardial effusion. She was first treated with diuretics for 6 weeks to allow fibrosis around the necrotic margins of the defect. Patch closure was then performed uneventfully on cardiopulmonary bypass.

Case 6

A 16-year-old motorcyclist lost control and sustained direct impact of the lower chest with a concrete gate post. Although there were no associated injuries, he became acutely dyspneic and shocked. He was transferred to a level 1 trauma center by helicopter where a loud continuous murmur was noted precordium. A plain chest radiograph showed distension of the cardiac shadow and bilateral pulmonary contusion under the contused chest wall. The sternum was intact and there were no rib fractures or pneumothorax. Two-dimensional echocardiography showed a fistula between the aortic root in the right coronary sinus and the right atrium (Fig 16.12a). The right atrium and right ventricle were enormously distended and the right ventricular free wall akinetic. The electrocardiogram showed right bundle branch block and ischemic changes over the right ventricle. In view of the extremely unusual appearances in the aortic root, an aortogram was performed which confirmed a post-traumatic fistula into the right atrium (Fig 16.12b).

Progressive hemodynamic deterioration prompted surgical exploration on cardiopulmonary bypass. The severity of the injury was such that the left side of the pericardium was lacerated (15 cm) with prolapse of the right atrium through the rent. There was hematoma around the aortic root and around the proximal right coronary artery. The right atrium and right ventricle were grossly distended with a right atrial pressure of 45 mmHg. When the aortic root was opened, there was a small laceration within the ostium of the right coronary artery. When the right atrium was opened, the appearances were remarkable with dehiscence of the crux of the heart extending vertically into the interventricular septum. The tricuspid valve annulus was split between anterior and septal leaflets and the right coronary artery had an irreparable longitudinal dehiscence for 1 cm, beginning at the origin and providing a fistula between the aortic root and the right atrium. The shredded right coronary was not repairable, and a vein graft was used to bypass the injury. The aortic root fistula was closed by oversewing the right coronary ostium. The right atrium was repaired directly and the

tricuspid valve replaced with a bioprosthesis. On discontinuing cardiopulmonary bypass, the contused right ventricle remained distended but the patient recovered with progressive improvement in ventricular function.

Case 7

A 38-year-old male motorcyclist was admitted unconscious to the emergency room with barely perceptible pulse and blood pressure. The history from paramedics was of a severe deceleration injury. He was intubated and ventilated but no source of bleeding was apparent. A plain chest radiograph showed both lungs to be contused but expanded. There was an unusual configuration of the cardiac shadow with the apex of the heart elevated. Intravenous infusion failed to increase the blood pressure and even vigorous cardiac massage was ineffective. Emergency room thoracotomy was therefore performed, and provided the reason for failure to resuscitate. The pericardium was lacerated in front of the left phrenic nerve with prolapse of left and right ventricles through the hole. This strangulated the heart in the atrioventricular groove and prevented the filling of the ventricles. There was obvious severe contusion at the point of impact over the right ventricle. Internal cardiac massage was commenced but failed to restore reactivity to fixed dilated pupils. The pericardium was opened further and the ventricles reduced to their normal position. However, with continued cardiac massage, the heart was still unable to sustain the circulation and the patient died. Post-mortem examination confirmed the presence of severe myocardial contusion in the interventricular septum and right ventricular free wall. There was a laceration at the base of the right coronary cusp of the aortic valve.

REFERENCES

1. Cicero J, Mattox KL. Epidemiology of chest trauma. *Surg Clin North Am* 1989; **69**: 15–19.
2. Mattox KL, Feliciano DV, Burch J, Beall AC, Jordan GL, Debakey ME. Five thousand seven hundred and sixty cardiovascular injuries in 4459 patients. *Ann Surg* 1989; **209**: 698–707.
3. Cane RD, Buchanan N. The electrocardiographic and clinical diagnosis of myocardial contusion. *Intensive Care Med* 1978; **4**: 99–102.
4. Saunders CR, Doty DB. Myocardial contusion. *Surg Gynecol Obstet* 1977; **144**: 595–603.
5. Snow N, Richardson JD, Flint LM. Myocardial contusion: implications for patients with multiple traumatic injuries. *Surgery* 1982; **92**: 744–50.

6. Parmley LF, Mannion WC, Mattingly TW. Non-penetrating traumatic injury of the heart. *Circulation* 1958; **18:** 375–396.

7. Al Kasab S, Westaby S, Al Zaibag A, Habbab M, Gunawardena KA, Al Fagih MR. Traumatic papillary muscle dysfunction: attempted mitral valve repair and eventual prosthetic replacement. *Eur Heart J* 1988; **9:** 1030–3.

8. Westaby S, Drossos G, Giannopoulos N. Post-traumatic coronary artery aneurysm. *Ann Thorac Surg* 1995; **60:** 712–13.

9. Manga P, King J. Trauma induced pseudoaneurysm of the right ventricle. Diagnosis by two-dimensional echocardiography. *Am J Cardiol* 1985; **55:** 195–6.

10. Westaby S. The injured heart. *Clin Intensive Care* 1990; **1:** 210–19.

11. Unterberg C, Buckwald A, Wiegard V. Traumatic thrombosis of the left main coronary artery and myocardial infarction caused by blunt chest trauma. *Clin Cardiol* 1989; **12:** 672–4.

12. Helling TS, Duke P, Beggs CW, Crouse LJ. A prospective evaluation of 68 patients suffering blunt chest trauma for evidence of cardiac surgery. *J Trauma* 1989; **29:** 961–6.

13. Ivatury RR, Shah PM, Ito F, Ramirez-Schon G, Suarez F, Rohnian M. Emergency room thoracotomy for the resuscitation of patients with 'fatal' penetrating injuries to the heart. *Ann Thorac Surg* 1981; **32:** 277–85.

14. Markiewicz W, Best LA, Burnstein S, Peleg H. Echocardiographic evaluation after blunt trauma of the chest. *Int J Cardiol* 1985; **8:** 269–74.

15. Kettunen P. Cardiac damage after blunt chest trauma, diagnosed using CKMB enzyme and electrocardiogram. *Int J Cardiol* 1984; **6:** 355–71.

17

Trauma to the chest wall and thoracic vertebrae

JOHN A ODELL

THE CHEST WALL

Lung hernia

Occasionally, because of traumatic injury, previous surgery or chest tube placement, a defect in the chest wall results and, on coughing or straining a soft tissue swelling will be seen to protrude. It is usually noticed some time after the injury or surgical procedure, but occasionally in the acute situation, where a chest wall laceration is present, lung may herniate through the defect and be entrapped.[1] It is presumably the result of damage or destruction of muscle layers. Occasionally bony irregularity and signs of inflammation may be seen and felt. The hernial orifice is usually easily palpated. The mass may spontaneously reduce with respiration or may be reduced using constant pressure. Radiographically, if the defect is profiled, lung will be seen outside the confines of the chest; a CT scan is diagnostic,[2] although in most instances this is unnecessary. The differential diagnosis includes soft neoplasms such as a lipoma or angioma, a communicating effusion or subcutaneous emphysema.

In most cases the hernia is asymptomatic and the patient needs only to be reassured of the benign nature of the abnormality and no surgical action is necessary. Occasionally, if there are symptoms, if the injury is acute with a large defect, if there is incarceration, or if the hernia bothers the patient, repair can be performed either by using autogenous tissue or artificial material such as a mesh or Gore-Tex sheet.[3]

The open chest wall defect

An open defect should be covered with an occlusive dressing. If the dressing is impervious, it should be occluded on three sides; the fourth side will act as a flap valve, allowing air to escape and preventing air entering. Definitive management is by tube thoracostomy and wound closure, which should be undertaken as soon as possible.

A large destructive chest wall injury usually requires prompt intubation and positive pressure ventilation. Once this has been instituted and the patient stabilized and resuscitated, he/she should be taken to the operating room. The help of a plastic surgeon experienced in the use of muscle flaps is advantageous. The thoracotomy incision should be planned to preserve muscle groups that may be necessary for wound coverage. A thorough debridement of devitalized tissue is necessary and if there is doubt the wound should be covered and inspected another day. Only when one is satisfied with viability should closure be undertaken. Prosthetic material should be avoided if possible, but polytetrafluoroethylene (PTFE), Marlex mesh and Teflon cloth have been used successfully[3] Autogenous tissue and advancement of ribs or portions of ribs may assist in stabilization of the chest. If the defect is low, the diaphragm may be transposed above the chest wall defect, converting the chest wall injury to an abdominal defect.[4]

Hematomas

A rich vascular network supplies the chest wall. The intercostal vein and artery located on the inner aspect of the rib are easily lacerated by rib fragments. Rib fractures may bleed from raw bone surfaces, muscles may tear and bleed and occasionally the lateral thoracic artery or branches may be lacerated. Significant amounts of blood can sequestrate in the soft tissues of

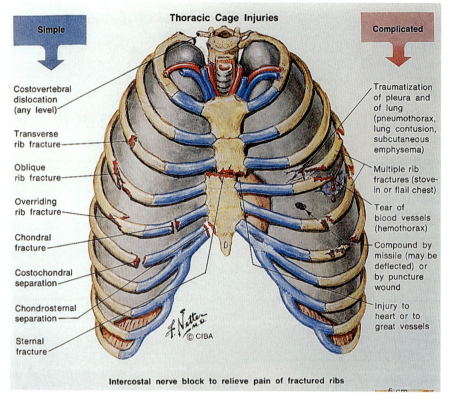

Figure 17.1 *The spectrum of chest wall injuries.*

the chest wall, particularly in the elderly where skin and subcutaneous tissue are lax. This may be sufficiently large to require transfusion; occasionally embolization of a bleeding vessel may be necessary.[5]

An extrapleural hematoma occurs in instances where bleeding is contained within the chest wall. It is commonly associated with rib fractures and it is presumed that a spicule of bone lacerates the closely applied intercostal artery. A breach of the pleura either does not occur or the pleura is adherent because of previous surgery to the chest or pleurisy, and a hemothorax does not result. The injury may follow transection of the internal thoracic artery.[6] The radiographic appearances are fairly typical – a lobulated opacity against the chest wall and close to a rib fracture, if visible. In those patients in whom the appearances are mistaken for a typical hemothorax and who have insertion of a chest tube, drainage is usually minimal, is often serous, and the chest radiograph remains unchanged. There is a higher risk of lung damage with attempted chest tube insertion. Usually no surgical intervention is necessary and the hematoma resolves with time. Occasionally surgical intervention is necessary – in a patient with internal thoracic artery injury continued bleeding requires surgical exploration.[6] In very rare circumstances, delayed life-threatening hemothorax associated with rib fractures can develop due to laceration of the intercostal artery.[7]

Rib fractures

Rib fractures constitute a major part of chest trauma (Fig 17.1). The fractures may be a marker of severe injury elsewhere or, if present as the sole injury, result in pain leading to secondary pulmonary insufficiency and prolonged convalescence.

INCIDENCE AND DIAGNOSIS

The exact incidence of rib fractures is unknown as many may be missed. Emphasis may be distracted towards ·management of more serious other injuries, not all patients are admitted, and not all rib fractures are detected on plain chest radiographs. In fact, up to 50% of rib fractures may not be detected on a chest radiograph.[8] Acute rib fractures are notoriously difficult to visualize using standard radiographic techniques, especially if undisplaced. Chest radiographs repeated a few weeks after the injury may show evidence of cortical new bone formation at the fracture site. In patients with persistent pain after trauma but without radiographically recognized rib fractures, nuclear scan imaging may confirm the diagnosis.[9] This investigative modality is extremely accurate with 90% of fractures detected at 72 hours.[9] In most patients the clinical diagnosis is usually accurate. Approximately 10% of a regional trauma center admissions will have rib fractures.[10]

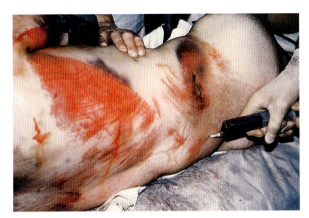

Figure 17.2 *Severe blunt injuries with extensive bruising, multiple rib fractures and a fractured lumbar spine. (SWTC.)*

MECHANISMS

The most common mechanism is a motor vehicle accident (Fig 17.2). The incidence of rib fractures in restrained and unrestrained occupants is almost identical.[11] Restraints, however, significantly reduce the number of severe injuries and the mortality rate is less.[11,12] Rib fractures can follow other forms of blunt trauma (Fig 17.3). Penetrating trauma is an uncommon cause, accounting for approximately 1% of patients with rib fractures.[10]

ASSOCIATED INJURIES

Only rarely do patients admitted to hospital have isolated rib fractures. In Ziegler and Agarwal's series only 6% had isolated fractures.[10] The associated injuries in this report are documented in Table 17.1 and are similar to the experience of others.[13–15]

MANAGEMENT

Clinicians should regard the presence of rib fractures as a marker for associated injuries and should carefully appraise their patient with this thought uppermost. The majority of patients require hospitalization, not only for

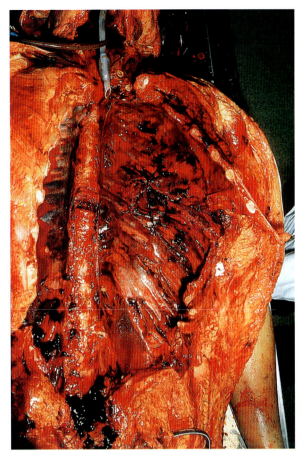

Figure 17.3 *Autopsy after a severe crush injury of the chest. There are multiple bilateral rib fractures each associated with blood loss of about 150 ml. There is a midthoracic spinal fracture which was not recognized before death. The patient died from acute respiratory failure through widespread bilateral lung contusion. (SWTC.)*

their associated injuries, but also for pain control and pulmonary complications. Approximately 30–40% develop pulmonary complications and of these patients approximately 5% die.[10] Pulmonary complications are the major cause of late death (see Fig 17.1). Not surprisingly, there is a correlation between increasing number of ribs fractured and severity of injury and mortality.[10,14,16]

Table 17.1 *Associated injuries*

Associated injuries	Number of patients	Percentage of patients	Mortality	Percentage
Hemothorax/pneumothorax	224	32	44	20
Lung contusions/lacerations	209	29	38	18
Thoracic aorta	31	2	11	85
Liver	75	11	30	40
Spleen	82	12	27	33
Kidney	61	9	12	20
Spinal cord	55	8	9	16
Cerebral	57	8	15	26
Diaphragm	16	2	8	50

Modified from Ziegler and Agarwal.[10] Some patients had more than one associated injury.

Deaths associated with rib fractures in the older extremes of life are associated with a lower injury severity score (ISS), suggesting that it takes a less severe injury to be lethal in the elderly. In the younger age group where ribs are more pliant, a rib fracture usually signifies greater trauma. It has been suggested that the presence of three or more rib fractures identifies a subgroup of patients who have a higher probability of serious injury.[16]

Blunt chest trauma that is not life-threatening (stable vital signs with no evidence of cardiac injury, solid or hollow viscus rupture, or fractures associated with significant blood loss) is a very common injury seen in emergency departments. Management of these patients is poorly defined and usually follows the clinical assessment of the patient and inclination of the clinician. Dubinsky and Low have attempted to define appropriate management.[17] In their group of patients they attempted repeat chest radiography 5–9 days after initial injury. The number of patients with sequelae was low and they recommended that investigation only be pursued if clinically justified because 'routine' radiological investigation is costly.

PAIN CONTROL

This is discussed in greater detail in Chapter 24. Because ribs cannot be immobilized, movement (breathing, coughing) is extremely painful and because of diminished tidal volumes, poor sputum mobilization and inactivity, the stage is set for pulmonary complications. Aggressive pain control and pulmonary toilet is necessary. This may take the form of intercostal blocks, patient-controlled analgesia, or epidural catheters.[18]

VENTILATION

In many patients with rib fractures the associated injury often dictates the need for intermittent positive pressure ventilation (IPPV). In some patients without complicated chest injuries IPPV may not be necessary (Fig 17.4).[19]

SURGICAL MANAGEMENT

Although this form of management does not receive broad support, there are advocates who suggest that the complications of IPPV outweigh the advantages of internal fixation of the chest wall.[20,21] In an effort to resolve this issue, Ahmed and Mohyuddin retrospectively compared two groups of patients: one managed by internal fixation (Fig 17.5) and the other by intubation and ventilation.[22] Although this was a retrospective study, the groups were similar in terms of age, sex, severity of chest wall and associated injury. Ventilation requirements and intensive care unit stay was less in the surgically stabilized group. Mortality rate was 8% in the surgically managed group versus 29% in the ventilator

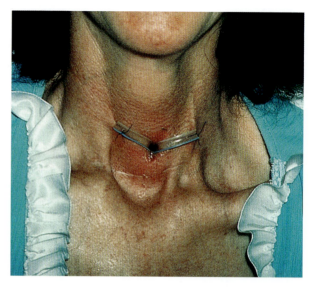

Figure 17.4 *Minitracheostomy in a patient with multiple rib fractures. This allowed regular tracheal suction and prevented the need for positive pressure ventilation. (SWTC.)*

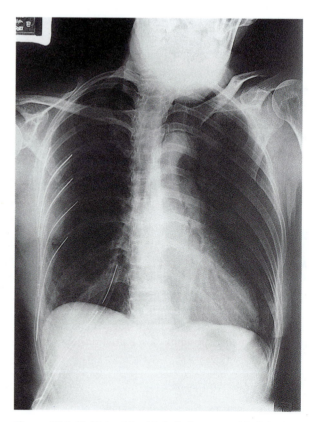

Figure 17.5 *Multiple right-sided rib fractures with flail chest treated surgically by pinning of the fractures. (SWTC.)*

managed group.[22] A number of techniques have been used. In larger ribs an intramedullary nail can be used, but this technique is not suitable for smaller ribs. In these circumstances, stainless steel struts with multiple holes, which can be curved and cut to appropriate shape and length, are sutured with non-absorbable sutures to

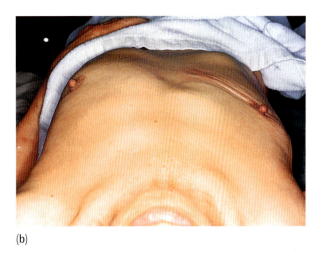

(a)   (b)

Figure 17.6 *(a, b) Young man with steering wheel impact to the right chest causing fractures to the costochondral junctions and deformity of the anterior chest wall. (SWTC.)*

the outside of the fractured ribs. The struts are tunneled and placed in position using small incisions. Where thoracotomy is needed for other reasons these can be placed at this time. In Ahmed and Mohyuddin's experience the ribs were internally fixed if an anesthetic was required for another indication such as an orthopedic procedure for other associated fractures. A particular place for internal fixation is the management of a traumatic thoracoplasty where the chest wall is depressed inwards (Fig 17.6).

Occasionally a patient with a history of previous rib fractures may have continued nagging pain and radiographic features of non-union. In the author's personal experience some of these patients have been managed elsewhere by resection of the bone ends with unsatisfactory results – the patient continues to have pain and it is often more severe. It is recommended that these patients be managed non-surgically. Occasionally patients are seen where the callus of the healing fracture impinges upon movement of the scapula: if persistent, the angulated, impinging area may be smoothed with a rasp.

SPECIFIC RIB FRACTURES

First rib

Fractures of the first rib are uncommon because it is one of the strongest, is the shortest rib and has a protected position. Mechanisms of fracture include: direct trauma, indirect trauma, sudden contracture of the neck musculature, and stress fracture because of repeated muscular pull.[23] Fracture of this rib indicates, in acute trauma, significant force and should alert the clinician to other associated injuries such as traumatic rupture of the aorta, brachial plexus injury and pulmonary contusion. Stress fracture may follow repetitive movements such as serving a volleyball[23] and usually occurs at the weakest point anatomically – the

groove for the subclavian artery where the rib is thinnest. It is at this point that the bone is subjected to upward traction by the scalene muscles and opposing traction by the serratus anterior, pectoralis major and intercostal muscles. Occasionally callus formation may result in brachial plexus involvement or the thoracic outlet syndrome.

Based on Richardson *et al.*'s paper published in 1974,[24] it has become accepted that fracture of the first rib is indicative of severe trauma. This was reinforced by a paper by Wilson *et al.*[25] who recommended large vessel angiography when the first or second rib was fractured. However, Woodring *et al.*[26] showed that other signs of mediastinal abnormality were of greater significance. When angiograms were reviewed, an arterial abnormality was found in 14.5% in those without and only 8% in those with first or second rib fracture.[26] Poole found a possible increased incidence of subclavian arterial injury with first or second rib fracture but no association with thoracic aorta injury, nor an association between multiple rib fractures and aortic trauma.[27] First rib fractures have a stronger association with injury to other organ systems, than with vascular injuries.[28]

The costal margin

There exists a condition that is infrequently recognized, described under synonyms of 'slipping ribs, clicking ribs, nerve entrapment and the rib tip syndrome', which may be associated either with a true traumatic incident or be perceived by the patient or the clinician as following trauma.[29–32] Prolonged retraction after upper abdominal surgery may also be a cause. The patient often complains of pain localized to the costal margin and hypochondrium. The pain may be intermittent and aggravated by bending or twisting. Often the patient is aware of a clicking sensation and can reproduce the pain by manipulation. The pain can be reproduced on

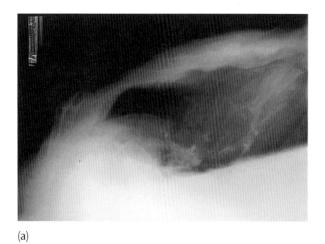

(a)

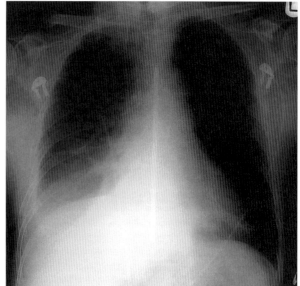

(b)

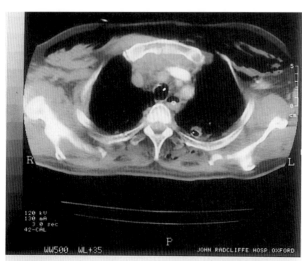
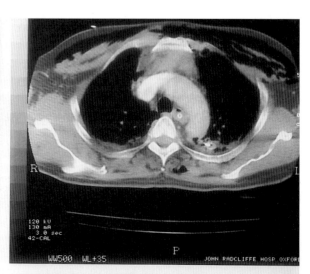
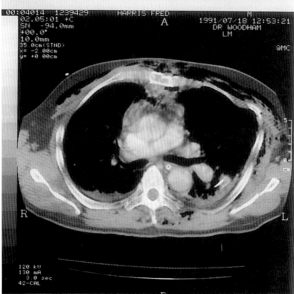
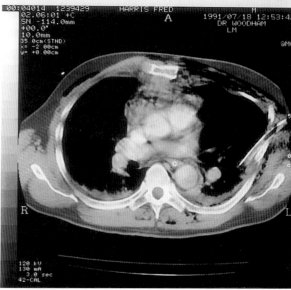

(c)

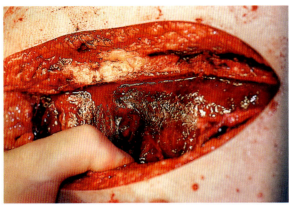

(d)

Figure 17.7 *(a) Painful overlapping sternal fracture treated by insertion of a Stineman pin through the sternal marrow and across the reduced fracture. (b) This relieves the pain of fractured sternum which may cause respiratory failure. (c) CT scan in this patient showed a widened mediastinum due to the anterior mediastinal hematoma. (d) Urgent median sternotomy in another patient with fractured sternum shows the anterior mediastinal hematoma in front of the pericardium. This patient had blunt traumatic rupture of the tricuspid valve. (SWTC.)*

examination by hooking the fingers under the costal margin and pulling up. There are no radiographic investigations that can confirm the diagnosis: the costal margin is translucent. Intercostal blocks are occasionally helpful in relieving the pain and may help in confirming the diagnosis. Occasionally removal of the affected costal cartilage may be necessary to relieve pain. This can be done with a short incision which is centered slightly more posteriorly than the maximum point of pain so that the cartilage can be excised (the pain is at the tip of the cartilage). The involved cartilage is easily recognized as the fibrous connections with the remainder of the costal margin are missing.

Sternal fractures

A 5-year retrospective study analyzing the natural history of sternal fractures in 66 patients has been reported by Wojcik;[33] a larger series has been reported by Hills and colleagues.[34] The most common mechanism was motor vehicle accidents (MVA) with the victim impacting the steering wheel (Fig 17.7). In Wojcik's series only one of the 39 patients involved in a MVA was wearing a restraint. Other causes are falls or direct blows. Rib fracture is the most common associated injury. There does not appear to be a significant association with life-threatening intrathoracic injuries such as myocardial contusion, thoracic aortic

rupture, tracheobronchial and esophageal rupture.[33,34] Sternal fractures are usually transverse (see Fig 17.1), are localized most commonly to the mid-body, followed by the manubrium and other areas of the body of the sternum. Occasionally manubriosternal joint disruption occurs.[35] Two types of manubriosternal dislocations are described. Type I is a backward displacement of the body caused by a direct force acting on the body directly. Type II is more common. In this situation the manubrium is displaced posteriorly and is believed to result from indirect forces and the strong ligamentous attachments of the first and second ribs. Women appear to have a higher frequency of sternal fracture, especially at an older age and a lower ISS than men. This is believed to represent osteoporosis and the relative skeletal strength.[34] Sternal fractures are poorly seen on the standard frontal or posterior chest radiograph and lateral or sternal views may be necessary. The fracture is easily seen on CT scans (see Fig 17.7).

MANAGEMENT

An issue raised whenever sternal fractures exist is that of myocardial contusion. Using generally accepted criteria, this is present in approximately 20% of patients with sternal fractures.[33,36,37] In Wojcik's series the incidence with localized sternal fractures was only 6% and none of the patients in the total group who had myocardial contusion developed life-threatening arrhythmias or required invasive monitoring or pharmacological support. They questioned whether in the isolated fracture patient myocardial contusion should be investigated and documented. In Hill's series only two patients (1.3%) had definite myocardial injury, but screening tests were not routinely performed.[34] The presence of a sternal fracture is not an indication for aortography.[34,38] An algorithm for management is presented in Fig 17.8.

Where deaths occurred in Hill's study, none could be contributed to the sternal fracture or its effect on the mediastinum.[34]

CLAVICULAR FRACTURES

These are common and usually of minimal consequence. Traumatic dislocation of the sternoclavicular joint is unusual because of the ligamentous attachments. Anterior dislocation is more common. If the dislocation is anterior, a prominent medial clavicular head is noticeable; if posterior, there is a hollow or a 'step-off' of the sternal edge. A fracture of the clavicle is usually managed with an arm sling. Open reduction and internal fixation are rarely necessary; when dislocation has occurred relocation under sedation or general anesthesia is indicated.

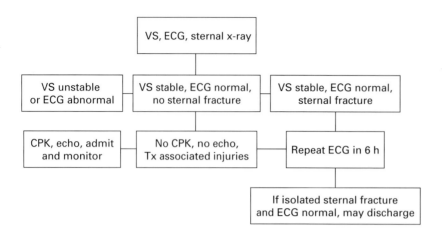

Figure 17.8 *Algorithm for patients with suspected myocardial contusion based on Chiu et al.'s figure.[45] Their approach is supported by others.[46] Patients with anterior chest wall bruising, sternal tenderness or deformity are considered. CPK, creatine phosphokinase isoenzyme; echo, echocardiogram; ECG, electrocardiogram; Tx, treatment; VS, vital signs.*

SCAPULAR FRACTURES

Scapular fractures are rare, as the scapula is sturdy and well protected by muscles. Their importance is a strong association with associated injuries. It is believed that most result from direct impact; patients have a high incidence of associated injuries to the ipsilateral lung and chest wall and to the ipsilateral shoulder girdle and its contained structures.[39] Impaction of the humeral head into the glenoid fossa is believed to induce many of the glenoid and glenoid neck fractures. The transmission of this force onto the clavicle is responsible for the high incidence of associated ipsilateral clavicular fracture with scapular fractures. Avulsive forces probably induce fractures of the coracoid and acromial process as well as some fractures of the superior border of the scapula. Fractures of the scapular body are the result of direct trauma. Occasionally, penetrating trauma may reach and fracture the thinner scapular body. Brachial plexus and arterial injuries occur more commonly with fractures of the body of the scapula in Thompson *et al.*'s experience;[39] in McGahan *et al.*'s experience peripheral nerve injuries were more common where injuries involved the acromion or acromioclavicular joint.[40] There has been one report of fracture of the scapula associated with intrathoracic penetration of a fracture fragment.[41] This was managed successfully by open reduction.

Most fractures can be diagnosed on the plain AP radiograph of the chest. An injury that is often associated and often unrecognized is posterior shoulder dislocation. Fractures of the body heal well and by themselves cause little morbidity; those involving the shoulder joint can result in long-term disability.

Although some have managed the fractures by open reduction, particularly if the articular surface of the glenoid is damaged, most are managed by conservative means. Simple immobilization continues until the acute pain has subsided, whereupon a range of motion exercise is emphasized.

Scapulothoracic dissociation

This is a rare injury which usually follows motor vehicle accidents – commonly motorcycle or snowmobile. The injury is essentially a forequarter amputation with preservation of the skin and soft tissues. A recent review of this injury[42] describes 11 patients. All had an absent radial pulse and complete motor and sensory loss below the shoulder. Some patients had Horner's syndrome. There was often a shoulder and chest wall hematoma. Although many extremities were pale and cold to the touch, most were not considered to have life-threatening ischemia. All patients had angiograms that demonstrated subclavian or axillary artery occlusion without extravastion of contrast. Roughly half the patients were revascularized; those that were not did not develop delayed hemorrhage nor a threatened limb. No patient had significant neurological recovery; all limbs were functionless without sensation. It was concluded that, because of the dismal functional outcome of the brachial plexus injury and the lack of hemorrhage and life-threatening ischemia, a conservative policy should be followed.

INTRATHORACIC DISPLACEMENT OF THE HUMERAL HEAD

This is a rare injury; a case report and review of the literature was reported recently by Kaar and colleagues.[43] Most have occurred following falls although one patient was involved in a motor vehicle accident. The mechanism is obscure; most believe that a single traumatic force is unlikely. Violent abduction is thought to cause initial anterior displacement of the head of the humerus – further violent abduction of the humerus against the ribs or direct trauma on the shoulder drive the displaced humeral head against the chest wall, result in local rib fractures and displacement within the chest.

The limited literature published on this subject appears to favor a conservative approach. Movement of the shoulder may be limited after recovery.

VERTEBRAL INJURIES

The author does not profess to be an expert in the surgical management of these injuries and will not attempt to advise on specific orthopedic and neurological management, but will instead concentrate on issues that may affect the thoracic surgeon. Occasionally, the hematoma associated with vertebral fractures may cause widening of the mediastinal silhouette and the issue of traumatic rupture of the aorta may be raised.

Subarachnoid-pleural fistula

Considering the frequency of blunt and penetrating chest trauma this is a rare occurrence. When Godley and colleagues reviewed the literature in 1995 only 18 cases had been reported.[44] Comments are made based on their review. The injury may occur secondary to either blunt or penetrating trauma. The mechanism of injury in blunt trauma may follow an acceleration–deceleration injury or, if thoracic spine fracture has occurred, follow combined laceration of the dura and pleura by a fragment of bone. Extreme extension of the spine results in tearing of the relatively immobile thoracic nerve roots leading to cerebrospinal fluid (CSF) leak; if pleural tearing is also present, a fistula results. Gunshot wounds are the commonest cause of penetrating trauma with direct injury to the dura and pleura. The leak is commonly into the pleural space, but the leak may track extrapleurally or into the mediastinum.

The rarity of the injury and insidious development of symptoms may lead to a delay in diagnosis. Symptoms of dyspnea or respiratory distress may accompany the significant volume of CSF that may collect in the pleural space. If chest drains are present, the volume of drainage may be large and persistent. Where leak is into the mediastinum or extrapleurally, the diagnosis may be difficult because of lack of symptoms. Symptoms of low CSF pressure such as headache, nausea and vomiting may occur. If a pneumothorax is present, a pneumocephalus may be present. This finding has been reported after thoracotomy, but has not been documented after trauma. Examination of the fluid is suggestive, but often inconclusive because of admixture with pleural fluid.

Water-soluble CT myelography has become the study of choice in confirming the diagnosis and defining the anatomy of the fistula. Occasionally radionuclide myelography has proved the diagnosis, but has not defined the anatomy.

Management options are influenced by symptoms, by the magnitude of the tear and the duration of the dural disruption. Conservative measures are reasonable and effective in patients with small acute dural injuries, but often this fails as the leak tends to remain open because of negative intrathoracic pressure. When non-operative management fails and clinical symptoms progress, or if there is concern regarding meningitis, then surgical intervention is indicated. Techniques for repair depend on the size of the dural tear and usually involve incorporation of autogenous tissue such as fat, muscle, pleura and fascia. All methods of repair reported have been effective without recurrence. An indwelling lumbar drain to maintain low CSF pressures is advantageous.

Thoracic duct injury

The thoracic duct, because of its protected position, is infrequently injured in blunt trauma. Traumatic hyperextension of the spine, with associated fracture-dislocation in some patients, has been postulated as the cause of thoracic duct injury.

The clinical presentation may be of excessive fluid drainage via chest tubes placed for associated pneumothorax or hemothorax. If the patient is fed orally, the typical appearance of chyle may be seen. Analysis will reveal chylomicrons, elevated triglycerides and lymphocytes. In some patients the leak is contained within the mediastinum, resulting in a contained mediastinal chyloma which may rupture into one or both pleural cavities a few days after the injury.

Once suspected, the diagnosis should be confirmed and the chest cavity drained. Drains tend to obstruct with gelatinous material and repeated new drains may be necessary. A short period (1 week) of conservative measures, utilizing discontinuation of oral feeding and intravenous nutrition, should be pursued in the hope of spontaneous closure. This situation occurs in approximately 50% of cases. Prolonged attempts at non-operative management should not be continued because of the debilitating effects, which result from the continued loss of protein and lymphocytes. The surgical approach is thoracotomy; the approach is usually on the side of the fluid collection. The thoracic duct is ligated at the level of the diaphragm where it is found between the azygos vein and aorta.

REFERENCES

1. Glenn C, Bonekat W, Cua A, Chapman D, McFall R. Lung hernia. *Am J Emerg Med* 1997; **15**: 260–2.
2. Sadler MA, Shapiro RS, Wagreich J, Halton K, Hecht A. CT diagnosis of acquired intercostal lung herniation. *Clin Imag* 1997; **21**: 104–6.

3. Flis V, Antonic J, Crnjac A, Zorko A. Air-to-surface missile wound of the thorax reconstructed with a polytetrafluoroethylene patch: case report. *J Trauma* 1993; **35:** 810–12.

4. Bender JS, Lucas CE. Management of close-range shotgun injuries to the chest by diaphragmatic transposition: case reports. *J Trauma* 1990; **30:** 1581–4.

5. Mayberry JC, Trunkey DD. The fractured rib in chest wall trauma. [Review] [75 refs]. *Chest Surg Clin North Am* 1997; **7:** 239–61.

6. Machin VG, Lau OJ. Extra-pleural haematoma secondary to blunt chest trauma. An unusual presentation. *Eur J Cardiothorac Surg* 1995; **9:** 109–10.

7. Ross RM, Cordoba A. Delayed life-threatening hemothorax associated with rib fractures. *J Trauma* 1986; **26:** 576–8.

8. Carrero R, Wayne M. Chest trauma. *Emerg Med Clin North Am* 1989; **7:** 389–418.

9. LaBan MM, Siegel CB, Schutz LK, Taylor RS. Occult radiographic fractures of the chest wall identified by nuclear scan imaging: report of seven cases. *Arch Phys Med Rehabil* 1994; **75:** 353–4.

10. Ziegler DW, Agarwal NN. The morbidity and mortality of rib fractures. *J Trauma* 1994; **37:** 975–9.

11. Newman RJ, Jones IS. A prospective study of 413 consecutive car occupants with chest injuries. *J Trauma* 1984; **24:** 129–35.

12. Kaplan BH, Crowley RA. Seatbelt effectiveness and cost of noncompliance among drivers admitted to a trauma center. *Am J Emerg Med* 1991; **9:** 4–10.

13. Shorr RM, Crittenden M, Indeck M, Hartunian SL, Rodriguez A. Blunt thoracic trauma. Analysis of 515 patients. *Ann Surg* 1987; **206:** 200–5.

14. Wilson RF, Murray C, Antonenko DR. Nonpenetrating thoracic injuries. *Surg Clin North Am* 1977; **57:** 17–36.

15. Poole GV Jr, Myers RT. Morbidity and mortality rates in major trauma to the upper chest. *Ann Surg* 1981; **193:** 70–5.

16. Lee RB, Bass SM, Morris JA Jr, MacKenzie EJ. Three or more rib fractures as an indicator for transfer to a Level I trauma center: a population-based study. *J Trauma* 1990; **30:** 689–94.

17. Dubinsky I, Low A. Non-life-threatening blunt chest trauma: appropriate investigation and treatment. *Am J Emerg Med* 1997; **15:** 240–3.

18. Mackersie RC, Karagianes TG, Hoyt DB, Davis JW. Prospective evaluation of epidural and intravenous administration of fentanyl for pain control and restoration of ventilatory function following multiple rib fractures. *J Trauma* 1991; **31:** 443–9.

19. Richardson JD, Adams I, Flint LM. Selective management of flail chest and pulmonary contusion. *Ann Surg* 1982; **196:** 481–7.

20. Paris F, Tarazona V, Blasco E, *et al.* Surgical stabilization of traumatic flail chest. *Thorax* 1975; **30:** 521–7.

21. Samarrai AR. Costosynthetic stabilization of massive chest wall instability. *Int Surg* 1990; **75:** 231–3.

22. Ahmed Z, Mohyuddin Z. Management of flail chest injury: internal versus endotracheal intubation and ventilation. *J Thorac Cardiovasc Surg* 1995; **110:** 1676–80.

23. Ochi M, Sasashige Y, Murakami T, Ikuta Y. Brachial plexus palsy secondary to stress fracture of the first rib: case report. *J Trauma* 1994; **36:** 128–30.

24. Richardson J, McElvein R, Trinkle J. First rib fracture: a hallmark of severe trauma. *Ann Surg* 1975; **181:** 251–4.

25. Wilson JM, Thomas AN, Goodman PC, Lewis FR. Severe chest trauma: morbidity implication. *Arch Surg* 1978; **113:** 846–9.

26. Woodring JH, Fried AM, Hatfield DR, Stevens RK, Todd EP. Fractures of the first and second ribs: predictive value for arterial and bronchial injury. *Am J Roentgenol* 1982; **138:** 211–15.

27. Poole GV. Fracture of the upper ribs and injury to the great vessels. *Surg Gynecol Obstet* 1989; **169:** 275–82.

28. Gupta A, Jamshidi M, Rubin JR. Traumatic first rib fracture: is angiography necessary? A review of 730 cases. [Review] [21 refs]. *Cardiovasc Surg* 1997; **5:** 48–53.

29. Spence EK, Rosato EF. The slipping rib syndrome. *Arch Surg* 1983; **118:** 1330–2.

30. Abbou S, Herman J. Slipping rib syndrome. *Postgrad Med* 1989; **86:** 75–8.

31. Copeland GP, Machin Dg, Shennan JM. Surgical treatment of the slipping rib. *Br J Surg* 1984; **71:** 522–3.

32. Parry WYN, Breckenridge I, Khalil YF. Bilateral clicking ribs. *Thorax* 1989; **44:** 72–3.

33. Wojcik JB. Sternal fractures – the natural history. *Ann Emerg Med* 1988; **17:** 912–14.

34. Hills MW, Delprado AM, Deane SA. Sternal fractures: associated injuries and management. *J Trauma* 1993; **35:** 55–60.

35. Schwagten V, Beaucourt L, Van SP. Traumatic manubriosternal joint disruption: case report. *J Trauma* 1994; **36:** 747–8.

36. Kumar AS, Puri K, Mittal VK, *et al.* Myocardial contusion following non-fatal blunt chest trauma. *J Trauma* 1983; **23:** 327–31.

37. Holliday RL. Myocardial contusion in chest trauma. *Can J Surg* 1983; **26:** 43–5.

38. Sturm JT, Luxenberg MG, Moudry BM, Perry JF Jr. Does sternal fracture increase the risk for aortic rupture? *Ann Thorac Surg* 1989; **48:** 697–8.

39. Thompson DA, Flynn TC, Miller PW, Fischer RP. The significance of scapular fractures. *J Trauma* 1985; **25:** 974–7.

40. McGahan JP, Rab GT, Dublin A. Fractures of the scapula. *J Trauma* 1980; **20:** 880–3.

41. Blue JM, Anglen JO, Helikson MA. Fracture of the scapula with intrathoracic penetration. A case report. *J Bone Joint Surg [Am]* 1997; **79:** 1076–8.

42. Sampson LN, Britton JC, Eldrup-Jorgensen J, Clark DE, Rosenberg JM, Bredenberg CE. The neurovascular outcome of scapulothoracic dissociation. *J Vasc Surg* 1993; **17:** 1083–8.

43. Kaar TK, Rice JJ, Mullan GB. Fracture-dislocation of the shoulder with intrathoracic displacement of the humeral head. [Review] [4 refs]. *Injury* 1995; **26:** 638–9.

44. Godley CD, McCabe CJ, Warren RL, Rosenberg WS. Traumatic subarachnoid-pleural fistula: case report.

[Review] [21 refs]. *J Trauma* 1995; **38:** 808–11.

45. Chiu WC, D'Amelio LF, Hammond JS. Sternal fractures in blunt chest trauma: a practical algorithm for management. *Am J Emerg Med* 1997; **15:** 252–5.

46. Heyes FL, Vincent R. Sternal fracture: what investigations are indicated? *Injury* 1993; **24:** 113–15.

18

Injury to the esophagus

CAMERON D WRIGHT AND HERMES C GRILLO

The etiology of esophageal injuries is diverse (Table 18.1) but the majority of injuries are iatrogenic in nature (Fig 18.1).[1] A recent review of 511 cases of esophageal perforation collected from several recent series indicated that 51% were iatrogenic, 19% were due to trauma and 16% were spontaneous.[1] The paucity of trauma as a cause reflects both the number of proce-

Table 18.1 *Etiology of esophageal injuries*

Instrumentation
• Esophagoscopy
• Dilation
• Pneumatic dilation for achalasia
• Esophageal tubes (nasogastric tubes, Sengstaken–Blakemore tubes, stents)
• Endotracheal tubes
Operative injury
• Spine surgery
• Thyroidectomy
• Mediastinoscopy
• Pulmonary resection
• Leiomyoma resection
• Aortic surgery
• Vagotomy
Trauma
• Penetrating
• Blunt
Barogenic (spontaneous)
• Postemetic (Boerhaave's syndrome)
• Other
Pneumatic
Foreign bodies
Caustic ingestion
• Acids
• Alkalis
• Pharmaceuticals

dures done on or around the esophagus and also the protection it enjoys deep in the chest.

Instrumentation is the most common cause of iatrogenic perforation. Esophagoscopy causes about one-third of all instrumental perforations and occurs in about 0.1% of all simple upper endoscopies (Fig 18.2).[1] The most common site of perforation at endoscopy is the cricopharyngeal area, the narrowest and tightest sphincter in the esophagus. Pneumatic dilatation for achlasia is occasionally (1–5%) complicated by perforation.[2] Bougienage dilatation of the esophagus is also occasionally (0.25–1%) complicated by perforation, especially in tighter angulated strictures. Any tube placed in the esophagus, whether intended or inadver-

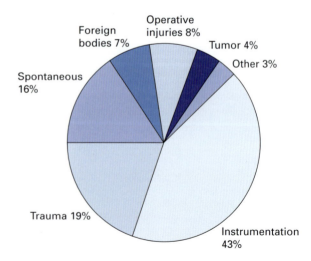

Figure 18.1 *The distribution of the causes of esophageal perforation. (Data from Jones WG, Ginsberg RJ. Esophageal perforation: a continuing challenge. Ann Thorac Surg 1992; 53: 534–43.)[1]*

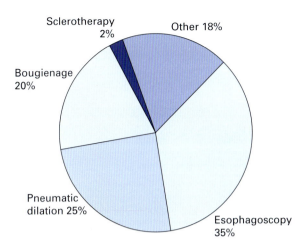

Figure 18.2 *The distribution of the causes of instrumental perforation of the esophagus. (Data from Jones WG, Ginsberg RJ. Esophageal perforation: a continuing challenge. Ann Thorac Surg 1992; 53: 534–43.)*[1]

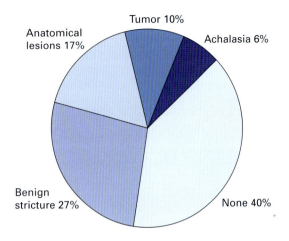

Figure 18.3 *The distribution of underlying diseases in cases of esophageal perforation. (Data from Jones WG, Ginsberg RJ. Esophageal perforation: a continuing challenge. Ann Thorac Surg 1992; 53: 534–43.)*[1]

tent, may cause a perforation. Not surprisingly, the majority of patients with esophageal perforation have underlying esophageal disease which either leads to the instrumentation or predisposes to a tear (Fig 18.3).[1] Operative injury to the esophagus may rarely occur during the course of any periesophageal surgery. Due to its intimate adherence to the spine, thyroid, trachea and aorta, the esophagus is at risk when operating on these structures. Cancer or severe inflammation around the esophagus can erode normal landmarks and enhances the possibility of an esophageal injury. If identified intraoperatively, prompt repair usually is without postoperative sequela. Not uncommonly, the injury is not detected until late postoperatively with resultant significantly increased morbidity.

Blunt trauma is a rare cause of esophagal injury.[1,3] The location of the esophagus deep within the rigid chest, together with the simplicity and strength of this muscular tube probably contribute to its relative freedom from injury. When blunt injury does occur, it occurs most often in the neck where there is less protection. Crushing, hyperextension and garroting-type injuries are the usual mechanisms of injury. The airway is often also injured, which complicates both diagnosis and treatment. Deceleration injuries and blunt abdominal trauma can also cause barogenic-type esophageal injuries due to excessive intraesophageal pressure against a closed glottis. These tears are similar in presentation to typical barogenic injuries with the low left intrathoracic esophagus commonly injured.

Barogenic or spontaneous perforations have a common mechanism, elevated intraesophageal pressure, which unites the apparently disparate causes. The term 'spontaneous perforation' is really a misnomer as they never occur spontaneously, but require forceful elevation of intraesophageal pressure to tear the esophagus.[4] The causes include vomiting (Boerhaave's

syndrome), childbirth, weightlifting and blunt abdominal trauma (Fig 18.4). The usual site for the tear is low on the left side and most are through the pleura. The reverse process has also been rarely reported, namely pneumatic rupture of the esophagus due to transoral insufflation of pressurized gas.[5] Experimental rupture of the esophagus occurs at an average pressure of 5 p.s.i. (34.5 kPa). Only 18 cases of pneumatic disruption of the esophagus have been reported. The esophagus can be ruptured anywhere along its length. The source of the compressed gas can be from a tire, a high pressure line, exploding air tanks or even from brewing beer in an unvented tank.

Foreign bodies can perforate the esophagus by direct puncture, by pressure necrosis or by attempted extraction.[6] Food foreign bodies frequently get stuck due to underlying esophageal obstruction, usually due to a stricture. Children frequently swallow foreign objects which, if large or irregular in shape, stay in the esophagus. Adults usually have bones or portions of dentures stuck in the esophagus. Patients in psychiatric hospitals and prisoners account for many of the adult patients with non-food foreign bodies (Fig 18.5).

Caustic injuries to the esophagus usually occur as a result of ingesting either strong acids or alkalis. Alkalis tend to cause liquefaction necrosis whereas acids tend to cause coagulation necrosis.[7] Either can produce full thickness necrosis of the esophagus. Ingestion tends to be accidental in children and intentional in adults who wish to commit suicide. Small batteries such as are used in calculators have a high concentration of strong alkalis and are commonly ingested by children. If the outer protective shell of the battery is breached, the alkali can leak out and cause severe injury to the esophagus. Various pharmaceuticals, including potassium chloride (tablets), some antibiotics and antiarrhythmics, may cause serious esophageal mucosal injury.[8] Sedated

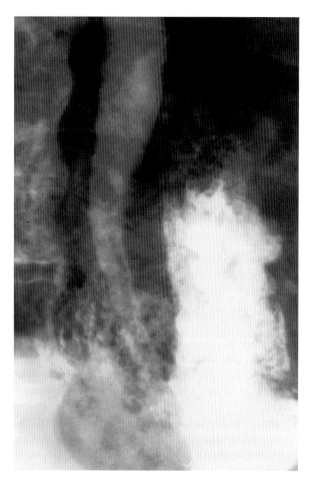

Figure 18.4 *Esophagogram of a patient who presented late after a barogenic perforation from vomiting (Borhaave's syndrome). Note extensive air in the mediastinum and large mediastinal collection of extravasated contrast. The patient had a successful outcome with buttressed primary repair.*

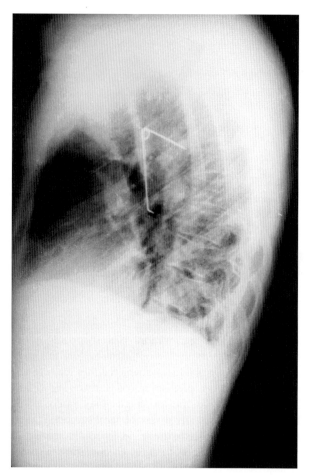

Figure 18.5 *Plain lateral chest radiograph demonstrating large open pin in the esophagus. The patient was psychotic and habitually swallowed foreign bodies. The pin was successfully removed by pulling it into a rigid esophagoscope. The minute perforation by the pin tip sealed itself.*

patients in the recumbent position in the intensive care unit (ICU) seem to be the most likely to be affected. Patients with pre-existing esophagitis and motility disorders or strictures are more likely to suffer injury. Esophagitis and stricture formation commonly result from these injuries but perforation has also been reported.

CLINICAL FEATURES

Manifestations differ in cervical and thoracic perforations (Fig 18.6).[9] In cervical perforations, subcutaneous emphysema is commonly present and is closely followed by pneumomediastinum. Pleural abnormalities and shock are less commonly seen than in thoracic perforations. Perforations of the thoracic esophagus are not usually associated with subcutaneous emphysema but have frequent pleural abnormalities and are more commonly associated with shock and dyspnea. Almost

all patients who have perforations have pain if they are conscious. Patients with barogenic perforations usually describe severe pain suddenly appearing after forceful vomiting. The pain in thoracic perforations is often localized to the subxiphoid region and thus attention is drawn away from the chest and esophagus. The differential diagnosis usually includes abdominal catastrophes such as pancreatitis or a perforated ulcer. Common misdiagnoses also include pneumonia, spontaneous pneumothorax, aortic dissection, and myocardial infarction. Patients with thoracic perforation usually appear gravely ill with the outward appearance of shock.

DIAGNOSIS

Early diagnosis of esophageal perforations is important as the mortality rate is a function of the time between perforation and treatment.[10,11] Perforations following

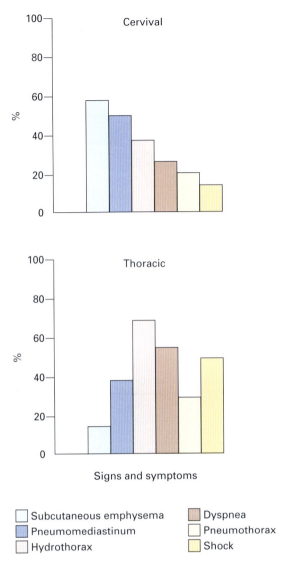

Signs and symptoms

☐ Subcutaneous emphysema		■ Dyspnea	
■ Pneumomediastinum		☐ Pneumothorax	
☐ Hydrothorax		☐ Shock	

Figure 18.6 *Differences in presentation between cervical and thoracic perforations. (Modified from Michel L, Grillo HC, Malt RA. Operative and nonoperative management of esophageal perforation. Ann Surg 1981; **194:** 57–63, with permission.)*[9]

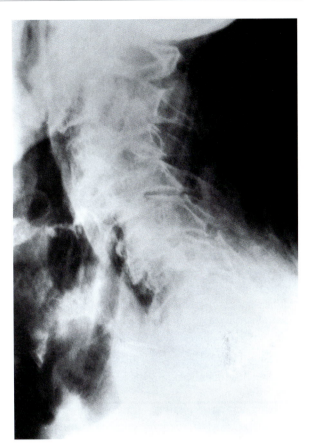

Figure 18.7 *Plain film of the lateral neck in a patient with neck pain following routine esophagoscopy. Extensive deep and subcutaneous emphysema is present. Treatment was by cervical drainage alone with a good result.*

instrumentation are often found sooner due to the heightened suspicions of medical personnel. The presence of neck, chest or abdominal pain after esophagoscopy should always be assumed to be due to a perforation until proven otherwise. Non-iatrogenic esophageal perforation is uncommon so the diagnosis is often not considered by emergency room physicians or cardiologists who often first see the patient.

The physical examination of patients with esophageal perforation is quite variable. Patients with cervical perforations initially often do not appear toxic. As previously mentioned, most patients with thoracic perforations are quite toxic and are readily diagnosed as appearing ill. Most patients will be febrile with a tachycardia. Patients presenting late will often be hypotensive. Patients with cervical perforations may have stiff necks with tenderness to palpation and readily evident cervical subcutaneous emphysema. Patients with extensive emphysema involving the head and neck often have a peculiar nasal quality to their voice which is easily recognized once it is first heard. Patients with thoracic perforations frequently have evidence of a pleural effusion on physical examination. Most patients with low thoracic perforations have upper abdominal tenderness and guarding which can initially confuse the examiner.

Plain film findings vary, depending on the location of the perforation and the time course of the perforation. Plain film findings include cervical or mediastinal emphysema, pneumothorax, pneumopericardium and pleural effusion (Fig 18.7). Computed tomographic (CT) findings of esophageal perforation include mediastinal emphysema, cavities adjacent to the esophagus and the mediastinum or pleural space and demonstration of a communication between the air- or contrast-filled esophagus and an adjacent mediastinal collection (Fig 18.8).

A contrast esophagogram is the standard diagnostic procedure used to confirm and localize an esophageal perforation. In addition, coexisting esophageal pathology is often delineated and the extent of contamination can be ascertained (Fig 18.9). Most radiologists use

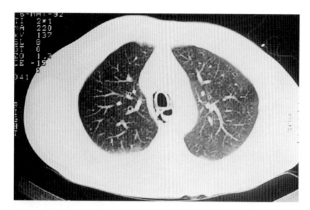

Figure 18.8 *CT of a patient with chest pain after vomiting. The plain chest film was normal and the treating emergency physician ordered this CT to investigate further. Air is present around both the trachea and esophagus. A subsequent esophagogram was negative for leak. Esophagoscopy confirmed a 4 cm long tear in the low esophagus, which was successfully repaired.*

a water-soluble contrast agent to avoid potential mediastinal contamination with barium. Some prefer dilute barium for enhanced mucosal detail and concerns about aspirating water-soluble contrast. Nevertheless, if a water-soluble contrast examination is negative and perforation is highly suspected, the esophagogram examination should be repeated with barium because of its higher accuracy. The false-negative rate of an esophogram for perforation approaches 10%.[1]

Esophagoscopy is useful in detecting esophageal perforation most commonly in the situation of trauma when it is not possible to perform an esophogram prior to proceeding to the operating room. In that situation, a careful endoscopic examination of the esophagus is very helpful in detecting and localizing perforations. The flexible endoscope is most useful for this purpose but the region around the cricoid is often poorly visualized due to the sphincter and lack of distensibility. For this one region, a rigid esophagoscopy is often preferable. However, an injury to the cervical spine should be excluded prior to proceeding to rigid esophagoscopy. Esophagoscopy is also useful in assessing non-traumatic perforation. The examination is best done with a flexible endoscope with minimal insufflation. It is particularly useful in cases where the esophagogram is negative or equivocal and in deciding which patients to select for conservative treatment. Information such as extent of tear, the condition of the mucosa and coexisting pathology can facilitate decision making.

TREATMENT

Treatment of esophageal perforation is individualized and depends on the presentation of the patient. Therapy

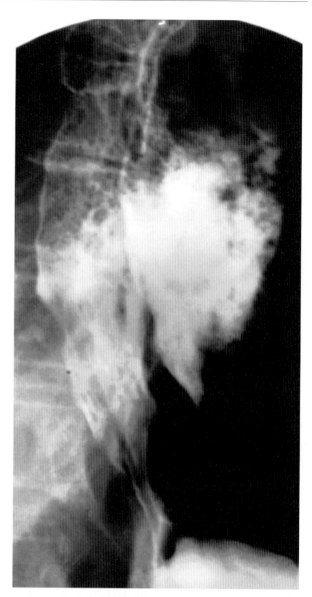

Figure 18.9 *Esophagogram of a patient with achalasia who suffered a tear during pneumatic dilatation. Note extensive extravasation of contrast and the dilated esophagus. A buttressed primary repair was performed as well as an esophagomyotomy on the opposite side with a successful result.*

is dependent upon the location of the perforation, the condition of the patient, the presence of underlying esophageal disease, time since perforation, and whether or not the perforation is free or contained. An algorithm for the treatment of esophageal perforation is detailed in Fig 18.10. Most, if not all, cervical perforations should be operatively explored and drained (Fig 18.11). Identifying and suturing the perforation is of secondary importance and is probably unnecessary in the majority of cases. The morbidity of this approach is extremely small whilst the benefits potentially are great. Several series have documented essentially no mortality with an aggressive operative approach whereas the non-

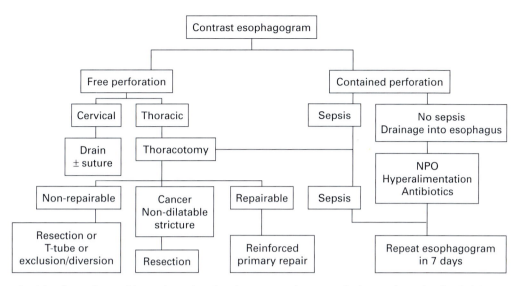

Figure 18.10 *Algorithm for patients with esophageal perforation. An esophagogram is the starting point for decision analysis.*

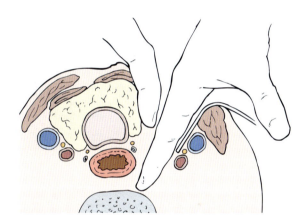

Figure 18.11 *Drainage of the cervical esophagus along the anterior border of the sternocleidomastoid muscle between the thyroid and carotid sheath.*

operative approach to a cervical perforation is occasionally followed by death.[1,11,12] Perforations are drained through the avascular plane between the carotid sheath and lateral border of the thyroid along the anterior border of the sternal cleidomastoid muscle. This approach provides entrance to the retrovisceral space with opportunity for irrigation and drainage of this space. Even if the perforation is not found, any resulting leak or fistula will soon close with good drainage (Fig 18.12).

The majority of thoracic perforations should be operated upon and the majority should be repairable. Pleural debridement and decortication are performed if necessary. This allows complete re-expansion of the lung to eliminate potential spaces and the possibility of postoperative empyema. The mediastinum is widely opened and debrided of all necrotic debris and tissue. By eliminating dead space, possible empyema and local-ized necrotic tissue, the possibility of secondary break-down of the esophageal repair is minimized. Usually the rent in the muscle of the esophagus is smaller than that of the mucosa so that the muscle must be more fully opened to expose the full extent of the mucosal tear (Fig 18.13). Failure to do so will lead to failure of the repair. The esophageal muscle is very often necrotic surrounding the tear so it must be debrided back to healthy muscle. It is uncommon for the mucosa to be necrotic or significantly destroyed. Nevertheless, the edges of the mucosa in long-standing perforations may have granulation tissue or poorly viable tissue and this must be debrided back to healthy tissue. The tear is then closed in two layers with fine interrupted sutures. Occasionally necrosis or induration of the muscle prohibits two-layer closure and only the mucosa can be closed. The mucosal layer is closed with an inverting technique, maintaining tension on the previously placed suture to facilitate mucosal inversion. A buttress is then carefully sewn over the repair. Intercostal muscle is most commonly used, but thickened pleura, stomach or omentum can also be used (Fig 18.14). The repair is tested by injection of air in a nasogastric tube with occlusion of the distal esophagus while under saline solution or by methylene blue injection.

Because this repair is performed in a contaminated field, buttressing of the repair is prudent. This provides an extra layer of protection to reduce the risk of a leak and if a leak should occur, contains it. Experimental evidence in animals and clinical series report a reduction in clinically significant leaks if repairs are buttressed.[13,14] Intercostal muscle is used preferentially due to its bulk, blood supply and arch of rotation. Omentum is useful in the late complicated situation.[15] Pleura and the fundus of the stomach can also be used as a buttress.[16] Pleura should not be used in early perforations due to its lack of substance and vascularity. With

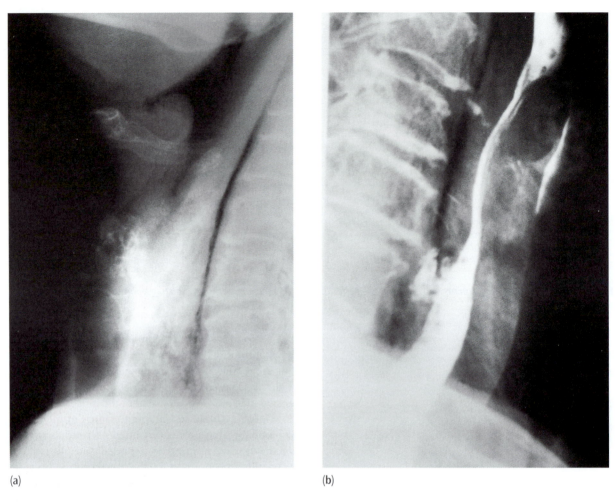

(a)

(b)

Figure 18.12 *(a) Plain film of the lateral neck in a patient who presented several days after an esophagoscopy with neck pain and dysphagia. Note air in visceral space and widening of space between trachea and spine. (b) Esophagogram of same patient confirming perforation. Successful result with drainage alone.*

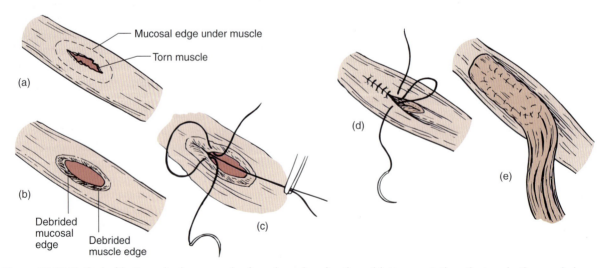

Figure 18.13 *Method of buttressed primary repair of esophageal perforations. (a) At presentation, the tear in the muscle is frequently not as large as the mucosal tear. (b) Both muscle and mucosa have been debrided back to healthy margins and all of the mucosal tear has been exposed. (c) Mucosal closure with fine interrupted inverting sutures. (d) Muscle closure (if possible). (e) Intercostal muscle flap used to buttress repair. The muscle is sutured circumferentially around the repair, not just tacked down. (From Wright CD, Mathisen DJ, Wain JC, et al. Reinforced primary repair of thoracic esophageal perforations. Ann Thorac Surg 1995; **60:** 245–49, with permission.)[10]*

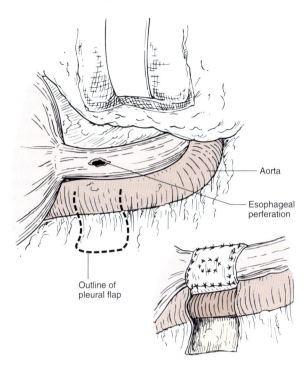

Figure 18.14 *Pleura can be used in chronic perforations after it has become thickened and well vascularized. The pedicle should be broad to preserve its blood supply. Pleura should not be relied upon in acute perforations when it is thin and flimsy. (From Grillo HC, Wilkens EW. Esophageal repair following late diagnosis of intrathoracic perforation. Ann Thorac Surg 1975; **20:** 387–99, with permission.)*[16]

time and inflammation, pleura can become quite robust and well vascularized and can then act as a reasonable buttress. Chest tubes are then placed in the gutter next to the repair and along the diaphragm. The chest cavity is thoroughly cleansed before closure. A separate small laparotomy is then made and a draining gastrostomy and feeding jejunostomy are performed. Enteral feeding by jejunostomy is begun as soon as bowel function returns. Adequate drainage of the stomach seems important to avoid reflux of gastric contents onto the repair. Broad spectrum antibiotics are administered, especially directed at mouth anaerobes and directed by culture results. A water-soluble contrast esophagogram is routinely performed on postoperative day 7 to check for leaks. If a leak does occur, it almost always is contained, asymptomatic and heals with observation only (Fig 18.15).[10] We believe this is due in large part to the additional buttress which is provided over the repair. Several authors including ourselves have reported good results with the results of primary repair of intrathoracic esophageal perforations regardless of whether they are early or late (Table 18.2).[10,14,17–19] Mortality is relatively low and remains concentrated in patients who present late after their perforations.

If any distal obstruction is present, the repair is at a greater risk of failure. Patients with dilatable strictures

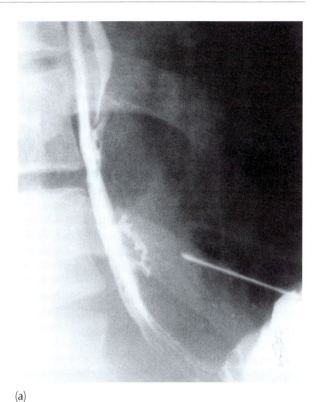

(a)

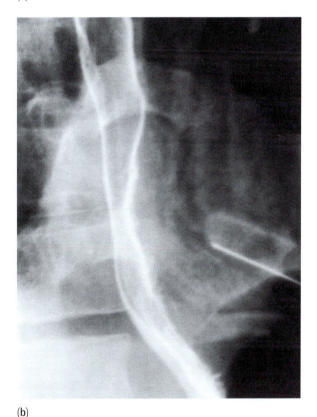

(b)

Figure 18.15 *(a) Esophagogram of a patient 1 week after buttressed repair of a postemetic perforation. The buttress used was intercostal muscle. A very small leak is seen which was asymptomatic. Fluoroscopy confirmed complete drainage of contrast back into the esophagus. (b) Esophagogram 1 week later confirms complete healing.*

Table 18.2 *Recent results with primary repair of intrathoracic esophageal perforations*

Author	Number	Iatrogenic (%)	Repair >24 h (%)	Leak rate (%)	Mortality (%)
Gouge	14	43	79	14	0
Ohri	9	55	55	30	10
Whyte	22	82	41	18	5
Wright	28	36	46	25	14
Wang	18	50	39	50	17

who are perforated during instrumentation, for example, should have completion of their dilatation performed intraoperatively followed by repair of the proximal perforation. Likewise, patients with achalasia who are perforated during pneumatic dilatation should have complete relief of their muscular obstruction with a myotomy carried down onto the stomach on the opposite side of the perforation (see Fig 18.9).[2]

Resection is necessary when there has been a perforation of a resectable cancer, a non-dilatable stricture or if the esophagus is not repairable.[20,21] When the diagno-

sis is made promptly and sepsis is not present, primary reconstruction of the gastrointestinal tract is undertaken with the standard mobilization and advancement of a gastric tube with esophagogastrostomy. When the diagnosis has been made late and especially if sepsis is present, reconstruction is usually best delayed and an end cervical esophagostomy is performed (Fig 18.16). The stomach is then drained with a gastrostomy and a jejunostomy is performed for feeding. Reconstruction is done at a later date, usually with the stomach.

Rarely, a perforation is present that is not readily repairable and the patient is not a candidate for a major operative procedure. In that case an esophageal T-tube has been used to convert the leak into a controlled fistula.[12] Upon adequate healing, the T-tube can be removed and the fistulous tract allowed to slowly close (Fig 18.17). It is important in these cases not to allow the T-tube to rest against the aorta to prevent a possible aortoesophageal fistula. Exclusion and diversion has been utilized by some authors for the treatment of the majority of esophageal perforations but most reserve it for the unusual case if the perforation is not amenable to primary buttressed repair.[22–25] Side or end cervical esophagostomy can be performed and the stomach

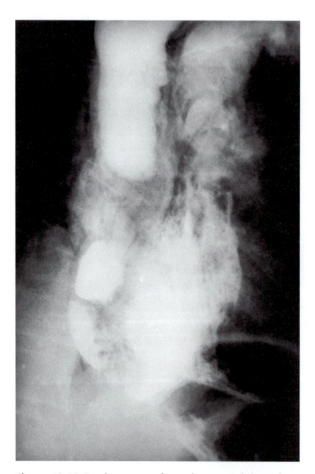

Figure 18.16 *Esophagogram of a patient several days after a postemetic perforation. The patient was in shock and renal failure. Content material widely extended into the mediastinum and pleura. Exploration revealed complete necrosis of the lower esophagus around the perforation so resection was performed. The patient survived and was later reconstituted with a substernal stomach reconstruction.*

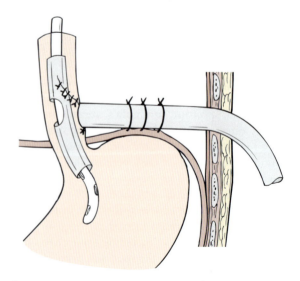

Figure 18.17 *T-tube placed through partially closed esophagus tear to convert to a controlled fistula. (From Bufkin BL, Miller JI, Mansour KA. Esophageal perforation: emphasis on management. Ann Thorac Surg 1996; **61**: 1447–52, with permission.)[12]*

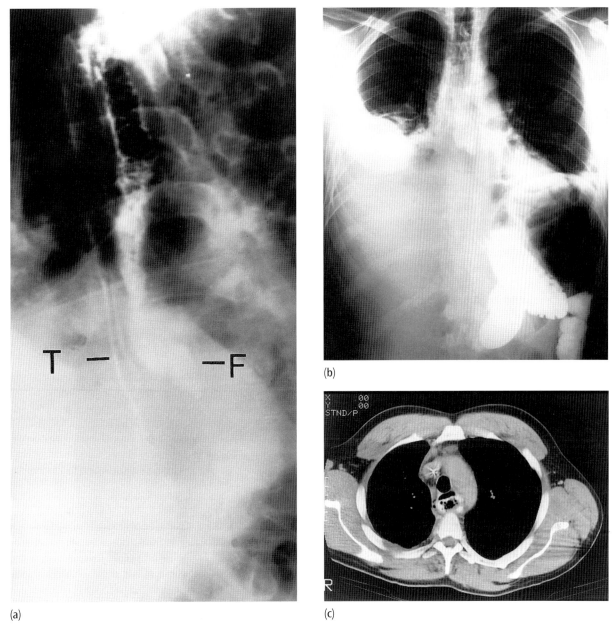

Figure 18.18 *(a) Patient with a dissection of the mucosa of the esophagus, an unusual variant of a 'contained' perforation. Oblique view of esophagogram demonstrating true (T) lumen to the left with contrast coating the esophagus distally and the false (F) lumen ending in a blind pouch within the esophagus. This patient previously underwent flexible esophagoscopy and insertion of the endoscope was noted to be difficult. He had severe pain and dysphagia after the procedure. Other views of the esophagogram confirmed the entry site of this dissection to be at the cricopharyngeal area. (b) Plain film of the chest in the same patient showing residual contrast in the false lumen and a loculated right pleural effusion. (c) CT scan of same patient demonstrating true lumen of esophagus anteriorly and false lumen (filled with air bubbles and contrast) posteriorly. The patient required a decortication of the empyema but did not require any procedure in the esophagus. Esophagogram in 1 week showed decreased size of false lumen and in 2 weeks was normal.*

contents can be excluded from the esophagus by various means including ligatures or staples around the esophagogastric junction. Following healing of the perforation and the return to wellbeing of the patient, the esophagostomy is reversed. Exclusion of the esophagus is reversed by removal of the ligature or bougienage of the occluding staples. Sometimes the esophagus cannot

be salvaged at that time necessitating esophageal replacement with either the stomach or colon. Endoesophageal stents are occasionally useful in the treatment of esophageal perforation, especially when a cancerous stricture has been dilated and perforated. If the perforation is contained, usually nothing need be done but if the perforation is uncontained an endoesophageal stent is usually the best treatment option. Surprisingly, this therapy, along with nutritional support and antibiotics, is frequently successful.

Non-operative therapy is not commonly employed in the treatment of esophageal perforations but is appropriate in certain highly selected circumstances. Limited contained esophageal perforations due to instrumentation that are diagnosed early are occasionally appropriate for this therapy as are perforations that present late with minimal symptoms and that have already weathered the test of time. There should not be distal obstruction present on the esophagogram and the patient should exhibit no signs of sepsis. The perforation should be well contained and the contrast material should promptly drain back into the esophagus and not stay within a large cavity. The perforation should not be intra-abdominal nor should it be adjacent to the aorta or trachea. Undrained perforations (or collections) adjacent to the aorta or trachea have not uncommonly fistulized to these two organs, resulting in a fatal outcome. Patients selected for this therapy are prohibited from eating or drinking and are usually hyperalimented since they will not be eating for at least 7–10 days. Broad spectrum antibiotics are administered. Careful clinical and radiological monitoring is necessary to ensure any complications or decline in clinical condition are rapidly dealt with. If non-operative therapy fails, prompt conversion to an operative approach is mandatory. In the presence of continued clinical improvement, a repeat esophagogram should be obtained prior to reinstitution of oral intake. The majority of 'leaks' after buttressed primary repair can be managed conservatively, secure in the knowledge that the leak is contained by a viable flap of covering tissue (see Fig 18.14).[10] An unusual type of perforation, that of the dissection of the mucosa away from the muscle wall in the submucosal plane, is shown in Fig 18.18. The mechanism of injury is usually either a tear at the cricopharyngeal area from insertion of an esophagoscope or a tear at the leading edge of a stricture during dilation. These dissection perforations usually heal without operation.

The initial focus of patients presenting with caustic ingestion injuries is identifying the agent and delineating the extent of injury. The majority of children who have a caustic ingestion immediately spit out the chemical due to its noxious taste. Accordingly, the damage tends to be mostly to the oropharynx with little involvement of the esophagus. Rare cases of sole esophageal involvement have been reported, so any history of ingestion should be fully investigated regardless of the presence or absence of oral burns. The larynx may be injured as well and occasionally may cause airway obstruction. Any hoarseness or stridor should be fully investigated and tracheostomy may be necessary. Adults who attempt suicide tend to drink much larger amounts of caustic agents and thus have more severe injuries.

Usually the treatment is supportive as long as there is no perforation or full thickness necrosis. Plain films can help localize perforations or suggest full thickness necrosis. Computed tomographic scans usually show extensive thickening of the affected organ with surrounding inflammatory changes. If a large amount of liquid has been ingested, insertion of a nasogastric tube may be helpful to assess the pH of the stomach contents. However, insertion of a nasogastric tube in a recently injured esophagus is not without risk and should be carefully assessed by the treating physician. Endoscopy is the mainstay of diagnosis and generally should be performed under general anesthesia so that optimal conditions are present.[26] Usually the flexible endoscope should be used but minimal insufflation is necessary to minimize the risk of perforation. Traditional teaching has been to stop once mucosal injury is reached for fear of perforation. We believe that careful endoscopy beyond the point of initial injury yields valuable information such as the depth of injury, the distal extent of injury and involvement of the stomach. A lumen must be carefully followed to prohibit undue pressure on the wall and the procedure should be terminated if passage is unclear due to the pathological process. The injury can be graded as follows:

- grade 1 – mucosal erythema
- grade 2 – non-circumferential deep mucosal burns/necrosis
- grade 3 – circumferential deep mucosal burns/necrosis.

Severe strictures invariably follow grade 3 injuries.

Treatment involves fluid resuscitation, antibiotics, prohibiting oral intake and nutritional support. Laparotomy is necessary for peritoneal signs, evidence of gastric perforation, or a persistent alkaline pH reading on the nasogastric tube aspirate. Esophagectomy is required for evidence of full thickness esophageal necrosis or perforation. Other organs (liver, spleen, pancreas, duodenum) may need to be resected or debrided if necrosis has extended to them. Restoration of gastrointestinal continuity is delayed until complete recovery occurs. Steroids used to be administered to ameliorate the expected esophageal stricture in instances of partial or full thickness esophageal injury. A recent prospective randomized study in pediatric patients concluded there was no benefit in steroid administration.[27] Since steroids have serious side-effects, their routine use is no longer recommended. The management of the anticipated esophageal stricture is usually expectant with early dilation. Other authors recommend immediate gastrostomy for passage of a string through the esophagus to facilitate future retrograde dilation or placement of an indwelling endoesophageal stent.[28]

Patients with esophageal foreign bodies are usually best managed by extraction with rigid esophagoscopy under general anesthesia.[29] Occasionally a fiberoptic

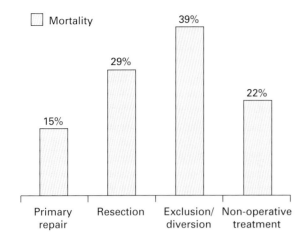

Figure 18.19 *Mortality rates according to treatment among 589 patients with esophageal perforation. (Data from Jones WA, Ginsberg RJ. Esophageal perforation: a continuing challenge.* Ann Thorac Surg *1992;* **53:***534–43.)*[1]

extraction is appropriate but the airway must be protected. A variety of forceps should be available and ideally practiced on an identical object prior to the extraction. Flexible snares are often helpful. Papain should not be used to 'dissolve' meat impactions in an effort to avoid esophagoscopy as perforation has been reported.[6] Sharp objects that perforate the esophagus should be thoughtfully removed as, rarely, they may perforate a vascular structure and require open removal.[30] An esophagogram should usually be obtained after extraction to check for perforation and define any underlying esophageal pathology.

RESULTS

A recent review of 13 collected series reporting on 589 patients reported an overall mortality of 22% for esophageal perforation (Fig 18.19).[1] Primary repair was associated with the lowest mortality although there was obvious selection bias present in the choice of therapy. Somewhat remarkable is the 22% mortality of patients treated non-operatively, emphasizing the necessity for careful selection for this approach. Recent reports have identified cause, location, delayed treatment, underlying disease and type of treatment as significant risk factors for death from esophageal perforation.[1] A trend towards earlier diagnosis and increasing survival has been noted in recent reports.[1,11] Iatrogenic injuries are more favorable than those due to barogenic mechanisms, probably due to the more limited injury with less contamination and to their earlier diagnosis. Barogenic perforations have a reported mortality rate of about 40%, whereas iatrogenic perforations usually result in a mortality rate of about 20%.[1]

Cervical esophageal perforations result in a mortality rate of only about 5%, whereas thoracic perforations usually result in a mortality rate of about 30%.[1] The reduced risk from cervical perforations is probably due to a combination of factors, including the confining anatomical tissue planes present in the neck, the rarity of coexisting disease in the cervical esophagus, and the absence of reflux of gastric contents.

Early diagnosis and treatment of esophageal perforation has long been recognized to be important to lead to a favorable result. Delay beyond 24 hours has been recognized as 'late' and is associated with higher complications, longer hospital stays and increased mortality.[1,10] In our experience, primary repair of early perforations yielded a mortality rate of 0, whereas those that were treated late had a mortality rate of 31%.[10] Patients who present with sepsis have an increased chance not only of leakage at the repaired site but also of death.

Patients with pre-existing esophageal disease appear to have an increased mortality, especially those with cancer. Lastly, the type of treatment is associated with different mortality rates. Reinforced primary repair is associated with the lowest mortality rates of any approach and is applicable in the majority of instances.[1]

REFERENCES

1. Jones WG, Ginsberg RJ. Esophageal perforation: a continuing challenge. *Ann Thorac Surg* 1992; **53:** 534–43.
2. Miller RE, Tiszenkel HI. Esophageal perforation due to pneumatic dilation for achalasia. *Surg Gynecol Obstet* 1988; **166:** 458–60.
3. Weiman DS, Walker WA, Brosnan KM, Pate JW, Fabian TC. Noniatrogenic esophageal trauma. *Ann Thorac Surg* 1995; **59:** 845–50.
4. Barrett NR. Spontaneous perforation of the oesophagus. *Thorax* 1946; **1:** 48–70.
5. Guth AA, Gouge TH, Depan HJ. Blast injury to the thoracic esophagus. *Ann Thorac Surg* 1991; **51:** 837–9.
6. Holsinger JW, Fuson RL, Sealy WC. Esophageal perforation following meat impaction and papain ingestion. *JAMA* 1968; **204:** 734.
7. Kirsh MM, Ritter F. Caustic ingestion and subsequent damage to the oropharyngeal and digestive passages. *Ann Thorac Surg* 1976; **21:** 74–82.
8. McCord GS, Clause RE. Pill-induced esophageal stricture: Clinical features and risk factors for development. *Am J Med* 1990; **88:** 512–18.
9. Michel L, Grillo HC, Malt RA. Operative and nonoperative management of esophageal perforations. *Ann Surg* 1981; **194:** 57–63.
10. Wright CD, Mathisen DJ. Wain JC, Moncure AC, Hilgenberg AD, Grillo HC. Reinforced primary repair of

thoracic esophageal perforation. *Ann Thorac Surg* 1995; **60:** 245–9.

11. Bladergroen MR, Lowe JE, Postlethwait RW. Diagnosis and recommended management of esophageal perforation and rupture. *Ann Thorac Surg* 1986; **42:** 235–9.

12. Bufkin BL, Miller JI, Mansour KA. Esophageal perforation: emphasis on management. *Ann Thorac Surg* 1996; **61:** 1447–52.

13. Bryant LR. Experimental evaluation of intercostal pedicle grafts in esophageal repair. *J Thorac Cardiovasc Surg* 1965; **50:** 626–33.

14. Gouge TH, Depan HJ, Spencer FC. Experience with the Grillo pleural wrap procedure in 18 patients with perforation of the thoracic esophagus. *Ann Surg* 1989; **209:** 612–19.

15. Mathisen DJ, Grillo HC, Vlahakes GJ, Daggett WM. The omentum in the management of complicated cardiothoracic problems. *J Thorac Cardiovasc Surg* 1988; **95:** 677–84.

16. Grillo HC, Wilkins EW. Esophageal repair following late diagnosis of intrathoracic perforation. *Ann Thorac Surg* 1975; **20:** 387–99.

17. Whyte RI, Iannettoni MD, Orringer MB. Intrathoracic esophageal perforation. *J Thorac Cardiovasc Surg* 1995; **109:** 140–6.

18. Wang N, Razzouk AJ, Safavi A, *et al.* Delayed primary repair of intrathoracic esophageal perforation: Is it safe? *J Thorac Cardiovasc Surg* 1996; **111:** 114–22.

19. Ohri SK, Liakakos TA, Pathi V, *et al.* Primary repair of iatrogenic thoracic esophageal perforation and Boerhaave's Syndrome. *Ann Thorac Surg* 1993; **55:** 603–6.

20. Orringer MG, Stirling MC. Esophagectomy for esophageal disruption. *Ann Thorac Surg* 1990; **49:** 35–43.

21. Salo JA, Isolauri JO, Heikkila LJ, *et al.* Management of delayed esophageal perforation with mediastinal sepsis. *J Thorac Cardiovasc Surg* 1993; **106:** 1088–91.

22. Urschel HC, Razzuk MA, Wood RE, *et al.* Improved management of esophageal perforation: exclusion and diversion in continuity. *Ann Surg* 1974; **179:** 587–91.

23. Chang CH, Lin PJ, Chang JP, *et al.* One-stage operation for treatment after delayed diagnosis of thoracic esophageal perforation. *Ann Thorac Surg* 1992; **53:** 617–20.

24. Bardini R, Bonavina L, Pavanello M. Temporary double exclusion of the perforated esophagus using absorbable staples. *Ann Thorac Surg* 1992; **54:** 1165–7.

25. Lee YC, Lee ST, Chun SH. New technique of esophageal exclusion for chronic esophageal perforation. *Ann Thorac Surg* 1991; **51:** 1020–2.

26. Zargar SA, Kochhar R, Mehta S, Mehta SK. The role of fiberoptic endoscopy in the management of corrosive ingestion and modified endoscopic classification of burns. *Gastrointest Endosc* 1991; **37:** 165–9.

27. Anderson KD, Rouse TM, Randolph JG. A controlled trial of corticosteroids in children with corrosive injury of the esophagus. *N Engl J Med* 1990; **323:** 637–40.

28. Mills LJ, Estrera AS, Platt MR. Avoidance of esophageal stricture following severe caustic burns by the use of an intraluminal stent. *Ann Thorac Surg* 1979; **28:** 60–5.

29. Webb WA. Management of foreign bodies of the upper gastrointestinal tract. *Gastroenterology* 1988; **94:** 204–16.

30. Yamada T, Sato H, Seki M, *et al.* Successful salvage of aortoesophageal fistula caused by a fish bone. *Ann Thorac Surg* 1996; **61:** 1843–5.

19

Airway trauma

EMILE A BACHA, DOUGLAS J MATHISEN AND HERMES C GRILLO

It is important for all surgeons involved in the care of trauma patients to understand the complexities of airway trauma. Even though an uncommon problem, it does occur with a relative and probably rising frequency.[1] The clinician must first recognize the injury, be aware of the common associated injuries, be familiar with the various techniques of airway management, and understand the principles of surgical repair of airway injuries. Successful management of airway injuries will not only save lives, but may also preserve the vocal cords and airway, precluding the need for lifelong tracheostomy.

HISTORICAL ASPECTS

One of the earliest descriptions of a tracheal injury was that of a sword wound treated by Ambroise Paré during the sixteenth century.[2] As initially reported by Seuvre in 1873, all cases of traumatic bronchial ruptures were thought to be uniformly fatal.[3] This view was rebutted by Krinitzki in 1927 when he reported the case of a young woman who survived 10 years following a complete right main stem rupture sustained after blunt chest trauma.[4] In 1931, Nissen described a 12-year-old girl with a delayed stricture at the site of a complete main stem bronchus rupture, and performed a subsequent successful pneumonectomy.[5] The first reported primary repair of a bronchial rupture resulting from blunt trauma was performed in 1947.[6] Repair of a total transection of the cervical trachea from blunt chest trauma was first reported in 1957.[7]

INCIDENCE

The true incidence of airway trauma is difficult to establish, because many patients sustaining trauma severe enough to cause such injuries die before reaching the hospital. Although it is a relatively rare injury, widespread mechanization and increased use of firearms have resulted in an increased incidence of airway injuries. Improved prehospital care has allowed more seriously injured patients to reach the hospital alive. In a classic treatise, Burke[1] reported a 10-fold increase in bronchial rupture between the first half of this century and the 1960s. Kemmerer and colleagues,[8] analyzing 585 deaths from traffic accidents over a 5-year period, found tracheobronchial transections in five patients (0.85%). Ecker et al.[9] reviewed tracheobronchial injuries over a 10-year period in Dallas County: only 105 patients were identified. Injury had resulted from penetrating trauma in 75 patients, and blunt trauma in 30. Eighty-one patients (70%) were dead on arrival. The cervical trachea was the most common location of injury in patients who survived, whereas among those who were dead on arrival the thoracic trachea was the most frequent site of injury. Most patients died from associated injury. Bertelsen and Howitz reviewed 1178 autopsies of blunt trauma victims and concluded that the incidence of tracheo-bronchial disruption was 2.8%, or 33 patients.[10] Of 33 patients, 27 died instantly, and 24 patients had severe associated injuries. Finally, Angood et al.[11] reported only 20 patients with injury to the larynx or cervical trachea out of more than 2000 patients with multisystem injuries treated at the Montreal General Hospital (Quebec, Canada) over a 10-year period.

ETIOLOGY

Blunt trauma

Damage from blunt cervical injury may occur in the airway at any level from the hyoid bone to the carina (Fig 19.1).[12–14] A sudden increase in airway pressure while the glottis remains closed can result in a linear rupture of the membranous trachea (Fig 19.1). Motor vehicle accidents resulting in rapid deceleration that causes the passenger to strike the extended neck against the dashboard or steering wheel produce the majority of laryngotracheal injuries ('padded dashboard syndrome'). Direct injury to the laryngotracheal area compresses the airway against the vertebral bodies, thereby resulting in a crushing injury. Hyperextension of the neck causes an avulsion injury by pulling the larynx away from the distal trachea, which is restricted in its excursion by surrounding tissue and the left main stem bronchus beneath the aortic arch. Striking the neck against an unseen wire or chain while riding a motorcycle or snowmobile accounts for a number of these injuries, the so-called clothesline injury (Fig 19.2).[12,15]

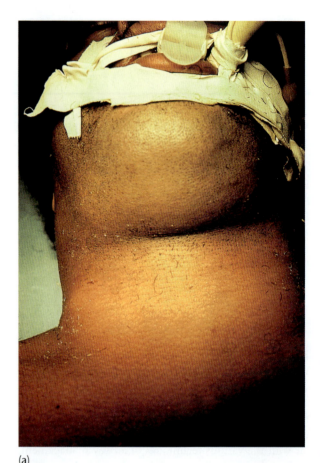

(a)

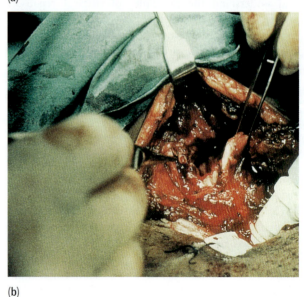

(b)

Figure 19.2 (a) Severe blunt trauma to the neck presenting with swelling stridor and hemoptysis. Urgent surgical intervention was required to establish an airway. This also revealed severe traumatic disruption of the larynx (b).

(a)

(b)

Figure 19.1 Schematic representation of transverse anterior injuries and linear tears of the membranous wall of the trachea.

Table 19.1 *Location of injuries*

	Blunt trauma			Penetrating trauma			Total
Cervical	28%	65	29%	77%	161	71%	226 (100%)
Thoracic trachea	27%	62	63%	17%	36	37%	98 (100%)
Bronchi	45%	105	90%	6%	12	10%	117 (100%)
Total	100%	232	–	100%	209	–	–

Compiled from references 9,12,14,16,17,20,23,37,46,48.

A direct blow to the chest or an acceleration/deceleration type injury produces sudden movement of the trachea around the relatively fixed points of the carina or cricoid, leading to shear forces that can result in transections, or linear tears of the membranous trachea.

Penetrating trauma

Penetrating trauma from stab wounds or gunshot wounds was thought to occur less frequently than blunt trauma (Table 19.1).[11,12] However, a steady increase in penetrating injuries to the trachea is noted, with gunshot wounds now predominating over stab wounds.[16,17] This is thought to be due to improved transportation of victims from the site of injury to medical facilities, and to the increased use of firearms.[16–18] Due to the intimate anatomical relationship of the airway to other neck structures, great vessels, lung and heart, there is a high incidence of serious associated injuries.

ANATOMY

The adult trachea measures 11 cm in average length from the inferior border of the cricoid cartilage to the carinal spur. There are 18–22 cartilaginous rings in the human trachea, with approximately two rings per centimeter.[19] The airway is elliptical in shape in the adult. The cricoid cartilage is the only complete cartilaginous ring, and the initial portion of the subglottic airway is intralaryngeal. The trachea courses from an immediately subcutaneous position in the neck anteriorly to a position against the esophagus and prevertebral fascia at the carinal level posteriorly. The membranous wall of the trachea is applied to the esophagus throughout its extent, with a plane of connective tissue between the two structures. The trachea is not a very extensible organ, and becomes more rigid with age. This explains why, with a closed glottis, a sudden increase in intraluminal airway pressure secondary to blunt trauma can result in longitudinal tears, usually along the weaker membranous wall. The most fixed points of the airway are the cricoid and the left main stem bronchus as it emerges under the aortic arch.

The relationships of the trachea to adjacent organs are fairly obvious. Anteriorly, the thyroid isthmus crosses the trachea at about the level of the second or third tracheal ring. The thyroid is fixed to the trachea laterally by connective tissue and vessels. Shortly below this the brachiocephalic artery courses obliquely across the anterior wall of the trachea. The brachiocephalic veins are anterior to this. The anterolateral surface below lies behind the aortic arch, which passes over the left main bronchus. The azygos vein arches over the right main stem bronchus and is adjacent to the tracheobronchial angle on that side. Laterally, the pleura is applied on the right with fibro-fatty node-containing tissue. The left recurrent nerve lies in close juxtaposition to the trachea along almost its entire length in the tracheoesophageal groove. It enters the larynx posterior to the cricoid cartilage at the level of the inferior cornu of the thyroid cartilage. On the right, the nerve approaches the trachea superiorly but ends in the same position.

The blood supply of the trachea and main bronchi is shared with the esophagus laterally. Above, the supply is from the inferior thyroid artery. The subclavian, supreme intercostal, internal thoracic, brachiocephalic, and superior and inferior bronchial arteries supply the remaining organ with fine lateral branches.

LOCATION OF INJURIES

Blunt trauma

Following blunt cervical trauma, the laryngotracheal junction, followed by the cervical trachea, is the most frequently injured area (Table 19.1).[11,12,20] After thoracic trauma, every level of the trachea and almost all the major bronchi have been reported to be involved. Most injuries occur within 2.5 cm of the carina.[21] In his evaluation of 130 cases of traumatic bronchial rupture, Burke[1] reported that injuries were equally divided between the right and left sides. The main stem bronchi were by far the most frequent sites of rupture. Eighty-six percent of the injuries involved the main bronchi. Those results were subsequently confirmed by Deslauriers *et al.* and Jones *et al.*[20,22]

Penetrating trauma

After penetrating trauma, the most commonly injured portion of the tracheobronchial tree is the cervical trachea (Table 19.1). One possible reason is that patients sustaining penetrating thoracic trauma are less likely to reach the hospital alive than patients with cervical penetrating trauma. In a large series from Charity Hospital and Tulane Medical Center, 106 patients with tracheobronchial injuries were admitted

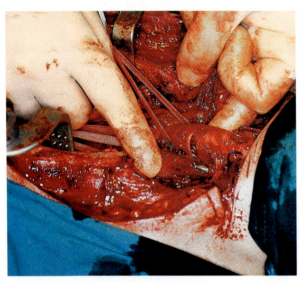

(a)

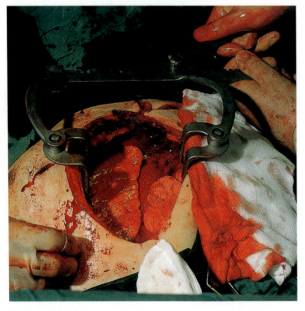

(b)

Figure 19.3 (a) Young female patient with multiple stab wounds to the chest and thoracic inlet. Median sternotomy has been performed to gain access to both sides of the chest (b). The principal injury was hemitransection of both the trachea and esophagus as shown.

over a 20-year period. One hundred patients had penetrating injuries, 78 of which involved the cervical trachea, 12 the thoracic trachea and 10 the major bronchi.[23] In a report describing 20 patients with penetrating tracheal trauma from Grady Memorial Hospital, 15 patients sustained injury to the cervical trachea (Fig 19.3).[17]

DIAGNOSIS

History and physical examination

INITIAL PRESENTATION

Airway trauma produces a spectrum of signs and symptoms that are often non-specific, and related to associated injuries. A high index of suspicion is imperative to avoid catastrophic consequences. Presentation may range from no visible external signs of trauma, to abrasion and contusion, to extensive laceration exposing cervical structures. The combination of the type of accident and the signs or symptoms of hemoptysis, localized pain, local contusion, subcutaneous emphysema, a change in voice, hoarseness, inspiratory stridor, or respiratory distress should alert the clinician to the possibility of airway injury. Sometimes, a crunching sound synchronous with the heart beat can be heard (Hamman's sign). Up to one-third of patients may be asymptomatic.[11] Early diagnosis is critical to avoid late complications. Injuries to the distal trachea and carina may present with these findings in addition to pneumothorax associated with a large air leak in which the lung fails to re-expand completely after placement of a chest tube (Fig 19.4). Dyspnea may sometimes worsen with suction. The presentation may be more subtle with a pneumothorax responding to pleural suction and cessation of air leak. Subcutaneous or mediastinal emphysema may be the only finding in injuries to the distal trachea. In a recent series, 85% of patients with tracheobronchial disruptions had subcutaneous emphysema, and 77% had dyspnea.[20] The airway itself may appear to be completely patent or be absent in an apneic patient. Some patients may have associated rib fractures or a flail chest segment.

LATE PRESENTATION

In 1959, Hood and Sloan[24] reviewed the literature and found that only 42% of bronchial injuries were diagnosed early (within 7 days), whereas 41% were diagnosed more than a month after injury. In a report by Taskinen et al., diagnosis was delayed in five of nine patients who presented with airway trauma.[25] All five developed dyspnea secondary to stricture formation at the site of injury. Delayed presentation following either

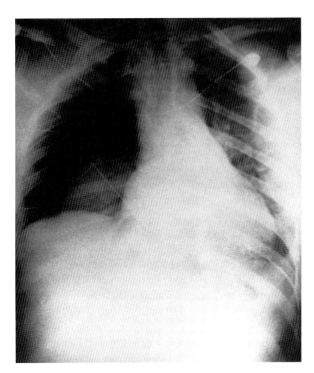

Figure 19.4 *Chest radiograph demonstrating large right-sided pneumothorax with the completely collapsed right lung lying in the cardiophrenic sulcus. This is a classic radiograph for a completely transected bronchus.*

initial management elsewhere or failure to diagnose was seen in 17 patients in a series from Massachusetts General Hospital (MGH).[12] Only one was due to a penetrating injury. The upper trachea was the most common location, and associated injuries consisted of esophageal injuries (three tracheoesophageal fistulae, one blind esophageal pouch), and vocal cord paralysis in 14 patients. All had symptomatic tracheal stenosis. In an effort to categorize patients presenting with airway trauma, Kirsh and associates distinguished between two groups of patients with a distinct clinical pattern.[21] In the first group, the site of disruption and the pleural space communicate freely (intrapleural rupture), and the classic signs of persistent lung collapse (Fig 19.4), large air leak, subcutaneous emphysema, and increased dyspnea with suction are seen. Hemoptysis may occur from disruption of a bronchial artery. The second group had little or no communication between the bronchus and the pleural space (extrapleural rupture), and hence, few symptoms were seen at the time of injury. Placement of a chest tube may re-expand the lung because the small communication between the lacerated airway and the pleural space can seal off with fibrin or blood clot. After chest tube removal, the lung may remain expanded. Initially, peribronchial tissues are firm enough to maintain airway continuity, and ventilation continues. The tear heals by granulation and epithelialization, which, in a matter of weeks, will obstruct the airway, rendering the lung atelectatic. A fibrous stricture then

develops. A favorable pathological condition occurs if the atelectatic lung remains uninfected, usually in cases of complete transections with complete occlusion and no communication with the proximal airway.[26] This condition offers the possibility of late reconstruction of the bronchus with salvage of the lung.[22] If the stricture results in partial bronchial obstruction, pulmonary infection and eventually irreversible pulmonary parenchymal destruction results.

Radiological findings

Radiological assessment is helpful, but excessive time should not be spent in preoperative studies because an apparently stable airway may acutely obstruct. Patients should never be left unattended while undergoing radiological evaluation. Plain radiographs of the neck may reveal distortion or disruption of the tracheal airway, hyoid bone elevation, or deep cervical emphysema, an early and reliable sign of airway injury. Radiographs of the cervical spine, contrast studies of the esophagus, and tomograms of the larynx and trachea may be helpful in evaluating less obvious injuries. In particular, a negative contrast study of the esophagus does not eliminate the need for a rigid esophagoscopy. A chest radiograph may reveal unilateral or bilateral pneumothorax, subcutaneous or mediastinal emphysema, peribronchial air, or fractured ribs. Mediastinal hematoma can indicate tracheobronchial injury, but could also be due to an aortic tear. With complete intrapleural bronchial separation, a so-called dropped lung can be seen, with the apex of the lung at the level of the hilum (Fig 19.4).[27]

Laboratory data

Patients with airway injuries often have low Pa_{O_2} values on arterial blood gases. Persistent hypoxia with oxygen administration or exacerbation of hypercapnia with mechanical ventilation should alert the clinician to the possibility of airway injury. A low hematocrit can be the result of associated injuries.

Computed tomography (CT)

CT has become the method of choice in the evaluation of laryngeal trauma and the planning of a reparative operation.[28] It is essential to accurately outline the type and degree of damage to the hyoid bone, arytenoids and the thyroid and cricoid cartilages.[28] However, it does not provide a functional assessment of vocal cord mobility. The role of CT scanning in the management of lower airway trauma is not well defined at this time.[29] In addition to findings usually depicted on the chest radiograph, such as rib fractures, pneumothoraces, mediastinal emphysema and pulmonary contusion, its greatest value lies in detecting a mediastinal hematoma, and associated injuries to the great vessels. An abrupt tapering of the ruptured main stem bronchus can be seen. A negative CT does not rule out airway trauma, nor does it obviate the need for bronchoscopy. Nuclear scans are used to assess long-term function after bronchoplastic repairs.[22]

ASSOCIATED INJURIES

Injuries of the magnitude sufficient to cause severe laryngotracheal or tracheobronchial damage may also cause injury to the esophagus, recurrent laryngeal nerves, larynx, cervical spine, or vascular structures. If time and circumstances permit, each patient should be carefully evaluated for these injuries.

Cervical spine

Cervical spine injuries may threaten the spinal cord and dictate the course of surgical management. The cervical spine must be stabilized initially following the standards set by the Advanced Trauma Life Support (ATLS) guidelines of the American College of Surgeons (Committee on Trauma, 1989). Extension or flexion of the neck to perform intubation, bronchoscopy, or esophagoscopy or to relieve tension on a tracheal anastomosis must be avoided in this situation, and urgent neurosurgical attention is mandatory. The airway can be assessed by flexible bronchoscopy (with an endotracheal tube passed over it), without neck flexion (Fig 19.5). Cervical spine radiographic series

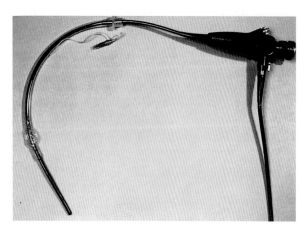

Figure 19.5 *A flexible bronchoscope with a small endotracheal tube threaded over. This is the best way to evaluate the airway when laryngotracheal trauma is suspected. If the bronchoscope can traverse the injured airway, it can serve as a guide to help advance the endotracheal tube.*

should be obtained in all cases, provided they do not delay an urgent surgical procedure. One series of 23 patients with tracheoesophageal injuries reported injuries to the cervicothoracic spinal cord in six patients.[13]

Esophagus

The cervical esophagus is frequently injured by accidents of this nature. In a recent series from MGH, six of 27 patients with laryngotracheal trauma were found to have an associated esophageal injury.[12] Other authors have had similar findings.[13,30] Contrast studies of the upper esophagus are helpful, but sometimes difficult to interpret. Esophagoscopy and direct inspection of the esophagus at the time of operation should be carried out when the possibility exists that the esophagus is involved. Esophageal injuries may be distant from the laryngeal or tracheal injury because of the distortion of tissue planes during traumatic impact. Direct insufflation of air through an esophagoscope while flooding the wound with saline for determination of leakage can be helpful in equivocal cases. Failure to recognize an esophageal injury may lead to mediastinal sepsis, tracheoesophageal fistula, and disruption of airway repair. When the esophagus has been injured, it should be repaired with a meticulous double-layer repair. It is imperative to interpose viable muscle, usually the detached sternohyoid, to prevent subsequent fistula formation (Fig 19.6). Of six patients with combined tracheoesophageal injuries from the MGH series, two patients had failed primary repair with interim development of tracheoesophageal fistula when no muscle flap was used (one patient underwent three attempts at closure). In 24 and six patients described, respectively, in reports from Tulane University School of Medicine[31] and MGH,[12] no tracheoesophageal fistulae developed when tracheal and esophageal suture lines were separated by muscle flaps. Identification of a tracheoesophageal fistula should be followed by prompt repair.

Vocal cords

Direct trauma to the vocal cords or recurrent laryngeal nerves may cause paralysis of one or both vocal cords. The nerves may be either completely transected or avulsed. They may, however, be intact and not functioning because of contusion. Subsequent recovery may follow. It is imperative that no effort be made to explore the traumatized wound to look for the recurrent nerves. They are very difficult to identify in such injuries, and damage may be caused. This is also true when seeing patients for delayed management. Vocal cord paralysis does not preclude successful reconstitution of the airway and achievement of a good functional voice. If division of the recurrent nerves is known or suspected, provisions must be made to secure the airway after repair of the tracheal injury. This can be done by an uncuffed endotracheal tube left in place for 48–72 hours. The patient should be taken to the operating room for subsequent evaluation. If a tracheostomy

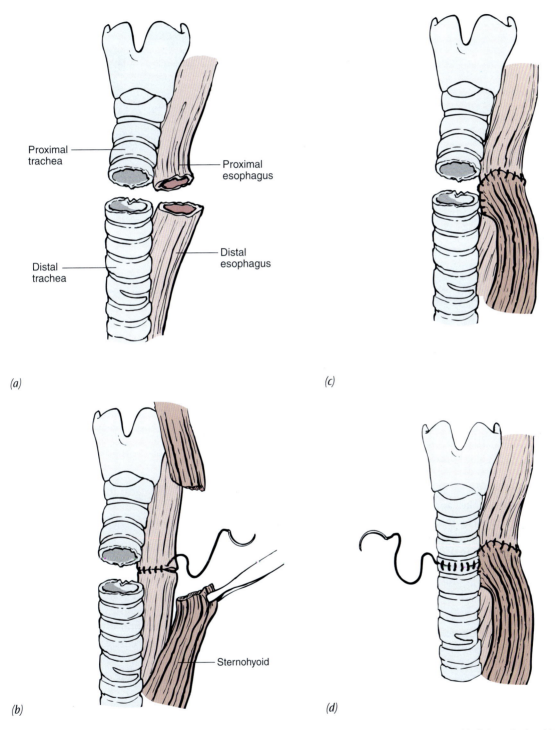

(a)

Proximal trachea

Proximal esophagus

Distal esophagus

Distal trachea

(b)

Sternohyoid

(c)

(d)

Figure 19.6 *(a–d) This diagram depicts (a) a completely transected trachea and esophagus. In this injury, it should be assumed both recurrent nerves are transected, thereby necessitating the need for a protecting tracheostomy after repair of the injuries. (b) The esophagus should be closed in two layers with fine suture material. (c) The sternohyoid is mobilized with its blood supply based inferiorly to cover the esophageal suture line and serve as a buttress between it and the tracheal suture line. (d) The trachea is repaired in the standard fashion using interrupted 4/0 absorbable suture material. Interrupted sutures are used for both anastomoses.*

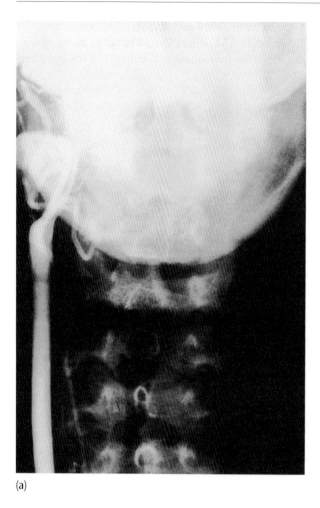
(a)

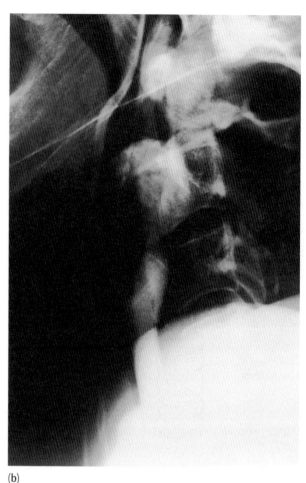
(b)

Figure 19.7 *An angiogram depicts a false aneurysm at the right carotid artery. This patient sustained blunt chest trauma and presented with delayed (2 weeks) tracheal stenosis and a bruit in the neck.*

is needed, it should be placed at least two rings away from the anastomosis. The anastomosis should be protected by a pedicled strap muscle. This can also be done at the time of surgical repair if it is elected to perform a tracheostomy at that time.

Laryngeal injuries

There has been an overall decrease in isolated laryngeal trauma secondary to the use of seat belts and air bags. However, laryngeal injuries occur frequently with blunt cervical tracheal trauma. Blunt laryngeal trauma can be classified into five categories:[32]

- group I: minor endolaryngeal trauma without fracture
- group II: moderate edema, hematoma with mucosal lacerations, no cartilage exposure or non-displaced fractures
- group III: severe edema, mucosal tears with exposed cartilage, and displaced fractures on CT

- group IV: severe endolaryngeal injury with unstable laryngeal framework
- group V: complete laryngotracheal separation.

Injuries involving the cricoid cartilage have a greater tendency toward immediate airway compromise than injuries to the thyroid cartilage.[33] Cases of very mild isolated laryngeal trauma that can be followed by repeated flexible fiberoptic bronchoscopies can be treated conservatively. Surgical exploration is indicated if airway obstruction, uncontrolled subcutaneous emphysema, extensive mucosal lacerations with exposure of cartilage, gross deformity or displaced fracture seen by CT scan are present.[32,33] Early repair, within 24–48 hours of injury, is preferable and associated with a better outcome.[33] Membranous and mucosal lacerations are meticulously reapproximated with absorbable sutures. Often, an open reduction of comminuted thyroid cartilage fractures is required through a midline thyrotomy. Stents are indicated in the presence of major mucosal injuries, comminuted fractures, and disruption of the anterior commissure. A tracheostomy is then always indicated.

Vascular injuries

Vascular injuries may occur to the carotid artery (Fig 19.7), the brachiocephalic artery (Fig 19.8), or the aorta itself. The tracheal injury is usually repaired first to allow adequate ventilation. A careful search should be made for differential pulses, localized bruits, or radiographic signs of aortic tears. Angiography is necessary to evaluate these lesions.

INITIAL AIRWAY MANAGEMENT

The initial and most important problem in acute laryngotracheal injury is to secure a satisfactory airway. If partial airway obstruction is present, attempts at oral intubation or intubation over a fiberoptic bronchoscope may be futile and may precipitate total obstruction. Repeated attempts at oral intubation must be avoided. Preparation for immediate cricothyroidotomy or tracheostomy must be made if intubation is attempted.

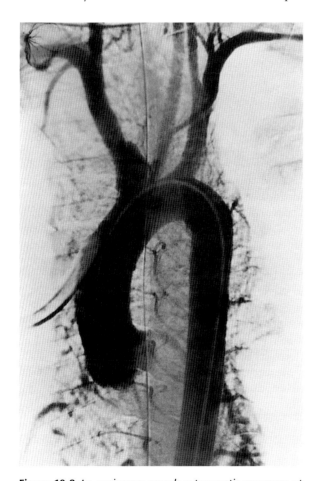

Figure 19.8 *An angiogram reveals a traumatic aneurysm at the base of the brachiocephalic artery. This patient presented following blunt chest trauma, a wide mediastinum, and bronchoscopic evidence of a linear tear of the membranous wall of the trachea.*

An emergency tracheostomy, when indicated, can be done under local anesthesia. A finger is used to locate the distal end of the completely transected trachea which often retracts into the mediastinum. The distal trachea is grasped by instruments and delivered into the wound where it can be secured and intubated with an endotracheal tube or tracheostomy tube. In the presence of a possible cervical spine injury (essentially every trauma patient), the patient's neck must be stabilized and kept in in-line traction. This will also help to maintain airway patency until definitive airway control can be achieved.[11] Large bore volume lines must be placed, and the patient rapidly but carefully evaluated for other life-threatening injuries. Associated intrathoracic hemorrhage due to great vessel laceration may demand an immediate thoracotomy in the emergency room. Direct digital occlusion of the tear and intubation under visual control may be performed prior to transporting the patient to the operating room for definitive repair. Immediate flexible bronchoscopy for control of the airway, diagnosis of bronchial or tracheal tears, and selective intubation of the right or left main stem bronchus is essential. Major intratracheal or intrabronchial hemorrhage may be controlled by selective intubation of one of the main stem bronchi. Bronchial blockers can also be used in this situation. A series[34] of nine patients with tracheobronchial disruptions found that flexible and rigid bronchoscopy, performed by trained cardiothoracic surgeons, was virtually 100% accurate in identifying those lesions. The liberal use of bronchoscopy cannot be overstated, and it has been a consistent finding by all investigators that bronchoscopy is the most useful and accurate method to confirm tracheobronchial injuries. In patients with multisystem trauma requiring immediate intubation as part of resuscitation, routine fiberoptic bronchoscopy on extubation or at the time of tracheostomy detected significant laryngeal and tracheal trauma in at least one series.[11]

Trauma patients with multiple system injuries frequently present a dilemma in terms of prioritization of indicated operative procedures. A secure airway, either by intubation across an injury, or selective intubation of a bronchus, may permit operative control of intra-abdominal or intracranial hemorrhage. We prefer to proceed to the definitive repair of the airway during the same session if the patient is hemodynamically stable. Otherwise, repair should be undertaken as soon as the patient's condition permits.

SURGICAL APPROACH

Acute injuries

Injuries to the upper airway can usually best be dealt with by a transverse collar incision, placed approximately 2 cm above the jugular notch. It gives excellent exposure of the cervical trachea and larynx, and allows a laryngeal or hyoid release when significant amounts of trachea have to be removed. A tracheostomy is to be avoided whenever possible, except when the area of injury can be used as a tracheostomy site, when injury to the recurrent nerves is suspected, or a severe laryngeal injury is present. If delayed repair of the airway is contemplated, a tracheostomy should not be placed through normal trachea so as to conserve as much viable trachea as possible for future reconstruction. On incising the neck, the surgeon will encounter a contused or disrupted trachea. A divided trachea usually retracts into the mediastinum. The finger is used to locate the divided end of the distal trachea. The trachea is grasped with a clamp and pulled into the operative field.[15] An endotracheal tube is inserted to provide a controlled airway. If primary repair is not contemplated, the end of the trachea should be secured to the skin as an end tracheostomy. The proximal end should also be brought out as a stoma, or it should be oversewn and a drain left in place. A primary anastomosis can be accomplished months later after scarring and inflammation have subsided. Conservation of viable trachea is mandatory in this circumstance. Once the airway has been stabilized, the extent of injury to the airway and adjacent structures must be determined. If distal exposure is needed, the upper third of the sternum can be divided. If the trachea and esophagus have been lacerated, access to the retracted anterior mucosa of the esophagus is facilitated by placing traction on the larynx to pull it down and away from the esophagus to allow better exposure. When trauma to the recurrent nerves is suspected, provision must be made to provide an airway at the completion of the repair. A small tracheostomy should be placed two rings below the level of the repair. The suture line should then be separated from the tracheostomy to prevent contamination with its danger of dehiscence or late stenosis. This can usually be done by reapproximating the thyroid gland or using local muscle flaps (see Fig 19.6). The tracheostomy should never be brought out through the suture line itself. Alternatively, a small, uncuffed endotracheal tube may be left in place at the end of the procedure. The patient should be returned to the operating room 2–3 days later and the tube removed so that the adequacy of the airway can be assessed. By this time, the anastomotic area should be sealed and the risk of contamination minimal. In most instances, a tracheostomy is preferable to prolonged endotracheal intubation.

Careful evaluation of the larynx is critical and should be done in conjunction with an otolaryngologist, if possible.[15,28] Endoscopic examination of the larynx should be undertaken to look for exposed or fractured cartilages, damage to the vocal cords, or other signs indicating damage to the larynx. Exposed cartilage

should be covered with mucosa to diminish the likelihood of chondritis. This can usually be done by resuturing the mucosa that has been avulsed from the larynx and remains attached to the distal airway. Fractures should be reduced and splinted, preferably over a mold, by an otolaryngologist competent in this type of reconstructive technique. Attempts to reduce and hold complex laryngeal fractures by multiple sutures alone may result in stenosis and malformation of the larynx. The shattered larynx is most easily molded when the injury is fresh. A badly fragmented site of tracheal division may require debridement. Little laryngeal tissue, if any, should be sacrificed. A protecting tracheostomy should be performed when a severe laryngeal injury is present.

Simple injuries of the trachea should be repaired with absorbable 4/0 Vicryl (polyglycolic acid polymer) sutures, using an interrupted technique. We have frequently reinforced these suture lines with local muscle flaps. Placement of a tracheostomy tube through a simple anterior laceration should be avoided unless prolonged intubation can be anticipated, in which case the injury can be treated as a tracheal stoma and allowed to close when the tracheostomy tube is removed.

Extensive injuries to the trachea require debridement of ragged edges and devitalized tissue. Conservation of viable trachea is imperative. Careful end-to-end approximation is done using interrupted absorbable 4/0 Vicryl sutures. The membranous portion is realigned, taking special care to reapproximate the junction between cartilaginous and membranous portions. Suture bites should be placed at about the same level from the cut edge. All sutures are placed and tagged individually first, and then tied down with the knots outside of the lumen. The repair is tested for air tightness under saline. Adjunctive hilar or laryngeal release maneuvers are seldom required. Small suction drains serve to remove accumulations of fluid. At completion of the operation, the patient's neck is flexed and secured by a stitch from the chin to the chest. This will avoid unnecessary tension on the repair.[35] An intrathoracic anastomosis should always be buttressed with a viable tissue flap, such as a pleural flap, pericardial fat pad or intercostal muscle.

Management of the airway in injuries to the distal trachea, carina, or proximal main stem bronchi can be difficult. Tears of the thoracic trachea or right bronchus are best approached through a right posterolateral thoracotomy by the way of the fourth intercostal space; when the left bronchus is transected, a left thoracotomy is required. Double-lumen tubes should be avoided because of the possibility of extending the injury. A long endotracheal tube can be positioned beyond the injury or into the appropriate main stem bronchus to provide single-lung ventilation (Fig 19.9). This should be done very carefully with a flexible bronchoscope to serve as a

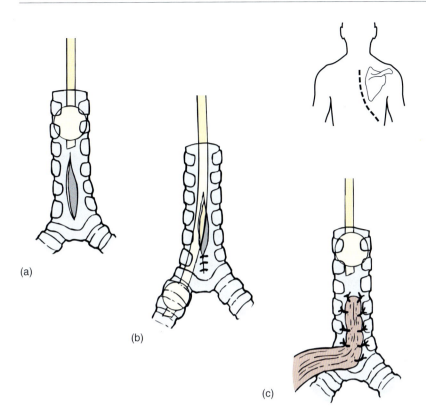

Figure 19.9 *Exposure for distal tracheal injuries is best achieved through a right posterolateral thoracotomy. (a) A long endotracheal tube should be placed over a flexible bronchoscope and carefully guided into place into the left main bronchus. (b) The injury is best repaired with 4/0 interrupted absorbable sutures. (c) The repair should be buttressed with a pleural, pericardial or pedicled intercostal muscle flap.*

(a)

(b)

(c)

guide and to check the final position. Great care must be taken not to extend the injury. A long, uncut endotracheal tube or preferably a more flexible Tovell tube with a proximal extension may allow the surgeon to manipulate the tube into the appropriate bronchus at the time of operation (see Fig 19.9). A high frequency jet ventilation catheter, if available, can be passed through an endotracheal tube and placed in proper position. For those situations where a long endotracheal tube is not used or cannot be positioned properly, a sterile flexible endotracheal tube (Tovell tube) with appropriate connecting tubing can be used to intubate the opposite lung across the operative field. The connecting tubing is passed from the operating field to the anesthetist. Repair of the injury is done by intermittently removing the endotracheal tube and individually placing sutures. After all sutures are placed, the tube is removed, the airway approximated, and ventilation continued through the original endotracheal tube. The suture line should be tested under saline, and reinforced with a pericardial, pleural, or pedicled intercostal muscle flap.[36] Depending on the severity of associated injuries, the patient is extubated as soon as possible, preferably at the completion of the procedure. A 'completion bronchoscopy' is always done. If intubation and ventilation are required, the endotracheal tube should be pulled back to a sufficient distance above the suture line. Ventilation pressures should be kept as low as possible.

Tracheobronchial rupture from blunt trauma usually occurs at a single spot and is transverse (74% of all cases). However, it may also be longitudinal (18%) or complex (8%), involving multiple segments of the tracheobronchial tree.[37] For extensive destruction of the carina and/or main bronchus, either with or without major vessel injury, consideration may be given to cardiopulmonary bypass.[37] This, however, must be weighed against the risk of heparinization in a trauma patient.[34,37] When a disrupted main bronchus is felt not to be reparable, sleeve resection can be performed in order to preserve lung tissue and avoid a pneumonectomy.[34,38]

Delayed management

LARYNGOTRACHEAL TRAUMA

Patients evaluated in a delayed fashion, either after initial failed repair or unrecognized injury, present special challenges. If stenosis is present and there is no tracheostomy, these patients should be handled as if the primary problem is tracheal stenosis. Of prime importance, the patient should no longer require mechanical ventilation, and associated injuries should have resolved. Careful radiological assessment is mandatory to determine the extent of injury and involvement of associated structures such as the esophagus. Functional assessment of the laryngeal airway requires evaluation by CT scan, stroboscopy and electromyography. The presence of paralyzed vocal cords does not preclude successful establishment of a patent airway and useful voice.[33,39] Various endoscopic microsurgical laryngeal procedures are now available to provide an adequate airway and a useful voice.[33,40,41] Glottic deficit can be corrected with collagen or fat implants. Unilateral vocal cord paralysis can be palliated by a medialization thyroplasty. If bilateral vocal cord paralysis persists, unilateral arytenoidectomy and lateralization of the vocal cord produces an adequate airway at the expense of some vocal function.[15] Several techniques of reconstruction using rib cartilage or local muscle flaps have been described for correcting loss of cartilaginous support.[33] It is important that laryngeal problems be corrected prior to any attempted tracheal repair. A sufficient period of time should elapse before tracheal reconstruction to allow for healing and to be certain that late stenosis does not occur. Failure to provide an adequate laryngeal airway will require a tracheostomy to be performed, which might jeopardize the repair. Furthermore, the larynx must be allowed sufficient time to heal so that it will be stable for a laryngotracheal anastomosis if that is necessary. Precise evaluation of the extent of injury is necessary. Measurements based on radiographic and endoscopic findings must be done to determine if adequate viable trachea exists to re-establish the airway. Inflammation and surrounding reaction should be minimal. A median of 5 months elapsed in our series[12] before definitive repair was undertaken. Silicone T-tubes can be a useful alternative to tracheostomy tubes if additional time is required.[42] Once the decision to proceed has been made, we prefer to evaluate these patients bronchoscopically at the time of the proposed operation. We prefer rigid bronchoscopy because flexible bronchoscopy may occlude the airway or precipitate airway obstruction. Critical airway stenosis (less than 6 mm) may require dilation through a series of increasingly larger rigid bronchoscopes or using Jackson dilators with great caution through a rigid bronchoscope. Dilating the stenotic airway permits the anesthesiologist to intubate the patient and control the airway. A cervical incision is employed, with division of the upper third of the sternum should additional exposure be required. Often the two ends of the trachea are separated, and the distal end retracts into the mediastinum. The dense scar joining the divided ends of the trachea may make dissection difficult. The distal trachea in this case should be identified and circumferential dissection carried out at this point. Care should be taken to avoid aspiration of blood into the tracheobronchial tree.

The injured area should be resected to well-structured trachea. Repair can then be accomplished using an 'open' technique with absorbable 4/0 sutures and removing the endotracheal tube as necessary to place sutures.[35] If previous repair has been attempted or extensive initial injury has occurred, approximation may be difficult. In addition to neck flexion, suprahyoid laryngeal release may be required to avoid anasto-

motic tension.[35] Injury to the cricoid cartilage or subsequent inflammatory stenosis at this level may require resection of the anterior half of the cricoid. Care must be taken to preserve the posterior plate because of the risk of injuring the recurrent nerves.[49] Removal of the cricoid in this oblique manner creates a larger subglottic airway. The distal trachea is divided in a gentle curve on either side. The midline of the thyroid cartilage is approximated to the midline of the peak of the 'prow', which has been fashioned in the most proximal trachea. The remainder of the repair is carried out in the standard manner.

TRACHEOBRONCHIAL TRAUMA

Delayed management of intrathoracic injuries encompasses many of the principles previously mentioned for acute and chronic cervical tracheal injuries. An unrecognized tracheobronchial tear usually results in a stricture. Unless there is irreversible loss of pulmonary parenchyma due to infection or bronchiectasis, an attempt should be made to preserve function with local resection and reimplantation of the bronchus, no matter how long it has been since the initial injury.[21,22] Several authors have reported good re-expansion, and near-normal lung function after delayed bronchial reconstruction.[22,26,43–45] Hilar release maneuvers may have to be performed to decrease anastomotic tension if end-to-end primary reconstruction is performed (sleeve resection). Tissue flaps are used in all cases to cover the anastomoses. If repair is impossible, pulmonary resection should be carried out to avoid further infection and pulmonary vascular shunting.

Conservative management

Highly selected patients with small tears of the airway may be managed non-operatively. These patients should be hemodynamically stable, have no major associated injuries, and require no positive airway ventilation. Bronchoscopy should demonstrate a small tear. Furthermore, if a pneumothorax was present, the lung should remain expanded with a single chest tube. Broad spectrum antibiotics should be given, and the patients carefully watched for signs of airway obstruction or mediastinal sepsis.

POSTOPERATIVE CARE

Basic postoperative management principles parallel those utilized after major airway resections and bronchoplastic procedures. Aggressive tracheobronchial toilet with chest physical therapy, early mobilization and frequent use of the flexible bronchoscope to suction out retained secretions are mandatory. All patients are placed on prophylactic broad spectrum parenteral antibiotics. Due to the high frequency of associated chest wall trauma, flail chest, rib fractures and pulmonary contusion, pain control is of paramount importance. This is usually achieved through a thoracic epidural catheter which can be placed postoperatively.

RESULTS

Simple isolated airway trauma generally results in excellent outcome. In our series,[12] all 10 patients managed after acute laryngotracheal trauma remain with an excellent airway. No delayed tracheal stenoses were noted. Two patients who initially presented with recurrent laryngeal nerve injuries have good functional voices that are somewhat husky. However, the prognosis is closely related to the associated injuries and the magnitude of the initial trauma, and the overall mortality after severe airway injury is high.[11] Thoracic injuries are usually more lethal as compared with cervical injuries (Table 19.2).[46,47] Kelly et al.[23] reported a 54% mortality rate for thoracic airway trauma (seven of 13 patients), and a 14% mortality rate for cervical airway trauma (11 of 80 patients). Based on the Pennsylvania Trauma Outcome Study,[47] the mortality rate adjusted for the Injury Severity Score Body Region was 50% if no other injuries were present, 65% if an extremity was involved, 76% if the head/neck region was injured, 81% if the abdomen was injured, and 100% if the T-spine was involved.

Outcome after delayed management, failure of initial management, or delayed diagnosis is somewhat less satisfactory. Dysphonia remains a significant late disability in patients who required late surgical repair of a laryngeal injury.[33] There is also a high incidence of vocal cord malfunction in patients presenting for delayed repair after laryngotracheal trauma. Among the 17 patients seen in a delayed fashion in our series, 16 have a good airway; one uses a tracheostomy intermit

tently.[12] Ten patients have a good voice. Three of them had unilateral and four, bilateral vocal cord paralysis. Six patients had a husky but very functional voice. Three of them had unilateral and three, bilateral paralyzed vocal cords. Only one patient is considered to have been a failure with respect to voice. Late bronchoplastic resection of bronchial strictures usually yields good results.[22]

CONCLUSIONS

Acute airway trauma can be successfully managed in the majority of patients by observation of certain principles of management:

- high level of suspicion
- proper airway management
- prioritization of definitive surgical care toward life-threatening injuries
- evaluation and exclusion of associated injuries such as esophageal injuries
- avoidance of searching for recurrent nerves
- separation of tracheal and esophageal suture lines
- conservation of viable trachea
- avoidance of tracheostomy through repair
- flexion of the neck to reduce tension.

Delayed recognition or failure of primary repair, even in the presence of a paralyzed larynx, concomitant esophageal injury, or completely atelectatic lung, can still be successfully managed in the majority of patients if certain principles are followed. These principles are the following:

- resolution of associated injuries
- removal of mechanical ventilation
- radiological and endoscopic evaluation
- repair of the larynx first
- resolution of scarring and inflammation
- separation of tracheal and esophageal suture lines
- general principles of tracheal surgery.

A paralyzed larynx does not preclude the reconstruction of the airway and voice, thereby saving those patients the necessity for lifelong permanent tracheostomy. Completely atelectatic lungs from stricture formation at the fracture site should be re-expanded by stricture resection and bronchial reanastomosis.

Table 19.2 Outcome of airway injuries

	No. of injuries	No. of deaths	Mortality (%)
Blunt			
Cervical	16	0	0
Thoracic trachea	14	2	14
Bronchial	32	8	25
Total	62	8	13
Penetrating			
Cervical	151	11	7
Thoracic trachea	31	11	35
Bronchial	11	3	27
Total	193	25	13

Compiled from references 9,11,12,14,16,17,20–23,34,37,46,48.

REFERENCES

1. Burke JF. Early diagnosis of traumatic rupture of the bronchus. *JAMA* 1962; **181**: 682–6.
2. Keyne G. *The Apologie and Treatise of Ambroise Pare.* London: Falcon Educational Books, 1951.

3. Seuvre M. Crushing injury from wheel of omnibus: rupture of right bronchus. *Bull Soc Anat Paris* 1873; **48:** 680.

4. Krinitzki SI. Zur Kasuistik einer vollstaendigen Zerreissung des rechten Luftroehrenastes. *Virschow Arch [Pathol Anat]* 1927; **266:** 815–919.

5. Nissen R. Classics in thoracic surgery: total pneumonectomy. *Ann Thorac Surg* 1980; **29:** 390–4.

6. Kinsella TJ, Johnsrud LW. Traumatic rupture of the bronchus. *J Thorac Cardiovasc Surg* 1947; **16:** 571–83.

7. Beskin CA. Rupture-separation of the cervical trachea following a closed chest injury. *J Thorac Surg* 1957; **34:** 392.

8. Kemmerer WT, Eckert WG, Gathright JB, Reemtsma K, Creech O Jr. Patterns of thoracic injuries in fatal traffic accidents. *J Trauma* 1961; **1:** 595–9.

9. Ecker RR, Libertini RV, Rea WJ, Sugg WL, Webb WR. Injuries of the trachea and bronchi. *Ann Thorac Surg* 1971; **11:** 289–92.

10. Bertelsen S, Howitz P. Injuries of the trachea and bronchi. *Thorax* 1972; **27:** 188–92.

11. Angood PB, Attia EL, Brown RA, Mulder DS. Extrinsic civilian trauma to the larynx and cervical trachea – important predictors of long-term morbidity. *J Trauma* 1986; **26:** 869–73.

12. Mathisen DJ, Grillo HC. Laryngotracheal trauma. *Ann Thorac Surg* 1989; **43:** 254–62.

13. Feliciano DV, Bitondo CG, Mattox KL, *et al*. Combined tracheoesophageal injuries. *Am J Surg* 1985; **150:** 710–15.

14. Grover FL, Ellestad C, Arom KV, Root HD, Cruz AB, Trinkle JK. Diagnosis and management of major tracheobronchial injuries. *Ann Thorac Surg* 1979; **28:** 384–91.

15. Sofferman RA. Management of laryngotracheal trauma. *Am J Surg* 1981; **141:** 412–17.

16. Symbas PN, Hatcher Cr Jr, Vlasis SE. Bullet wounds of the trachea. *J Thorac Cardiovasc Surg* 1982; **83:** 235–8.

17. Symbas PN, Hatcher CR Jr, Boehm GAW. Acute penetrating tracheal trauma. *Ann Thorac Surg* 1976; **22:** 473–7.

18. Beall AC Jr, Noon GP, Harris HH. Surgical management of tracheal trauma. *J Trauma* 1967; **7:** 248–56.

19. Grillo HC, Dignan EF, Miura T. Extensive resection and reconstruction of mediastinal trachea without prosthesis or graft: an anatomical study in man. *J Thorac Cardiovasc Surg* 1964; **48:** 741.

20. Jones WS, Mavroudis C, Richardson JD, Gray LA, Howe WR. Management of tracheobronchial disruption resulting from blunt trauma. *Surgery* 1984; **95:** 319–22.

21. Kirsh MM, Orringer MB, Behrendt DM, Sloan H. Management of tracheobronchial disruption secondary to nonpenetrating trauma. *Ann Thorac Surg* 1976; **22:** 93–101.

22. Deslauriers J, Beaulieu M, Archambault G, Laforge J, Bernier R. Diagnosis and long-term follow-up of major bronchial disruptions due to nonpenetrating trauma. *Ann Thorac Surg* 1982; **33:** 32–9.

23. Kelly JP, Webb WR, Moulder PV, Everson C, Burch BH, Lindsey ES. Management of airway trauma. I: Tracheobronchial injuries. *Ann Thorac Surg* 1985; **40:** 551–5.

24. Hood RM, Sloan HE. Injuries of the trachea and major bronchi. *J Thorac Surg* 1959; **38:** 458.

25. Taskinen SO, Salo JA, Halttunen PE. Tracheobronchial rupture due to blunt chest trauma: a follow up study. *Ann Thorac Surg* 1989; **48:** 846–9.

26. Benfield JR, Long ET, Harrison RW, *et al*. Should a chronic atelectatic lung be reaerated or excised? *Dis Chest* 1960; **37:** 67.

27. Klumpe DH, Sang OHK, Wayman SA. A characteristic finding in unilateral complete bronchial transection. *AJR Radium Ther Neck Med* 1970; **110:** 704–5.

28. Myers EM, Iko BO. The management of acute laryngeal trauma. *J Trauma* 1987; **27:** 448–52.

29. Weir IH, Muller NL, Connell DG. CT diagnosis of bronchial rupture. *J Comput Assist Tomogr* 1988; **12:** 1035–6.

30. Pate JW. Tracheobronchial and esophageal injuries. *Surg Clin North Am* 1989; **69:** 111–23.

31. Kelly JP, Webb WR, Moulder PV, Moustouakas NM, Lirtzman M. Management of airway trauma. II: Combined injuries of the trachea and esophagus. *Ann Thorac Surg* 1987; **43:** 160–3.

32. Fuhrman GM, Stieg FH, Buerk CA. Blunt laryngeal trauma: classification and management. *J Trauma* 1990; **30:** 87–92.

33. Chagon FP, Mulder DS. Laryngotracheal trauma. *Chest Surg Clin North Am* 1996; **6:** 733–48.

34. Baumgartner F, Sheppard B, de Virgilio C, *et al*. Tracheal and main bronchial disruptions after blunt chest trauma: presentation and management. *Ann Thorac Surg* 1990; **50:** 569–74.

35. Grillo HC. Surgery of the trachea. *Curr Probl Surg* 1970; **July:** 3–59.

36. Grillo HC, Mathisen DJ. Surgical management of tracheal strictures. *Surg Clin North Am* 1988; **68:** 511–24.

37. Symbas PN, Justicz AG, Ricketts RR. Rupture of the airways from blunt trauma: treatment of complex injuries. *Ann Thorac Surg* 1992; **54:** 177–83.

38. McCarthy JF, Claffey LP, O'Donovan F, Guiney EJ, Luke DA. Emergency sleeve lobectomy after blunt chest trauma in a child. *J Trauma* 1996; **41:** 892–4.

39. Potter CR, Sessions DG, Ogura JH. Blunt laryngotracheal trauma. *Otolaryngology* 1978; **86:** 909–23.

40. Montgomery WW. Management of glottic stenosis. *Otolaryngol Clin North Am* 1979; **12:** 841–7.

41. Sessions DG, Ogura JH, Heeneman H. Surgical management of bilateral vocal cord paralysis. *Laryngoscope* 1976; **86:** 559–66.

42. Gaissert HA, Grillo HC, Mathisen DJ, Wain JC. Temporary and permanent restoration of airway continuity with the tracheal T tube. *J Thorac Cardiovasc Surg* 1994; **107:** 600–6.

43. Campbell TC, Swindell HV, Dominy DE. Delayed repair of rupture of the bronchus. *J Thorac Cardiovasc Surg* 1962; **43:** 320.

44. Gomez-Engler HE, Barker AF, Klein R, *et al.* Post traumatic bronchial stenosis and acute respiratory insufficiency. *J Thorac Cardiovasc Surg* 1980; **79:** 864–7.

45. Nonoyama A, Masuda A, Kasahara K, Mogi T, Kagawa T. Total rupture of the left main bronchus successfully repaired nine years after injury. *Ann Thorac Surg* 1976; **21:** 445–8.

46. Mulder DS, Barkun JS. Injury to the trachea, bronchus and esophagus. In: Mattox KL, Moore EE, Feliciano DV, eds. *Definitive Trauma Care.* New York: Appleton-Century-Crofts, 1986: 343–54.

47. Campbell DB. Trauma to the chest wall, lung, and major airways. *Semin Thorac Cardiovasc Surg* 1992; **4:** 234–40.

48. Mills SA, Johnston FR, Hudspeth AS, Breyer RH, Myers RT, Cordell AR. Clinical spectrum of blunt tracheo-bronchial disruption illustrated by seven cases. *J Thorac Cardiovasc Surg* 1982; **84:** 49–58.

49. Grillo HC, Mathisen DJ, Wain JC. Laryngotracheal resection and reconstruction for subglottic stenosis. *Ann Thoracic Surg* 1992; **53:** 54–63.

20

Blunt injury to the lung

ROBERT B WAGNER AND JOHN M CHO

DEFINITION

Most textbooks and multiple papers define pulmonary contusion as a 'bruise of the lung', including microscopic interstitial hemorrhage and edema, without laceration. The 'pulmonary contusion regimen'[1] of fluid restriction, diuretics, and steroids is based upon this standard definition. However, our differing interpretation of pulmonary contusion is based on experience with blunt lung injury studied by CT scan, hemodynamics, and microscopy of injured lung. As a result of these studies, begun in 1983, we conclude that the lesion known as pulmonary contusion is a pulmonary laceration contiguous with intraparenchymal, intraalveolar hemorrhage.[2-5]

Pulmonary parenchymal injury, i.e. pulmonary contusion, may occur with or without chest wall fracture; physiological disturbances may be significant or may be inconsequential. In these patients a complete clinical assessment of the lesion may require combined radiologic and physiologic evaluations for management.

We classify four types of pulmonary contusions/lacerations based on the mechanism of injury and CT findings.[2,4] We grade the contusion by quantifying the percentage of air-space filling and requirements for assisted ventilation.[3,4] By utilizing this information, we have successfully managed patients without fluid restriction, steroids and diuretics. As pulmonary contusion can progress, successful management of larger lesions requires physiological monitoring with possible ventilator support. An early CT scan of the chest can be useful in the initial evaluation of this lesion and on occasion will reveal occult pathology requiring surgical attention.

DIAGNOSIS

Diagnosis of pulmonary contusion

- History of blunt chest trauma
- Radiologic pulmonary density (CT more sensitive, but not always available)
- Increase in alveolar-arterial oxygen gradient
- Moist rales on auscultation

Traditionally, the diagnosis of pulmonary contusion is based on the following criteria:

- a history of non-penetrating chest trauma
- radiological pulmonary density
- increase in alveolar-arterial oxygen tension gradient
- moist rales on auscultation
- evidence of intrapulmonary hemorrhage.[6,7]

We strongly believe that CT of the chest, specifically of the lungs, is more sensitive in diagnosing blunt injury of the lung. The CT scan demonstrates that a pulmonary laceration is the primary underlying injury in the majority of cases of blunt trauma causing lung injury. Exceptions occur when blood or serum fills small lacerations or when atelectasis compresses and obscures the laceration. The pulmonary laceration is the basic component of the pulmonary contusion. Air-space filling (radiodensity seen on the chest film) is

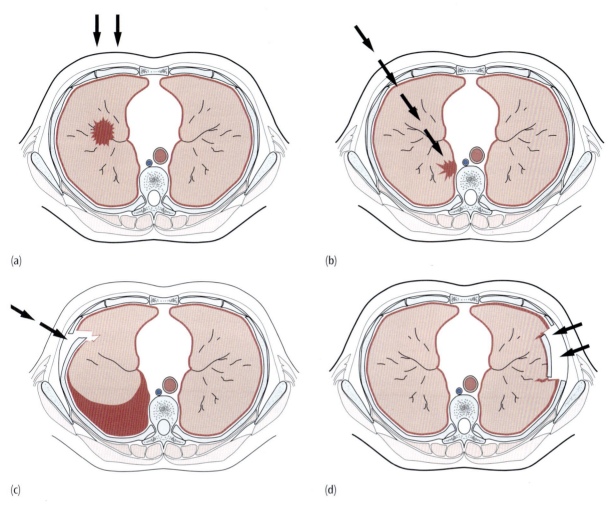

Figure 20.1 *(a) Schematic drawing of type 1 injury. The chest wall has been compressed inward. The underlying air-filled lung is restricted as the glottis reflexly closes with injury. This results in rupture of pulmonary parenchyma. The laceration, which may be irregular initially, is almost immediately converted into a spherical shape by the elasticity of the surrounding lung tissue. If the laceration extends through the visceral pleura, a pneumothorax results. (b) Schematic drawing of type 2 injury. The lower (more cartilaginous) chest wall has been severely compressed pushing the air-filled lung over the rigid vertebral body or aorta. This results in a shearing effect on the lung. (c) Schematic drawing of a rib fracture with the sharp edge of the rib penetrating the adjacent lung (type 3 laceration). If the hole is large enough, a pneumothorax results. Even a small laceration will result in a significant pneumothorax if the patient is placed on a ventilator. (d) Schematic drawing of a type 4 laceration. The lung is adherent to the parietal pleural. When the chest wall is rapidly compressed, such as occurs with a flail chest, the pleural adhesions in the non-depressed lung will not allow that portion of the lung to drop away. This results in tearing of the lung.*

dependent on contiguous intra-alveolar hemorrhage secondary to the lung tear. In the rare patient who requires operative resection of lung parenchyma, histological examination of these sections demonstrates intra-alveolar hemorrhage without interstitial injury.

Although controversy remains as to the utilization of CT scans in chest trauma, several studies demonstrate the efficacy of CT over plain films.[2,8–12] In patients with a history of significant chest trauma, three times as many lesions can be seen on CT scan versus chest radiograph.[2] Although many findings may have no clinical significance, early diagnoses of pneumothoraces and hemothoraces allow for immediate and correct management, thus avoiding complications. In our original series of patients with a history of severe chest trauma who had negative plain films, CT studies demonstrated pulmonary parenchymal injuries in a significant percentage (four of eight).[2]

ETIOLOGY AND MECHANISM OF PULMONARY LACERATION/CONTUSION

The mechanisms of pulmonary contusion in non-blast, non-penetrating chest trauma include:

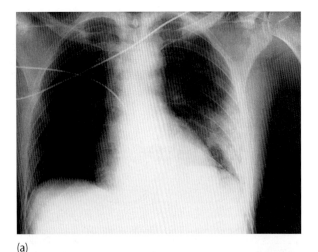

(a)

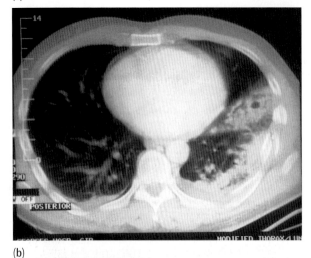

(b)

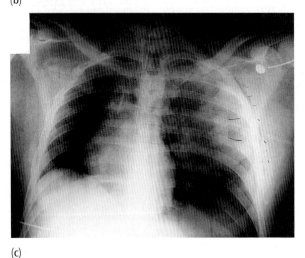

(c)

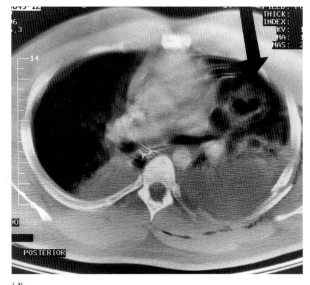

(d)

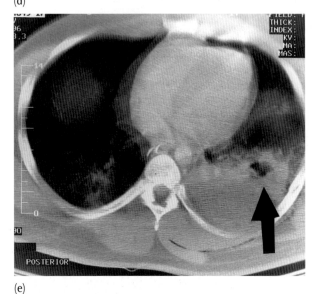

(e)

Figure 20.2 *(a) Admission AP portable chest film. A fluffy radiodensity is seen in the left lateral lung field. Several minimally displaced rib fractures are seen laterally. (b) CT reveals a small type 1 laceration in left upper lobe laterally. The laceration is surrounded by blood-filled alveoli. The fissure is well demonstrated by the blood-filled alveoli above, and the air-filled alveoli below. Some blood has spilled over into the left lower lobe posteriorly, and laterally. A small amount of blood has also spilled over the carina into the posterior basal segment of the right lower lobe. (c) Admission AP film. A large left subpulmonic pneumothorax is present. The heart and mediastinum are shifted to the right. Subcutaneous air is seen along the left chest wall. A hazy density is seen in the left upper lung field. (d) CT scan after placement of a chest tube demonstrates a large type 1 laceration in the left upper lobe. A second type 1 laceration is seen just proximal to the major fissure. The left lower lobe is filled with blood as is the medial basal segment of the right lower lobe. (e) Same patient, lower cut. Within the left lower lobe a large type 1 laceration is seen within the air space (arrow).*

- sudden chest wall compression with rupture of lung parenchyma
- chest wall compression with a shearing effect against the vertebral body or aorta
- rib fracture with penetration of the underlying lung by displaced ribs
- chest wall displacement where the underlying lung is adherent to the parietal pleura.

On the basis of CT pattern, mechanism of injury, location of the associated rib fracture, and surgical findings, we have classified pulmonary lacerations into four types (Fig 20.1).[2] The pattern of the contusion, i.e. air-space filling by blood, is determined strictly by gravity, as can be demonstrated by the CT. The volume of air-space filling plays a paramount role in the requirement for ventilator support of the injured patient.[3,4]

RADIOGRAPHIC FINDINGS

The radiographic plain film diagnosis of pulmonary contusion has been based on the classic findings of a pulmonary infiltrate seen within hours of trauma. The radiological findings may be:

1. irregular, coarse nodular densities that may be discrete or confluent
2. homogeneous consolidation
3. a combination of changes of both of the above
4. diffuse, often patchy infiltration of the lung that diminishes and usually disappears completely within a few days.[13–15]

The opacities resulting from lung contusions are said to differ from those of incipient bronchopneumonia (e.g. by aspiration) in that they are not confined within the anatomical limits of the various segments and lobes.[16]

CT APPEARANCE

Classification of pulmonary lacerations

We have classified pulmonary lacerations into four types on the basis of CT pattern, mechanism of injury, location of associated rib fracture, and surgical findings.[2,4]

Type 1 lesions appear on CT scan as an air-filled cavity or air-fluid level in an intraparenchymal cavity (Fig 20.2). Frequently, the laceration may result in a pneumothorax by extending through the visceral pleura. In this case, the laceration may be seen as a linear tear, seen on CT scans as an air-containing line through the parenchyma that does not follow an anatomical bronchial distribution (Fig 20.3). Type 1 lacerations result from sudden compression of a pliable chest wall. With sudden chest compression the glottis reflexively closes, thus creating a closed system in which the lung may be likened to an air-filled paper bag that is suddenly and violently compressed, causing the lung to rupture.

The CT appearance of type 2 lacerations (contusions) is that of an air-containing cavity or intra-

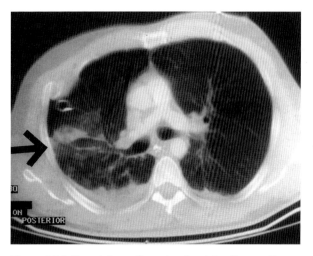

Figure 20.3 *Type 1 laceration extending laterally as a linear tear, right upper lobe.*

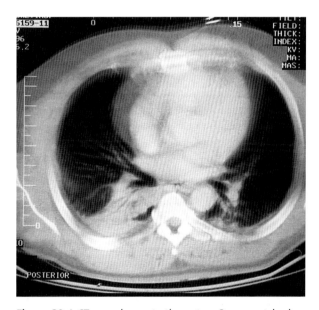

Figure 20.4 *CT scan demonstrating a type 2 paravertebral laceration with blood-filled alveoli immediately adjacent to the laceration. In Figure 20.5(b) the lung immediately lateral is atelectatic. The laceration is partially filled with blood as seen by the air-fluid level.*

parenchymal air–fluid level within the paravertebral lung (Fig 20.4). Type 2 lacerations occur when the more pliable lower chest wall is acutely and severely compressed, causing the lower lobe to shift suddenly across the vertebral body or aorta. This results in a shearing-type injury.

A type 3 laceration (contusion) appears as a small peripheral cavity or peripheral linear radiolucency that is always contiguous to a fractured rib (Fig 20.5). This type of laceration results from the lung being penetrated by the sharp ends of the displaced fractured rib or ribs (Fig 20.6).

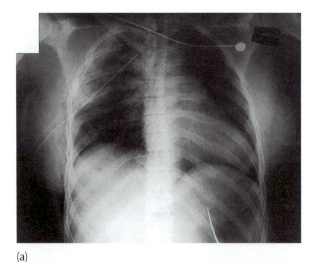

(a)

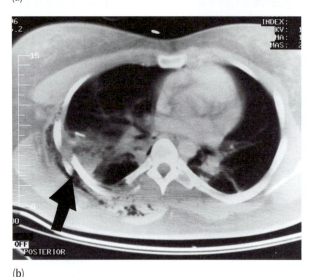

(b)

Figure 20.5 *(a) Admission AP chest film. A chest tube is in place. There is a radiodensity in the right upper lobe field. The seventh rib is fractured. (b) CT scan, same patient at level of seventh rib. The fractured rib can be seen at the edge of the lung parenchyma. The area of lung penetration is surrounded by air-space filling (blood). The chest tube (linear radiodensity) is just above the air-space filling.*

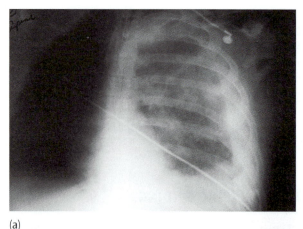

(a)

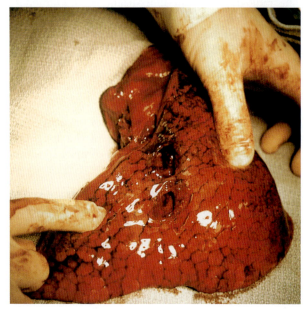

(b)

Figure 20.6 *(a) Admission AP chest film. The entire left lung field is hazy. There is a lateral hemothorax. Multiple left ribs are fractured. (b) Left upper lobe resected because of massive air leak and bleeding. Two deep holes in the lung can be clearly seen to have been caused by adjacent penetrating fractured ribs.*

Type 4 lacerations result from avulsion of previously formed, firm pleuropulmonary adhesions and sudden chest wall compression. The lung is torn from abrupt movement of the chest wall inward (Fig 20.7).

With rare exceptions, all patients who sustain compressive injuries (types 1 and 2) are younger than 40 years of age, when older costal cartilages and costovertebral joints lose flexibility or calcify. Some patients sustain multiple lacerations that may be of different types (Fig 20.8).

Considerable confusion remains in the literature as to the correct nomenclature for blunt lung injury (Table 20.1). Confusion arises from not appreciating that the basic injury is a pulmonary laceration. In

what is commonly designated pulmonary contusion on a plain film, the laceration is usually obscured by surrounding air-space filling. If the laceration is clearly seen on the plain film, it is called a *traumatic lung cyst* or *pseudocyst*. If the laceration is filled with blood, clot, or eventually fibrosis, and the surrounding blood filled parenchyma has cleared, then the lesion is called a *pulmonary hematoma* (Fig 20.9). Pulmonary hematomas have occasionally been subjected to a thoracotomy as solitary pulmonary nodules.

Pulmonary laceration

- → pulmonary contusion – when surrounded by intra-alveolar hemorrhage

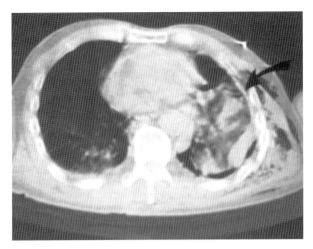

Figure 20.7 *Type 4 laceration. Chest CT scan of a patient who previously had undergone a left upper lobectomy. Pleural adhesions are present. The depressed ribs have torn the adherent underlying lung, resulting in multiple tears and air-space filling. A circumferential pneumothorax is seen around the lobe which is non-adherent.*

- → pulmonary hematoma – when cavity filled with blood; when cavity has scarred down
- → traumatic pulmonary cyst; pseudocyst – when as a pulmonary cavity.

Pattern of injury

Pulmonary lacerations result in varying degrees of intraparenchymal hemorrhage, which is the obvious abnormality seen on the plain chest film. Blood, as does any other liquid bronchial aspirate, flows dependently and the pattern of air-space filling is determined by gravity and bronchial anatomy. The pattern of air-space

Table 20.1 *Nomenclature for blunt lung injury (pulmonary laceration)*

Without visualization of cavity
- Pulmonary laceration
- Pulmonary contusion
- Pulmonary concussion
- Traumatic pneumonia

With visualization of cavity
- Traumatic pneumatocele
- Traumatic cyst
- Rupture of lung
- Pulmonary laceration
- Pulmonary cavitation
- Post-traumatic pulmonary pseudocystic hematoma
- Traumatic pulmonary pseudocyst
- Post-traumatic pulmonary abscess

With cavity filled by blood or scar
- Pulmonary hematoma

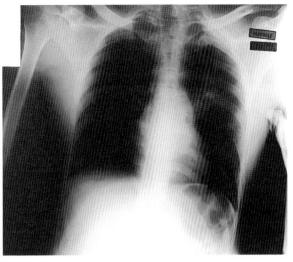

(a)

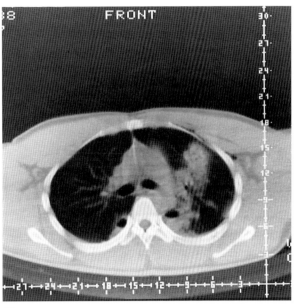

(b)

Figure 20.8 *(a) Admission AP chest. Slightly overpenetrated, but a haziness is seen in the left upper lung field. (b) Same patient. CT of chest reveals a small type 1 laceration in the left upper lobe surrounded by air-space filling and bilateral type 2 lacerations adjacent to the vertebrae (right) and descending aorta (left).*

filling visualized on the CT scan is determined by anatomy comparable to that pointed out by Brock in his classic monograph on pulmonary abscess.[17] Traumatized patients are usually placed in the supine position. Accordingly, if the laceration occurs within the right upper lobe, blood will drain posteriorly within the right upper lobe and then via the lower lobe bronchus into the right lower lobe posteriorly, and perhaps some will spill over into the left lower lobe posteriorly. In general, the blood will bypass the anatomically anterior bronchus of the middle lobe. In

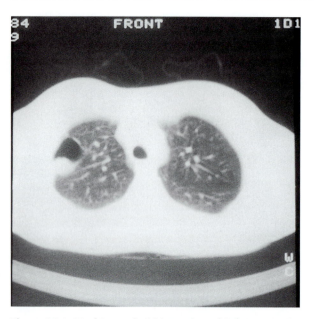

Figure 20.9 *CT of 2-month-old laceration with hematoma in posterior aspect of residual laceration.*

the majority of the population the minor fissure is incomplete. This continuity of lung tissue between the right upper and middle lobes explains why, occasionally, air-space filling will be found in the adjacent middle lobe, or in the case of a middle lobe injury, some blood may be seen within the right upper lobe. Lacerations occurring in the left upper lobe will drain blood into the left lower lobe or into the right lower lobe.

If either lower lobe is lacerated, resultant hemorrhage will flow further dependently within the parenchyma (the posterior and lateral basal segments receiving the largest measure of the drainage). Most of the blood that does reach the bronchial tree will be coughed out, suctioned out, or sometimes spill over the carina into the opposite (dependent) lower lobe (Fig 20.10).

A characteristic finding of air-space filling by blood, particularly in upper lobe injury, is that the consolidation is limited by the adjacent fissure (see Fig 20.2b). This finding helps to confirm that the air-space filling represents spillover blood and not interstitial injury (contusion) that would not be limited by a fissure.

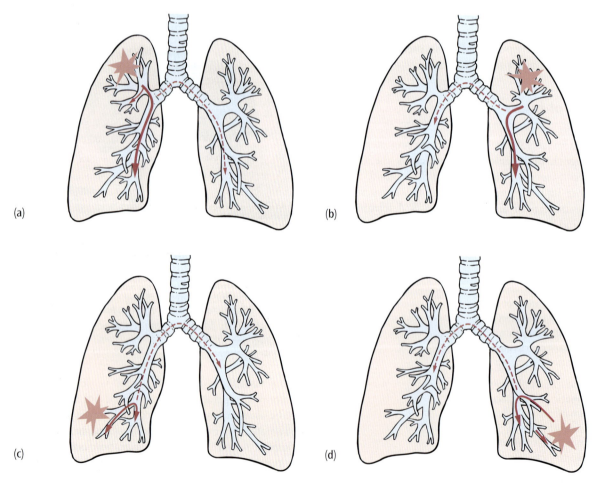

Figure 20.10 *Schematic diagrams representing the pattern of spillover hemorrhage from laceration within (a) the right upper lobe, (b) left upper lobe, (c) right lower lobe, (d) left lower lobe. (From Wagner RB, Crawford WO Jr, Schimpf PP et al. Quantitation and pattern of parenchymal lung injury in blunt chest trauma: diagnostic and therapeutic implications. CT: J Comput Tomogr 1988;* **12:** *270–281.)*[3]

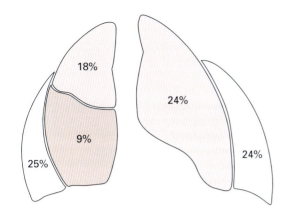

Figure 20.11 *Schematic diagram demonstrating the percentages of the individual lobes of the lung.*

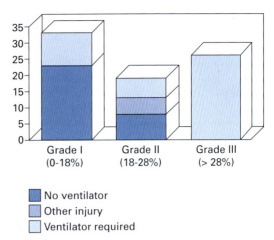

Figure 20.12 *Air-space filling disease compared with ventilator requirement (for pulmonary insufficiency). Note that all patients with greater than 28% air-space filling disease required ventilator support for pulmonary insufficiency, whereas no patient with less than 18% of air-space filling disease required ventilator support for pulmonary insufficiency. 'Other' injuries were primarily central nervous system injuries or surgery for abdominal trauma requiring intubation for anesthesia. (Adapted from Wagner RB, Jamieson PM. Pulmonary contusion: evaluation and classification of computed tomography. Surg Clin North Am 1989; **69**: 31–40.)[4]*

The air-space filling is dynamic; hemorrhage from the laceration may continue, stop, or restart. The patient may cough out significant amounts of blood, thus diminishing air-space filling seen on an earlier radiograph or CT scan. An initial negative chest film may later show significant air-space filling; however, we have never seen a patient with a negative chest CT examination later develop findings consistent with a pulmonary laceration/contusion.

Quantification of pulmonary contusion

We have quantified and graded the parenchymal lung injury in blunt chest trauma by estimating the percentage of air-space filling of each lobe of the lungs as seen on CT scan.[3,4] Based on the average of two previously published studies of individual lobe and lung volumes, the lobes are assigned standard percentages of total lung volume, with the left lung containing 48% of the total lung volume, 24% in the lower lobe and 24% in the upper lobe.[18,19] The right lung, which contains 52% of the total lung volume, is subdivided into the right upper lobe (18%), middle lobe (9%), and the lower lobe (25% of the total lung volume) (Fig 20.11).

Each lobe is evaluated individually. The concept is very simple. For example, if one-half of the right upper lobe is consolidated, then this would represent half of 18% or 9% of the total lung volume. The estimated air-space filling percentages of each of the five lobes are then added, and the sum is termed the total air-space filling for that injury (Fig 20.12). We have found that patients with injuries with 18% or less air-space filling will not require ventilatory support and have termed these grade I injuries. By contrast, patients with total air-space filling of greater than 30% will require ventilatory support; we have termed these grade III injuries. Patients with injuries from 19% to 30% are intermediate with those closer to 30% more likely to require

ventilatory support. These injuries we have called grade II injuries.[3,4]

This technique is easy both to learn and to apply, and readings by different observers are generally within a few percentage points. We believe that quantification and grading are useful in that patients with grade I injuries can be managed easily outside the intensive care unit, whereas grades II and III injuries must be admitted to an intensive care unit or equivalent.

Although we have come to appreciate the reliability of the grading system, we have never used CT quantification as the sole indication for patient intubation. Rather, we have continued to rely on standard physiological data as described below. On the other hand, when a patient has greater than 30% air-space filling on admission, that patient is admitted to the intensive care unit and monitored carefully as he/she invariably requires ventilatory support within the next 24 hours.

Another potential advantage of injury grading is morbidity and mortality reporting. Patients with grade I and grade II injuries rarely die primarily from the lung injury and morbidity will be relatively low, whereas those with grade III injuries, by definition more severe, have a higher complication rate. In our experience, all deaths attributable to lung injuries occurred with grade III injuries. The cause of death was more often the result of associated injuries than pulmonary contusion.

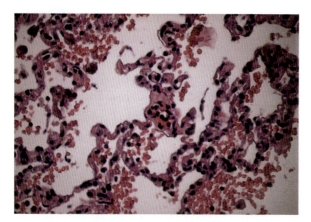

Figure 20.13 *Photomicrograph from a resected pulmonary contusion lobe (H & E × 100). There is intra-alveolar hemorrhage with no evidence of interstitial hemorrhage.*

Table 20.2 *Complications directly attributable to pulmonary contusion/laceration*

- Air leak (bronchopleural or alveolo-pleural fistula)
- Pneumothorax
- Hemothorax
- Subcutaneous emphysema
- Mediastinal emphysema
- Pulmonary hematoma
- Air embolism
- Hemoptysis
- Pulmonary cavitation
- Hypoxemia
- High shunt fraction
- Acute pulmonary hypertension
- Low pulmonary compliance (stiff lungs)

Pulmonary hemodynamics

As demonstrated histologically, the air-space filling seen on the chest film or CT examination in pulmonary contusion is primarily intra-alveolar blood (Fig 20.13). The resulting pulmonary hemodynamic changes are a manifestation of the resultant hypoxic pulmonary vasoconstriction. In our studies of the pulmonary hemodynamics of pulmonary contusion, in which shunt fractions and pulmonary vascular resistance index were compared with specific air-space injury percentages, we found that pulmonary vasoconstriction frequently occurs after pulmonary contusion. In patients whose pulmonary vascular tree reacts to air-space filling, the pulmonary vascular resistance index (PVRI) climbs directly relative to the size of the lung injury. However, in these patients, the shunt fraction is not predictable, although the shunt fraction almost always remains below 30%. This reactive vasoconstriction most probably represents a compensatory mechanism to limit perfusion of traumatized parenchyma, thereby minimizing increases in shunt fraction. Patients who do not demonstrate this response, non-reactors, have an unchecked increase in shunt fraction that is related directly to the size of the injury (air-space filling).[5]

Other phenomena, which occur subsequent to traumatic lung injury, include bronchosconstriction and atelectasis secondary to bronchial obstruction by blood clots.[20,21] Ventilation/perfusion mismatching has been demonstrated in pulmonary contusion.[22]

Much of the experimental work on animals with pulmonary contusion was performed by creating blast injuries. In the most commonly quoted work, which creates a true interstitial injury and capillary leak, a 0.38 special revolver with blank cartridges was fired against coins taped to the animal's chest wall.[1] We believe that this resulting lung contusion is more analogous to a blast wound and not to civilian blunt chest trauma, such as results from an automobile accident. However, it was from this animal model that the 'pulmonary contusion regimen' of fluid restriction, diuretics and steroids was conceived.[1]

COMPLICATIONS

Table 20.2 lists all complications attributable to the lung laceration and the laceration's accompanying spillover hemorrhage. Parenchymal laceration extending through the visceral pleura usually results in pneumothorax and hemothorax. Subcutaneous emphysema occurs when air from the pneumothorax escapes through the torn parietal pleura and intercostal muscle into the subcutaneous tissues or when the air extends upward via the mediastinum into the soft tissues. Mediastinal emphysema is usually secondary to barotrauma in which intraparenchymal alveoli rupture and air dissects through perivascular sheaths into the mediastinum; it may also occur secondary to a traumatic laceration. The entity generally described as *pulmonary cavitation, pneumatocele, or post-traumatic pulmonary cyst* is actually the pulmonary laceration itself. The roughly spherical shape of intraparenchymal lacerations is attributable to the normal elastic elements of the lung pulling centrifugally in all directions on the disrupted area.[2,23] A *pulmonary hematoma* is the pulmonary laceration filled with blood, clot, or fibrous tissue (see Fig 20.9).[2] Although air embolism may occur without positive pressure ventilation, it occurs most frequently with assisted ventilation during which the air or air–oxygen mix is more easily forced into open pulmonary venules. Gross hemoptysis is infrequent; however, when patients with contusions/lacerations are bronchoscoped early, blood is seen in the tracheobronchial tree in over 90% of these cases.[24] Low pulmonary compliance or stiff lung which diminishes the elasticity of the lung is a manifestation

Table 20.3 *Complications indirectly attributable to pulmonary contusion/laceration*

- Atelectasis
- Pneumonia
- Empyema
- Sepsis
- Adult respiratory distress syndrome (ARDS)
- Pulmonary abscess
- Delayed hemoptysis
- Barotrauma

of a blood-filled lobe or lobes. High shunt fractions or acute pulmonary hypertension with resultant hypoxemia are manifestations of air-space filling, as described previously.

The indirect complications attributable to pulmonary contusions/lacerations are listed in Table 20.3. They are readily explained as untoward sequelae of the pulmonary laceration. Atelectasis is a secondary complication resulting from residual endobronchial blood with resorption of air from the distal pulmonary parenchyma. Blood-filled alveoli or an inadequately drained hemothorax are excellent culture media for bacteria that can cause pneumonia or empyema and sepsis. Inadequately treated sepsis, whether it is from the lung or elsewhere, is the primary etiology of ARDS. The pulmonary hematoma may become infected, leading to a pulmonary abscess, which in turn may cause delayed hemoptysis. When the blood-filled lung parenchyma causes diminished pulmonary compliance, the requirement for increased airway pressures during mechanical ventilation may result in pulmonary barotrauma.

Mortality

Since the 1960s, published mortality rates from pulmonary contusion have varied between 0% and 45%. These extremes are due in part to reporting methods, selection of patients, and also to improvements in therapy, particularly the addition of positive end-expiratory pressure (PEEP) to the armentarium. Most deaths with pulmonary contusion result from head and other associated injuries. In our series of 144 patients, our mortality rate was 9.1% (13 patients) with 2.8% (four patients) dying as a direct result of their pulmonary parenchymal injury.[25]

Table 20.4 *Indications for intubation with blunt lung injury*

- A Pa_{O_2} level <60 Torr (8 kPa) on room air or 80 Torr (10.6 kPa) on oxygen inhalation
- A Pc_{O_2} >50 Torr (6.6 kPa)
- Serious non-thoracic injuries
- Patients undergoing general anesthesia
- Airway obstruction

MANAGEMENT OF PULMONARY CONTUSION

- Resuscitate and physical examination proceed simultaneously
- If respiratory difficulties are noted, maintain airway
- Oxygen is given by mask or intubation if necessary
- Support the circulation with adequate i.v. fluids as required
- If patient is responding to resuscitation, perform chest radiograph
- If shock continues, attend to life-threatening situations, e.g. tension pneumothorax, cardiac tamponade, abdominal hemorrhage, etc.
- If stable, chest CT
- Monitor O_2 Sats, blood gases, Swan–Ganz catheter, if injury warrants
- Manage identified *direct* complications of injury (see complications of injury)
- Admit to appropriate ward
- Prevent *indirect* complications: relief of chest pain; maintain good pulmonary toilet, bronchoscopy if necessary; if on ventilator, keep airway pressures low

The goals in managing pulmonary contusion are prevention of complications and management of complications when they occur. Good pulmonary toilet is mandatory. Antibiotics for pulmonary contusion are not warranted but can be instituted when indicated for other reasons. We believe that the 'pulmonary contusion regimen' frequently described as fluid restriction, diuretics and steroids has no place in the management of this injury. These patients, more often than not, have multiple serious injuries that require aggressive fluids, blood replacement therapy and antibiotics. Steroids would seldom be of value in the patient with a contaminated wound.

Although we believe that the volume of air-space filling is the ultimate determinant as to whether or not ventilator support is required, we rely primarily on physiological data (Table 20.4) for determining when it is appropriate to ventilate. On the other hand, most patients with pulmonary contusions have other serious injuries requiring intubation.

Monitoring

Any patient presenting to a modern emergency room with a significant chest injury should at least have a baseline measurement of the oxygen saturation. If the oxygen saturation is low, and particularly if the patient may require ventilator support, a blood gas should be drawn and consideration given for a radial artery cannula. If the patient does require ventilator support, it is useful to monitor pulmonary compliance as 'effective compliance,' i.e. tidal volume in ml/airway pressure in cmH_2O. When used sequentially, this is a valuable guideline for monitoring the progress, or lack thereof, of the injured lung.[26] Swan–Ganz catheters may be required in the larger grade III injuries or in any patient who is clinically deteriorating after appropriate initial management.

Individual management

The management of patients with pulmonary contusion should be individualized. With monitoring, pulmonary toilet, and anesthesia techniques to reduce pain, many patients can be safely managed without a ventilator. This is particularly true in patients with trauma limited to the chest. However, we have found that patients with pulmonary contusions of air-space filling of greater than 30% will ultimately require ventilator support, whether they have a flail chest or not.

The physiological criteria for the institution of ventilator support have been well established (Table 20.4) and includes patients with:

- a PaO_2 level less than 60 Torr (8 kPa) on room air or 80 Torr (10.6 kPa) on oxygen inhalation
- serious non-thoracic injuries
- a need for general anesthesia
- airway obstruction.[27,28]

PEEP is of great value, particularly in the larger lesions. The risk of air embolization with high PEEP should be kept in mind, particularly where there is a large laceration. Recently, transesophageal echocardiography[29] has been utilized in the diagnosis of air embolism. High frequency oscillatory ventilation may be of value when hypoxemic respiratory failure is associated with an ongoing air leak.[30] In the rare case of severe unilateral contused lung, which cannot be managed by the usual methods, independent lung ventilation[31,32] or resectional surgery may be required.[33]

By nature, the typical trauma patient will have relatively healthy lungs. However, if the trauma victim is older or if the pretraumatized lungs are diseased, a lesser injury will require ventilatory support.

Treatment of direct complications

If complications (see Table 20.2) develop, early appropriate therapy must be instituted. Pneumothorax, hemothorax, and air leak, the most common complications, are easily controlled by tube thoracostomy.

Hemoptysis and atelectasis may require therapeutic bronchoscopy to prevent significant atelectasis. Subcutaneous or mediastinal emphysema rarely requires specific therapy unless it is truly massive. Should this complication occur, repositioning the chest tube or tubes, or decreasing positive pressure on the ventilator may be useful. The pulmonary laceration and/or pulmonary hematoma, which is a laceration filled with blood, require no special treatment. Unless the laceration becomes infected, it will ultimately heal. A pulmonary laceration may not heal when the cavity is in a lobe adjacent to the site of a previously resected lobe. In this instance, the residual lobe will hyperinflate, thereby increasing the elastic pull on the cavity. With large contusions, i.e. 50% air-space filling, one must be concerned with the possibility of high shunt fractions or the potential development of acute pulmonary hypertension with right heart failure. These patients require Swan–Ganz monitoring. Rarely, pulmonary resection is necessary to correct the underlying pathophysiology.[34,35]

Treatment of indirect complications

Besides atelectasis, which is easily treated by removal of clot or secretions from the involved bronchus, and barotrauma, which may arise from diminished pulmonary compliance, indirect complications of pulmonary contusion are caused by infection (see Table 20.3). Empyema requires drainage, preferably early tube drainage; pneumonia should be treated with culture-directed antibiotics. Successful treatment for the pulmonary abscess that occurs in an infected laceration may be achieved with CT-directed catheter drainage,[36] but some cases may require thoracotomy. ARDS, the most dreaded complication, is relatively rare in the properly treated pulmonary contusion and occurs most commonly secondary to an infection in another system.

Surgery for pulmonary contusion/laceration

Fewer than 5% of patients with pulmonary contusions will require an urgent thoracotomy to control air leak, massive hemorrhage, hemoptysis, air embolism or severe unrelenting hemodynamic abnormality (high shunt fraction or acute pulmonary hypertension; Table 20.5). When urgent thoracotomy is required, the mortality rate is relatively high.[25,37,38] Prior to the utilization of CT, pulmonary laceration was considered to be a rather rare phenomenon, most often diagnosed at thoracotomy or autopsy. In 1971, Moghissi reported that in 182 patients with blunt chest injury only eight pulmonary lacerations were found, an incidence of only 4.4%.[37] Similarly, Hankins et al. in 1977, reviewed a 3.5-

Table 20.5 *Indications for urgent thoracotomy in blunt lung injury*

- Massive air leak
- Massive hemothorax (1500 ml initially, then 200 ml/h)
- Massive hemoptysis
- Major air embolism
- Life-threatening progressive high shunt fraction with localized contusion
- Life-threatening progressive right heart failure with localized contusion

year experience at the University of Maryland and found a 3.7% incidence of pulmonary laceration.[38] The majority of the patients from both series underwent thoracotomy because of major hemorrhage or massive air leak. These reports led to the impression that pulmonary laceration is a dramatic event with major life-threatening clinical manifestations that, in most instances, would require thoracotomy for optimal treatment. Based on our CT findings, it is clear that only a small percentage of pulmonary lacerations require surgery. In our series, only five of 144 patients (3%) were operated on for their pulmonary parenchyma injury. Another five patients underwent urgent thoracotomy for other intrathoracic injuries and four patients underwent delayed thoracotomy for complications of their pulmonary parenchymal injury.[25]

Surgical fixation of the flail chest has been recommended intermittently for years.[39] Our experience with operative management is limited to those few patients who require operative intervention for another reason, such as massive air leak or hemorrhage.

Follow-up studies

There are few series that examine the late sequelae of pulmonary contusion. The data that exist are mixed, one study suggesting only moderate decreases in objective pulmonary function studies[40] and another reporting significant reduction in the functional residual capacity.[41] This disparity could be due possibly to not stratifying patients into severity (grade) of pulmonary injuries. Follow-up CT scans of the injured lungs demonstrate fibrous changes at the site of injury.[2,41]

REFERENCES

1. Trinkle JK, Furman RW, Hinshaw MA, *et al.* Pulmonary contusion: pathogenesis and effect of various resuscitative measures. *Ann Thorac Surg* 1973; **16:** 568–73.

2. Wagner RB, Crawford WO Jr, Schimpf PP. Classification of parenchymal injuries of the lung. *Radiology* 1988; **167:** 77–82.

3. Wagner RB, Crawford WO Jr, Schimpf PP, Jamieson PM, Rao KCVG. Quantitation and pattern of parenchymal lung injury in blunt chest trauma. CT. *J Comput Tomogr* 1988; **12:** 270–81.

4. Wagner RB, Jamieson PM. Pulmonary contusion: evaluation and classification by computed tomography. *Surg Clin North Am* 1989; **69:** 31–40.

5. Wagner RB, Slivko B, Jamieson PM, Dills MS, Edwards FH. Effect of lung contusion on pulmonary hemodynamics. *Ann Thorac Surg* 1991; **52:** 51–8.

6. Hankins JR, Attar S, Turney SZ, *et al.* Differential diagnosis of pulmonary parenchymal changes in thoracic trauma. *Am Surg* 1973; **39:** 309–18.

7. Shin B, McAslan TC, Hankins JR, *et al.* Management of lung contusion. *Am Surg* 1979; **45:** 168–75.

8. Toombs BD, Sandler CM, Lester RG. Computed tomography of chest trauma. *Radiology* 1981; **140:** 733–8.

9. Toombs BD, Lester RG, Ben-Menachem Y, Sandler CM. Computed tomography in blunt trauma. *Radiol Clin North Am* 1981; **19:** 17–35.

10. Greene R. Lung alterations in thoracic trauma. *J Thorac Imaging* 1987; **2:** 1–11.

11. McGonigal MD, Schwab CW, Kauder DR, Miller WT, Grumbach K. Supplemental emergent chest computed tomography in the management of blunt torso trauma. *J Trauma* 1990; **30:** 1431–5.

12. Karaaslan T, Meuli R, Androux R, Duvoisin B, Hessler C, Schnyder P. Traumatic chest lesions in patients with severe head trauma: a comparative study with computed tomography and conventional chest roentgenograms. *J Trauma* 1995; **39:** 1081–6.

13. Williams JR, Stembridge VA. Pulmonary contusions secondary to nonpenetrating chest trauma. *Am J Roentgenol* 1964; **91:** 284–90.

14. Stevens E, Templeton AW. Traumatic nonpenetrating lung contusion. *Radiology* 1965; **85:** 247–52.

15. Crawford WO Jr. Pulmonary injury in thoracic and non-thoracic trauma. *Radiol Clin North Am* 1973; **11:** 527–41.

16. Besson A, Saegesser FA. *A Colour Atlas of Chest Trauma and Associated Injuries.* Vol. 1. Weert, Netherlands: Wolfe, 1982.

17. Brock RC. *Lung Abscess.* Oxford: Blackwell Scientific, 1952.

18. Pierce RJ, Brown DJ, Denison DM. Radiographic, scintigraphic, and gas-dilution estimates of individual lung and lobar volumes in man. *Thorax* 1980; **35:** 773–80.

19. Horsfield K. Morphologhy of the human bronchial tree. MD Thesis. University of Birmingham, 1967, quoted by Pierce *et al.*[18]

20. Mosely RV, Doty DB, Pruitt BA Jr. Physiologic changes following chest injury in combat casualties. *Surg Gynecol Obstet* 1969; **129:** 233–42.

21. Mosely RV, Vernick JJ, Doty DB. Response to blunt chest injury: a new experimental model. *J Trauma* 1970; **10**: 673–83.

22. Van Eeden SF, Klopper JF, Alheit B, Bardin PG. Ventilation-perfusion imaging in evaluating regional lung function in nonpenetrating injury to the chest. *Chest* 1989; **95**: 632–8.

23. Moolten SE. Mechanical production of cavities in isolated lungs. *Arch Pathol* 1938; **19**: 825–32.

24. Joka T, Obertacke U, Herrmann J. Early diagnosis of pulmonary contusion by means of bronchoscopy. *Unfallchirurg* 1987; **90**: 286–91.

25. Jamieson PM, Schimpf PP, Wagner RB. Clinical findings in pulmonary laceration (contusion): correlation with trauma score and computed tomography grading. Presented at the 1989 meeting of the Washington, DC Academy of Surgery, January 19, 1989.

26. Bendixen HH, Egbert LD, Hedley-Whyte J, Laver MB, Pontoppidan H. *Respiratory Care*. St Louis: CV Mosby, 1965; 147.

27. Trinkle JK, Richardson JD, Franz JL, *et al.* Management of flail chest without mechanical ventilation. *Ann Thorac Surg* 1975; **19**: 355–63.

28. Barone JE, Pizzi WF, Nealon TF, *et al.* Indications for intubation in blunt chest trauma. *J Trauma* 1986; **26**: 334–8.

29. Saada M, Goarin JP, Riou B, *et al.* Systemic gas embolism complicating pulmonary contusion. *Am J Respir Crit Care Med* 1995; **152**: 812–15.

30. Dallessio JJ, Markley MA, Lohe A, Kuluz JW, Oiticica C, McLaughlin GE. Management of a traumatic pulmonary pseudocyst using high-frequency oscillatory ventilation. *J Trauma* 1995; **39**: 1188–90.

31. Hurst JM, DeHaven CB, Branson RD. Comparison of convential mechanical ventilation and synchronous independent lung ventilation (SILV) in the treatment of unilateral lung injury. *J Trauma* 1985; **25**: 766–70.

32. Siegel JH, Stoklosa JC, Borg U, *et al.* Quantification of asymmetric lung pathophysiology as a guide to the use of simultaneous independent lung ventilation in posttraumatic and septic adult respiratory distress syndrome. *Ann Surg* 1985; **202**: 425–39.

33. Khan FA, Phillips W, Khan A, Seriff NS. Unusual unilateral blunt chest trauma without rib fractures leading to pulmonary laceration requiring pneumonectomy. *Chest* 1974; **66**: 211–14.

34. Fisher RP, Geiger JP, Guernsey JM. Pulmonary resections for severe pulmonary contusions secondary to high-velocity missile wounds. *J Trauma* 1974; **14**: 293–302.

35. Wagner RB. In discussion of: Wagner RB, Slivko B, Jamieson PM, Dills MS, Edwards FH. Effect of lung contusion on pulmonary hemodynamics. *Ann Thorac Surg* 1991; **52**: 58.

36. Moore FA, Moore EE, Haenel JB, Waring BJ, Parsons PE. Post-traumatic pulmonary pseudocyst in the adult: pathophysiology, recognition, and selective management. *J Trauma* 1989; **29**: 1380–5.

37. Moghissi K. Laceration of the lung following blunt trauma. *Thorax* 1971; **26**: 223–8.

38. Hankins JR, McAslan TC, Shin B, *et al.* Extensive pulmonary laceration caused by blunt trauma. *J Thorac Cardiovasc Surg* 1977; **74**: 519–27.

39. Moore BP. Operative stabilization on nonpenetrating chest injuries. *J Thorac Cardiovasc Surg* 1975; **70**: 619–30.

40. Svennevig JL, Vaage J, Westheim A, Hafsahl G, Refsum HE. Late sequelae of lung contusion. *Injury* 1989; **20**: 253–6.

41. Kishikawa M, Yoshioka T, Shimazu T, Sugimoto H, Yoshioka T, Sugimoto T. Pulmonary contusion causes long-term respiratory dysfunction with decreased functional residual capacity. *J Trauma* 1991; **31**: 1203–8.

part 4

General considerations

21

Acute respiratory distress syndrome

JEFFREY LIPMAN AND ROGER SAADIA

The acute (inaccurately referred to as 'adult') respiratory distress syndrome (ARDS) is a clinical condition of rapid onset associated with a mortality of over 50%. It is frequently encountered nowadays in intensive care units (ICUs) and trauma centers. It was first described as a distinct clinical entity by Ashbaugh and colleagues in 1967;[1] it had been less precisely identified previously but, since then, its definition has been based generally on four criteria (hypoxemia, diffuse pulmonary infiltrates on the chest radiograph, decreased lung compliance and absence of left-sided heart failure) occurring on the background of an appropriate antecedent history.

DEFINITION

Ever since its description, ARDS has been beset by difficulties in the adoption of a universal definition; this is not surprising, given the heterogeneity of the pathological conditions underlying this syndrome. Uniform diagnostic criteria are necessary if one is to compare different studies or test a management modality. Different authors chose different criteria to define, for example, hypoxemia or the maximal value of the pulmonary artery wedge pressure. More confusion was caused by uncertainties about the relationship between ARDS and other relatively loosely defined clinical entities such as fat embolism (Fig 21.1), acute neurogenic edema or barotrauma (Fig 21.2). A lung injury score was proposed to quantify the severity of the pulmonary insult;[2] this was based on the grading of four components: radiographic extent of alveolar consolidation, degree of hypoxemia, pulmonary compliance and

amount of positive end-expiratory pressure (PEEP) used. More recently, the American-European Consensus Committee on ARDS recommended the following defining criteria for ARDS:[3]

1. an acute onset
2. a level of oxygenation determined by the partial pressure of arterial oxygen (PaO_2) to the fraction of inspired oxygen (FIO_2) ratio equal to or less than 200 mmHg (26.6 kPa) (regardless of PEEP level)
3. bilateral infiltrates on the the frontal chest radiograph
4. pulmonary artery wedge pressure (PAWP) equal to or less than 18 mmHg (2.4 kPa) (when measured) or no clinical evidence of left atrial hypertension.

The Committee further proposed that ARDS be seen to be located at the severe end of a spectrum of disease termed 'acute lung injury'. This is defined by the same criteria as ARDS except for the oxygenation [PaO_2 to FIO_2 ratio equal to or less than 300 mmHg (40 kPa)].

PATHOPHYSIOLOGY

ARDS begins with damage at either the air–lung interface (epithelial injury) or the blood–lung interface (endothelial injury), eventually involving the alveolar–capillary membrane (Fig 21.3). This dual injury results in the filling of the alveolar air space and the expansion of the interstitium by an inflammatory exudate rich in plasma proteins and containing red blood cells, platelets and leukocytes (predominantly neutrophils).[4] Alveolar obliteration together with surfactant inactivation are responsible for an early

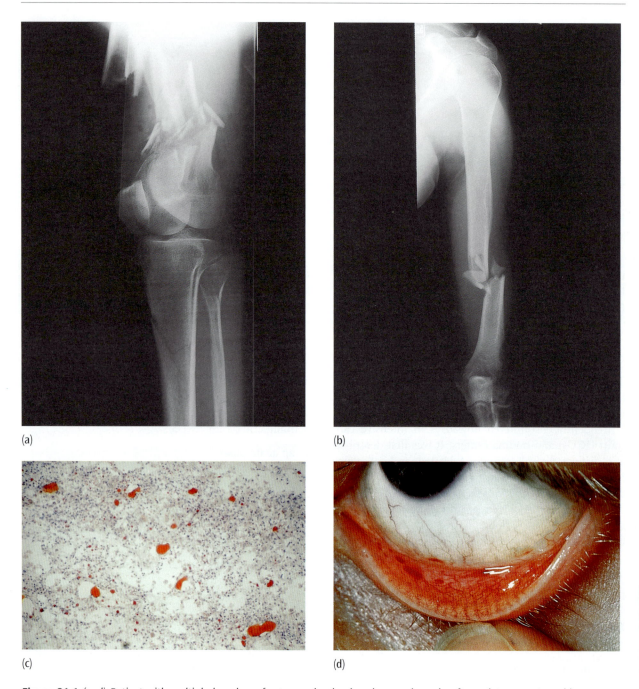

(a)

(b)

(c)

(d)

Figure 21.1 *(a–d) Patient with multiple long bone fractures who developed severe hypoxia after polytrauma. Lung biopsy showed widespread fat embolism with occlusion of the pulmonary capillaries (c). Fat embolism was also evident in the conjunctivi.*

shunt effect resulting from the perfusion of unventilated alveoli. In addition to these events at the air–lung interface, endothelial damage is caused by microvascular thrombosis with aggregates of platelets and leukocytes.[5] The patency of the pulmonary microvasculature is compromised, resulting in increased dead space as more lung parenchyma is ventilated but not perfused. The pulmonary circulation responds to hypoxemia by vasoconstriction around the obliterated alveoli, thereby diverting venous blood flow to well ventilated alveoli.

This hypoxic pulmonary vasoconstriction predisposes to pulmonary hypertension, which results in increase of the right ventricular afterload and worsening of the pulmonary edema.[6] These pathological changes are aggravated by the formation, a few days later, of a granulation tissue followed by fibrosis which occupies the alveolar air space previously obliterated by edema and microatelectasis.[7] There is thus a chronological succession of three phases: 'exudative', 'proliferative' and 'fibrotic'; commonly however, there is some overlap

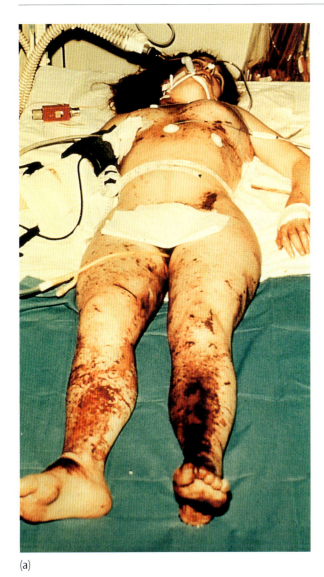

(a)

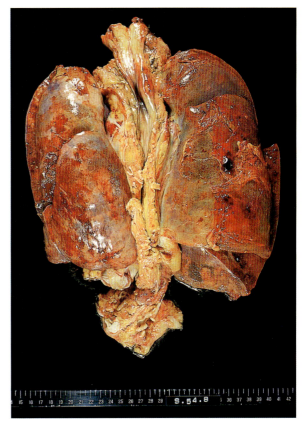

(b)

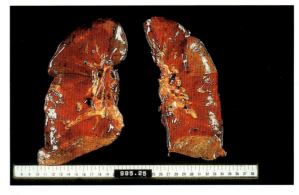

(c)

Figure 21.2 *Bomb blast injury in a restricted space. The victim suffered severe pulmonary barotrauma (a). A subsequent post mortem showed extensive hemorrhage and consolidation throughout both lungs, section through the lungs showed them to be airless with the consistency of liver (b and c).*

between these phases. Alveolar edema and subsequent pulmonary fibrosis may result in markedly decreased pulmonary compliance.

A systemic inflammatory response accompanies the acute lung injury and may determine its progression. Both cellular and humoral factors are involved. Margination and activation of leukocytes play a central role, resulting in the release of cytotoxic free radicals and cytokines.[8] It is believed that leukocyte priming sets the stage for subsequent cytokine release that may be triggered by a variety of clinical events. Several homeostatic systems are also activated: the complement and kinin systems, the cyclooxygenase and leukotriene pathways, the coagulation cascade and the nitric

oxide–cyclic guanosine monophosphate pathway. Knowledge about the precise sequence and relative importance of these biochemical events is currently lacking.

PREDISPOSING CONDITIONS

The lung's response to acute injury of various etiology proceeds along a series of common pathways; there is a large heterogenous group of clinical conditions or toxic agents responsible for the development of acute lung injury and ARDS. It is useful to relate the predisposing

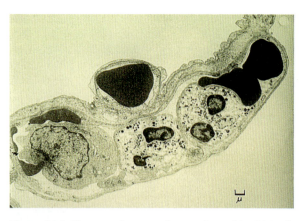

Figure 21.3 *Electron microscopy in a patient with ARDS. The pulmonary microvasculature is filled with activated neutrophils. Protease enzymes and oxygen free radicals released through neutrophil activation increase the permeability of the alveolar–capillary barrier, causing pulmonary edema.*

Table 21.1 *Common etiologies of ARDS*

Surgical	Medical
Direct lung injury	
Aspiration	Aspiration
Nosocomial pneumonia	Community-acquired and nosocomial pneumonia
Thoracic trauma	Pneumonitis (drug-induced, toxic inhalation, oxygen, radiation)
Fat embolism	Near-drowning
Distant injury	
Extrapulmonary sepsis	Extrapulmonary sepsis
Severe inflammation, necrosis	Severe inflammation, necrosis
Severe extrathoracic trauma	
Burns	
Shock	Shock
Multiple transfusions	
DIC	DIC
Acute pancreatitis	
Cardiopulmonary bypass	

DIC, diffuse intravascular coagulation.

conditions to one of two pathogenic pathways: the direct effect of an insult on lung parenchyma or the indirect result of an acute systemic inflammatory response (Table 21.1). Traumatic lung contusion or aspiration of gastric contents are examples of the former, while necrotizing pancreatitis or extrapulmonary sepsis are causative factors associated with the latter. The incidence of each etiological factor varies according to the ICU population under study; in a medical ICU, infectious pneumonia is the predominant cause of ARDS, whereas trauma and abdominal sepsis are more commonly incriminated in a surgical facility.

ARDS AND THE TRAUMA SURGEON

ARDS is a common complication of severe trauma, but it is not always easy to ascribe its development to a particular risk factor. Thus, in a severe blunt polytrauma patient, any of the following, singly or in combination, may be responsible: aspiration, head trauma, direct lung contusion, massive blood transfusion, disseminated intravascular coagulation, fat embolism, or a septic complication (pneumonia, occult intra-abdominal abscess). At other times, however, the underlying pathological condition is easily identified: fat embolism occurring 48 hours after trauma in a hitherto well patient with a mid-shaft femoral fracture; or postoperative deterioration of the respiratory function in a patient in whom a septic abdominal focus is demonstrated at a relook laparotomy.

Trauma is frequently complicated by sepsis and multiple organ dysfunction (MOD), of which ARDS is usually the first manifestation. In patients with ARDS and a clinical picture of sepsis, the two most common

sources of infection are the abdominal cavity and the lung.[9] The time sequence of clinical sepsis and ARDS may provide a clue to the source of infection: when sepsis precedes ARDS, an abdominal septic focus is most likely; a nosocomial pneumonia is, however, most commonly incriminated if the septic syndrome develops after the onset of ARDS.[10] In one study, the presence of bacteremia was frequently associated with an abdominal source of infection, whereas sterile blood cultures occurred more commonly with a pulmonary source.[11]

ARDS and MOD may complicate trauma in at least two different patterns. A massive tissue injury with profound hypovolemic shock may trigger an exaggerated systemic inflammatory response without infection resulting in early ARDS and MOD, a scenario referred to as 'one-hit'. Alternatively, in the 'two-hit' model, less severely injured patients enter a state of moderate inflammatory response; delayed ARDS and MOD are subsequently caused by one or several secondary insults (abdominal sepsis, pneumonia, repeated surgery, transient bacteremia from invasive monitoring, and others).[12] These insults may be responsible for release of cytokines. The characterization of MOD as early or late rests, however, on clinical observation and precise biochemical correlation is lacking.

The prognosis of post-traumatic ARDS varies widely, according to the underlying pathology. An isolated lung contusion in a previously healthy subject carries a relatively good prognosis; similarly, fat embolism following a long bone fracture is rarely fatal if appropriately treated. Conversely, survival is markedly decreased in ARDS occurring after severe multiple trauma, especially if associated with sepsis. In this particular context, the mortality of ARDS is accounted for by the severity of the underlying injury complex; in addition, ARDS with sepsis is often a component of MOD, the prognosis of which is closely dependent on the number of organs in failure.

MANAGEMENT

Prevention of ARDS is possible by limiting the incidence and severity of acute lung injury. This can be achieved, particularly in the trauma patient, by adherence to sound surgical principles and provision of high quality immediate care. In established ARDS, treatment rests principally on correction of the underlying cause, expert ventilatory support and judicious hemodynamic management. A number of adjunctive therapeutic measures are currently being investigated.

Prevention and treatment of the underlying condition

Several management interventions play an important role in the prevention of acute lung injury. Optimal airway management of the trauma victim, starting at the roadside and continuing throughout the initial resuscitation in the emergency room, will prevent aspiration. Skilful airway management in the ICU is essential. In this setting, the administration of sucralfate in preference to antacid therapy, as a prophylaxis against stress ulceration, has been advocated as a means to prevent gastric bacterial overgrowth,[13] but it has not be shown to decisively protect against nosocomial pneumonia and ARDS. Similarly, selective decontamination of the gut by non-absorbable antibiotics has not lived up to earlier expectations in the prevention of microbial aspiration into the tracheobronchial tree or in survival benefit.[14] The aggressive management of hypovolemic shock has been identified as a key factor in the prevention of delayed ARDS and MOD; this is supported by work in the laboratory animal as well as clinical observations in trauma victims, even though the sequence of pathological events linking trauma to MOD is not yet completely elucidated. A great deal of controversy still surrounds the timing of fracture fixation and its influence on the incidence of fat embolism; current opinion favors early fixation (within 24–48 hours) but with the recommendation that this policy be implemented with a degree of discrimination based on the clinical condition of the patient.[15] It is noteworthy that the application of prophylactic PEEP in trauma patients at risk for ARDS is of no benefit.[16] Transfused human leukocyte antibodies (HLA) have been implicated in the pathogenesis of transfusion-related acute lung injury: the combination of these antibodies with the host's marginated pool of granulocytes activates the complement pathway and generates a systemic inflammatory response; there may be merit in preventive donor selection, as multiparous women and previously transfused subjects are more likely to donate HLA antibodies.[17] Early drainage of abscesses and thorough debridement of devitalized tissues or burn eschars will decrease the incidence of sepsis-triggered MOD. In severe abdominal sepsis or massive trauma, the conventional, once-for-all laparotomy is often inadequate. It is often replaced nowadays by a policy of electively staged relook laparotomies every 48–72 hours until the peritoneal cavity is deemed clean: the rationale for this policy is to anticipate the formation of septic collections and to preclude, before they have become clinically apparent, their deleterious systemic effects in the form of incipient MOD.

In established ARDS, active search for the cause is a critical management step. In the surgical setting, this revolves mainly around the identification of a possible occult septic focus, usually intra-abdominal. In the patient who has already undergone a laparotomy as part of the initial treatment, it is often difficult to exclude the possibility of a complication in the form of an intra-abdominal abscess. The CT scan is a useful diagnostic modality, but a relook laparotomy, 'on demand', is often undertaken at a very low threshold of clinical suspicion. However, the drainage of such a septic focus does not always result in the reversal of established MOD. The problem is further complicated by the fact that, in over a third of trauma patients with ARDS and MOD, no discrete focus of infection is present; and it is well accepted now that the systemic inflammatory response syndrome and the ensuing MOD are not always caused by a septic source.[18] Massive tissue injury alone may trigger the cytokine cascade.

Principles of mechanical ventilation

Optimal mechanical ventilatory support in ARDS aims at the provision of adequate oxygenation and carbon dioxide clearance; at the same time, the possibility of further pulmonary injury, particularly in the form of barotrauma, pulmonary infections and possibly oxygen toxicity must be given serious consideration. As a low mixed venous oxygen concentration is a cause of hypoxemia, the appropriate Pa_{O_2} should be achieved while maintaining an adequate cardiac output. To this end, it is necessary to adjust the FI_{O_2} and the patient's functional residual capacity (FRC).

In patients with ARDS, ventilation at low lung volumes results in alveolar collapse. Increased alveolar shear forces are required on reopening, with the potential for lung damage.[19] It is therefore preferable to maintain alveolar patency (and at the same time the FRC) throughout the ventilatory cycle. Sophisticated monitoring (proximal airway pressure–volume curves) may be needed to optimize the ventilatory support, but most ICUs use arterial blood gases as a surrogate end point instead.

The use of positive end-expiratory pressure (PEEP) has been a cornerstone in the treatment of ARDS.[20] Physiologically, PEEP enhances lung volume by recruiting collapsed alveoli and increasing functional residual capacity; extravascular lung water is redistributed from the air space to the interstitium, with a consequent increase of the alveolar surface available for gas exchange and reduction of the shunt effect. PEEP is an essential adjunct in allowing adequate oxygenation with less toxic levels of F_{IO_2}. Above a certain level, however, PEEP decreases venous return by increasing intrathoracic pressure; this may reduce significantly cardiac output and tissue oxygen delivery. In addition, PEEP may compress the capillaries around the distensible alveoli, resulting in impaired oxygenation and increased pulmonary vascular resistance.

Tidal volumes of 10–15 ml/kg have been recommended for patients receiving mechanical ventilation. More recently, large tidal volumes and high peak airway pressures have been recognized as causes of lung injury.[21] In patients with ARDS, computed tomography has revealed the inhomogeneous distribution of the areas of consolidation: these predominate in the dependent portions of the lung. Furthermore, it was demonstrated by traditional physiological analysis that these areas of radiological consolidation have a marked reduction in compliance, whereas lung regions that appear normally aerated have a normal compliance.[22] Thus, the lung tissue available for gas exchange in ARDS is markedly reduced in volume but normal in compliance (hence the concept of 'baby lung'); in these patients, traditional tidal volumes may overdistend the aerated alveoli and compound the pre-existing lung injury. Smaller tidal volumes of 5–10 ml/kg seem therefore more appropriate in this setting.

With peak airway pressures rising above 40 cmH$_2$O, alveolar rupture as evidenced by pulmonary interstitial emphysema was observed. It is now widely believed that a rise in the partial pressure of arterial carbon dioxide (P_{aCO_2}) is less hazardous than high airway pressures. In patients with adequate oxygenation but excessively elevated airway pressures, reductions in the tidal volume and minute ventilation may decrease airway pressure at the price of hypercapnia; this strategy is referred to as controlled hypoventilation with permissive hypercapnia.[23] The P_{aCO_2} may be allowed to rise up to 100 mmHg (13.3 kPa) and the pH to fall to 7.20; these abnormalities are well tolerated and can be metabolically compensated over 2–3 days in the setting of a normal renal function. Either sodium bicarbonate or tris(hydroxymethyl)aminomethane (THAM) are occasionally necessary to maintain an adequate pH. Permissive hypercapnia is contraindicated in the presence of an elevated intracranial pressure.

Inverse ratio ventilation represents another variation of conventional ventilation in which an inspiratory:expiratory ratio >1 is applied.[24] The prolonged inspiratory time results in increased mean airway pressures but helps maintain acceptable peak airway pressures. The longer application of inspiratory positive pressure aims at recruiting collapsed alveoli; yet, the abbreviated period of expiration is adequate for carbon dioxide clearance. It has also been suggested that sustained inpiratory pressures may have a beneficial effect on the non-functional areas of the pulmonary parenchyma. Improvements in gas exchange may take several hours to occur. Inverse ratio ventilation usually requires heavy sedation or neuromuscular blockade which, if prolonged, may cause protracted weakness and paralysis. Sometimes, with these long inspiratory times (or with high rates), there is intrathoracic gas retention leading to the phenomenon of intrinsic PEEP ('auto-PEEP'); if severe, this effect may lead to marked reduction of cardiac output and even electromechanical dissociation.

Pressure-controlled ventilation may be administered either with conventional inspiratory:expiratory ratio or inverse ratio ventilation.[25] It consists of the application of a fixed or preset pressure to the airway for a given time. Consequently, the tidal volume depends on airway resistance and lung compliance. Pressure-controlled with inverse ratio ventilation has the advantage of producing a rapid pressure rise, allowing time for redistribution of gas into the alveoli that are slow to open, while limiting the peak airway pressure to a predetermined level.

Because lung infiltrates predominate in the dependent pulmonary regions, changes in position may improve oxygenation; the prone position in particular has been advocated.[26] While its efficacy remains to be proven, the technique is difficult to implement in the ICU and requires meticulous attention to detail on the part of the medical and nursing team; the access to and security of the airway may be threatened, intravenous lines may be dislodged; in addition iatrogenic complications such as nerve or muscle compression, venous stasis, pressure sores and limited diaphragmatic excursion may occur.

Fluid therapy and hemodynamic monitoring

This is a controversial area in the management of ARDS.[27] There are two general approaches to fluid management:

1. maintenance of a relatively normal intravascular volume
2. marked fluid restriction and support of blood pressure and cardiac output with vasopressor drugs

if necessary, in order to minimize the fluid leakage into the interstitium and alveoli.

In some retrospective studies of survival, there is evidence in favor of a reduction in extravascular lung water. On the other hand, a decrease of the preload from a negative fluid balance will reduce cardiac output and oxygen delivery to the tissues; this strategy will also decrease the renal and splanchnic perfusion; in combination, these effects may predispose to MOD. It is likely that no single policy is successfully applicable to the whole spectrum of ARDS patients. An isolated lung contusion in a patient with good renal function is probably best treated with fluid restriction and diuretics. Conversely, adequate fluid repletion may be necessary in the patient with multiple trauma, potential for recurrent hemorrhage, sepsis, incipient MOD and indication for several trips to the operating room.

The practice of 'supranormal' hemodynamic management with fluids and vasopressors has been advocated as a means of optimizing cardiac output and oxygen delivery. Patients are treated prophylactically to increase oxygen delivery to above a level of 600 ml/min/m^2. This strategy is based on the premise that the prognosis of critically ill patients is adversely affected by a hidden tissue oxygen debt and that oxygen consumption seems to depend, at least to some extent, on oxygen delivery. This concept remains yet to be validated.[28]

The use of colloid in patients with leaky pulmonary (and possibly systemic) capillaries is another area of debate. Any colloids administered early in the course of ARDS are likely to leak out of the intravascular space across an incompetent alveolar–capillary membrane;[29] they are therefore unlikely to result in increased intravascular oncotic pressure or decreased tissue edema.

The role of pulmonary artery catheters remains to be accurately defined in ARDS. Potential complications, unproven benefit for survival and cost argue against their routine insertion in all patients. These catheters may be necessary as a diagnostic tool in distinguishing between cardiogenic pulmonary edema and acute lung injury. They may also be useful, in some patients, in monitoring the effect of PEEP on cardiac output and tissue oxygen delivery. They are particularly helpful in the implementation of the strategy of fluid restriction with vasopressors. In any case, their use seems particularly justified in the early management of the more unstable patients.

Pharmacological intervention

Several clinical trials have tested the broad anti-inflammatory properties of corticosteroids in the treatment of early sepsis and the prevention or treatment of ARDS.

No beneficial effect was found; indeed, there was sometimes a greater mortality in the treated group. More recent experience suggests, however, that corticosteroid 'salvage' therapy may be useful in the late fibroproliferative phase of the disease (15 days after onset), particularly in patients refractory to conventional treatment.[30,31] Another possible indication for corticosteroid therapy, in medical patients, is the presence of a high number of eosinophils in the blood or on bronchoalveolar lavage.[32] Systemic infection must be ruled out or treated before the institution of steroid therapy.

Pharmacological blockade of the mediators of the inflammatory response has been evaluated in critically ill patients with sepsis and MOD (including patients with ARDS). Monoclonal antibodies against endotoxin or cytokines as well as cytokine receptor antagonists have been studied. The results of prospective randomized trials have so far been disappointing.[33]

A number of other drugs have been used in ARDS with as yet no proven benefit: ketoconazole (a potent inhibitor of thromboxane synthesis), pentoxifylline (an inhibitor of neutrophil chemotaxis and activation), non-steroidal anti-inflammatory agents such as ibuprofen and indomethacin (inhibitors of prostaglandin pathways), acetylcysteine (an antioxidant scavenger of oxygen free radicals), and others.

Novel therapeutic modalities

Replacement therapy with exogenous lung surfactant has been highly successful in neonatal ARDS. In adult patients, surfactant is dysfunctional rather than deficient. The expected benefits of exogenous surfactant include a greater stability of the alveolar space with improved ventilation and antibacterial properties causing a reduction in the incidence of nosocomial pneumonia. The role of surfactant therapy is still under investigation in the adult patient.[34]

As an alternative to the high airway pressure generated by conventional techniques in ARDS, alternative strategies have been tested. High frequency oscillation has found some protagonists, especially in pediatric ARDS.[35] Extracorporeal respiratory support has been evaluated in severe ARDS. There are two forms: extracorporeal membrane oxygenation by means of a venoarterial bypass[36] and extracorporeal carbon dioxide removal utilizing a venovenous bypass. The latter modality has been developed more recently and combined with low frequency positive pressure ventilation;[37] the advantages of the technique are a reduction of the respiratory rates and peak airway pressures. Carbon dioxide is eliminated extracorporeally while most of the oxygenation occurs through the lungs. Compared to venoarterial bypass, venovenous bypass preserves the pulmonary arterial blood flow and decreases the tendency for pulmonary ischemia. The need for systemic heparinization and the frequent development of thromcytopenia greatly limit the use of extracorporeal support in the surgical patient. There is as yet no convincing evidence of survival benefit with these techniques.

Inhaled nitric oxide is a powerful vasodilator, reversing the pulmonary hypoxemia-induced vasoconstriction. Having diffused into the blood vessels, nitric oxide binds readily to hemoglobin and is precluded from causing systemic vasodilatation. The selective vasodilatation of the pulmonary vasculature in the well ventilated portions of the lung improves the ventilation-to-perfusion matching.[38] Results of large randomized trials of nitric oxide inhalation are awaited.

Liquid ventilation with intratracheal administration of perfluorocarbon has shown great promise in animal models of lung injury. Encouraging results have also been demonstrated in severe pediatric respiratory failure. Perfluorocarbon has a low surface tension and a high solubility for oxygen and carbon dioxide. It enhances the recruitment of poorly ventilated dependent lung regions, improves the matching of ventilation to perfusion and assists in airway secretion clearance.[39]

CONCLUSION

ARDS is a severe form of acute respiratory failure of various etiologies. Despite major advances in intensive care, it still carries a prohibitive mortality, although there may be some evidence that the prognosis has somewhat improved over the past few years in certain subgroups of patients, particularly the young adult, in the setting of direct lung damage and without severe sepsis. Conceptual progress has taken place recently to bring clarity and uniformity to the definition of acute lung injury and ARDS. In addition, great strides are being made in understanding the physiopathology of this syndrome. As a result, rational therapeutic modalities have evolved on multiple fronts: prevention, elimination of the underlying cause, ventilatory and fluid management, pharmacological interventions, and others. While the evidence for their efficacy is compelling in some, proof of benefit is presently being sought, in others, by means of large multi-institutional randomized trials. Until these find clinical relevance, the management of ARDS is largely supportive, whilst limiting further complications.

REFERENCES

1. Ashbaugh DG, Bigelow DB, Petty TL, Levine BE. Acute respiratory distress in adults. *Lancet* 1967; **2**: 319–23.

2. Murray JF, Matthay MA, Luce JM, Flick MR. An expanded definition of the adult respiratory distress syndrome. *Am Rev Respir Dis* 1988; **138**: 720–3. (Erratum: *Am Rev Respir Dis* 1989; **139**: 1065).

3. Bernard GR, Artigas A, Brigham KL, *et al*. The American-European Consensus Conference on ARDS. Definitions, mechanisms, relevant outcomes and clinical trial coordination. *Am J Respir Crit Care Med* 1994; **149**: 818–24.

4. Bachofen M, Weibel ER. Structural alterations of lung parenchyma in the adult respiratory distress syndrome. *Clin Chest Med* 1982; **3**: 55–6.

5. Tomashefski JF. Pulmonary pathology of the adult respiratory distress syndrome. *Clin Chest Med* 1990; **11**: 593–619.

6. Zapol WM, Jones R. Vascular components of ARDS: clinical pulmonary hemodynamics and morphology. *Am Rev Respir Dis* 1987; **136**: 471–4.

7. Marinelli WA, Henke CA, Harmon KR, Hertz MI, Bitterman PB. Mechanisms of alveolar fibrosis after acute lung injury. *Clin Chest Med* 1990; **11**: 657–72.

8. Brigham KL, Meyrick B. Endotoxin and lung injury. *Am Rev Respir Dis* 1986; **133**: 913–27.

9. Seidenfeld JJ, Pohl DF, Bell RC, Harris JD, Hohansen WG. Incidence, site and outcome of infections in patients with the adult respiratory distress syndrome. *Am Rev Respir Dis* 1986; **134**: 12–16.

10. Montgomery AB, Stager MA, Carrico CJ, Hudson LD. Causes of mortality in patients with the adult respiratory distress syndrome. *Am Rev Respir Dis* 1985; **132**: 485–9.

11. Bell RC, Coalson JJ, Smith JD, Johansen WG. Multiple organ system failure and infection in adult respiratory distress syndrome. *Ann Intern Med* 1983; **99**: 293–8.

12. Moore FA, Moore EE. Evolving concepts in the pathogenesis of postinjury multiple organ failure. *Surg Clin North Am* 1995; **75**: 257–77.

13. Cook DJ, Reeve BK, Guyatt GH, *et al*. Stress ulcer prophylaxis in critically ill patients. Resolving discordant meta-analyses. *JAMA* 1996; **275**: 308–14.

14. Atkinson SW, Bihari DJ. Selective decontamination of the gut. *Br Med J* 1993; **306**: 1480–1.

15. Reynolds MA, Richardson JD, Spain DA, Seligson D, Wilson MA, Miller FB. Is the timing of fracture fixation important for the patient with multiple trauma? *Ann Surg* 1995; **222**: 470–81.

16. Pepe PE, Hudson LD, Carrico CJ. Early application of positive end-expiratory pressure in patients at risk for the adult respiratory distress syndrome. *N Engl J Med* 1984; **311**: 281–6.

17. Florell SR, Velasco SE, Fine PG. Perioperative recognition, management and pathologic diagnosis of transfusion-related acute lung injury. *Anesthesiology* 1994; **81**: 508–10.

18. Saadia R, Lipman J. Multiple organ failure after trauma. *Br Med J* 1996; **313**: 573–4.

19. Lachmann B. Open up the lung and keep the lung open. *Intensive Care Med* 1992; **18**: 319–21.

20. Marini JJ. Positive end-expiratory pressure and adult respiratory distress syndrome: what are we missing? *J Crit Care* 1992; **7**: 137–41.

21. Gammon RB, Shin MS, Buchalter SE. Pulmonary barotrauma in mechanical ventilation: patterns and risk factors. *Chest* 1992; **103**: 568–72.

22. Gattinoni L, Pesenti A, Avalli L, Rossi F, Bombino M. Pressure-volume curve of the total respiratory system in acute respiratory failure: computed tomographic scan study. *Am Rev Respir Dis* 1987; **136**: 730–6.

23. Hickling KG, Henderson SJ, Jackson R. Low mortality associated with low volume pressure limited ventilation with permissive hypercapnia in severe adult respiratory distress syndrome. *Intensive Care Med* 1990; **16**: 372–7.

24. Marcy TW, Marini JJ. Inverse ratio ventilation in ARDS: rationale and implementation. *Chest* 1991; **100**: 494–504.

25. Lain DC, DiBenedetto R, Morris SL, Nguyem AV, Saulters R, Causey D. Pressure controlled inverse ratio ventilation as a method to reduce peak inspiratory pressure and provide adequate ventilation and oxygenation. *Chest* 1989; **95**: 1081–8.

26. Ryan DW, Pelosi P. The prone position in acute respiratory distress syndrome. *Br Med J* 1995; **312**: 860.

27. Schuster DP. The case for and against fluid restriction and occlusion pressure reduction in adult respiratory distress syndrome. *New Horizons* 1993; **1**: 478–88.

28. Gattinoni L, Brazzi L, Pelosi P, *et al.* A trial of goal-oriented hemodynamic therapy in critically ill patients. *N Engl J Med* 1995; **333**: 1025–32.

29. Sibbald WJ, Short AK, Warshawski FJ, Cunningham DG, Cheung H. Thermal dye measurements of extravascular lung water in critically ill patients. *Chest* 1985; **87**: 585–92.

30. Meduri GU, Chinn AJ, Leeper KV, *et al.* Corticosteroid rescue treatment of progressive fibroproliferation in late ARDS. Patterns of response and predictors of outcome. *Chest* 1994; **105**: 1516–27.

31. Biffl WL, Moore FA, Moore EE, Haenel JB, McIntyre RC, Burch JM. Are corticosteroids salvage therapy for refractory acute respiratory distress syndrome? *Am J Surg* 1995; **170**: 591–6.

32. Allen JN, Pacht ER, Gadek JE, Davis WB. Acute eosinophilic pneumonia as a reversible cause of noninfectious respiratory failure. *N Engl J Med* 1989; **321**: 569–74.

33. Bernard G. Sepsis trials. Intersection of investigation, regulation, funding and practice. *Am J Respir Crit Care Med* 1995; **152**: 4–10.

34. Jobe AH. Pulmonary surfactant therapy. *N Engl J Med* 1993; **328**: 861–8.

35. Arensman RM, Statter MB, Bastawrous AL, Madonna MB. Modern treatment modalities for neonatal and pediatric respiratory failure. *Am J Surg* 1996; **172**: 41–7.

36. Zapol WM, Snider MT, Hill JD, *et al.* Extracorporeal membrane oxygenation in severe acute respiratory failure. *JAMA* 1979; **242**: 2193–6.

37. Gattinoni L, Pesenti A, Mascheroni D, *et al.* Low-frequency positive pressure ventilation with extracorporeal CO_2 removal in severe acute respiratory failure. *JAMA* 1986; **256**: 881–6.

38. Bigatello LM, Hurford WE, Kacmarek RE, Roberts JD, Zapol WM. Prolonged inhalation of low concentrations of nitric oxide in patients with severe adult respiratory distress syndrome. Effects on pulmonary hemodynamics and oxygenation. *Anesthesiology* 1994; **80**: 761–70.

39. Hirschl RB, Pranikoff T, Gauger P, Schreiner RJ, Dechert R, Bartlett RH. Liquid ventilation in adults, children and full-term neonates. *Lancet* 1995; **346**: 1201–2.

FURTHER READING

Bigatello LM, Zapol WM. New approaches to acute lung injury. *Br J Anaesth* 1996; **77**: 99–109.

Kollef MH, Schuster DP. The acute respiratory distress syndrome. *N Engl J Med* 1995; **332**: 27–37.

Marinelli WA, Ingbar DH. Diagnosis and management of acute lung injury. *Clin Chest Med* 1994; **15**: 517–46.

22

Scoring systems in the assessment of the trauma patient: are they worthwhile?

DAVID J J MUCKART

Purpose of objective systems

- Triage
- Prediction of outcome
- Provide information to relatives
- Audit
- Facilitate research
- Epidemiological data

Scoring systems were designed to objectively quantify the severity of injury and overcome the variability inherent with subjective assessment. Numerous objective methods are now available for use in both prehospital triage and in-hospital management, an indication that none is ideal. Although systems for triage are designed to determine which level of care is required, they are indirectly performing the same function as in-hospital systems, namely assessment of mortality risk and therefore prediction of outcome.

An accurate method of predicting outcome would be of immense value to patients, their families and clinicians. Treatment could be guided, futility minimized, and research facilitated. A lack of effective treatments, especially in critical illness or following major injury, made prognostication easier for the ancient physicians and reputations were gained by the art of subjective prediction. Advances in medicine now make this a complex process, and the belief has arisen that more objective methods are necessary.[1] Furthermore, survival or death are no longer adequate endpoints and additional information is required in survivors with

respect to morbidity and quality of life.[2] Most clinicians are familiar with the common objective systems; few realize the complex basis of subjective prediction. Both methods have certain advantages and limitations,[3,4] and an understanding of these is essential when evaluating their roles.

SUBJECTIVE PREDICTION OF OUTCOME

Prediction of outcome using clinical judgment is prone to error in a number of ways.[3,5] First, even under identical circumstances, the individual metabolic response to an injury is variable and it has become increasingly clear that this is genetically determined.[6] In moderation, the metabolic response is a prerequisite for survival but if uncontrolled it results in the systemic inflammatory response syndrome (SIRS),[7] which may precipitate multiple organ dysfunction syndrome (MODS).[8] This was recognized 200 years ago by John Hunter[8] based on his military experience when he wrote:

> There is a circumstance attending accidental injury which does not belong to disease, namely that the injury done has in all cases a tendency to produce both the disposition and the means of cure.

There is little indication, however, of the likely course of the metabolic response in the early post-injury phase, especially following major trauma.

The second source of error concerns the psychological basis of decision making in medicine which is relevant to outcome prediction. Clinical judgment is based on information theory and there is an inherent tendency towards systematic error.[3] The human capacity for rational thought is limited (the psychological principle of bounded or limited rationality). As a result, certain mental shortcuts are adopted by clinicians to compensate for these deficiencies, especially when available information is incomplete. The method used most commonly is hypothetico-deductive reasoning.[9] This strategy necessitates forming an initial hypothesis which becomes the cornerstone to support or refute further evidence. Although designed to aid decision making, it is also flawed. The number of hypotheses that the human can consider at one time is small. In order to avoid the need to formulate new hypotheses, negative data that do not fit the initial hypothesis tend to be discounted, and positive findings may be weighted inappropriately. Based upon an initial hypothesis and the available evidence, a probability of outcome is then estimated. This may later be adjusted in the light of new information, but such alterations are usually biased in favor of the original probability value (adjustment and anchoring),[3,5] and tend to err on the side of a favorable prediction. Clinicians also suffer from hindsight bias. This consists of the erroneous belief that even after an event has occurred it could have been predicted beforehand. Such bias may have negative consequences on future decision making.

Pitfalls in subjective prediction of outcome
- Variable individual metabolic response to trauma

Errors in subjective decision making
- limited or bounded rationality
- hypothetico-deductive reasoning
- adjustment and anchoring
- availability
- hindsight bias
- poor calibration

The probability of an event occurring (e.g. expected outcome) is judged by the ease with which similar events are recalled (availability).[3–5] Although limited experience with the injury in question will obviously restrict judgmental ability, factors other than frequency affect availability and result in bias. Outstanding or unusual outcomes are more easily retrievable and may thus appear mistakenly to have occurred more frequently.

In the present economic climate of cost containment, a conflict may arise between expensive therapeutic options in both time and money[10] and possible futility, which includes not only mortality but also morbidity and quality of life. In situations of high demand but limited resources, the triage maxim of save the greatest number of lives applies. Context and contingency, which are dictated by the working environment, must therefore be considered in decision making and outcome prediction.[2,3,11] This is not addressed by objective systems. Although subjective prediction exhibits good discrimination (the ability to predict death or survival in an individual) and has been reported to compare favorably with objective scoring systems,[12–14] calibration (prediction of outcome for the entire range of risk), and reproducibility are poor.[4] This has led to the development of objective methods of outcome prediction.

OBJECTIVE PREDICTION OF OUTCOME

The ideal objective system

- User friendly – limited variables
- Variables are independently associated with outcome
- System is applicable to all environments
- System is applicable to all injuries
- Accurate prediction of mortality and morbidity

The ideal objective system must fulfil a number of criteria that relate to the system itself, the patient and the desired endpoint.[2] The system must employ a limited number of predictor variables which are collected routinely and are independently associated with outcome. It must be relevant to all working environments and as such, validated by independent researchers. There should be no restriction to specific diseases or injuries, and it should predict not only survival or death, but also possible morbidity or quality of life in an individual patient. To date, no such utopian system has been designed.

From the early 1970s both trauma-specific and general objective systems have evolved.[15–29] The former encompass all phases of trauma management, whereas the latter have predominantly addressed outcome in the critically ill using variables collected within the first 24 hours of intensive care unit (ICU) admission. The majority of injured patients do not require intensive care and the trauma-specific systems are therefore of limited use in the critically ill. The reverse is true of ICU systems. Cerebral injury, either direct or indirectly as a result of hypoxia, is the commonest cause of trauma deaths.[30] Consequently, both systems include either the Glasgow Coma Scale (GCS) or the presence of coma and heavily weight this component. In patients without head injury the GCS is unrelated to outcome and this seriously affects system accuracy.[31] Head injured patients rarely die from MODS[32] and it is therefore highly unlikely that a single objective system will gain universal acceptance.

TRAUMA-SPECIFIC OBJECTIVE SYSTEMS

Although the extent of anatomical disruption is frequently used to measure the severity of injury, its limitations were postulated more than 60 years ago by Sir David Cuthbertson[33] when he wrote:

> An injury such as the dislocation of an ankle might produce as great a disturbance of metabolism as the splintering of both bones of a leg. It may be that future work will indicate that our conception of the degree of severity of an injury is at fault.

This prophecy remained largely ignored until the realization dawned that the anatomical disruption *per se* does not predict outcome and this led to the incorporation of a physiological component into most trauma predictive systems.[28,29]

Initially designed for blunt injury, the anatomical Abbreviated Injury Score (AIS)[24] and subsequent Injury Severity Score (ISS)[25] have been upgraded to incorporate penetrating trauma. This, in combination with the physiological Trauma Score (TS)[26] or Revised Trauma Score (RTS),[27] age and injury mechanism resulted in the TRISS[28] method. Multivariate analysis and logistic regression were used to calculate a predictive equation, but unlike general systems the probability of survival (*Ps*) is calculated rather than the risk of death (*R*). TRISS is the currrent adopted gold standard for major trauma outcome studies (MTOS) which involve four categories of patient: those requiring hospital admission, specialist care, ICU admission, and within each of these areas, those who die. It has been designed as an audit mechanism to assess overall performance of trauma care systems and identify patients with unexpected outcomes for further scrutiny. As such, it is not a useful tool for the day-to-day basis of patient management. Furthermore, problems exist with the nature, timing and completeness of data collection. As with the general systems, categoric weighting is used for age and mechanism of injury and a decision criterion of *Ps* = 0.5 distinguishes survivors from non-survivors. The possible combinations of age and injury mechanism produce four Ps_{50} isobars in a plot of ISS versus RTS (Fig 22.1). This is important to realize if the method is to be applied correctly and although it is alluded to in the text of the original TRISS article, only one isobar is illustrated. The RTS component is retrieved early from paramedical or emergency room observations, with the anatomical scaling following exact identification of injuries. Although the initial physiological derangment is expected to be at its worst prior to management, this is not necessarily true. For

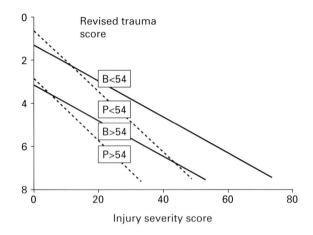

Figure 22.1 *The four possible Ps_{50} isobars for TRISS (B, blunt; P, penetrating; 54, years of age).*

example, a patient with rib fractures and a pulmonary contusion managed initially with epidural analgesia and a continuous positive airway pressure (CPAP) system may become progressively hypoxic and require intubation and positive pressure ventilation. If injuries are overlooked, the ISS will be erroneously low. In those who die, forensic data will verify anatomical assessment but this may not be possible in those whose missed injury is non-fatal. Furthermore, it has been suggested that the ISS may not distinguish poor care from severe injuries.[34]

Systems designed and validated in one environment may not be applicable to others.[31,35] This pertains to both anatomical nature and mechanism of injury, and geographical location. As already mentioned, death from head injury is related mainly to the magnitude of brain trauma and not the metabolic derangement. Although the triphasic mortality distribution is relevant to urban centers with sophisticated prehospital services, as emphasized by Trunkey,[35] it may not be the same in other areas. The distribution in Durban for penetrating torso trauma[36] underlines this fact (Fig 22.2). This patient group involves predominantly young males and age is not an independent predictive variable. Many of these patients suffer multiple injuries to a single anatomical zone, either the chest or abdomen. Calculation of the ISS entails scoring only the most extensively damaged organ within an individual anatomical compartment. This is problematic because the outcome from multiple injuries is worse than single organ injury although the ISS may be identical.[37] For example, in an analysis of patients with cardiac injury in the Durban metropolitan area,[38] associated pleural breech carried a significantly higher mortality rate than isolated cardiac injury with tamponade but the ISS was identical. This shortcoming has been addressed by the authors of the original ISS who have proposed a modified format, the New Injury Severity Score (NISS), whereby the three most severe injuries are scored regardless of their

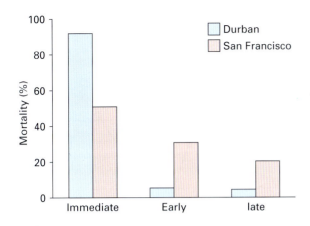

Figure 22.2 *Triphasic trauma mortality distribution for the two metropolitan areas of San Francisco[3] and Durban.[36]*

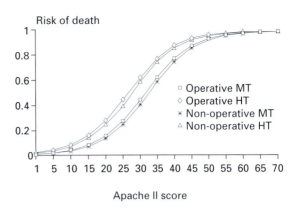

Figure 22.3 *Apache II score versus the predicted risk of death for operative and non-operative head trauma (HT) and multiple trauma (MT).*

anatomical location.[39] This system has been validated in centers in the USA but requires further evaluation.

GENERAL OBJECTIVE SYSTEMS

One of the main criticisms of general objective systems is that they are not relevant to an individual patient but only to diagnostic groups.[40] It must be emphasized, however, that at no time have the authors of these systems suggested that they be applied on an individual basis. This statement notwithstanding, it must be considered as one of the major disadvantages.

The term 'objective' is, in fact, a misnomer. In many of the commonly used scoring systems, the predictor variables were selected either by the authors or consensus amongst selected physicians.[15,16,21] Categoric weighting of variables was likewise subjective. In an attempt to improve performance, the more recent scoring systems were developed using statistical modeling techniques to select and weight the variables.[17-20] Although each selected variable was independently assessed for the association with hospital mortality, the variables were still chosen using clinical judgment. No system is therefore truly objective; there is only subjective objectivity. As with the earlier systems, multiple logistic regression analysis was applied to produce an equation for the risk of death (R). If the system uses a regression equation, plotting R versus the score produces a sigmoid curve regardless of the system used (Fig 22.3). This highlights graphically an inherent deficiency. Within intermediate ranges of R the score changes little, the opposite being true at extremes of risk. Using the Apache II system and the diagnostic category of multiple trauma as an example, within the decile of risk 0–0.1 the score changes by 17 points whereas the subsequent 17 points are spread across the next five deciles of risk. The system is therefore inefficient in the very area where clinical judgment is most

difficult. Furthermore, equivalent scores do not carry the same risk of death (Fig 22.3), which is also dependent on the four possible diagnostic categories for trauma (operative or non-operative head and multiple trauma). An equivalent Apache II score in these groups may result in up to a 20% difference in predicted mortality rate. The trauma-specific ASCOT system[29] has attempted to address these problems by excluding from analysis those patients with either devastating or minor injuries based on ISS and RTS. Although statistical analysis shows little difference in discriminatory power, the authors suggest that it may be a more appropriate system for MTOS analysis.[41]

Despite claims that these systems have improved with each phase of development,[17,19,42] the overall sensitivity (ability to predict death) remains largely unaltered using a decision criterion of $R = 0.5$, and approximates 50%. It should be noted that sensitivity and specificity are sometimes reported in reverse. Sensitivity describes the proportion of patients with the condition who have a positive test. For systems designed to predict R, this means the number of patients correctly predicted to die divided by the total number of deaths, and for systems designed to predict Ps it means the number of correctly predicted survivors divided by the total number of survivors. Comparing the corrected sensitivities, each of the systems have little more than a 50:50 chance of predicting death correctly. This highlights the problem of using a 50% decision criterion to predict outcome. Reducing the R cutoff value increases sensitivity but reduces specificity. It is also clinically impractical to suggest that an R value of 0.05 has the same risk as that of 0.49 although both patients would fall into the expected survival category. Even with these shortcomings would the predicted risk of death influence treatment decisions? An R value of 0.8 for a diagnostic category certainly implies an unfavorable outcome in the majority of patients, but one in every five will potentially survive. Even in systems with perfect calibration the problem lies in identifying that individual who will defy statistical probability within each decile of risk. The anonymous quote '...probability is only one factor to be taken into account when making a decision. Statistics should be used as a drunken man uses the lampost – for support rather than illumination'[43] must surely apply in such situations and clinical judgment and time remain of paramount importance.

PITFALLS IN OBJECTIVE SYSTEMS

> **Pitfalls in objective systems**
>
> - Subjective selection of variables
> - Categoric cut-point analysis
> - Decision criterion of Ps or $R = 0.5$
> - Timing of data collection
> - Bias
> - Missed injuries

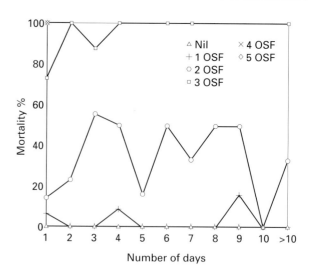

Figure 22.4 *Mortality rate versus number of days of concurrent organ failures for critically injured patients without head trauma in the Surgical ICU, King Edward VIII Hospital, Durban.*

Despite the low reported sensitivities, objective systems have gained acceptance because of the high correct classification rates. This is a seriously flawed mathematical concept and is dependent on sample size and mortality rate.[44] If the latter is low (e.g. <10%), and all patients are predicted to survive, the correct classification rate will automatically equal survival rate (>90%). The systems, however, are designed to predict death and not survival.

Most systems are designed to be used within 24 hours of admission to intensive care. The poor performance and sensitivities may be explained by the errors and bias which may occur with such brevity. Preadmission treatment (lead-time bias), imprecise diagnosis (selection bias), and incomplete data collection (detection bias) may confound predictive ability.[4] Lead-time bias refers to treatment started prior to ICU admission which may impact on predictor variables. For example, inotropic support instituted during surgery may normalize mean arterial pressure but this is not accounted for when calculating the score in the ICU and R will automatically be falsely low. Although the wrong diagnosis is uncommon in trauma patients, missed injuries impact significantly on outcome[45] and their effects may not be apparent within the first 24 hours when the score is calculated. Variables which are not recorded are assumed to be normal and those systems incorporating numerous parameters may increase the risk of detection bias. Furthermore, most systems use a categoric (cutpoint) method to weight the predictor variables. This is removed from the clinical situation where a physiological continuum of derangement occurs.

It is difficult to believe that on the basis of such a fleeting assessment a predicted risk of death would influ-ence management. Suggestions that a daily risk evaluation in the light of further data could guide therapy[17,20] may introduce expectation bias and influence treatment decisions in both a positive and negative direction.[46] Even if, for any combination of predictor variables over time, the estimated and observed mortality rate is 100%, statistical analysis is not absolute. It simply indicates that survival to date is unprecedented in such situations.[47] If organ dysfunction over time is used to predict outcome, at extremes of dysfunction the expected outcome is usually clinically obvious. This is exemplified by plotting outcome versus the number of concurrent organ failures (Fig 22.4). Patients with less than two concurrent organ failures for any length of time have high survival rates, whereas those with three or more for more than 72 hours do not survive. The problem lies in the intermediate zone of two concurrent organ failures where the outcome is extremely variable regardless of their duration. Neither objective nor subjective methods are accurate and survival or futility cannot be predicted.

Claims that objective scoring systems have potential advantages over clinical judgment because of reproducibility and a database larger than any one clinician's experience remain unsubstantiated. Objective risk estimates need further comparison with clinical judgment.

There is one confounding factor that is common to subjective and both general and trauma-specific objective systems. Unforseen complications and errors in management have a significant effect on outcome,[48,49] and trauma patients have been identified as a high risk category for these events.[50] These are usually clinically obvious and should be addressed in unit or hospital morbidity and mortality meetings. An objective system is not required for this purpose.

Not one system, either subjective or objective, predicts long-term survival or quality of life in survivors of critical injury. Mortality rates in patients discharged from hospital only approximate age-matched controls after 3 years[51] and quality of life may be reduced significantly.[52] As emphasized by Buist,[2] however, who judges quality of life – clinicians or patients – and by what means is this assessed? Although a number of quality of life scales have been devised, there may be no correlation between measured functional status and patients' perceptions.[53]

Objective scoring systems undoubtedly have a major role in stratifying severity of critical illness for the purpose of clinical research and audit. They alleviate the concern of possible dissimilarity between study and control groups. It is essential, however, that the system used has been validated for that environment and nature of injury. They cannot, however, be used to deny admission, predict outcome, or dictate management on an individual basis.[40] The answer to the question posed in the title of this chapter may be found in the advice of Hippocrates[54] iterated 2000 years ago:

It is unwise to prophesy either death or recovery in acute disease.

REFERENCES

1. Watts CM, Knaus WA. The case for using objective scoring systems to predict intensive care unit outcome. *Crit Care Clin* 1994; **10:** 73–90.
2. Buist M. Intensive care unit resource allocation. *Anaesth Intensive Care* 1994; **22:** 44–60.
3. Goldman GM. Judgmental error in intensive care practice. *J Int Care Med* 1990; **5:** 93–103.
4. Cowen JS, Kelly MA. Errors and bias in using predictive scoring systems. *Crit Care Clin* 1994; **10:** 53–72.
5. Tversky A, Khaneman D. Judgment under uncertainty: heuristics and biases. *Science* 1974; **185:** 1124–31.
6. Guillou PG. Biological variation in the development of sepsis after surgery or trauma. *Lancet* 1993; **342:** 217–20.
7. Members of the American College of Chest Physicians/Society of Critical Care Medicine Consensus Conference Committee. Definitions for sepsis and organ failure and guidelines for the use of innovative therapies in sepsis. *Crit Care Med* 1992; **20:** 864–74.
8. Hunter J. *Treatise on the Blood, Inflammation, and Gunshot Wounds.* London: Nicol, 1794.
9. Kassirer JP, Gorry AG. Clinical problem solving: a behavioural analysis. *Ann Intern Med* 1978; **89:** 245–55.
10. Oye RK, Bellamy PE. Patterns of resource consumption in medical intensive care. *Chest* 1991; **99:** 685–9.
11. Teres D. Civilian triage in the ICU: the ritual of the last bed. *Crit Care Med* 1993; **21:** 598–606.
12. Brannen AL, Godfrey LJ, Goether WE. Prediction of outcome from critical illness. *Arch Intern Med* 1989; **149:** 1083–6.
13. Kruse JA, Thill-Baharozian MC, Carlson RW. Comparison of clinical assessment with Apache II for predicting mortality risk in patients admitted to a medical intensive care unit. *JAMA* 1988; **260:** 1739–42.
14. Poses RM, Bekes C, Winkler RL. Are two (inexperienced) heads better than one (experienced) head? Averaging house officers' prognostic judgments for critically ill patients. *Arch Intern Med* 1990; **150:** 1874–8.
15. Knaus WA, Zimmerman JE, Wagner DP, Draper EA, Lawrence DE. Apache – acute physiology and chronic health evaluation: a physiologically based classification system. *Crit Care Med* 1981; **9:** 591–7.
16. Knaus WA, Draper EA, Wagner DP, Zimmerman JE. Apache II: a severity of disease classification system. *Crit Care Med* 1985; **13:** 818–29.
17. Knaus WA, Wagner DP, Draper EA, *et al.* The Apache III prognostic system. *Chest* 1991; **100:** 1619–36.
18. Teres D, Lemeshow S, Avrunin JS, Pastides H. Validation of the mortality prediction model for ICU patients. *Crit Care Med* 1987; **15:** 208–12.
19. Lemeshow S, Teres D, Avrunin JS, Gage RW. Refining intensive care unit outcome prediction by using changing probabilities of mortality. *Crit Care Med* 1988; **16:** 470–7.
20. Lemeshow S, Teres D, Klar J, Avrunin JS, Gehlbach SH, Rapoport J. Mortality probability models (MPM II) based on an international cohort of intensive care unit patients. *JAMA* 1993; **270:** 2478–86.
21. Le Gall J-R, Loirat P, Alperovitch A, *et al.* A simplified acute physiology score for ICU patients. *Crit Care Med* 1984; **12:** 975–7.
22. Le Gall J-R, Lemeshow S, Saulnier F. A new simplified acute physiology score (SAPS II) based on a European/North American multicenter study. *JAMA* 1993; **270:** 2957–63.
23. Teasdale G, Jennet B. Assessment of coma and impaired consciousness. A practical scale. *Lancet* 1974; **2:** 81–4.
24. Association for the Advancement of Automotive Medicine. *The Abbreviated Injury Scale.* Des Plaines, IL: AAAM, 1990.
25. Baker SP, O'Neill B, Haddon W, *et al.* The Injury Severity Score: a method for describing patients with multiple injuries and evaluating emergency care. *J Trauma* 1974; **14:** 187–96.
26. Champion HR, Sacco WJ, Carnazzo AJ, *et al.* The Trauma Score. *Crit Care Med* 1981; **9:** 672–6.
27. Champion HR, Sacco WJ, Copes WS, *et al.* A revision of the Trauma Score. *J Trauma* 1989; **29:** 623–9.
28. Boyd CR, Tolson MA, Copes WS. Evaluating trauma care: the TRISS method. *J Trauma* 1987; **27:** 370–8.
29. Champion HS, Copes WS, Sacco WJ, *et al.* A new characterization of injury severity. *J Trauma* 1990; **30:** 539–46.

30. Trunkey DD. Torso trauma. *Curr Probl Surg* 1987; **24:** 215–65.

31. Muckart DJJ, Bhagwanjee S, Neijenhuis PA. Prediction of the risk of death using the Apache II scoring system in critically ill trauma patients without head injury. *Br J Surg* 1996; **83:** 1123–7.

32. Moore FA, Moore EE. Evolving concepts in the pathogenesis of postinjury multiple organ failure. *Surg Clin North Am* 1995; **75:** 257–77.

33. Cuthbertson DP. Observations on the disturbance of metabolism produced by injury to the limbs. *Q J Med* 1932; **1:** 233–46.

34. Rutledge R. The Injury Severity Score is unable to differentiate between poor care and severe injury. *J Trauma* 1996; **40:** 944–50.

35. Trunkey DD. Trauma. *Sci Am* 1983; **249 (August):** 20–7.

36. Muckart DJJ, Meumann C, Botha JBC. The changing pattern of penetrating torso trauma in KwaZulu/Natal – a clinical and pathological review. *S Afr J Med* 1995; **85:** 1172–4.

37. Muckart DJJ, Bhagwanjee S. The ACCP/SCCM Consensus Conference definitions of the systemic inflammatory response syndrome and allied disorders in critically injured patients. *Crit Care Med* 1997; **25:** 1789–95.

38. Campbell NC, Thomson SR, Muckart DJJ, *et al.* A review of 1198 cases of penetrating cardiac trauma. *Br J Surg* 1997; **84:** 1737–40.

39. Osler T, Baker SP, Long W. A modification of the Injury Severity Score that both improves accuracy and simplifies scoring. *J Trauma* 1997; **43:** 922–6.

40. Suter P, Armaganidas A, Beaufils F, *et al.* Predicting outcome in ICU patients. *Intensive Care Med* 1994; **20:** 390–7.

41. Champion HR, Copes WS, Sacco WJ, *et al.* Improved predictions from a severity characterization of trauma (ASCOT) over Trauma and Injury Severity Score (TRISS): results of an independent validation. *J Trauma* 1996; **40:** 42–9.

42. Castella X, Artigas A, Bion J, Kari A. A comparison of severity of illness scoring systems for intensive care unit patients: results of a multicenter, multinational study. *Crit Care Med* 1995; **23:** 1327–35.

43. Anonymous. TPN and Apache II. *Lancet* 1986; **1:** 1478.

44. Ruttiman UE. Statistical approaches to development and validation of predictive models. *Crit Care Clin* 1994; **10:** 19–35.

45. Muckart DJJ, Thomson SR. Undetected injuries: a preventable cause of increased morbidity and mortality. *Am J Surg* 1991; **162:** 457–60.

46. Murray LS, Teasdale GM, Murray GD, *et al.* Does prediction of outcome alter patient management? *Lancet* 1993; **341:** 1487–91.

47. Knaus WA, Draper EA, Wagner DP, Zimmerman JE. Prognosis in acute organ system failure. *Ann Surg* 1985; **202:** 685–93.

48. Muckart DJJ, Bhagwanjee S, Aitchison JM. Adverse events in the surgical intensive care unit: a cause of increased mortality. *S Afr J Surg* 1994; **32:** 69–73.

49. Davis JW, Hoyt DB, McArdle MS, *et al.* The significance of critical care errors in causing preventable death in trauma patients in a trauma system. *J Trauma* 1991; **31:** 813–19.

50. Brennan TA, Leappe LL, Laird NM, *et al.* Incidence of adverse events and negligence in hospital patients. *N Engl J Med* 1991; **324:** 370–6.

51. Ridley S, Penderleith L. Survival after intensive care. *Anaesthesia* 1994; **49:** 933–5.

52. Ridley SA, Wallace PG. Quality of life after intensive care. *Anaesthesia* 1990; **45:** 808–13.

53. Patrick DL, Danis M, Southerland LI, Hong G. Quality of life following intensive care. *J Gen Intern Med* 1988; **3:** 218–23.

54. Silverstein ML. Prediction instruments and clinical judgment in critical care. *JAMA* 1988; **260:** 1758–9.

FURTHER READING

Civetta JM. Scoring systems: do we need a different approach? *Crit Care Med* 1991; **19:** 1460–1.

Demetriades D, Chan LS, Velmahos G, *et al.* TRISS methodology in trauma: the need for alternatives. *Br J Surg* 1998; **85:** 379–84.

Hunt JP, Meyer AA. Predicting survival in the intensive care unit. *Curr Probl Surg* 1997; **34:** 525–600.

Schuster DP, Kolleff MH. Predicting intensive care unit outcome. *Crit Care Clin* 1994; **10:** 1–246.

23

The use of antibiotics in chest trauma

BRIDGET L ATKINS AND DEREK W M CROOK

Infection is an important cause of late morbidity and mortality following trauma. Antibiotics are commonly used in the hope of preventing such infections. This chapter deals with the role of antibiotics in prophylaxis and the treatment of established infections.

PROPHYLAXIS

General principles of antibiotic prophylaxis in surgery

The role of antibiotic prophylaxis for elective and urgent operations has been validated by many prospective randomized clinical trials.[1,2]

TIMING, DOSAGE AND ROUTE OF ADMINISTRATION

Clinical studies, in addition to animal experiments, indicate that the timing of antibiotic administration is important. In patients undergoing elective surgical procedures, the incidence of postoperative infection is significantly reduced when antibiotics are given in the 2 hours before surgery compared to when antibiotics are given before or after this time.[3] Adequate levels of antibiotic should be maintained throughout the surgical procedure. The risk of postoperative infection is increased in patients who have low serum antibiotic levels at the close of surgery.[4] Antibiotics with a short half-life (<1 hour) should be readministered for every 2–3 hours of operative time.[2] In all but elective colonic procedures, intravenous administration of antibiotic is the preferred route for prophylaxis. When given in a small volume over a short period of time, high levels in serum and tissues can be expected.

CHOICE OF ANTIBIOTIC

No single antibiotic agent or combination should be relied on for effective prophylaxis in all operations. If efficacy data from clinical trials are not available, the agent(s) chosen should be active against the organisms likely to cause infectious complications in each procedure. The safety and cost of the antibiotic must also be taken into account. The cephalosporins (a class of β-lactam antibiotic) are the group most commonly used for surgical prophylaxis (see below).

DURATION

The goal in prophylaxis with β-lactam agents is to maintain serum levels of free drug above the minimum inhibitory concentration (MIC) for common contaminating pathogens during the entire surgical procedure and for a sufficient interval after wound closure.[5] For most surgical procedures the necessary duration of prophylaxis would be less than 24 hours. Table 23.1 provides a summary of suggested recommendations for antibiotic prophylaxis in chest trauma.

Prophylaxis of thoracotomy, sternotomy or clean elective surgery

The organisms likely to cause postoperative thoracic wound infections following clean surgery are skin flora such as *Staphylococcus* spp. and *Streptococcus* spp. Rarely, Gram-negative bacilli such as *Escherichia coli* may cause wound infections. Therefore antibiotic prophylaxis is designed to be effective against these organisms. As the local antibiotic susceptibilities of these organisms may vary over time or from center to center, the choice of antibiotic(s) used for prophylaxis will vary accordingly.

Table 23.1 *Suggested recommendations for antimicrobial prophylaxis*

Clinical situation	Antibiotic recommendation (dose)	Duration
Thoracotomy, sternotomy or clean elective surgery	Cefuroxime 1.5 g or cefonicid 1 g or cefamandole 1 g	Immediately preoperatively with a second dose of cefuroxime or cefamandole if surgery > 4 hours
Blunt chest trauma requiring drain	Cefuroxime 1.5 g t.d.s. or cefonicid 1 g o.d. or cefamandole 1 g q.d.s.	24 hours
not requiring drain	None	
Penetrating trauma	Cefuroxime 1.5 g t.d.s. or cefonicid 1 g o.d. or cefamandole 1 g q.d.s.	24 hours
Suspected aspiration	Cefuroxime 1.5 g t.d.s. or cefonicid 1 g o.d. or cefamandole 1 g q.d.s. ± metronidazole 400 mg t.d.s. p.o.	None or 3–5 days
Esophageal perforation	Cefuroxime 1.5 g t.d.s. or cefonicid 1 g o.d. or cefamandole 1 g q.d.s. ± metronidazole 400 mg t.d.s. p.o.	24 hours (assuming early operative repair)
High risk of MRSA	Add glycopeptide such as vancomycin 1 g (single dose) to above	
Cephalosporin-allergic patients Anaphylaxis	Gentamicin 5 mg/kg i.v. (single dose) + clindamycin 300 mg	As above
Rash	Co-amoxiclav 1 g (or as in anaphylaxis)	As above

Early trials using penicillin (the first β-lactam antibiotic) alone, in thoracic surgery, showed a reduction in wound infection compared to placebo.[6,7] Based on these clinical trials, antibiotic prophylaxis has been widely adopted. Since these studies, newer antibiotics have been developed and antibiotic resistance has increased so the choice of antibiotic has changed. World wide, the cephalosporins (a class of β-lactam antibiotic) are the most commonly used antibiotics for surgical prophylaxis.[8] The choice of a cephalosporin reflects recognition that a single drug in this class has activity against the likely infecting organisms, negating the need for combinations of antibiotics. In a recent survey of UK cardiac surgeons, it was found that the use of single agent prophylaxis rather than combination therapy is increasing.[9]

Cephalosporins vary in their spectrum of activity depending on a classification into 'generations' or on their antipseudomonal activity. First generation cephalosporins (e.g. cephalothin) have greater activity for Gram-positive organisms such as staphylococci and streptococci than second generation (e.g. cefuroxime) or third generation cephalosporins (e.g. ceftriaxone or the antipseudomonal drug ceftazidime). However, activity for Gram-negative bacilli increases progressively up the generations. The main potential limitation of cephalosporins in prophylaxis is the increasing prevalence of methicillin-resistant *Staphylococcus aureus* (MRSA), which is resistant to all β-lactams including cephalosporins.

Trials of cephalothin in elective thoracic surgery do not agree on whether there is benefit over placebo.[10–12] Cefazolin (a first generation cephalosporin) at induction followed by cephalothin postoperatively had no benefit compared with placebo.[13] The statistical power of all these studies, however, was insufficient to detect even moderate differences in infection rates, thus limiting the interpretation of the results. Antibiotic prophylaxis trials comparing first and second generation cephalosporins in cardiothoracic surgery show that the second generation cephalosporins (e.g. cefuroxime, cefamandole and ceforanide) are significantly better than first generation cephalosporins (e.g. cephalothin and cefazolin).[14–16]

It is important to be aware of local antimicrobial susceptibilities when choosing prophylaxis regimens; for example, a unit with a high incidence of MRSA infection should use an agent, such as a glycopeptide (e.g. vancomycin), known to be active against MRSA.

Antimicrobial prophylaxis in trauma

In surgery, antibiotics can be administered before potential contamination of tissues. In trauma, however, there may be bacterial contamination of wounds before admission to hospital and then further potential contamination during surgery. In order to maximize prophylaxis, ideally antibiotics should be administered just prior to contamination. This is usually not possible in

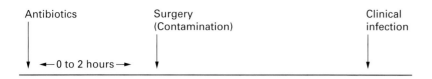

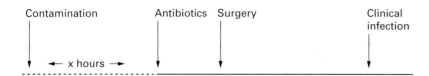

Figure 23.1 *Schematic representation of the timing of antibiotic administration in relation to tissue contamination in (a) non-trauma (i.e. elective) and (b) trauma surgery.*

trauma cases. Animal models, however, show that the incidence and severity of infections can be reduced by the administration of antibiotics during a finite period following bacterial contamination of tissues.[17,18] This could be represented schematically (Fig 23.1). Prophylactic efficacy diminishes and then disappears as the time interval between contamination and antibiotic administration (x) increases beyond 3–6 hours.[1,2]

DURATION OF ANTIBIOTICS

Some regard antibiotics in contaminated trauma as early presumptive treatment and, therefore, not prophylaxis. Treatment implies a duration of antibiotic administration of approximately 5 days. However, the majority of cases of trauma on presentation do not have established infection. Trauma cases fall in the grey area between antibiotic prophylaxis and antibiotic treatment.[19] Trial data on the ideal duration of antibiotics in

trauma are not clear. The initial animal studies used a single dose of antibiotic (within 3 hours of contamination). Published trials use a range of durations from one dose to 14 days. When the duration of the antibiotic administration has been the subject of comparative clinical trials, the shorter duration has been consistently as effective as longer duration prophylaxis.[4,19,20]

There is no convincing clinical trial evidence for the role of antibiotics in thoracic trauma other than for chest drain insertion (for a discussion of prophylaxis for chest drains see below). The experience in other areas can be used to develop an approach for chest trauma. In a review of the role of antibiotic prophylaxis in penetrating abdominal trauma and open fractures it was felt that there was clear benefit with administering antibiotics.[19] Investigations reported in this review surprisingly did not show an effect of either the interval from trauma to starting prophylaxis or duration of prophylaxis on the risk of developing post-traumatic infection.

Table 23.2 *Prospective randomized controlled clinical trials of antibiotic prophylaxis for chest drain insertion*

Year	Author	Antibiotic/Duration	Chest injury	All infections Antibiotic	Control	Sig*	Empyema Antibiotic	Control	Sig*
1977	Grover[20]	Clindamycin – until drain removal or 5 days (whichever shorter)	Penetrating	.4/38	13/37	Yes	1/38	6/37	Yes
1981	Stone[21]	Cefamandole – until drain removal	Both and spontaneous pneumothorax	1/60	8/60	No	1/60	3/60	No
1985	LeBlanc[22]	Cephapirin – until drain removal	Both and spontaneous pneumothorax	2/39	7/46	No	0/39	1/46	No
1985	Mandal[23]	Doxycycline – until drain removal	Penetrating	0/40	1/40	No	0/40	1/40	No
1986	LoCurto[24]	Cefoxitin – until drain removal	Both	0/30	8/28	Yes	0/30	5/28	Yes
1990	Brunner[25]	Cefazolin – until drain removal	Both	1/44	9/46	Yes	0/44	6/46	Yes
1993	Cant[26]	Cefazolin – 24 hours	Penetrating		0/57		5/56		Yes
1994	Nichols[27]	Cefonicid – until drain removal	Both (most penetrating)	1/63	6/56	Yes	0/63	3/56	Yes

*Shows a significant benefit of antibiotic over placebo.
Studies of Cant, Nichols, Grover and Stone were double blinded.

Despite the lack of antibiotic prophylaxis studies in chest trauma, it is reasonable to administer prophylactic antibiotics in cases of penetrating trauma or open fractures of the chest. The same antibiotics used for elective surgery should be used.

Antibiotic prophylaxis of chest drains

Eight clinical trials have addressed the issue as to whether antibiotic prophylaxis is of benefit when a chest drain is inserted. The trials are summarized in Table 23.2. None of these trials addresses the issue of antibiotic duration. In a further trial, a single dose of ampicillin prior to chest drain insertion, versus giving antibiotics until drain removal, showed no difference in infection rates, both being 3%.[28] This study had approximately 90 patients in each group and is the only study addressing the duration of antibiotic prophylaxis. The study was, however, still too small to detect moderate differences in infection rate. Two meta-analyses were done in 1992[29] and 1995.[30] These both examined the first six studies in Table 23.2 and both concluded that antibiotics were beneficial; however, it was not possible to determine the optimal duration required. Though these studies purport to specifically address the issue of antibiotic prophylaxis for chest drain insertion, they investigate the effect of prophylactic antibiotics on both penetrating trauma and chest drain insertion. There is no evidence for a benefit of antibiotics in patients requiring a chest drain for non-traumatic reasons[31] and they should not be used in this situation as a routine.

On the basis of the above discussion, our recommendation would be to give a single large dose of an antibiotic such as a cephalosporin (see section on thoracotomy above) prior to chest drain insertion for chest trauma. This will also act as general prophylaxis for the traumatic wound. Prolongation of prophylaxis beyond 24 hours is unlikely to be of any benefit.

Esophageal perforation

There are no clinical trials that examine the role of antibiotic prophylaxis in esophageal perforation. This again is a grey area between prophylaxis and early presumptive therapy of infection. With perforation, there will be passage of upper intestinal organisms into the mediastinum and possibly the pleural space. Antibiotics may be effective for a short period in preventing systemic spread of infection from the mediastinum or a closed pleural space. However, the flora leaking from the esophageal perforation will substitute rapidly to multi-resistant nosocomial organisms in hospitalized patients on antibiotics. It is common clinical practice to administer antibiotics for long periods of time, particularly in patients treated non-surgically.[32,33] Our personal practice is to use brief courses of antibiotics, most of the emphasis being on achieving surgical repair and drainage. Duration of initial antibiotics will depend on whether mediastinal sepsis is established or not. In cases treated early with surgery, antibiotic treatment will be brief, but in patients with mediastinitis, antibiotic treatment may be prolonged (see treatment of mediastinitis).

Aspiration

In cases of chest trauma there may be suspicion of oropharyngeal or gastric fluid aspiration. The infectious complications that occur secondary to aspiration are as follows:[34]

- Pneumonitis (acid, infective or both)
- Necrotizing pneumonia (multiple cavitations <1 cm in diameter)
- Lung abscess (one or more cavities >1 cm diameter that communicate with a bronchus)
- Empyema.

The organisms in normal oral flora are anaerobes such as *Fusobacterium* spp., *Prevotella* spp. and aerobes such as 'hemolytic streptococci'.[35,36] In addition to this flora, alcoholics and chronically ill patients are often colonized with Gram-negative aerobic bacilli (e.g. *E. coli*). Development of clinical infection can be insidious and sometimes takes up to 1–2 weeks.

There are no clinical trials that examine the impact of prophylaxis or very early antibiotic treatment in cases with aspiration. Some practitioners would use a single dose or no antibiotics, monitoring the patient carefully and treating infection when it occurs. This approach is easier in intubated and ventilated patients where microbial analysis of bronchoalveolar lavage fluid can be readily used to diagnose infection (see below) and specific antibiotic treatment used. It is also reasonable practice to use empiric antibiotics early for 3–5 days. If this is done, agents that cover the common oral flora should be used. Most community-acquired pneumonias secondary to aspiration are caused by organisms sensitive to the β-lactam antibiotics such as the penicillins and cephalosporins. A cephalosporin, such as cefuroxime or cefamandole, or a penicillin, such as Augmentin (co-amoxiclav) would also cover the majority of community-acquired Gram-negative bacilli and would be a reasonable choice for early treatment or prophylaxis. Many practitioners prefer to use or add agents with anaerobic activity which explains the frequent addition of metronidazole to antibiotic regimens.

TREATMENT OF ESTABLISHED INFECTIONS

Pneumonia

Patients with a reduced conscious level, with traumatic injuries to the chest or the critically ill, requiring ventilation, are highly susceptible to pneumonia. In the majority of cases, this will be hospital-acquired. In a one-day prevalence study of 10 038 patients on intensive care units (ICUs) across Europe the prevalence of infection was 44.8%, of which 46.9% had pneumonia. The most frequently reported organisms were aerobic Gram-negative bacilli (e.g. *E. coli*), *S. aureus* (including MRSA), *Pseudomonas aeruginosa*, coagulase-negative staphylococci and fungi.[37] Conventional criteria for diagnosing nosocomial pneumonia include fever, leukocytosis, purulent sputum and the appearance of new or progressive infiltrates on chest radiography. All these criteria are non-specific in the ICU patient. Sputum specimens have no value in the diagnosis of pneumonia on ICU. The protected specimen brush (PSB) or bronchoalveolar lavage (BAL) provide a means of examining lung bacterial flora.[38] When the above clinical criteria of pneumonia are met, a growth of 10^3 c.f.u./ml (c.f.u. = colony forming unit) from PSB or 10^5 c.f.u./ml from BAL is considered a diagnostic level of organisms consistent with pneumonia.

Identification of the infecting bacterial flora allows rational and specific antimicrobial therapy. There are no placebo-controlled trials proving that antimicrobial treatment of pneumonia in ventilated pneumonia affects outcome. However, inappropriate antibiotic therapy is associated with increased mortality[39] and it is widely believed that antimicrobial therapy is beneficial. However, it has been shown that prior antibiotic use not only predisposes to bacterial colonization but also leads to pneumonia caused by less susceptible organisms such as *P. aeruginosa* and MRSA.[40,41] It is, therefore, important to treat patients only when they satisfy microbiological and clinical criteria for pneumonia, avoiding inappropriate prescribing.

Various empiric regimens are used to treat nosocomial pneumonia. A combination of an antipseudomonal β-lactam with an aminoglycoside offers broad cover, with synergy against *Pseudomonas* spp. Antistaphylococcal antibiotics should be added if there are staphylococci on Gram stain of BAL fluid. If MRSA is a possible cause of infection, then a glycopeptide such as vancomycin should be added to the treatment regimen. When the results of PSB or BAL cultures are ready, the therapy can be modified to a specific agent. The duration of antibiotic therapy is usually 7 days. Anaerobic or staphylococcal lung abscesses may require up to 4 weeks.

Mediastinitis

Mediastinitis is a risk following rupture of the esophagus, large airways or surgery involving the mediastinum, particularly sternotomy. Once established, the management is a combination of surgery and antibiotics. There are a number of approaches, none of which has been validated by clinical trials. The essential elements are to achieve thorough drainage and administer high dose appropriate antibiotics. Detection of the etiological agent is critical to choosing appropriate specific antibiotic treatment. Surface swabs have no value in diagnosing the presence of mediastinal infection. Reliable samples of pus or infected tissue by surgery or diagnostic aspiration should be obtained before starting empiric antibiotics in order to plan rational antibiotic therapy. Empiric treatment varies, depending on the likely source of mediastinitis. Post-sternotomy infection is usually caused by *S. aureus*, but occasionally a wide range of nosocomial pathogens may be the cause. Initially the choice should be a broad spectrum agent with antistaphylococcal activity, and if MRSA is prevalent should include a glycopeptide. There are many broad spectrum regimens and an in-depth discussion of them is beyond the scope of this chapter (see Table 23.4 for general guidelines). Practitioners should refer to infection specialists or specialist tests for guidance and specific recommendations. Mediastinitis early after rupture of the esophagus or large airway should be caused by susceptible nasopharyngeal flora and treatment with a second generation cephalosporin such as cefuroxime should be effective therapy. However, later after hospitalization, persistent leak from a hollow viscus leads to infection with multiresistant nosocomial flora. In these circumstances, empiric therapy should be with broad spectrum drugs as above for post-sternotomy infection. Culture of reliable samples usually reveals the pathogen(s) and, based on susceptibility tests, specific therapy can be confidently chosen.

Empyema

The risk of post-traumatic pleural empyema is much less than it was a few decades ago because of modern surgical techniques and antibiotics. In 1535 chest casualties in the Korean war, 952 had hemothoraces and of these 26% became infected.[42] Recent series put the risk at between 0.5% and 5%.[43–47] The presence of a hemopneumothorax increases the risk of infection in chest trauma. The risk of empyema is greatest when the pleural space is incompletely drained and when thoracic drains are in place for a prolonged period.[47]

The bacteriology of post-traumatic empyema differs from that of spontaneous empyema (Table 23.3). The high number of anaerobic infections reported by Bartlett[49] is due to better anaerobic culture techniques and is particularly a feature of spontaneous empyema, empyema following rupture of a hollow viscus or strangulated bowel herniating through a ruptured diaphragm. *S. aureus* is the commonest cause of post-traumatic empyema followed by aerobic Gram-negative bacilli (e.g. *E. coli*), then *Pseudomonas* spp.

The management of empyema follows the principles of the management of any deep purulent collection. The

Table 23.3 *The bacteriology of post-traumatic and spontaneous empyema*

	Post-traumatic	Both	Spontaneous	
	Caplan[46] 31 cases	Lemmer[48] 70 cases	Bartlett[49] 83 cases	Ferguson[50] 119 cases
Staphylococcus aureus	45%	24%	20%	13%
Streptococcus pneumoniae	0%	6%	6%	24%
Other streptococci	10% (β-haemolytic)	23% not speciated; 16% enterococci	20%	30% (all *Streptococcus milleri*)
Enterobacteriaceae	39%	7%	23%	9%
Pseudomonas spp.	19%	11%	12%	4%
Anaerobes	10%	13%	76%	31%
Others		40%	7%	13%

Table 23.4 *Possible antibiotic regimens for empiric treatment of serious infections (e.g. aspiration pneumonia, mediastinitis, empyema) prior to results of microbiological cultures*

Clinical situation	Recommendation
Early community-acquired infection (within 3 days of admission)	Cefuroxime 1.5 g t.d.s. + metronidazole 400 mg t.d.s. p.o. or clindamycin 600 mg t.d.s. i.v. + ciprofloxacin 400 mg b.d. i.v. (+ gentamicin* 5 mg/kg o.d. i.v. (one or two doses only) if severe systemic sepsis)
Late hospital-acquired infection (broad spectrum therapy)	Tazocin 4.5 g t.d.s. or meropenem 1 g t.d.s. i.v. (+ gentamicin* 5 mg/kg o.d. i.v. (one or two doses only) if severe systemic sepsis)
High MRSA risk	Add glycopeptide such as vancomycin* 1 g b.d. to above

*The doses of vancomycin and gentamicin should be adjusted according to renal function.

pus should be drained, a sample should be cultured, and empirical antibiotics started. Surgical drainage is critical and must be complete; antibiotics have an adjunctive role.

Recommended empiric antibiotics vary, depending on the likely source of infection. A cephalosporin with good antistaphylococcal activity plus an anaerobic agent such as metronidazole is a satisfactory initial regimen for most cases. However, if the local prevalence of MRSA is high, then a glycopeptide such as vancomycin should be added to this regimen. For clinically septic patients who have acquired the infection in hospital, broad spectrum therapy with antipseudomonal activity should be chosen (see Table 23.4 for summary of recommendations). As soon as accurate microbiological results are available, specific antibiotic therapy should be used.

The duration of antibiotic therapy follows general infection principles. No clinical trials have been done to show any regimen to be superior to another. Intravenous therapy is continued by most practitioners until the patient is clearly afebrile and improving clinically, appropriate oral therapy is then continued for prolonged periods. Certain specific pathogens, such as *S. aureus*, are treated with more prolonged intravenous therapy.

REFERENCES

1. Kaiser AB. Antimicrobial prophylaxis in surgery. *N Engl J Med* 1986; **315**: 1129–38.

2. Nichols RL. Surgical antimicrobial prophylaxis. *Med Clin North Am* 1995; **3**: 509–22.

3. Classen DC, Scott-Evans R, Pestonik SL, Horn SD, Menlove RL, Burke JP. The timing of prophylactic administration of antibiotics and the risk of surgical-wound infections. *N Engl J Med* 1992; **326**: 281–6.

4. Goldmann DA, Hopkins CC, Karchmer AW, *et al.* Cephalothin prophylaxis in cardiac valve surgery. A prospective, double-blind comparison of two-day and six-day regimens. *J Thorac Cardiovasc Surg* 1977; **73**: 470–9.

5. Redington J, Ebert SC, Craig WA. Role of antimicrobial prophylaxis and pharmacodynamics in surgical prophylaxis. *Rev Infect Dis* 1991; **13(Suppl 10)**: s790–9.

6. Citron KM. Controlled trial of prophylactic penicillin in thoracic surgery. *Thorax* 1965; **20**: 418–50.

7. Fridmodt-Moller N, Ostri P, Krough Pederson IB, Poulson SR. Antibiotic prophylaxis in pulmonary surgery. A double blind study of penicillin vs placebo. *Ann Surg* 1982; **195**: 444–50.

8. Gorbach SL. The role of cephalosporins in surgical prophylaxis. *J Antimicrob Chemother* 1989; **23(suppl D)**: 61.

9. Parry GW, Holden SR, Shabbo FP. Antibiotic prophylaxis for cardiac surgery: current United Kingdom practice. *Br Heart J* 1993; **70**: 585–6.

10. Ilves R, Cooper JD, Todd TRJ, Griffith Pearson FG. Prospective, randomised, double blind study using prophylactic cephalothin for major, elective, general thoracic operations. *J Thorac Cardiovasc Surg* 1981; **81**: 813–17.

11. Bryant LR, Dillon ML, Mobin-Uddin K. Prophylactic antibiotics in noncardiac thoracic operations. *Ann Thorac Surg* 1975; **19**: 671–6.

12. Cameron JL, Imbembo A, Kieffer RF, Spray S, Baker RR. Prospective clinical trial of antibiotics for pulmonary resections. *Surg Gynecol Obstet* 1981; **152**: 156–8.

13. Truesdale R, D'Alessandri R, Manuel V, Daicoff G, Kluge RM. Antimicrobial vs placebo prophylaxis in noncardiac thoracic surgery. *JAMA* 1979; **241**: 1254–6.

14. Slama TG, Sklar SJ, Misinski J, Fess SW. Randomized comparison of cefamandole, cefazolin and cefuroxime prophylaxis in open heart surgery. *Antimicrob Agents Chemother* 1986; **29**: 744–7.

15. Kaiser AB, Petracek MR, Lea JW, *et al*. Efficacy of cefazolin, cefamandole and gentamicin as prophylactic agents in cardiac surgery. Results of a prospective randomized trial in 1030 patients. *Ann Surg* 1987; **206**: 791–7.

16. Platt R, Munoz A, Stella J, VanDevanter S, Koster JK. Antibiotic prophylaxis for cardiovascular surgery. *Ann Intern Med* 1984; **101**: 770–4.

17. Miles AA, Miles EM, Burke J. The value and duration of defence reactions of the skin to the primary lodgement of bacteria. *Br J Exp Pathol* 1957; **38**: 79–96.

18. Burke JF. The effective period of preventative antibiotic action in experimental incisions and dermal lesions. *Surgery* 1961; **50**: 161–8.

19. Dellinger EP. Antibiotic prophylaxis in trauma: penetrating abdominal injuries and open fractures. *Rev Infect Dis* 1991; **13(Suppl 10)**; S847–57.

20. Grover FL, Richardson JD, Fewel JG, Arom KV, Webb GE, Trinkle JK. Prophylactic antibiotics in the treatment of penetrating chest wounds. A prospective double blind study. *J Thorac Cardiovasc Surg* 1977; **74**: 528–36.

21. Stone HH, Symbas PN, Hooper A. Cefamandole for prophylaxis against infection in closed tube thoracostomy. *J Trauma* 1981; **21**: 975–7.

22. LeBlanc KA, Tucker WY. Prophylactic antibiotics and closed tube thoracostomy. *Surg Gynecol Obstet* 1985; **160**: 259–63.

23. Mandal AK, Montano J, Thadepalli H. Prophylactic antibiotics and no antibiotics compared in penetrating chest trauma. *J Trauma* 1985; **25**: 639–43.

24. LoCurto JJ, Tischler CD, Swan KG, *et al*. Tube thoracostomy and trauma – antibiotics or not? *J Trauma* 1986; **26**: 1067–72.

25. Brunner RG, O'Neal Vinsant G, Alexander RH, Laneve L, Fallon WF. The role of antibiotic therapy in the prevention of empyema in patients with an isolated chest injury(ISS 9–10): a prospective study. *J Trauma* 1990; **30**: 1148–54.

26. Cant PJ, Smyth S, Smart DO. Antibiotic prophylaxis is indicated for chest stab wounds requiring closed tube thoracostomy. *Br J Surg* 1993; **80**: 464–6.

27. Nichols RL, Smith JW, Muzik AC, *et al*. Preventative antibiotic usage in traumatic thoracic injuries requiring closed tube thoracostomy. *Chest* 1994; **106**: 1493–7.

28. Demetriades D, Breckon V, Breckon C, *et al*. Antibiotic prophylaxis in penetrating injuries of the chest. *Ann R Coll Surg Engl* 1991; **73**: 348–51.

29. Fallon WF, Wears RL. Prophylactic antibiotics for the prevention of infectious complications including empyema following tube thoracostomy for trauma: results of meta-analysis. *J Trauma* 1992; **33**: 110–17.

30. Evans JT, Green JD, Carlin PE, Barrett LO. Meta-analysis of antibiotics in tube thoracostomy. *Am Surg* 1995; **61**: 215–19.

31. Neugebauer MK, Fosburg RC, Trummer MJ. Routine antibiotic therapy following pleural space intubation. A reappraisal. *J Thorac Cardiovasc Surg* 1971; **6**: 882–4.

32. Bufkin BL, Miller JI, Mansour KA. Esophageal perforation: emphasis on management. *Ann Thorac Surg* 1996; **61**: 1447–52.

33. Weiman DS, Walker WA, Brosnan KM, Pate JW, Fabian TC. Noniatrogenic oesophageal trauma. *Ann Thorac Surg* 1995; **59**: 845–50.

34. Finegold SM. Aspiration pneumonia. *Rev Infect Dis* 1991; **13(Suppl 9)**: S737–42.

35. Johanson WG Jr, Harris GD. Aspiration pneumonia, anaerobic infections and lung abscess. *Med Clin North Am* 1971; **50**: 510–20.

36. Finegold SM. *Anaerobic Bacteria in Human Disease*. New York: Academic Press, 1977.

37. Vincent JL, Bihari DJ, Suter PM, *et al*. The prevalence of nosocomial infection in intensive care units in Europe. Results of the European Prevalence of Infection in Intensive Care (EPIC) Study. *JAMA* 1995; **274**: 639–44.

38. Garrad CS, Crook DWM. Nosocomial pneumonia in the critically ill. *Curr Anaesth Crit Care* 1991; **2**: 155–60.

39. Torres A, Aznar R, Gatell JM, *et al*. Incidence, risk and prognosis factors of nosocomial pneumonia in mechanically ventilated patients. *Am Rev Respir Dis* 1990; **142**: 523–8.

40. Rello J, Ausina V, Ricart J, Castella, Pratts G. Impact of previous antimicrobial therapy on the aetiology and outcome of ventilator associated pneumonia. *Chest* 1993; **104**: 1230–5.

41. Niederman MS. Gram-negative colonization of the respiratory tract: pathogenesis and clinical consequences. *Semin Resp Infect* 1990; **5**: 173–81.

42. Valle AR. Management of war wounds of the chest. *J Thorac Surg* 1952; **24**: 457–81.

43. Oparah SS, Mandal AK. Penetrating wound of the chest: experience with 200 consecutive cases. *J Trauma* 1976; **16**: 868–72.

44. Graham JM, Mattox KL, Beall AC Jr. Penetrating trauma of the lung. *J Trauma* 1979; **19**: 665–9.

45. Helling TS, Gyles NR, Eisenstein CL, Soracco CA. Complications following blunt and penetrating injuries in 216 victims of chest trauma requiring tube thoracostomy. *J Trauma* 1989; **29**: 1367–70.

46. Caplan ES, Hoyt NJ, Rodriguez A, Adams Cowley R. Empyema occurring in the multiply traumatized patient. *J Trauma* 1984; **24**: 785–9.

47. Craig Eddy A, Luna GK, Copass M. Empyema thoracis in patients undergoing emergent closed tube thoracostomy for thoracic trauma. *Am J Surg* 1989; **157:** 494–7.

48. Lemmer JH, Botham MJ, Orringer MB. Modern management of adult thoracic empyema. *J Thorac Cardiovasc Surg* 1985; **90:** 849–55.

49. Bartlett JG, Gorbach SL, Thadepalli H, Finegold SM. Bacteriology of empyema. *Lancet* 1974; **1:** 338–40.

50. Ferguson AD, Prescott RJ, Selkon JB, Watson D, Swinburn CR. The clinical course and management of thoracic empyema. *Q J Med* 1996; **89:** 285–9.

FURTHER READING

American Thoracic Society. Hospital-acquired pneumonia in adults: diagnosis, assessment of severity, initial antimicrobial therapy and preventative strategies. A consensus statement. *Am J Respir Crit Care Med* 1995; **153:** 1711–25.

Fiore AE, Joshi M, Caplan ES. Approach to infection in the multiply traumatised patient. In: Mandell GL, Bennett JE, Dolin R, eds *Mandell, Douglas and Bennett's Principles and Practice of Infectious Diseases*, 4th edn. New York: Churchill Livingstone, 1995; 2756–61.

International Symposium on Perioperative Antibiotic Prophylaxis. *Rev Infect Dis* 1991; **13(Suppl 10):** S779–890.

Kernodle DS, Kaiser AB. Post-operative infections and antimicrobial prophylaxis. In: *Mandell, Douglas and Bennett's Principles and Practice of Infectious Diseases*, 4th edn. New York: Churchill Livingstone, 1995; 2742–56.

Pain management in chest trauma

TIM J LAMER

Numerous studies have demonstrated that pain following trauma and surgery has been a neglected and often poorly managed aspect in the care of the hospitalized patient.[1,2] Furthermore, trauma and surgery introduce a cascade of adverse physiological events which can be attenuated by appropriate analgesic techniques. Aggressive pain management is indicated following trauma, not only for humanitarian and ethical reasons but also to facilitate recovery following trauma and surgery.

Table 24.1 *Physiological responses to pain and trauma*

Pulmonary
    Reduced lung volumes and flow parameters
    Poor cough
    Secretion retention and atelectasis

Cardiac
    Tachycardia (increases myocardial oxygen consumption)
    Hypertension (increases myocardial oxygen consumption)

Vascular
    Vasoconstriction
    Reduced extremity blood flow
    Enhanced venous thrombosis

Endocrine
    Altered protein metabolism
    Fluid and electrolyte changes
    Hyperglycemia

Gastrointestinal/Genitourinary
    Urine retention
    Impaired bowel motility

Hematological
    Hypercoagulable state
    Impaired immunity

ADVERSE EFFECTS OF POST-TRAUMATIC PAIN

Pain and the stress response following trauma and surgery contribute to a number of changes in organ system function, many of which are detrimental to the patient's wellbeing and recovery (Table 24.1).

Pulmonary effects

Pulmonary dysfunction and pneumonitis are major sources of morbidity following chest trauma and surgery. The severe pain accompanying rib fractures or thoracotomy often leads to splinting, hypoxia, hypoventilation, atelectasis, and pulmonary infection.[3,4] The frequency and severity of post-traumatic pulmonary complications can be significantly reduced by effective analgesia[4,5]

Cardiac effects

Acute pain activates the sympathetic nervous system which leads to tachycardia, increased systemic vascular resistance and increased afterload. Each of these factors increases myocardial oxygen demand and can promote myocardial ischemia in vulnerable patients. Effective analgesia blunts this response and recent evidence indicates that segmental thoracic epidural analgesia using a local anesthetic can markedly diminish myocardial work and improve the ischemic myocardium.[6]

Vascular effects

Pain and the accompanying sympathetic nervous system activation leads to peripheral vasoconstriction and may initiate a cascade of events that produce a hypercoagulable state. Attenuation of this stress response with aggressive epidural analgesia using a local anesthetic may prevent peripheral vasoconstriction, improve peripheral blood flow, and diminish the occurrence of post-traumatic hypercoagulability, thereby decreasing the potential for post-traumatic and postoperative thromboembolic complications.[7,8]

Gastrointestinal effects

Pain and the stress response promote decreased gastrointestinal motility and a catabolic state. Post-traumatic ileus is a leading cause of prolonged hospitalization and a significant catabolic state may lead to poor wound healing, fatigue and muscle weakness. Appropriate analgesic intervention can hasten the return of normal gastrointestinal function.[9–11]

INTRODUCTION TO ANALGESIC TECHNIQUES FOR CHEST TRAUMA

It is possible to block the transmission of pain signals at many sites along the pain pathway from the peripheral tissues to the central nervous system (Fig 24.1). Coincidental blockade of afferent input from the periphery into the spinal cord using local anesthetic agents will blunt the stress response.[12,13] Often, it is advantageous to block pain transmission at more than one site along the pathway.[13,14] This multi-modal approach has the advantage of providing superior analgesia while using lower doses of analgesic agents than if a single agent was used. In many cases this also reduces the frequency of side-effects. For example, one of the most efficacious analgesic techniques following chest trauma is to use a combination of a local anesthetic nerve block (epidural or intercostal), a neuraxial (epidural or intrathecal) opioid, and a systemic anti-inflammatory agent (non-steroidal or corticosteroid anti-inflammatory agent). In the following discussions of individual analgesic techniques, it is important to keep in mind the concept of multi-modal analgesia.

SYSTEMIC OPIOIDS

Systemic opioids form the cornerstone of analgesic therapy and are the basis of comparison for other analgesic techniques. Routes of administration include transcutaneous, oral, subcutaneous, rectal, intramuscular and intravenous. For the trauma patient with severe, acute pain the intravenous route is preferred. Currently available transcutaneous analgesics (e.g. transdermal fentanyl) have a very slow onset, achieving peak blood levels 15–20 hours following application, which makes timely dosage titration impossible. Oral, intramuscular and rectal administration have erratic and unpredictable absorption and are also difficult to titrate to a suitable level of analgesia. In patients who are alert and communicative, patient-controlled analgesia is the preferred technique for administering intravenous opioid analgesia.

Patient-controlled analgesia (PCA)

Patient-controlled analgesia (PCA) is the administration of an analgesic agent, usually an opioid, by any route (usually intravenous), in an amount sufficient to produce analgesia. In practice, the technique is usually performed using one of the many commercially available PCA infusion devices. The use of a PCA machine allows the practitioner to tailor the analgesic regimen to a variety of clinical conditions.

Management of five key variables will determine the success of the technique:

1. Loading dose
2. Continuous infusion rate
3. Demand dose
4. Lock-out period
5. Maximum 4-hour dose.

The success of PCA can be undermined by the same attitudes that limit the effectiveness of conventional intramuscular analgesia, that is, deliberate underdosing by setting unreasonably low demand doses or exces-

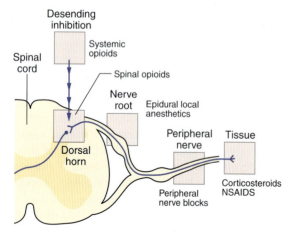

Figure 24.1 *Anatomical sites most commonly blocked by analgesic techniques.*

Table 24.2 *Guidelines for opioid PCA*

Drug	Relative potency	Demand dose (mg)	Lock-out (min)	Basal infusion* (mg/h)
Meperidine	1	10–30	5–10	Not recommended
Morphine	7–10	0.5–3.0	5–10	1.0–2.0
Hydromorphone	70–100	0.1–0.4	5–10	0.1–0.3

*Basal infusion is not recommended for routine use (see text).

sively long lock-out periods. Table 24.2 provides general guidelines for a variety of opioids. Elderly or debilitated patients may require less and patients who have tolerance from long-term opioid exposure may require considerably more medication. The routine use of the same demand dose and lock-out interval for every patient (e.g. on preprinted orders) is to be discouraged. Appropriate nursing assessment is essential to ensure that the selected variables are appropriate. If not, then the dosage or lock-out settings need to be changed.

Continuous infusion

The use of a basal or continuous infusion in conjunction with the demand feature is not recommended for routine management. Most patients can be managed with appropriately programmed demand doses. The addition of a basal infusion does not necessarily increase efficacy but it may increase the likelihood of side-effects.[15] Patients with high opioid dosage requirements and patients who fall asleep and then awaken with pain that does not readily respond to a demand dose are good candidates for the addition of a background infusion (Table 24.2).

Drug selection

Any opioid can be used for PCA. It is best to be very familiar with two or three agents. Morphine, meperidine (pethidine) and hydromorphone are most commonly used in the USA. If a patient has a drug sensitivity or side-effect with one agent, switching to another agent will usually correct the problem.

The practitioner should be aware that morphine and meperidine have active metabolites. Normeperidine (norpethidine), a metabolite of meperidine, is a CNS stimulant and is excreted by the kidneys. Patients with renal dysfunction who receive large doses of meperidine can develop seizures due to normeperidine accumulation. Morphine-6-glucuronide is an active metabolite of morphine that is also renally excreted. Accumulation of this metabolite in patients with renal dysfunction can lead to respiratory depression. Hydromorphone does not have any known active metabolites and is an ideal agent to use in patients with renal dysfunction.

Table 24.3 *Possible adverse effects of systemic opioids*

- Nausea and vomiting
- Sedation
- Impaired gastrointestinal motility
- Suppresses cough reflex
- Urinary retention
- Respiratory depression
- Pupillary constriction

Side-effects

Problems and side-effects from PCA may be drug or equipment related. Most mechanical problems are related to equipment misprogramming. Other less common problems include patients gaining access to the locked program button and the extremely rare runaway drug delivery due to equipment malfunction. Patient overdose may occur when PCA becomes family-controlled analgesia. Patient and family members should be advised that only the patient is to activate the PCA device. Other problems are related to opioid side-effects (Table 24.3).

ANTI-INFLAMMATORY DRUGS

Anti-inflammatory drugs can be administered by oral, rectal, intravenous or intramuscular routes. For the thoracic trauma patient the intravenous route is preferred. The two major classes of anti-inflammatory drugs are non-steroidal anti-inflammatory drugs (NSAIDs) and corticosteroids. Ketorolac is currently the only NSAID available for intravenous use in the USA.

Ketorolac

Ketorolac, like other NSAIDs, blocks the synthesis of prostaglandins peripherally and exerts additional prostaglandin-independent peripheral and central analgesic and anti-inflammatory effects. It is an effective analgesic when used alone but is most effective when combined with a systemic opioid or spinal analgesia. Its major attraction is the ability to produce analgesia without causing respiratory depression or impaired gastrointestinal motility.[16]

Ketorolac is indicated for short-term (<5 days) treatment of moderate to severe pain. The recommended dose for healthy patients less than 65 years old with normal renal function is 30 mg i.v. or i.m. every 6 hours. When combined with an opioid or spinal analgesia, the dose can often be decreased to 15 mg. For patients older than 65 years, the recommended dose is 15 mg every 6 hours. This is also the appropriate dose for patients with mild to moderate renal dysfunction, however, this drug should be used only with extreme caution and appropriate monitoring of renal function in these patients.

Possible side-effects are similar to other NSAIDs and include gastropathy, coagulopathy, and nephropathy. A recent post-marketing surveillance study comparing more than 10 000 courses of parenteral ketorolac with more than 10 000 courses of parenteral opioids revealed only a very small increase in the risk of gastrointestinal or operative site bleeding with ketorolac.[17] Use in patients younger than 65 at an average of 105 mg/day or lower for less than 5 days was not associated with increased risk.

Renal toxicity may occur unexpectedly. Risk factors include pre-existing renal impairment, hypovolemia, patients over 65 years, and heart failure. Ketorolac should be avoided or used only very sparingly in hypovolemic patients.

Contraindications for the use of ketorolac and other NSAIDs include active peptic ulcer disease, aspirin allergy, and patients whose clinical condition will not permit the use of an agent with antiplatelet effects (e.g. intracranial hemorrhage).

Corticosteroids

Corticosteroids are potent analgesic and anti-inflammatory agents. Recent studies have demonstrated that adding a parenteral corticosteroid to a postoperative analgesic regimen improves pain relief, improves pulmonary function, and reduces the postoperative hyperthermic response.[13,18] Confirmatory studies are needed to determine the role of corticosteroids following surgery and trauma; however, mounting evidence supports the concept of adding a potent anti-inflammatory analgesic to the postoperative analgesic regimen.

EPIDURAL ANALGESIA

Anatomy

The spinal cord descends in the spinal canal from the foramen magnum and ends at the L1–L2 area. It is

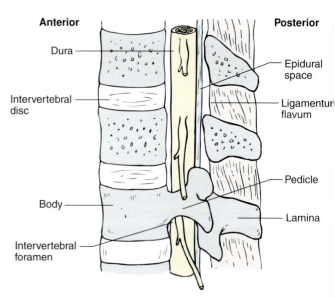

Figure 24.2 *Anatomy of the epidural space. The epidural space is a narrow space composed of adipose tissue, epidural blood vessels, and nerve roots. Posteriorly, it is situated between the ligamentum flavum and the thecal sac.*

surrounded by cerebrospinal fluid (CSF) which is enclosed within the dura mater (dura).

The epidural space lies just superficial to the dura (Fig 24.2) and it contains adipose tissue, blood vessels, and the spinal nerve roots as they pass from the spinal canal toward the intervertebral foramen.

Local anesthetics injected into the epidural space diffuse cephalad and caudad from the site of the injection. The extent of diffusion is controlled by the volume and dosage of the injectant. Epidural local anesthetics block nerve conduction by interfering with nerve impulse propagation at the level of the nerve roots.

The smaller diameter pain and autonomic nerve fibers are more susceptible to local anesthetic blockade than are the larger sensory and motor fibers. The extent of sensory and motor block depends on the concentration and dosage of the anesthetic injected.

Opioids injected into the epidural space diffuse across the dura and into the spinal cord. Opioids bind with opioid receptors located within the dorsal horn of the spinal cord to produce a potent analgesic effect. Opioid receptor binding effects only analgesia. There are no significant effects on the autonomic or motor fibers (Table 24.4).

Epidural opioids

Since the first report of spinal opioid analgesia appeared in 1979, hundreds of subsequent studies have demonstrated that epidural opioids provide analgesia that is superior to systemic opioids (p.o., i.m., i.v.).[19] Opioids can be delivered to the epidural space via intermittent

Table 24.4 *Effects of epidural local anesthetic compared with epidural opioid*

Physiological effect	Epidural opioid	Epidural local anesthetic
Site of action	Dorsal horn	Nerve roots
Pain relief	Yes	Yes
Extremity motor block	No	Dose-related
Sensory block	No	Dose-related
Sympathetic block	No	Yes
Urine retention	Often	Often

Table 24.5 *Epidural opioid dosage guidelines*

Opioid	Loading dosage	Infusion dosage
Fentanyl	1.0–1.5 µg/kg	0.75–1.0 µg/kg/h
Morphine	0.03–0.07 mg/kg	0.005–0.0075 mg/kg/h
Meperidine	0.5–1.0 mg/kg	0.15–0.25 mg/kg/h

bolus injection or continuous infusion. For pain control following thoracic surgery or trauma, the use of a continuous infusion via an indwelling epidural catheter is the preferred technique as it allows easy dosage titration to optimize analgesia and minimize side-effects. The main advantage of epidural opioid analgesia over many other techniques is the ability to provide intense analgesia without producing sensory, motor, or sympathetic blockade. Epidural opioids are most effective for relieving sharp, well localized body wall pain and are not as effective for cutaneous pain and pain from nerve damage.

Several investigators have demonstrated significant improvement in ventilatory function and in many cases, avoidance of mechanical ventilation when epidural analgesia was compared to conventional systemic analgesia in patients with blunt chest trauma and multiple rib fractures or flail chest.[20–22] Similarly, many studies involving post-thoracotomy patients have demonstrated superior analgesia, improved pulmonary function, and reduced pulmonary morbidity with epidural analgesia instead of conventional systemic opioid analgesia.[4,19,23,24]

Any opioid can be used for epidural analgesia but the greatest clinical experience has been with morphine and fentanyl. The major clinical differences between these two drugs are due to their different solubility properties. Morphine is more water soluble and once it gets into the CSF it will ascend the spinal axis as the CSF circulates within the spinal canal and it is more likely than fentanyl to reach upper thoracic and cervical dermatomes. Fentanyl is more lipid soluble (approximately 800 times more soluble than morphine) and is rapidly taken up into the spinal cord and blood vessels after it is injected. Not as much drug is available to ascend the spinal axis within the CSF. Therefore, fentanyl provides a more segmental analgesic block whereas morphine provides a more diffuse or widespread block. From a practical standpoint, lipid-soluble drugs such as fentanyl need to be administered reasonably close to the desired area of analgesia whereas morphine can be administered at a site more distant from the area of desired analgesia.[25] For thoracic analgesia, epidural fentanyl is best administered via a thoracic epidural catheter or injection while morphine can

provide excellent pain relief via a lumbar catheter or injection. The downside of morphine's propensity to spread more within the CSF is a higher frequency of side-effects. Table 24.5 lists general dosage guidelines for epidural analgesia.

Side-effects of epidural opioids are usually nuisance problems which are easily managed and are listed in Table 24.6.[26] Urine retention occurs in 30–60% of patients with epidural opioid analgesia. Since most patients who require epidural analgesia following major trauma and surgery also require an indwelling urinary catheter, this is seldom a significant clinical problem. Nausea, vomiting and pruritis occur in 10–20% of patients and are easily managed by the interventions outlined in Table 24.6.

The most feared complication of epidural opioid analgesia is respiratory depression and it is more common with morphine than fentanyl, again, due to morphine's CSF solubility and its propensity to ascend the spinal axis and reach brainstem respiratory center receptors. Careful monitoring protocols can minimize the occurrence of this complication (Table 24.7). Hypersomnolence is a harbinger of respiratory depres-

Table 24.6 *Side-effects of epidural opioids*

Side-effect	Management
Excessive somnolence and/or bradypnea	Reduce rate of infusion or temporarily stop infusion Change to a different drug Low dose naloxone infusion* Nalbuphine†
Pruritis	Try diphenhydramine (25 mg i.v./i.m.) first Nalbuphine† Low dose naloxone infusion*
Urine retention	Indwelling catheter Intermittent catheter Nalbuphine† or naloxone*
Nausea and vomiting	Phenothiazine or butyrophenone antiemetic (e.g. droperidol 0.625 mg i.v./i.m.) Ondansetron 4 mg i.v. Nalbuphine† or naloxone*

*Naloxone infusion: 5–10 µg/kg/h titrated to reduce side-effects and maintain analgesia.
†Nalbuphine: 5 mg i.v. will reduce side-effects and maintain analgesia.

Table 24.7 *Epidural opioid monitoring protocol*

Do not administer other sedative, hypnotic, or analgesic agents without prior discussion with the Anesthesiology Service.

Maintain an indwelling intravenous catheter.

Monitor respiratory rate and level of consciousness every 15 min for 2 h and then every hour for 22 h, then every 4 h until discontinuing therapy.

Respiratory rate less than 10: call Anesthesiology Service.

Respiratory rate less than 8 or acute deterioration in level of consciousness: stimulate the patient to breathe
- administer 100% oxygen by mask
- naloxone 0.1 mg i.v. stat and may repeat in 3–5 min
- stop epidural infusion
- arterial blood gas
- call Anesthesiology Service.

sion and careful assessment of respiratory rate and level of consciousness and arousal are the keys to prevent clinically significant respiratory depression.[27,28] Treatment depends on the degree of compromise and may include i.v. naloxone, mask ventilation or intubation and positive pressure ventilation.

Intrathecal opioids

In some situations epidural catheters for pain control may not be feasible or may be contraindicated. A single dose of preservative-free morphine injected directly into the lumbar CSF via a small gauge (22–27 gauge) spinal needle can provide profound analgesia. A 0.25 mg dose can provide 15–24 hours of pain relief.[29]

Epidural local analgesia

Like epidural opioid analgesia, the administration of a local anesthetic into the epidural space can provide potent analgesia. The mechanism of action, physiological effects, and side-effects are markedly different. Most of the currently available local anesthetics are suitable agents but bupivacaine is the most commonly used agent for continuous infusion epidural local analgesia.

Epidural local anesthetics block nerve roots just before they enter the spinal cord. Administration of large doses will block sensory, motor, and autonomic fibers. Fortunately, pain fibers are more susceptible to anesthetic block whereas the larger sensory and motor fibers are more resistant. By adjusting the concentration and dosage of anesthetic, it is usually possible to successfully block pain fibers while minimizing the degree of motor block. Autonomic fibers are very susceptible to blockade. This is a good news–bad news effect. The bad news is that extensive sympathetic

blockade may lead to hypotension, especially in the volume-depleted patient. The good news is blockade of sympathetic nerves supplying the lower extremities improves lower extremity blood flow and significantly reduces the likelihood of venous thromboembolic complications.[7,8] Blockade of sympathetic fibers supplying the gastrointestinal tract may improve motility and hasten the recovery of gastrointestinal function following major trauma and surgery.[9–11]

The key to providing successful analgesia while minimizing side-effects is to produce a segmental block whenever possible. For pain control following thoracic surgery or trauma, this is accomplished by placing a catheter in the thoracic epidural space as close as possible to the dermatome, myotome and sclerotome levels involved. A segmental block can then be accomplished with bupivacaine concentrations ranging from 0.10% to 0.25% at an infusion rate of 6–8 ml/h. On the other hand, trying to achieve thoracic local analgesia from the lumbar epidural space requires a larger dose and volume of anesthetic and will increase the chance of hypotension and lower extremity weakness.

Side-effects of epidural local analgesia are of two major varieties, those related to the physiological effects of local anesthetic blockade (hypotension, lower extremity block, urine retention, loss of sensation) and those related to accidental placement of the anesthetic into a site other than the epidural space. Accidental injection of a large dose of local anesthetic into the intrathecal space instead of the epidural space can lead to profound neural blockade and in some cases, total CNS neural blockade which leads to significant hypotension and respiratory arrest. Provided timely and appropriate resuscitation occurs, this complication will resolve without sequelae as the anesthetic wears off. Accidental injection into an epidural blood vessel can result in a seizure, cardiovascular collapse and even fatal cardiac arrhythmias. Again, prompt resuscitative maneuvers will usually lead to an uneventful recovery. It is best to prevent these complications by careful aspiration for blood or CSF, incremental injection of local anesthetic rather than injection of a large bolus, and use of an epinephrine (adrenaline) containing a local anesthetic test dose.

Epidural local and opioid combinations

Most of the side-effects of epidural analgesia are dose related. Lower dosages of local anesthetics will reduce the severity and frequency of hypotension, motor block and urine retention. Lower dosages of opioids will reduce the severity and frequency of pruritus, urine retention, nausea and respiratory depression.

Many studies have demonstrated the analgesic effects of the combination of an epidural opioid and a local anesthetic to be additive or even synergistic. Such a

Table 24.8 *Combination opioid and anesthetic epidural analgesia*

Analgesic agents	Concentration	Comment
Bupivacaine/ fentanyl	0.05%/5 µg/ml	Requires segmental placement for optimal result (see text). This low concentration of bupivacaine minimizes motor block
Bupivacaine/ fentanyl	0.125%/5 µg/ml	Higher concentration bupivacaine is beneficial when muscle spasm is a significant pain problem
Bupivacaine/ morphine	0.05–0.10%/ 0.05 mg/ml	Morphine provides more extensive analgesia than fentanyl but also produces a higher frequency of side-effects

Table 24.9 *Commonly used local anesthetics*

Anesthetic agent	Concentration	Duration of analgesia*
Ropivacaine	0.75%	6–8 hours
	0.5%	4–6 hours
Bupivacaine	0.5%	8–12 hours
	0.25%	6–8 hours
Mepivacaine	1.5%	3–6 hours
	1.0%	2–4 hours
Lidocaine	2.0%	3–5 hours
	1.0%	2–3 hours
Chloroprocaine	3.0%	1–2 hours

*The duration may be extended by up to 50% for some agents by adding epinephrine to a final concentration of 1:200 000.

combination allows each agent to be used in dosages lower than are required for either agent alone.[19] The result is analgesia that is equal or superior to a single agent with fewer side-effects. Table 24.8 lists some commonly used epidural analgesic combinations. Unless there is a contraindication, a combination of a local anesthetic agent plus an opioid should be used when epidural analgesia is chosen for pain control following thoracic trauma or surgery.

REGIONAL NERVE BLOCKS

Regional nerve blocks offer the advantage of providing analgesia without the systemic side-effects associated with systemic or epidural analgesic techniques. Nerves can be blocked by physical or chemical modalities. Physical modalities include heat- or cold-induced lesions. For example, cryoanalgesia utilizes a special probe placed next to the nerves to be blocked. The probe cools the nerve to approximately −20°C. The resulting block lasts for 2–4 weeks; however, the analgesia is inferior to that provided by epidural analgesia and there is a small risk of post-block neuroma formation which can produce a chronic neuralgia.[30,31] Similarly, radiofrequency analgesia utilizes a special probe which heats the adjacent nerve and has drawbacks that are similar to cryoanalgesia.

Local anesthetic nerve blocks are preferable to physical modalities for neural blockade following surgery or trauma. The most common techniques for thoracic analgesia are intercostal nerve block, paravertebral nerve block and intrapleural analgesia. The practitioner should become familiar with a short- and a long-acting anesthetic agent (Table 24.9). Mepivacaine and lidocaine (lignocaine) are the two most commonly used short-acting anesthetics. Intercostal nerve block with these agents provides 2–6 hours of pain relief depending on the concentration used. The addition of epinephrine at a concentration of 1:200 000 will increase the duration. Bupivacaine currently is the long-acting agent of choice. Intercostal nerve block with bupivacaine will provide 6–12 hours of pain relief. Ropivacaine is a new local anesthetic with a duration of action similar to that of bupivacaine. It has less cardiovascular toxicity than bupivacaine and may be used for nerve blocks that require large doses of anesthetic.

Anatomy

The second through twelfth thoracic spinal nerves supply motor, sensory and sympathetic fibers to the skin and all layers of the thoracic and abdominal body wall including the parietal pleura and peritoneum (Fig 24.3). Upon exiting the intervertebral foramina, the thoracic nerves divide into dorsal or posterior rami and ventral or anterior rami. The dorsal rami innervate the vertebrae, vertebral ligaments and paravertebral muscle and skin. The ventral rami course between the ribs. Approximately 2–3 cm beyond the foramen, the nerve courses between the internal intercostal muscles and the innermost intercostal muscles. At this point the nerve assumes its position as the intercostal nerve as it courses just inferior to each rib accompanied by an intercostal artery and vein. There is considerable overlap of truncal dermatomes and myotomes. Blocking a single thoracic nerve root or intercostal nerve may not always lead to an appreciable area of anesthesia. It is usually necessary to block two or more adjacent nerves.

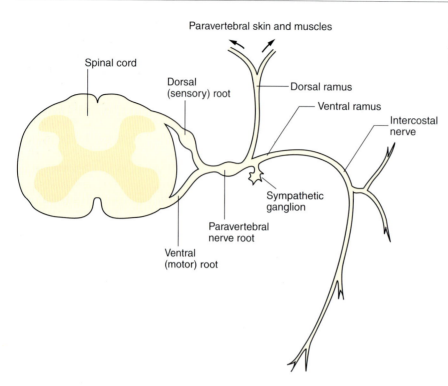

Figure 24.3 *Anatomy of a thoracic spinal nerve including schematic representation of paravertebral nerve root and intercostal nerve.*

Paravertebral nerve block

Paravertebral nerve block (PNB) involves blocking the thoracic nerve (or nerves) just after it exits the intervertebral foramen and is performed as follows. After appropriate sterile preparation, skin and subcutaneous anesthesia are performed with 1% lidocaine. A 22 gauge, 6–8 cm needle is inserted perpendicular to the skin through a point 3.0–3.5 cm from the midline and immediately lateral to the spinous process one level cephalad to the level to be blocked (Fig 24.4). For example, if the fifth thoracic nerve

root is to be blocked, the tip of the fourth thoracic spinous process is identified. The needle is advanced to contact the transverse process (average depth is 2.5–3.0 cm). After contacting the transverse process, a point is marked on the needle 1.5 cm beyond the skin. The needle is withdrawn 1.5–2 cm and repositioned to aim approximately 10° caudally. The needle is advanced to slip past the lamina and transverse process to the previously marked point on the needle. If a paresthesia is encountered, the needle is withdrawn 2 mm.

After aspiration for air, blood and CSF is negative, 5 ml of local anesthetic is injected. Bupivacaine 0.25% with 1:200 000 epinephrine will provide 6–8 hours of analgesia. If long-term analgesia is desired, a large bore (17–18 gauge) needle can be placed as described above and a 22 gauge catheter can be threaded through the needle. The needle is removed and the catheter is secured. The catheter can be managed with intermittent injections or with a continuous infusion of 0.25% bupivacaine at 4–6 ml/h.

Paravertebral block at a single level will most often lead to anesthesia and analgesia of several adjacent levels. Several studies have demonstrated that the injectant will spread along the paravertebral space to one or more levels above and below the level of injection.[32,33]

Possible side-effects and complications are as follows:

- Pneumothorax. In inexperienced hands the frequency of this complication can be quite high. It can be performed safely in patients who have a chest tube in place.
- Epidural spread. Local anesthetics injected near the intervertebral foramen can spread centrally along the

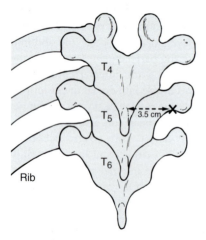

Figure 24.4 *Anatomy of thoracic paravertebral nerve block. In this example, the fifth thoracic nerve is blocked by identifying a point 3.5 cm from the midline of the fourth thoracic vertebral spinous process (see text for full explanation).*

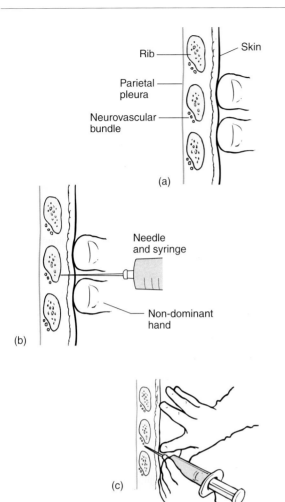

Figure 24.5 *Intercostal nerve block. (a) The index and middle finger of the non-dominant hand bracket the rib corresponding to the nerve to be blocked. (b) The dominant hand advances a needle and prefilled syringe down to the rib surface. (c) The non-dominant hand stabilizes the needle and syringe unit as it is 'walked' off the inferior margin of the rib and advanced 2–3 mm beyond the rib margin (see text for full explanation).*

nerve root, into the epidural space. Extensive epidural spread may lead to hypotension.[33]

- Systemic local anesthetic toxicity.
- Nerve root trauma. One should never inject directly into a nerve root.
- Hematoma. This procedure should be avoided in a patient with a coagulopathy or on anticoagulant therapy.

Intercostal nerve block

Intercostal nerve block (ICB) involves blocking the nerve (or nerves) as it courses underneath the rib in the

intercostal groove and is performed as follows. The ipsilateral arm is raised above the head to rotate the scapula. The rib or ribs of the corresponding nerve(s) to be blocked are identified 5–7 cm from the middle of the spine. The index and middle finger of the non-dominant hand bracket the rib (Fig 24.5). The dominant hand advances the needle attached to a prefilled syringe until the rib is contacted (a 23 gauge 2.5–4 cm needle is used). The non-dominant hand is then removed from the skin and grasps the syringe to stabilize the needle and syringe unit. The operator then carefully 'walks' the needle inferiorly across the rib surface. As the needle tip slides off the inferior surface of the rib, it is advanced 2–3 mm in order to position the tip next to the nerve in the intercostal groove. After negative aspiration, 3–5 ml of local anesthetic agent (usually 0.25% or 0.5% bupivacaine) is injected. This block also can be performed under direct vision with the chest cavity opened during thoracotomy. Side-effects and complications of ICB, like PNB, include pneumothorax, nerve trauma, systemic anesthetic toxicity, hematoma and epidural spread.

Intercostal and paravertebral nerve blocks provide effective analgesia following thoracotomy and rib fractures. Intercostal nerve block is an excellent anesthetic technique prior to chest tube insertion. Analgesia is usually superior to systemic opioid analgesia but is not as effective as epidural analgesia.[34–37] The combination of intercostal nerve block(s) supplemented with PCA opioid analgesia is an effective technique for patients who are not suitable candidates for epidural analgesia.

Intrapleural analgesia

An indwelling catheter placed into the pleural space between the visceral and parietal pleura and injected with a local anesthetic can provide excellent thoracic analgesia.[38–40] Anesthetics injected into the pleural space distribute in a gravity-dependent fashion to the most dependent area of the pleural space (Fig 24.6). The patient should be positioned to distribute the anesthetic along the posterior paravertebral area of the intercostal space where the intercostal nerves are covered by only the pleura, endothoracic fascia and internal intercostal membranes.[41] The local anesthetic agent diffuses across these tissue layers and can anesthetize the intercostal nerves and the thoracic sympathetic trunk on the affected side.

Intrapleural analgesia is most commonly performed as a continuous anesthetic infusion through an indwelling catheter. The catheter can be placed intra-operatively following an open chest procedure or percutaneously using an epidural catheter kit. After appropriate skin preparation and local anesthesia, a 17–18 gauge, 9 cm Tuohy-type styletted needle is

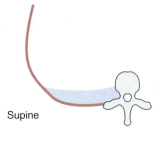

Supine

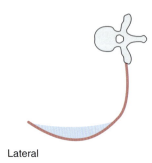

Lateral

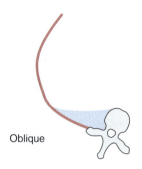

Oblique

Figure 24.6 *Spread of intrapleural local anesthetic in a gravity-dependent fashion. The anesthetic is represented by the shaded area. It is obvious why the supine and painful-side-up oblique positions are preferred.*

advanced down to the sixth or seventh rib at approximately the posterior axillary line. When the rib is contacted, the stylet is removed and a 5 ml syringe with the plunger removed is attached to the needle and then filled with 3 ml of saline. The needle is slowly advanced superiorly over the top of the rib and when the needle enters the pleural space, the saline water column in the syringe will be drawn into the pleural space. The needle is fixed at this position, the syringe quickly removed, and the 22 gauge epidural catheter is quickly threaded through the needle, 4–5 cm beyond the needle tip. The needle is removed, the catheter is fixed to the skin and an injection port is connected to the catheter.

The patient is then positioned supine with the painful side up in a slightly oblique position; 20 ml of 0.5% bupivacaine with 1:200 000 epinephrine injected in 5 ml increments over 3–5 minutes will provide 4–8 hours of analgesia. Alternatively, a continuous infusion of 0.25% bupivacaine at 6–10 ml/h will provide analgesia.

Side-effects and complications are as follows:[42]
- Pneumothorax. This complication is quite rare if the technique is performed exactly as described.
- Local anesthetic systemic toxicity. This is most likely to occur if a bolus of 0.5% bupivacaine is injected too quickly or in patients with significant pleural disease or inflammation which will hasten the vascular uptake of anesthetic injected into the pleural space.
- Lung trauma.
- Inadequate analgesia. This is most likely due to improper patient positioning or unrecognized catheter placement outside of the pleural space.

This technique is not recommended for open chest cases which will require postoperative thoracostomy tube drainage as significant anesthetic lost through the chest tube will diminish the effectiveness.[43,44]

SUMMARY

Various techniques are available to provide analgesia following thoracic trauma or surgery. The appropriate

Table 24.10 *Summary of analgesic techniques for thoracic trauma*

Clinical problem	Suggested techniques
Chest tube related pain	Intercostal block
	Systemic opioid plus NSAID
	Local anesthetic instilled into chest tube (if not contraindicated)
Thoracotomy	Thoracic epidural coadministration of opioid plus anesthetic (plus NSAID when needed)
	Intercostal block(s) plus systemic opioid
	Paravertebral block(s) plus systemic opioid
	Systemic opioid plus NSAID
Thoracoabdominal surgery	Thoracic epidural coadministration of opioid plus anesthetic (plus NSAID when needed for breakthrough)
	Systemic opioid plus NSAID
Chest wall trauma (including rib fracture)	Thoracic epidural analgesia
	Paravertebral or intercostal blocks plus systemic opioid
	Intrapleural analgesia plus systemic opioid
	Systemic opioid plus NSAID
The hemodynamically unstable patient	Epidural or systemic opioids
	Regional nerve blocks where appropriate
	Avoid epidural local anesthetics
The septic patient	If possible, avoid indwelling catheter techniques as the catheter could serve as a focus for infection

technique(s) will depend on the extent of the injury and the patient's underlying medication condition, especially the hemodynamic and cardiopulmonary status. Table 24.10 lists some of the most commonly used techniques for a variety of painful conditions.

REFERENCES

1. Donovan M, Dillon P, McGuire L. Incidence and characteristics of pain in a sample of medical-surgical inpatients. *Pain* 1987; **30:** 69–73.
2. Watt-Watson JH. Nurse's knowledge of pain issues: a survey. *J Pain Symptom Manage* 1987; **2:** 207–11.
3. Lutz LJ, Lamer TJ. Management of postoperative pain: review of current techniques and methods. *Mayo Clin Proc* 1990; **65:** 584–90.
4. Shulman M, Sandler AN, Bradley JW, Young PS, Brebner J. Post thoracotomy pain and pulmonary function following epidural and systemic morphine. *Anesthesiology* 1984; **61:** 569–75.
5. Cuschieri RJ, Morran CG, Howie JC, McArdle CS. Postoperative pain and pulmonary complications with comparison of three analgesic regiments. *Br J Surg* 1985; **72:** 495–8.
6. Kock M, Blomberg S, Emanuelsson H, Lomsky M, Stromblad S-O, Ricksten S-E. Thoracic epidural anesthesia improves global and regional left ventricular function during stress-induced myocardial ischemia in patients with coronary artery disease. *Anesth Analg* 1990; **71:** 625–30.
7. Tuman KJ, McCarthy RJ, March RJ, Delaria GA, Patel RV, Ivankovich AD. Effects of epidural anesthesia and analgesia on coagulation and outcome after major vascular surgery. *Anesth Analg* 1991; **73:** 696–704.
8. Bowler GMR, Lamont MC, Scott DB. Effect of extradural bupivacaine or I.V. diamorphine on calf blood flow in patients after surgery. *Br J Anaesth* 1987; **59:** 1412–15.
9. Ahn H, Bronge A, Johansson K, Ygge H, Lindhagen J. Effect of continuous postoperative epidural analgesia on intestinal motility. *Br J Surg* 1988; **75:** 1176–8.
10. Udassin R, Eimerl D, Schiffman J, Hastel Y. Epidural anesthesia accelerates the recovery of post ischemic bowel motility in the rat. *Anesthesiology* 1994; **80:** 832–6.
11. Wattuil M, Thoren T, Hennerdal S, Garvil J-E. Epidural analgesia with bupivacaine reduces postoperative paralytic ileus after hysterectomy. *Anesth Analg* 1989; **68:** 353–8.
12. Weissman C, Hollinger I. Modifying systemic responses with anesthetic techniques. *Anesthesiol Clin North Am* 1988; **6:** 221–35.
13. Schulze S, Miller IW, Bang U, Rye B, Kehlet H. Effect of combined prednisone, epidural analgesia and indomethacin on pain, systemic response and convalescence after cholecystectomy. *Acta Chir Scand* 1990; **156:** 203–9.
14. Bisgaard C, Mouridsen P, Dahl JB. Continuous lumbar epidural bupivacaine plus morphine versus epidural morphine after abdominal surgery. *Eur J Anaesth* 1990; **7:** 219–25.
15. Catling JA, Pinto DM, Jordan C, Jones JG. Respiratory effects of analgesia after cholecystectomy: comparison of continuous and intermittent papaveretum. *Br Med J* 1980; **281:** 478–81.
16. Dahl JB, Kehlet H. Non-steroidal anti-inflammatory drugs: rationale for use in severe postoperative pain. *Br J Anaesth* 1991; **66:** 703–12.
17. Strom BL, Berlin JA, Kinman JL, *et al.* Parenteral ketorolac and risk of gastrointestinal and operative site bleeding: a postmarketing surveillance study. *JAMA* 1996; **275:** 376–82.
18. Korman B, McKay RJ. Steroids and postoperative analgesia. *Anaesth Intensive Care* 1985; **13:** 395–8.
19. Kavanagh BP, Katz J, Sandler AN. Pain control after thoracic surgery: a review of current techniques. *Anesthesiology* 1994; **81:** 737–59.
20. Mackesie RC, Shackford SR, Hoyt DB, Karagaines TG. Continuous epidural fentanyl analgesia: ventilatory function improvement with routine use in treatment of blunt chest injury. *J Trauma* 1987; **27:** 1207–12.
21. Diltman M, Keller R, Wolff G. A rationale for epidural analgesia in the treatment of multiple rib fractures. *Intensive Care Med* 1978; **4:** 193–7.
22. Rankin APN, Comber REH. Management of fifty cases of chest injury with a regimen of epidural bupivacaine and morphine. *Anaesth Intensive Care* 1984; **12:** 311–14.
23. Benzon HT, Wong HY, Belavic AM, *et al.* A randomized double-blind comparison of epidural fentanyl infusion versus PCA with morphine for post thoracotomy pain. *Anesth Analg* 1993; **76:** 316–22.
24. Logas WG, El-Baz N, El-Ganzouri A, *et al.* Continuous thoracic epidural analgesia for postoperative pain relief following thoracotomy: a randomized prospective study. *Anesthesiology* 1987; **67:** 787–91.
25. Sawchuk CW, Ong B, Unruth HW, Horan TA, Greengrass R. Thoracic versus lumbar epidural fentanyl for post thoracotomy pain. *Ann Thorac Surg* 1993; **55:** 1472–6.
26. Cousins MJ, Mather LE. Intrathecal and epidural administration of opioids. *Anesthesiology* 1984; **61:** 276–310.
27. Ready LB, Loper KA, Nessly M, Wild L. Postoperative epidural morphine is safe on surgical wards. *Anesthesiology* 1991; **75:** 452–6.
28. Morgan M. The rational use of intrathecal and extradural opioids. *Br J Anaesth* 1989; **63:** 165–88.
29. Gray JR, Fromme GA, Nauss LA, Wang JK, Ilstrup DM. Intrathecal morphine for post-thoracotomy pain. *Anesth Analg* 1986; **65:** 873–6.
30. Keenan DJM, Cave K, Langdon L, Lea RE. Comparative trial of rectal indomethacin and cryoanalgesia for control of early post thoracotomy pain. *Br Med J* 1983; **287:** 1335–7.

31. Conacher ID, Locke T, Hilton C. Neuralgia after cryo-analgesia for thoracotomy (letter). *Lancet* 1986; **1**: 277.

32. Gilbert J, Hultman J. Thoracic paravertebral block: a method of pain control. *Acta Anaesthesiol Scand* 1989; **33**: 142–5.

33. Tenicela R, Pollan SB. Paravertebral–peridural block technique: a unilateral thoracic block. *Clin J Pain* 1990; **6**: 227–34.

34. Bigler D, Dirkes W, Hansen R, Rosenberg J, Kehlet H. Effects of thoracic paravertebral block with bupivacaine versus combined thoracic epidural block with bupivacaine and morphine on pain and pulmonary function after cholecystectomy. *Acta Anaesthesiol Scand* 1989; **33**: 561–4.

35. Toledo-Pereyra LH, DeMuster TR. Prospective randomized evaluation of intrathoracic intercostal nerve block with bupivacaine on postoperative ventilatory function. *Ann Thorac Surg* 1979; **27**: 203–5.

36. Engberg G, Wiklund L. Pulmonary complications after upper abdominal surgery: their prevention with inter-costal blocks. *Acta Anaesthesiol Scand* 1988; **32**: 1–9.

37. Faust RJ, Nauss LA. Post-thoracotomy intercostal block: comparison of its effects on pulmonary function with those of intramuscular meperidine. *Anesth Analg* 1976; **55**: 542–6.

38. Rocco A, Reiestad F, Gudman J, McKay W. Intrapleural administration of local anesthetics for pain relief in patients with multiple rib fractures. *Reg Anaesth* 1987; **12**: 10–14.

39. Reiestad F, Stromskag KE. Interpleural catheter in the management of postoperative pain. *Reg Anaesth* 1986; **11**: 89–91.

40. vanKleef JW, Logeman A, Burm AGL, deVoogt JWH, Mooren RAG, vanKleef-Mannot IM. Continuous interpleural infusion of bupivacaine for postoperative analgesia after surgery with flank incisions: a double-blind comparison of 0.25% and 0.5% solutions. *Anesth Analg* 1992; **75**: 268–74.

41. Stromskag KE, Hauge O, Stern PA. Distribution of local anesthetics injected into the interpleural space, studied by computerized tomography. *Acta Anaesthesiol Scand* 1990; **34**: 323–76.

42. Stromskag KE, Minor B, Steen PA. Side effects and complications related to interpleural analgesia: an update. *Acta Anaesthesiol Scand* 1990; **34**: 473–7.

43. Ruffin L, Fletcher D, Sperandio M, *et al.* Interpleural infusion of 2% lidocaine with 1:200 000 epinephrine for post thoracotomy analgesia. *Anesth Analg* 1994; **94**: 328–34.

44. Ferrante FM, Chan VWS, Arthur G, Rocco AG. Interpleural analgesia after thoracotomy. *Anesth Analg* 1991; **72**: 105–9.

25

Lung function following traumatic ARDS

STEVE G PETERS

Nearly 30 years after the description of adult respiratory distress syndrome (ARDS), this condition remains a frequent and often fatal complication of trauma or shock from any cause. Overall mortality is approximately 40–50% and may approach 80–90% in patients with multiorgan system failure. However, it has been noted with optimism that survivors of ARDS may recover almost fully over several weeks or months following injury. This chapter reviews the course and patterns of pulmonary function in survivors of ARDS.

PATHOPHYSIOLOGY

Acute respiratory distress syndrome is characterized by alveolar inflammation, exudation of fluid and fibrin, and a fibroproliferative phase lasting days to weeks. Despite the wide variety of injuries and conditions leading to ARDS, the findings of diffuse alveolar damage, capillary leak, and non-hydrostatic pulmonary edema are by definition characteristic. Acute lung injury may occur as isolated organ failure, but evidence suggests the presence of a systemic inflammatory response in most cases, especially those associated with trauma and/or sepsis.[1–3] The proposed pathogenesis attributes a key role to the activation of complement by a variety of injuries associated with ARDS, including shock and trauma. Neutrophil recruitment follows, with release of proteolytic enzymes and toxic oxygen species. Further elaboration of cytokines perpetuates the acute lung injury and promotes a systemic inflammatory response. A variety of inflammatory mediators including interleukins (IL-1, IL-6, IL-8), complement C3a, prostaglandins, and thromboxane have been measured in serum from patients with traumatic ARDS.[2–4] During the acute illness, persistent elevation in the serum of IL-1β and IL-6 have been associated with increased mortality.[4] Studies of bronchoalveolar lavage (BAL) fluid from patients with ARDS have shown elevated numbers of neutrophils and inflammatory cytokines. Persistent neutrophilic alveolitis and the continued presence of proinflammatory cytokines in BAL have been associated with poor outcome.[5–8] A decrease in these mediators typically parallels clinical recovery. Signs of activation of the coagulation cascade and disseminated intravascular coagulation have also been associated with the development of ARDS and multiorgan dysfunction in trauma patients.[9,10]

Extensive proliferation of fibrous tissue is associated with mortality in the late stages of ARDS.[11] In recovering patients, scarring may occur. Cystic changes and pneumatocele formation have been attributed to barotrauma. However, severe interstitial fibrosis is rarely observed in patients surviving ARDS.

PULMONARY FUNCTION

Physiologically, ARDS is characterized by decreased lung volumes, reduced compliance, and intrapulmonary shunting. Remarkable resolution of these abnormalities occurs in the majority of patients surviving ARDS. Early studies of small groups of survivors found nearly normal pulmonary function or mild restrictive disease in most patients.[12–17] Limitations of these studies include small numbers of patients, uncontrolled patient selection, loss of follow-up of many individuals, variable timing of pulmonary function tests (PFTs), and absence of PFT data prior to the onset of ARDS.[18,19] More recent studies have attempted to measure lung function at consistent intervals following ARDS and to identify risk factors for persistent impairment.[20-25]

Outcome following ARDS: overview

- Overall mortality approximately 40–50%
- In survivors, PFTs return toward normal over 3–6 months
- Residual impairment typically mild restrictive pattern with decreased lung volumes and diffusing capacity

---

In a study of pulmonary function following recovery from ARDS, Klein et al. observed mild reductions in lung volumes, static compliance and diffusing capacity in eight patients who had developed ARDS following trauma.[13] Of note, ARDS was complicated by lung contusion in five patients, rib fractures in four, hemothorax in two, and multiple extrathoracic injuries in six subjects. For the trauma patient, injuries involving the major airways, chest cage, pleura, or diaphragm might be expected to affect the course of recovery of respiratory function. These factors have not been studied systematically. Nevertheless, in assessing respiratory impairment in a patient surviving traumatic ARDS, consideration should be given to injuries beyond the lung parenchyma. Vocal cord paralysis and/or tracheal stenosis may present with inspiratory obstruction, especially evident on the inspiratory limb of a flow–volume loop. Restrictive abnormalities of the chest wall and pleura can lead to decreased lung volumes, usually with preserved gas exchange. Phrenic nerve injury and diaphragm weakness are characterized by decreased vital capacity, relatively increased residual volume, and decreased maximal inspiratory pressure.

Potential coexisting injuries in patients with traumatic ARDS

Upper airway
   Vocal cord dysfunction
   Tracheal stenosis
Chest wall
   Rib cage, sternum
Pleura
   Hemothorax, empyema
Phrenic nerve, diaphragm

Other early studies of ARDS survivors assessed subjects at varying time intervals from 1 month to 4 years after hospital discharge.[14-17] Nearly all patients were asymptomatic in initial reports. However, these studies appear to have selected groups with relatively mild disease. Approximately 10–50% of patients in

recent series have noted dyspnea with exertion. Ghio and colleagues, using American Thoracic Society criteria, documented physiological impairment during the first year following ARDS.[25] Of 27 patients, 18 showed impairment at 1 year; changes were mild in 13 (72%), moderate in four (22%), and severe in one (5.6%). Eighty-four percent of patients reported symptoms of dyspnea, cough, or sputum production. Of note, there was no association between symptoms and the degree of impairment by pulmonary function tests.

Lung volumes (total lung capacity, vital capacity) typically are markedly decreased during the acute phase of ARDS. Survivors usually show rapid improvement in lung volumes over 1–3 months. Approximately 80% of patients show normal or mildly reduced volumes by 6 months.[22-27] Ten to fifteen percent of patients have shown moderately decreased lung volumes, and a minority show severe reduction. Studies have consistently demonstrated that most of the recovery occurs in the first 3 months following hospitalization. McHugh et al. evaluated a prospectively identified cohort at regular intervals for one year following ARDS.[22] Lung volumes approached predicted values by 3 months, with little additional improvement at 6 months, and no further increase at 12 months. These authors suggested that clinical follow-up and assessment of residual impairment be scheduled approximately 6 months after extubation.

Although reduced static lung compliance is a criterion for the diagnosis of ARDS, increased resistance to airflow has also been documented.[28] A subset of patients has been reported to show airway obstruction following ARDS, with some improvement in airflow following inhaled bronchodilators.[12,17] Simpson and colleagues also found three of nine patients with airway hyperreactivity documented by methacholine challenge.[17] However, these studies included a majority of smokers, and data regarding airway reactivity and the degree of obstructive lung disease prior to ARDS were limited. Airway disease has not been observed frequently in other series with the exception of major airway lesions (e.g. tracheal stenosis) or peripheral airway disease (e.g. bronchiolitis associated with toxic inhalation or viral pneumonia).

Measurements of gas exchange in survivors of ARDS have shown gradual improvement in alveolar–arterial oxygen gradient, with resting Pa_{O_2} near predicted values. However, mild oxygen desaturation with exercise may be demonstrated in approximately 50–80% of survivors. The most consistently observed abnormality of gas transfer is a mild reduction in carbon monoxide diffusing capacity (D_{LCO}). D_{LCO} averages approximately 50–80% of predicted values at 6–12 months following ARDS, even in the presence of normal lung volumes. The carbon monoxide diffusing capacity is reported to be the best single predictor of impairment.[25] While hypoxemia results from ventila-

Table 25.1 *Patterns of pulmonary function in survivors of ARDS*

Measurement	Average values (relative to predicted)
Lung volumes (TLC, VC)	Normal to slight decrease
Airflow (FEV$_1$/FVC)	Usually normal
Lung compliance	Mild decrease
Diffusing capacity (DLCO)	Mild to moderate decrease
Oxygenation	Normal to slight decrease at rest Mild O$_2$ desaturation with exercise
Alveolar ventilation	
Dead space, V_D/V_T	Normal to slight increase
PaCO$_2$	Usually normal

tion/perfusion mismatch and intrapulmonary shunting, decreased DLCO has been linked to decreased capillary blood volume.[29]

Alveolar ventilation and PaCO$_2$ typically are normal following recovery from ARDS. Dead space to tidal volume ratios (V_D/V_T) may be slightly increased at rest or with exercise; compensatory hyperventilation can maintain normal PaCO$_2$. Rarely, patients have persistent elevations in dead space and may be hypercapnic.

Recognizing that wide individual variability may be observed, Table 25.1 summarizes typical PFT patterns in survivors of ARDS.

PREDICTORS OF IMPAIRMENT FOLLOWING ARDS

A number of recent studies have sought to identify risk factors for persistent impairment in ARDS survivors.[23–25] Age, underlying diagnosis and smoking history have not shown significant correlations, although relatively small numbers of patients have been analyzed. A variety of markers of severity of the acute illness have been associated with subsequent PFT abnormalities. Peters *et al.* found that decreased DLCO after recovery was related to increased alveolar–arterial gradient, elevation of pulmonary artery pressures, and severity of chest radiographic abnormalities on days 4 through 7 of the acute phase of ARDS.[24] Reduced forced vital capacity (FVC) after recovery was related to acute increases in pulmonary vascular resistance and levels of positive end-expiratory pressure (PEEP) during mechanical ventilation. Patients with sepsis also showed a slightly greater degree of impairment. Ghio *et al.* correlated the severity of impairment on serial PFTs with maximal pulmonary artery pressure, lowest thoracic compliance and highest level of PEEP during the acute phase.[25] Elliott and colleagues found the best correlation for decreased DLCO with the duration of treatment with inspired oxygen fraction (FIO$_2$) greater than 0.60.[23]

> **Factors associated with persistent impairment of lung function following ARDS**
> Prior lung disease, e.g. COPD, fibrosis
> Severity of illness
>   Decrease in vital capacity
>   Lowest static compliance
>   Highest mean pulmonary artery pressure
>   Elevated airway pressures
>   Level of PEEP
>   Duration of FIO$_2$ > 0.6

Although mechanical ventilation with high airway pressures, PEEP, tidal volumes, and inspired O$_2$ concentrations may contribute to lung injury, no controlled studies have been carried out to assess the effects of ventilation management on long-term outcome following ARDS. The association of long-term abnormalities in pulmonary function with levels of PEEP and inspired oxygen concentrations during the acute phase may simply reflect severity of illness rather than toxicity of the therapeutic interventions. In trauma patients, studies of barotrauma are complicated by the primary injuries. Miller and colleagues found pneumothoraces in 29 of 40 (73%) of trauma patients treated with PEEP $\geq$15 cmH$_2$O, but pneumothorax was felt to be due to the initial trauma in all but three patients.[30] Any attempt to minimize barotrauma and O$_2$ toxicity must be weighed against the adverse consequences of persistent hypoxemia and shunting.[31–33] It is anticipated that prospective, controlled studies will soon begin to evaluate strategies for mechanical ventilation in ARDS.

Specific pulmonary function studies can be tailored to the clinical findings and recovery of individual patients. If the patient has improved rapidly and has become asymptomatic within days to weeks of hospitalization, early testing with spirometry, diffusing capacity and oxygen saturation may confirm satisfactory recovery. If symptoms and/or physiological impairment persist, it is recommended that pulmonary function be retested after 3–6 months.[19–22] Lung volumes (e.g. total lung capacity, vital capacity, functional residual capacity, residual volume) are best measured by plethysmography, since non-homogeneous areas of lung disease and air trapping may lead to falsely low volumes measured by washout techniques. Spirometry will assess the forced vital capacity and airflow (FEV$_1$/FVC). If abnormalities exist, maximal voluntary ventilation (MVV, l/min) should be reduced in proportion to the decrease in FEV$_1$. A disproportionate decrease in MVV suggests poor effort, muscle weakness, or inspiratory obstruction. In this setting or if stridor is present, an inspiratory flow–volume loop can identify cases of upper airway obstruction. Measurement of maximal inspiratory and expiratory pressures can identify diaphragm injury and/or muscle weakness. Arterial blood gases at rest and with exercise can be used to quantify residual ventilation/perfusion mismatch.

SUMMARY

ARDS following trauma is characterized by severe physiological derangement and high mortality. However, for patients surviving the acute injury, the prognosis for significant recovery of lung function is excellent. Mild reductions in lung volumes and diffusing capacity are most commonly observed 3–6 months after injury. Other thoracic injuries may complicate the course. Symptoms of dyspnea may be out of proportion to changes in lung volumes and spirometry. In such patients, arterial blood gases and exercise testing may identify additional abnormalities.

REFERENCES

1. Kreuzfelder E, Joka T, Keinecke HO, et al. Adult respiratory distress syndrome as a specific manifestation of a general permeability defect in trauma patients. Am Rev Resp Dis 1988; **137:** 95–9.

2. Meade P, Shoemaker WC, Donnelly TJ, et al. Temporal patterns of hemodynamics, oxygen transport, cytokine activity, and complement activity in the development of adult respiratory distress syndrome after severe injury. J Trauma 1994; **36:** 651–7.

3. Rivkind AI, Siegel JH, Guadalupi P, Littleton M. Sequential patterns of eicosanoid, platelet, and neutrophil interactions in the evolution of the fulminant post-traumatic adult respiratory distress syndrome. Ann Surg 1989; **210:** 355–72.

4. Meduri GU, Headley S, Kohler G, et al. Persistent elevation of inflammatory cytokines predicts a poor outcome in ARDS. Plasma IL-1 beta and IL-6 levels are consistent and efficient predictors of outcome over time. Chest 1995; **107:** 1062–73.

5. Steinberg KP, Milberg JA, Martin TR, Maunder RJ, Cockrill BA, Hudson LD. Evolution of bronchoalveolar cell populations in the adult respiratory distress syndrome. Am J Respir Crit Care Med 1994; **150:** 113–22.

6. Baughman RP, Gunther KL, Rashkin MC, Keeton DA, Pattishall EN. Changes in the inflammatory response of the lung during acute respiratory distress syndrome: prognostic indicators. Am J Respir Crit Care Med 1996; **154:** 76–81.

7. Meduri GU, Kohler G, Headley S, Tolley E, Stentz F, Postlethwaite A. Inflammatory cytokines in the BAL of patients with ARDS. Persistent elevation over time predicts poor outcome. Chest 1995; **108:** 1303–14.

8. Donnelly SC, Strieter RM, Reid PT, et al. The association between mortality rates and decreased concentrations of interleukin-10 and interleukin-1 receptor antagonist in the lung fluids of patients with the adult respiratory distress syndrome. Ann Intern Med 1996; **125:** 191–6.

9. Alberts KA, Noren I, Rubin M, Torngren S. Respiratory distress following major trauma. Predictive value of blood coagulation tests. Acta Orthop Scand 1986; **57:** 158–62.

10. Gando S, Nakanishi Y, Tedo I. Cytokines and plasminogen activator inhibitor-1 in posttrauma disseminated intravascular coagulation: relationship to multiple organ dysfunction syndrome. Crit Care Med 1995; **23:** 1835–42.

11. Meduri GU, Chinn AJ, Leeper KV, et al. Corticosteroid rescue treatment of progressive fibroproliferation in late ARDS. Patterns of response and predictors of outcome. Chest 1994; **105:** 1516–26.

12. Lakshminarayan S, Stanford RE, Petty TL. Prognosis after recovery from adult respiratory distress syndrome. Am Rev Respir Dis 1976; **113:** 7–16.

13. Klein IJ, van Haeringen JR, Sluiter HJ, Holloway R, Peset R. Pulmonary function after recovery from the adult respiratory distress syndrome. Chest 1976; **69:** 350–5.

14. Yernault JC, Englert M, Sergysels R, Degaute JP, De Coster A. Follow-up of pulmonary function after 'shock lung'. Bull Eur Physiopathol Respir 1977; **13:** 241–8.

15. Douglas ME, Downs JB. Pulmonary function following severe acute respiratory failure and high levels of positive end-expiratory pressure. Chest 1977; **71:** 18–22.

16. Rotman HH, Lavelle TF, Dimcheff DG, FandenBelt RJ, Weg JG. Long-term physiologic consequences of the adult respiratory distress syndrome. Chest 1977; **72:** 190–2.

17. Simpson DL, Goodman M, Spector SL, Petty TL. Long-term follow-up and bronchial reactivity testing in survivors of the adult respiratory distress syndrome. Am Rev Respir Dis 1978; **117:** 449–54.

18. Hudson LD. What happens to survivors of the adult respiratory distress syndrome? Chest 1994; **105(3 Suppl):** 123S–6S.

19. Elliott CG. Pulmonary sequelae in survivors of the adult respiratory distress syndrome. Clin Chest Med 1990; **11:** 789–800.

20. Elliott CG, Morris AH, Cengiz M. Pulmonary function and exercise gas exchange in survivors of adult respiratory distress syndrome. Am Rev Respir Dis 1981; **123:** 492–5.

21. Suchyta MR, Elliott CG, Jensen RL, Crapo RO. Predicting the presence of pulmonary function impairment in adult respiratory distress syndrome survivors. Respiration 1993; **60:** 103–8.

22. McHugh LG, Milberg JA, Whitcomb ME, Schoene RB, Maunder RJ, Hudson LD. Recovery of function in survivors of the adult respiratory distress syndrome. Am J Respir Crit Care Med 1994; **150:** 90–4.

23. Elliott CG, Rasmusson BY, Crapo RO, Morris AH, Jensen

RL. Prediction of pulmonary function abnormalities after adult respiratory distress syndrome (ARDS). *Am Rev Respir Dis* 1987; **135:** 634–8.

24. Peters JI, Bell RC, Prihoda TJ, Harris G, Andrews C, Johanson WG. Clinical determinants of abnormalities in pulmonary functions in survivors of the adult respiratory distress syndrome. *Am Rev Respir Dis* 1989; **139:** 1163–8.

25. Ghio AJ, Elliott CG, Crapo RO, Berlin SL, Jensen RL. Impairment after adult respiratory distress syndrome. An evaluation based on American Thoracic Society recommendations. *Am Rev Respir Dis* 1989; **139:** 1158–62.

26. Hert R, Albert RK. Sequelae of the adult respiratory distress syndrome. *Thorax* 1994; **49:** 8–13.

27. Alberts WM, Priest GR, Moser KM. The outlook for suvivors of ARDS. *Chest* 1983; **84:** 272–4.

28. Wright PE, Bernard GR. The role of airflow resistance in patients with the adult respiratory distress syndrome. *Am Rev Respir Dis* 1989; **139:** 1169–74.

29. Buchser E, Leuenberger P, Chiolero R, Perret C, Freeman J. Reduced pulmonary capillary blood volume as a long-term sequel of ARDS. *Chest* 1985; **87:** 608–11.

30. Miller RS, Nelson LD, DiRusso SM, Rutherford EJ, Safcsak K, Morris JA. High-level positive end-expiratory pressure management in trauma-associated adult respiratory distress syndrome. *J Trauma* 1992; **33:** 284–90.

31. DiRusso SM, Nelson LD, Safcsak K, Miller RS. Survival in patients with severe adult respiratory distress syndrome treated with high-level positive end-expiratory pressure. *Crit Care Med* 1995; **23:** 1485–96.

32. Hurst JM, Branson RD, DeHaven CB. The role of high-frequency ventilation in post-traumatic respiratory insufficiency. *J Trauma* 1987; **27:** 236–42.

33. Laghi F, Siegel JH, Rivkind AI, *et al.* Respiratory index/pulmonary shunt relationship: quantification of severity and prognosis in the post-traumatic adult respiratory distress syndrome. *Crit Care Med* 1989; **17:** 1121–8.

26

Thoracic trauma in children

PAUL ROUX

Thoracic injuries are relatively infrequent in children, but are potentially lethal and often compound consequences of other associated injuries.

This chapter presents an approach to the diagnosis and management of chest injuries. Clues to diagnosis are highlighted as they present during the first assessment in the emergency room. Information necessary for rapid and adequate pediatric resuscitation is provided. Techniques for emergency procedures are described as adapted for children. Once the child is relatively stable, frequent reassessment and vigilance are necessary to detect and diagnose complications and respiratory injuries which present subacutely.

INTRODUCTION

Injuries are the leading cause of death in children between 1 and 14 years of age[1] and a cause of permanent disability to many. Whereas most injuries to children occur in the home, serious and life-threaten-

ing injuries are most frequently the result of motor vehicle accidents (MVAs) in which children are involved as passengers, pedestrians or cyclists (Table 26.1).[2] Boys are injured more frequently than girls and the age group under 6 years is most at risk of pedestrian MVAs.[1] Falls affect a younger population and cause less severe injuries overall. Penetrating injuries as a result of interpersonal violence are less common in children. Child abuse should be considered where the history does not fit the injuries.

Between 4.5% and 10% of all childhood injuries involve the chest, of which 10–25% will be significant. In these patients, thoracic trauma is a reliable indication of injury severity[3] although the primary cause of death is most often associated head injury.[4] Motor vehicle accidents are the most frequent cause;[4] penetrating trauma, the result of gunshot and stab wounds, is more frequent in certain North American cities.[5]

EMERGENCY ROOM ASSESSMENT AND RESUSCITATION

Children with significant injuries have generally suffered multiple trauma. The causes of early death in this group are airway compromise, hypovolemic shock and injury to the central nervous system (CNS), all of which threaten CNS function. The immediate goal of primary assessment is to identify life-threatening respiratory, circulatory and central nervous system failure and the goal of of resuscitation is to safeguard the CNS supply of oxygenated blood. Cardiopulmonary respiration (CPR) proceeds in the same sequence as in adult patients, but distinctive features in the anatomy and

Table 26.1 *The pattern of chest injury in children*

- Chest injuries represent between 5% and 10% of all childhood injuries.
- Between 10% and 20% of children admitted to a trauma center will have chest injuries.
- Blunt chest injury predominates.
- Most injuries are MVA-related.
- Multiple trauma is the rule if the chest is injured in an MVA.
- Stabs and gunshot injuries predominate in some North American urban communities.

physiology of children require specialized equipment and knowledge for optimal resuscitation.

The airway

A cervical spine injury is always assumed to be present when assessing and securing the airway. Because of the relative size of the occiput, a small child lying supine on a flat surface will have a slightly flexed head. The neutral position requires support below the shoulders to keep the head in the 'sniffing' position. Performing the jaw thrust maneuver elevates the tongue off the back of the pharynx. This simple procedure, and suction of blood and secretions from the pharynx, will restore an airway in most patients. Oxygen and bag ventilation will be life supporting until a decision is made to intubate or until a person with the necessary skill can assist.

> If the airway is clear and the chest is moving, bag ventilation with oxygen is life saving and as good as endotracheal intubation.

Oropharyngeal airways are rarely useful in children. In those with an intact gag reflex they may be a stimulus to choking, laryngospasm and vomiting, whereas those without a gag reflex generally need an endotracheal tube to safeguard the airway.

Unless intubation is a life-dependent emergency, the child should be bag ventilated with oxygen before starting intubation. Intubation should be carried out by a skilled operator if possible. Equipment for suction, intubation and ventilation of children should be checked and ready in every trauma unit.

Oro- or nasotracheal intubation should be performed in unconscious children with poor respiratory drive, in cases of head injury with respiratory distress, chest injury or hypoxia, in patients with extensive injury to the face and neck, for flail chest and where a stable airway cannot otherwise be ensured.

The laryngoscope with the largest blade to fit the patient's mouth will provide the best view. Straight-bladed laryngoscopes are generally used in children under 1 year of age and curved blades in older children. The light should be checked before using the 'scope and a back-up instrument should be available.

Cuffed endotracheal tubes and the shouldered Cole's tube for newborn babies should not be used in children. Both can cause subglottic pressure necrosis and post-intubation stenosis. A tube appropriate in size and length for the patient's age should be chosen. In malnourished children, height age (the age at which the child's current height would lie on the 50th percentile for age) is more appropriate than chronological age.

The appropriate size for an endotracheal tube may be estimated as follows (see also Table 26.2):

Oral tube:
Internal diameter (mm) = (Age/4) + 4
Length (cm) = (Age/2) + 12 for an oral tube;
Nasal tube:
Length (cm) = (Age/2) + 15

Nasotracheal tubes are better anchored and more easily secured than oral tubes and therefore preferred in children, particularly if the patient is restless or likely to be moved.

The laryngoscope is an instrument for the left hand. The flange is designed to displace the tongue to the left and the blade is there to raise the tongue and mandible anteriorly. Any effort to induce extension of the head with the blade will take the pharynx out of alignment with the glottic opening, and will make intubation more difficult.

Before passing the tube, the supraglottic area, the vocal chords and the upper trachea are inspected for injury and foreign bodies.

The endotracheal tube is most easily passed with the patient's head in the 'sniffing' position, as described above. Magill's forceps may be necessary to lift a nasotracheal tube anteriorly through the glottis and cricoid pressure will better align the trachea with the path of the tube. It is not necessary to visualize the cords when intubating through the nose: the distortion of tissue necessary to see a child's cords elevates the glottis anterior to the 'normal' path of the tube and makes intubation more difficult. It is sufficient to identify the midline while passing the tube. After the tube is passed, a visual inspection is done to confirm that it lies between the cords.

Intubation of the right main bronchus with an over-long tube is more common in children. Breath sounds should be checked after passing a tube to ensure they are bilaterally equal. Children needing prolonged ventilation should have an audible leak back past the tube in the positive phase of the ventilatory cycle. If there is no leak, the tube diameter may be too large and may result

Table 26.2 *Endotracheal tube sizes in children*

Age (years)	Prem	0	0.5	1	2	3	4.5	6	9	12
Internal diameter (mm)	2.5	3.0	3.5	4.0	4.5	5.0	5.5	6.0	7.0	8.0
Length (orotracheal) (cm)	8.5	9.5	10.5	12	13	13.5	14	15	16	18
Length (nasotracheal) (cm)		11.5	12.5	14	1.5	15.5	16	17	19	21

Table 26.3 *Signs of respiratory distress in children*

* Tachypnea (see Table 26.4)
* Intercostal recession
* Use of accessory muscles
* Flaring alae nasi
* Grunting

Table 26.4 *Vital signs at different ages: approximate normal range*

Age (years)	Respiratory rate (breaths/min)	Pulse rate (beats/min)	Blood pressure (mmHg)
<1	30–40	110–160	80/50
2–5	25–30	95–140	90/60
5–12	20–25	80–120	100/60
>12	15–20	60–100	110/70

in subglottic pressure necrosis with post-intubation stenosis. In all patients, confirmation of correct tube length should be made on a follow-up chest radiograph.

Breathing

Once the airway is secure, breathing is assessed. A child with multiple injuries is likely to have sustained intrathoracic trauma, with serious effects on respiration. Head injury may cause depression of respiratory drive.

A rapid, thorough assessment of respiratory function is performed, checking for the features of respiratory distress (Table 26.3); the chest is examined for expansion, breath sounds and appropriate abdominal wall excursion; and the effects of hypoxia and hypercapnia on other organ systems are sought. Poor respiratory effort is an indication for ventilation, which can be given by bag and mask, but which will require a mechanical device in the long term. Normal respiratory rates in children vary with age and are given in Table 26.4, together with normal values for the other vital signs.

Respiratory insufficiency is suggested by a reduction in breath sounds, poor chest wall expansion and reduced or paradoxical chest or abdominal wall excursion. A reduced respiratory rate is seen in severely injured children as a preterminal event and should be interpreted as a grave and late sign of respiratory failure.

A depressed level of consciousness is a sign of hypoxia in the child (Table 26.5). Hypoxic children may initially appear agitated or drowsy and progress to increasing drowsiness and eventual coma. Grunting respiration may indicate hypoxia, but is also caused by the pain of breathing with a bruised chest wall or fractured ribs. Hypoxic children are pale, rather than cyanosed. Cyanosis is a near terminal sign and a normal skin color is often seen in hypoxic children. Older

Table 26.5 *Signs of hypoxia in the child*

* Depressed consciousness, agitation, coma
* Tachycardia
* Grunting respiration
* Pallor
* Cyanosis (late)

children may have a tachycardia, but shock, pain and anxiety may produce the same effect.

> Cyanosis is an extremely late sign of hypoxia in the child.

Respiration can be controlled with a stable airway and positive pressure ventilation in most chest trauma, but not if tension pneumothorax, massive hemothorax and bilateral hemopneumothorax are present. Asymmetric chest wall motion, reduced breath sounds, mediastinal shift away from a unilateral lesion and increased or decreased resonance to percussion in a hypoxemic, hypotensive patient indicate these serious complications. Urgent decompression of the pleural space is life saving.

> Respiratory function cannot be normalized without management of tension pneumothorax and massive hemothorax.

An urgent upright chest radiograph is ideal prior to needle thoracentesis, but is not essential. A 12 gauge intravenous catheter on a syringe is inserted into the third or fourth intercostal space in the midclavicular line on the affected side. An escape of air under pressure is usually followed by improved oxygenation and perfusion. A positive thoracentesis is followed by tube thoracostomy as soon as is practical. A chest radiograph is done in the stable patient, to decide the caliber of and best position for the chest tube. For isolated pneumothorax, a small caliber tube is placed in the third intercostal space and directed towards the head. The presence of intrapleural blood requires a large bore tube (as big as the intercostal space will allow) in the fifth or sixth intercostal space in the anterior axillary line, directed as far posteriorly as possible.

The volumes of air and blood draining from the chest provide clues to the extent and nature of the underlying injury. Massive exsanguinating blood loss is an indication for emergency thoracotomy, to identify and manage major vessel injury. Persistent high volume air leak suggests injury to the bronchial tree and indicates bronchoscopy.

Any patient with respiratory distress requires initial oxygen supplementation, whether or not ventilatory support is required. High flow oxygen should be provided, to avoid rebreathing hypercapnia. In small children a translucent head box is useful because it allows the child some movement, does not have the agitating effect of a face mask and allows observation of the face. Inspired oxygen tensions can be measured exactly.

Arterial oxygen saturation measured by pulse oximetry is sufficient to determine pulmonary ability to oxygenate blood. Arterial blood gas analysis is necessary for adequate assessment of children in hypercapnic ventilatory failure or in shock. Inspiratory oxygen tension and corresponding arterial oxygen saturation should be recorded. Change in the a/A gradient over time is a very good index of clinical progress.

Circulation

A rapid assessment of heart rate, pulse, blood pressure, peripheral temperature, respiratory rate and level of consciousness will identify significant blood loss. Brachial pulses, the carotids and femoral pulses should be checked for clues to intrathoracic injury to the aorta or a major vessel. Emergency aortography may be required. An arrhythmia suggests cardiac contusion.

Shock with evidence of raised pressure in the neck veins suggests cardiac tamponade either because of injury to the heart and pericardium, or because of tension pneumothorax. In either case, pulsus paradoxus by palpation or sphygmomanometry will be present.

In older children presenting with cardiac arrest, external cardiac massage is performed using the same technique as in adults. Children under the age of 2 years respond optimally to a technique directed at intermittent increase in intrathoracic pressure rather than to intermittent anteroposterior pressure as in the adult. Efficacy of both mechanisms is assessed by feeling for an impulse in the carotid or brachial artery. Infants are not at risk of rib fracture from cardiac massage.[6] Cardiac arrest after trauma carries a very poor prognosis and the results of external cardiac massage, which are dismal, are not improved by open chest massage.[7]

Apart from the obvious causes of blood loss and hypovolemic shock in multiple trauma, chest injuries can add to circulatory failure in children. Occult hemothorax is a common cause of shock. The blood volume of a child is approximately 80 ml/kg. The average weight of a 3-year-old is 14 kg and of a 5-year-old approximately 20 kg. An acute blood loss of 200 ml and 300 ml, respectively, will cause hypovolemic shock in each. Tension pneumothorax is a cause of shock in the child, because of cardiac tamponade. Acute gastric dilation in association with diaphragmatic rupture may have the same effect.

Venous access may present problems in the management of circulatory collapse. Percutaneous venipuncture, using the largest catheter possible, should be attempted once airway and breathing are established. If this fails, saphenous vein cutdown at the ankle and intraosseous cannulation are alternatives. Jugular and subclavian venous puncture should be avoided in the child because of the high complication rate.

For intraosseous infusion, an 18 gauge or larger needle with a stylet is used. Spinal needles or bone marrow aspiration needles are appropriate. Fluid will need to be infused at a higher hydrostatic pressure than usual. Complications of fat embolism and osteitis limit this technique to situations of absolute necessity only. Laboratory assays of blood aspirated from marrow yield valid results for hemoglobin concentration, sodium, chloride, potassium, urea creatinine and standard bicarbonate, but not for platelet count, white cell count or carbon dioxide and oxygen tensions.[8]

Resuscitation volume is calculated as 25% of blood volume and given as crystalloid (Ringer's lactate or normal saline) in the acute phase. Aliquots of 25% of the blood volume are repeated until intravascular volume is restored. Evidence for improvement will be a fall in the heart rate, improved peripheral circulation and an increase in blood pressure.

Children who do not respond to intravenous resuscitation should be reassessed for signs of pneumothorax or tamponade. A chest drain or pericardiocentesis may be indicated. An urgent chest radiograph should be performed.

Disability

In the head-injured or shocked child a rapid assessment of CNS function records the level of consciousness as: Alert, responsive to Voice, responsive to Pain, or Unresponsive (AVPU). The unresponsive head-injured child will require endotracheal intubation and ventilation, regardless of respiratory status.

A depressed level of consciousness in a child with respiratory signs but no head injury means reduced cerebral oxygen delivery until proved otherwise. Urgent management of shock and possible hypoxia is required.

A depressed level of consciousness is a sign of hypoxia in the child.

Exposure

In the child, as in the adult, the entire body is examined so as not to miss clues to underlying injury. Roadside hypothermia is treated and further exposure prevented. Because of a high ratio of body surface to size, children are more likely to suffer exposure hypothermia than are adults. Measure core and surface temperatures on admission with a low range thermometer. Hypothermia may contribute significantly to a poor outcome.

SPECIFIC ASSESSMENT OF THE RESPIRATORY SYSTEM

History

Information about the accident from the parents or an observer is invaluable. Any child with a history of a fall from a height, having been rolled over by the wheel of a vehicle or crushed in any other way must be assumed to have internal injury to the chest, regardless of the absence of external signs. The pliability of the pediatric chest means that external signs of blunt force may be absent.

An observer may confirm events around an MVA. Children involved in pedestrian MVAs classically present with injuries to the trunk, lower limbs and head. This is the so-called 'Waddle's triad'. The vehicle's leading fender makes the first impact, with trauma to the trunk and the lower limbs. The child is then propelled bodily in the direction of the major force of impact and head injury is caused by deceleration as it hits the road surface. In a taller child, the triad of injuries may occur when the child's head impacts on the bonnet of the vehicle, as the primary force causes the body to jack-knife. In either event, significant chest injury is likely, regardless of external appearances. In the absence of any information regarding the accident, assume that chest injury has occurred.

> Chest injury is assumed in any child with multiple injuries from an MVA.

In cases where children have fallen from moving vehicles, injuries depend in extent on the velocities involved, and may resemble those which occur in falls from a height. Injuries to cyclists may be similar to those seen in pedestrian MVAs, especially if the cyclist was without a helmet. Injuries incurred by children who are passengers depend on deceleration forces. Chest wall abrasions are useful indications of underlying injury in these children. Lower limb injuries are less frequent in this group than in adults, or in children involved in pedestrian MVAs. Evidence of blunt or penetrating abdominal injury is an indication for careful examination of the chest. Any child with liver or splenic injury requires a chest radiograph.

General examination

Skin abrasions, lacerations or contusion over the chest are always significant in the context of blunt trauma, and indicate the need for further investigation. Petechial hemorrhages of the skin over the chest and neck are frequently present in crush injuries. Surgical emphy-sema of the neck and chest suggests significant injury to the major airways. Lacerations may penetrate to the pleural space and should be closely examined for the passage of air. The management of a sucking chest wound is an emergency.

Examination of the respiratory system

Once the injured child is stable, a careful, detailed, and complete examination of the respiratory system is central to further management.

INSPECTION

The normal respiratory rates at different ages are given in Table 26.4. The significance of the rate and charac-ter of respiration has been discussed.

Inspection of the chest wall will identify a unilateral lesion. Reduced ipsilateral chest wall motion will be present in unilateral pneumothorax, hemothorax, pulmonary contusion and multiple rib fracture. Increased chest wall motion will be present in flail chest, in which case chest wall motion will be paradoxical, and in diaphragmatic paralysis, in which case abdominal wall motion during the respiratory cycle will be ipsilaterally paradoxical. If reduced chest wall motion is missed on inspection, auscultatory signs will be misinterpreted.

Intercostal recession (indrawing) indicates reduced pulmonary compliance, or an obstructed airway. Airway obstruction is best assessed by auscultation at the mouth, where stertor and stridor indicate upper airway compromise. In the absence of evidence for airway obstruction or trauma involving the pleural space, intercostal recession during inspiration suggests pulmonary contusion.

Paradoxical abdominal wall motion indicates diaphragmatic injury or a phrenic nerve palsy. The diagnosis is best confirmed by fluoroscopy or ultra-sonography.

Gastric distension is common in traumatized children (Fig 26.1). Aerophagy while crying may lead to acute gastric dilation. In the child with a chest injury, gastric dilation may be a critical factor in respiratory compromise and requires immediate decompression by nasogastric tube. In the patient with diaphragmatic rupture or paralysis, the massively distended stomach may herniate into the chest, causing symptoms similar to those of tension pneumothorax.[9]

PALPATION

Superficial palpation of the skin over the chest and neck will detect the fine crepitus of subcutaneous emphy-sema. In the traumatized child this is a sign of major airway injury and indicates specific and urgent manage-ment. Coarse crepitus may indicate rib fracture, but this

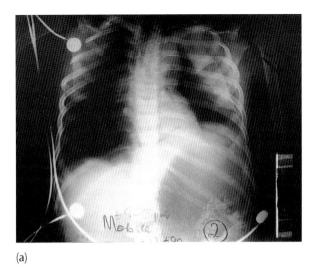

(a)

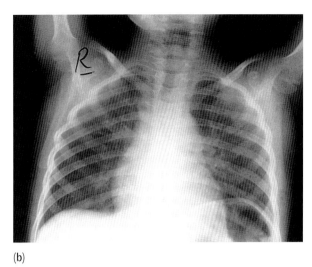

(b)

Figure 26.1 *(a) Acute gastric dilation in a 4-year-old injured in a pedestrian MVA. This boy had a head injury, fractured mandible and femur and a left hemopneumothorax. Note the elevated left hemidiaphragm. The patient required ventilation for the head injury, tube thoracostomy and gastric decompression with a large bore nasogastric tube. (b) Persistent elevation of the left hemidiaphragm 2 months after trauma. Paradoxical abdominal wall motion during respiration and poor movement of the diaphragm on screening indicated phrenic nerve injury.*

is less common in children than in adults, because the child's ribs are pliable and fractures are more likely to be of the 'greenstick' variety, or undisplaced.

Palpation may support the visual impression of reduced chest wall motion, but is less informative than observation, because the traditional palpation with a hand on each side of the chest in the child serves to obscure rather than illuminate.

Tracheal deviation is an important sign of mediastinal shift, but in young children with easily displaced tissue, the left-sided aortic arch tends to cause a slight deviation of the trachea to the right in the normal child, generally best appreciated on the chest radiograph. The cardiac apical impulse should be located to confirm tracheal and mediastinal shift. In the child this is normally in the fifth left intercostal space and in the midclavicular line. Palpation of the liver more than 2 cm below the right costal margin in the midclavicular line suggests possible caudad displacement of the liver by an intrathoracic process.

PERCUSSION

Unilateral stony dullness to percussion indicates hemothorax, as in an adult. In the child, as discussed below, hemothorax suggests underlying pulmonary contusion. Since there is often no other clinical indication of contusion, dullness to percussion has added importance.

Percussion may also give the clues to gastric dilation and to right-sided pneumothorax, when the upper border of the liver is displaced downwards from the fifth intercostal space.

AUSCULTATION

Unless examination of the child's chest has been carried out in an organized way, and the examiner has already established whether the injury is unilateral before reaching for a stethoscope, auscultation will be misleading. The normal bronchovesicular breath sounds of a child are loud to the ear of a person used to adult breath sounds. For this reason, normal signs may be misinterpreted as pathological, and reduced breath sounds on the side of a unilateral injury, as heard over a hemothorax or a pneumothorax, might be thought to be

Table 26.6 *Physical clues to underlying chest trauma in the child with multiple injuries*

- Bruises, lacerations, or abrasion of the chest wall
- Petechial hemorrhages of chest wall and skin over the neck
- Subcutaneous emphysema
- Head injury plus fractured femur (Waddle's triad)
- Fractured humerus
- Injury to the liver or spleen
- Asymmetrical chest wall motion
- Flail chest
- Respiratory distress: tachypnea, recession, grunting, flaring alae nasi
- Paradoxical abdominal wall motion
- Cyanosis
- Abdominal distension
- Shock
- Absent pulses
- Arrhythmia

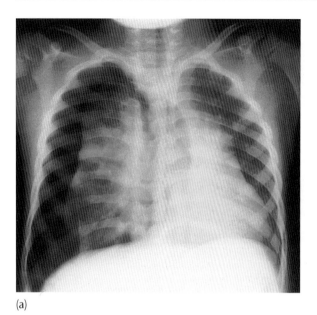
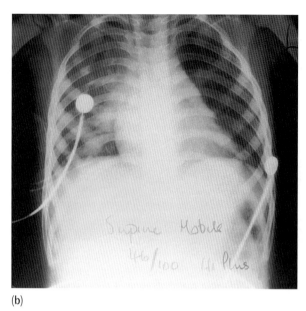

(a)   (b)

Figure 26.2 *(a) A 3-year-old injured in a pedestrian MVA suffered a head injury, fractured right femur and a tension hemopneumothorax. Note the transmediastinal herniation of pleural air under pressure. The supine radiograph did not show a 250 ml hemothorax. (b) Intercostal drainage has restored the mediastinum to the midline and revealed some patches of presumed pulmonary contusion. No rib fractures were visible on this or follow-up radiographs.*

normal. In other respects, careful auscultation will elicit the same data as it would in the adult patient.

Any clues to an underlying chest injury (Table 26.6) gained from the history and the examination, should prompt a chest radiograph.

ASSESSMENT AND MANAGEMENT OF THORACIC INJURIES

Upper airway obstruction

Traumatic obstruction due to laryngotracheal fracture or contusion is rare in children. If the child is unconscious, obstruction is the result of loss of pharyngeal 'stenting' by muscles normally under autonomic control. Management of the upper airway is described above.

Tension pneumothorax

Clinical features and management have been described previously (Fig 26.2).

If the patient is in extremis, radiographic confirmation of the diagnosis is not awaited and the patient is treated as an emergency. Emergency management is decompression by venous catheter as described above, followed by tube thoracostomy. An intercostal drain is placed as described above. An underwater seal is used without suction. The duration of drainage in the child

depends on the duration of positive pressure ventilation (usually for head injury) and drainage of any associated hemothorax or post-traumatic effusion. Persistent air leak via the chest drain suggests tracheal or bronchial injury. If the entry wound of the chest drain is airtight, bronchoscopic evaluation should be considered.

Pneumothorax

Sucking chest wounds are rare in childhood.

Isolated simple pneumothorax is unusual in the child with multiple injuries, but may occur as a result of a fall, or injury during play. If pleural air accounts for less than 30% of volume in the affected hemithorax and associated with moderate trauma, the child is observed. If the respiratory rate increases, an erect chest radiograph must be obtained.

Mediastinal shift and persistent tachypnea are indications for tube thoracostomy.

Apparent simple pneumothorax following blunt chest injury in a child with other injuries suggests underlying pulmonary contusion. Such a patient is also likely to have a post-traumatic pleural effusion, which might readily be missed on the supine chest radiograph taken in the emergency room.[4]

Hemothorax

Massive hemothorax is rare in children, because blunt trauma predominates and rarely causes bleeding from major intrathoracic arteries. Injury to a major artery is more likely in children with first rib fracture.[10]

Massive hemothorax presents with respiratory distress and mediastinal shift with ipsilateral dullness to percussion. Neck veins are not distended as in tension pneumothorax. Shock precedes respiratory failure.

Injury to a major intrathoracic vessel must be assumed when tube thoracostomy produces total blood loss in excess of 20% of blood volume or an ongoing blood loss in excess of 1–2 ml/kg/h. Such losses indicate thoracotomy for control of bleeding. The small absolute blood volumes in the child necessitate great vigilance and rapid reaction to this injury.

Active hemorrhage in the chest of a child injured by gunshot is reported to have been visible on computed tomography (CT) of the chest.[11] CT evidence of active hemorrhage depends on brisk extravasation of contrast-enhanced blood. Scans in such cases are therefore not recommended, because of the risk of exsanguination during the procedure.

A sero-sanguinous post-traumatic effusion is frequently associated with pulmonary contusion. The effusion appears to be dynamic, since early removal of the chest drain may lead to reappearance of an intrapleural collection and an increase in respiratory distress. Placement of a chest drain in the management of blunt chest injury in children is not an indication for prophylactic antibiotic therapy.

Cardiac tamponade

Because children rarely suffer stabs to the chest, cardiac tamponade is rare in pediatric trauma. Occasionally a tension pneumopericardium following blunt trauma may occur.[12] The clinical diagnosis depends on recognition of pulsus paradoxus, a small pulse pressure, distended neck veins and muffled heart sounds. Echocardiography is diagnostic of pericardial fluid. Definitive treatment may require thoracotomy and direct repair.

Myocardial contusion

The frequency with which myocardial contusion is identified depends on the criteria for diagnosis. It is reported to occur in up to to 40% of adult patients with anterior chest trauma[13] and is significantly more frequent in patients with a high Injury Severity Score (ISS).

Although it may occur frequently, the condition does not appear to be of clinical significance in pediatric trauma. When screened for by serial measurements of creatine-phosphokinase isoenzyme (CPK-MB) levels, electro- and echocardiography, cardiac contusion may be diagnosed in up to 14% of pediatric blunt chest

injuries:[14] in this study, none of the children with contusion had evidence of cardiac failure or arrhythmia at any time after their injury.

Patients suspected of having myocardial contusion should be managed with a cardiac monitor. Baseline CPK-MB levels should be measured to facilitate longitudinal assessment. Echocardiography should be carried out in cases where signs of cardiac failure develop.

Rib fractures

The pliable thoracic wall of a child can absorb the kinetic energy of a moderate force without significant injury, and rib fractures are generally rare in pediatric trauma. In severely injured children rib fractures are common.[4] Children with rib fractures are significantly more severely injured than those without, and multiple rib fractures are a marker of a more severe injury pattern. Mortality risk increases in proportion to the number of ribs fractured.[15] Increased mortality relates to associated head injury, but rib fractures may also be an external marker of severe intrathoracic injury.

Rib fractures may cause severe pain with breathing, but pain can be difficult to identify in a small child. There may be grunting respiration, tachypnea and splinting of the involved side of the chest. These signs are also seen with other forms of thoracic injury and are not specific.

Management of rib fractures requires control of pain as the first priority (Table 26.7). Opioid narcotic analgesia is appropriate and a continuous morphine infusion is of great benefit to some patients. Analgesia enables the child to cough better and also helps with physiotherapy. The consequences of adequate pain control are fewer complications due to mucus plugging and atelectasis, shorter periods of ventilation and therefore fewer episodes of secondary respiratory infection.

Intercostal nerve anesthetic blocks are recommended by some authorities, in preference to parenteral opioids.

Most children with rib fractures will also have pulmonary contusion, post-traumatic pleural effusion, pneumothorax, hemothorax or hemopneumothorax.[4]

Chest wall strapping is of no benefit to children with chest injuries. Restricting chest wall motion decreases

Table 26.7 *Pain control in children with rib fractures*

Morphine by continuous infusion	0.05 mg/kg/h
Intermittent intra-venous morphine	0.1 mg/kg every 2–3 h
Tilidine drops	1 per year of age + 1 every 3–4 h

- *Write a regular dosage schedule for analgesia. Do not write 'as required'.*

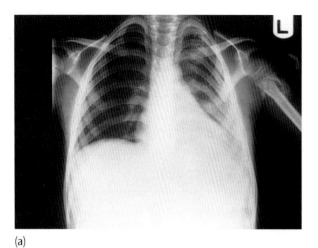

(a)

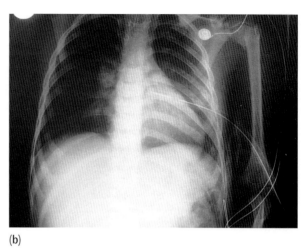

(b)

Figure 26.3 *(a) First chest radiograph of a 5-year-old injured in a pedestrian MVA. He suffered head injury, rupture of the medial capsule of the knee and abrasions to the trunk. Flail chest was evident. The chest radiograph shows a fracture of the left humeral neck, fractures to ribs 3–8 on the left and reduced left lung volume. A left hemothorax is suspected. (b) The patient has been intubated and tube thoracostomy has been performed. Note the re-expansion of the left lung with IPPV and positive end-expiratory pressure.*

airway clearance and increases the frequency of mucus plugging and secondary infection.

> Strapping up the chest wall is detrimental to recovery from chest injury.

Lower rib fractures raise the possibility of trauma to the kidneys, liver and spleen and are an indication for further assessment if abdominal injury has not already been identified.

First rib fractures

First rib fractures are infrequently described in children, but when present, identify a group of patients at high risk of major intrathoracic vascular injuries.

Children with first rib fracture on chest radiograph, with or without hemothorax, who have loss or diminution of upper limb pulses, require emergency investigation by aortography, to detect injury to major vessels.[10] These patients are at high risk of exsanguinating intrathoracic hemorrhage, which may first be identified by blood loss through a chest tube. Successful repair of major vessel rupture is reported, but a high rate of immediate roadside mortality is likely and most children die before reaching hospital.[16]

Flail chest

Flail chest occurs when the integrity of the rib cage is lost due to multiple fractures of two or more adjacent ribs and a segment of the chest wall moves paradoxically during the respiratory cycle. Children tolerate the resultant diminution in respiratory efficiency poorly.

Because the forces that cause flail chest are large, associated injury is common. Associated head injury results in a reduction in respiratory drive and airway control, underlying pulmonary contusion contributes to hypoxemia and intra-abdominal injury impairs diaphragmatic function.

Initial management of flail chest consists of airway control supplemental oxygen, pain control, and decompression of acute gastric dilation. Stabilization of respiratory function may depend on parallel management of associated head and intra-abdominal injuries. Severe flail chest will require intubation with positive pressure ventilation and positive end-expiratory pressure (PEEP) for 'internal splinting' of the chest wall (Fig 26.3).

Pulmonary contusion

Pulmonary contusion is the most common injury seen after blunt chest trauma in children.[4,17] After pedestrian MVAs the majority of cases will have associated rib fractures visible on chest radiograph, but a third will not. This injury often occurs in association with pneumothorax and hemothorax or post-traumatic serosanguinous effusion (Fig 26.4).[4] Radiologically, contusion may worsen over the first 24–48 hours after injury or appear after a similar delay.

Management of contusion is centered on the maintenance of oxygenation. Supplemental oxygen should be given from the outset. Requirements as assessed by pulse oximetry or blood gas analysis may increase over the first 24 hours after injury. Severe contusion in a

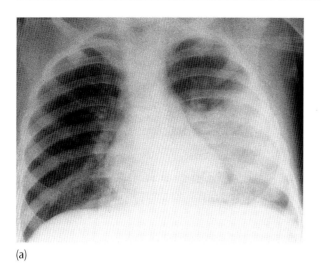

(a)

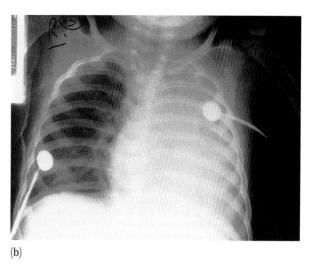

(b)

Figure 26.4 *(a) A 2-year-old passenger in an MVA sustained a head injury, liver lacerations, fracture of the left radius and ulna and blunt chest injury. The initial radiograph shows fractures of ribs 2–4 on the left and left-sided pulmonary contusion. (b) A radiograph taken the following day showed a pleural effusion. This radiograph, taken 48 hours after the accident, shows further accumulation of fluid, clinically associated with increasing tachypnea. A serosanguinous effusion was drained over the following 3 days. Symptomatic improvement was immediate.*

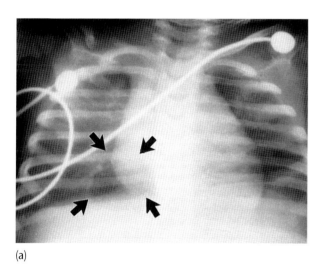

(a)

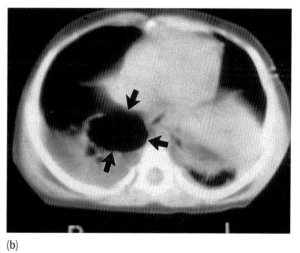

(b)

Figure 26.5 *(a) Chest radiograph showing post-traumatic pneumatocele in a child with blunt chest injury. There is surrounding contusion. A left hemopneumothorax has been drained. (b) The computerized tomographic scan shows bilateral pulmonary contusion and a left-sided hemopneumothorax in the same child. The chest drain site is evident on the left.*

non-ventilated patient will require mask PEEP if inspiratory oxygen concentrations in excess of 40% are required to sustain an adequate arterial oxygen tension. Intubation with positive pressure ventilation is rarely required and should be avoided if possible, since intubation is associated with secondary infection. Tube thoracostomy is indicated for associated post-traumatic effusion or pneumothorax.

The goal of therapy is to prevent progression to the adult respiratory distress syndrome (ARDS). Steroid therapy and prophylactic antibiotics are not indicated. Steroids used for associated head injury have been noted to increase infectious complications.

Traumatic pneumatocele

Spontaneous pulmonary pseudocysts may be observed in an area of contusion (Fig 26.5). No specific treatment is required. They should be distinguished from infectious abscesses and congenital cystic lesions. Spontaneous resolution occurs over weeks.[18]

Tracheal and bronchial disruption

Tracheobronchial injuries are rare but potentially fatal. They occur as a result of blunt and penetrating trauma[19]

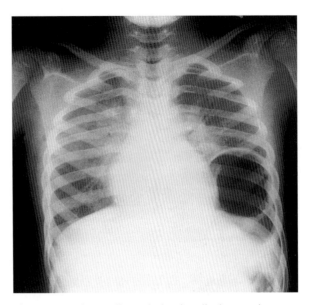

Figure 26.6 *Chest radiograph showing diaphragmatic rupture. This 6-year-old boy had a head injury, from which he died 2 days after the accident. He also had a laceration to the left lobe of the liver, a tear to the transverse colon and a ruptured urethra, associated with a pelvic fracture.*

and have been reported in children as a complication of foreign body inhalation.[20]

Patients may present early with pneumomediastinum or with persistent air leak through a thoracostomy tube; or late with persistent atelectasis and recurrent lower respiratory tract infection.[21] In both scenarios, bronchoscopy is diagnostic. Computed tomography of the chest may be useful in cases with an insidious and late presentation.[22]

Surgical repair is generally successful and uncomplicated. Post-surgical stenosis responds to dilatation.

Diaphragmatic injuries

Diaphragmatic paralysis should be suspected following chest trauma if there is paradoxical abdominal wall motion during spontaneous respiration. The diagnosis may be obscured by other injuries and is revealed when the child ventilated for other reasons proves difficult to wean. An elevated hemidiaphragm on the chest radiograph suggests the injury (see Fig 26.1). Radiographic diagnosis is confirmed by screening. This is a rare injury in children. Complete recovery after prolonged ventilation for bilateral paralysis has been reported.[23]

Diaphragmatic rupture occurs in 3–5% of children with blunt abdominal trauma and in 10–15% of those with penetrating injuries to the lower chest.[24] Damage may be missed because of the severity of associated injuries. The diagnosis should be suspected if the diaphragm is abnormally elevated, persistently obscured

(in the absence of effusion or lower lobe atelectasis), or immobile on inspiratory and expiratory films, with an abnormal gas pattern in the chest (Fig 26.6), atypical 'pneumothorax', or if the nasogastric tube is displaced.[24]

Diagnosis is reliably made by peritoneal lavage, if this is used in conjunction with chest radiography.[25] Complications are limited by early recognition. Even the smallest defect must be repaired.

Traumatic esophageal rupture

This injury is extremely rare in children and requires trauma which will generate high intraesophageal pressures.[26] Rupture leads to mediastinitis with secondary infection and may be fatal.

The clue to diagnosis is a pneumomediastinum on the chest radiograph. Bronchoscopic evaluation is mandatory. Antibiotics should cover Gram-negative, Gram-positive and anaerobic organisms.

Penetrating trauma

Most penetrating chest wounds to children which result from domestic accidents are of moderate severity and readily managed following protocols for adults.

Penetrating injuries from stab and gunshot wounds tend to occur in male adolescents.[27,28] Techniques for the management of adults are appropriate in these patients, with the proviso that the relatively smaller blood volumes are taken into account during cardiovascular resuscitation.

REFERENCES

1. Rivara FP. Traumatic deaths of children in the United States: currently available prevention strategies. *Pediatrics* 1985; **75**: 456–62.
2. Peclet MH, Newman KD, Eichelberger MR, *et al.* Patterns of injury in children. *J Pediatr Surg* 1990; **25**: 85–91.
3. Peclet MH, Newman KD, Eichelberger MR, Gotschall CS, Garcia VF, Bowman LM. Thoracic trauma in children: an indicator of increased mortality. *J Pediatr Surg* 1990; **25**: 961–6.
4. Roux P, Fisher RM. Chest injuries in children: an analysis of 100 cases of blunt chest injuries from motor vehicle accidents. *J Pediatr Surg* 1992; **27**: 551–5.
5. Meller JL, Little AG, Shermetta DW. Thoracic trauma in children. *Pediatrics* 1984; **74**: 813–19.
6. Spevak M, Kleinman PK, Belanger PL, Primack C, Richmond JM. Cardiopulmonary resuscitation and rib fractures in infants. A postmortem radiologic–pathologic study. *JAMA* 1994; **272**: 617–18.

7. Sheikh A, Brogan T. Outcome and cost of open- and closed-chest cardiopulmonary resuscitation in pediatric cardiac arrests. *Pediatrics* 1994; **93**: 392–8.

8. Ummenhofer W, Frei FJ, Urweiler A, Drewe J. Are laboratory values in bone marrow aspirate predictable for venous blood in paediatric patients? *Resuscitation* 1994; **27**: 123–8.

9. Worthy SA, Kang EY, Hartman TE, Kwong JS, Mayo JR, Muller NL. Diaphragmatic rupture: CT findings in 11 patients. *Radiology* 1995; **194**: 885–8.

10. Harris GJ, Soper RT. Pediatric first rib fractures. *J Trauma* 1990; **30**: 343–5.

11. Taylor GA, Kaufman RA, Sivit CJ. Active haemorrhage in children after thoracoabdominal trauma: clinical and CT features. *Am J Roentgenol* 1994; **162**: 401–4.

12. McDougal CB, Mulder GA, Hoffman JR. Tension pneumopericardium following blunt chest trauma. *Ann Emerg Med* 1985; **14**: 167–70.

13. Fabian TC, Mangiante EC, Patterson RC, Payne LW, Isaacson ML. Myocardial contusion in blunt trauma: clinical characteristics, means of diagnosis, and implications for patient management. *J Trauma* 1988; **28**: 50–7.

14. Larger JC, Winthrop AL, Weisson DE, *et al.* Diagnosis and incidence of cardiac injury in children with blunt thoracic trauma. *J Pediatr Surg* 1989; **24**: 1091–4.

15. Garcia VF, Gotschall CS, Eichelberger MR, Bowman LM. Rib fractures in children: a marker of severe trauma. *J Trauma* 1990; **30**: 695–700.

16. Bergman K, Spence L, Wesson D, Bohn D, Dykes E. Thoracic vascular injuries: a postmortem study. *J Trauma* 1990; **30**: 604–6.

17. Smyth BT. Chest trauma in children. *J Pediatr Surg* 1979; **14**: 41–7.

18. Blane CE, White SJ, Wesley JR, Coran AG. Immediate traumatic pulmonary pseudocyst formation in children. *Surgery* 1981; **90**: 872–5.

19. Barmada H, Gibbons JR. Tracheobronchial injury in blunt and penetrating chest trauma. *Chest* 1994; **106**: 74–8.

20. Burton EM, Riggs W, Kaufman RA, Houston CS. Pneumomediastinum caused by foreign body aspiration in children. *Pediatr Radiol* 1989; **20**: 45–7.

21. Hancock BJ, Wiseman NE. Tracheobronchial injuries in children. *J Pediatr Surg* 1991; **26**: 1316–19.

22. Palder SB, Shandling B, Manson D. Rupture of the thoracic trachea following blunt trauma: diagnosis by CAT scan. *J Pediatr Surg* 1991; **26**: 1320–2.

23. Commare MC, Kurstjens SP, Barois A. Diaphragmatic paralysis in children: a review of 11 cases. *Pediatr Pulmonol* 1994; **18**: 187–93.

24. Brandt NI, Luks FI, Spigland NA, DiLorenzo M, Laberge J-M, Ouimet A. Diaphragmatic injury in children. *J Trauma* 1992; **32**: 298–301.

25. Troop B, Myers RM, Agarwal NN. Early recognition of diaphragmatic injuries from blunt trauma. *Ann Emerg Med* 1985; **14**: 97–101.

26. Ben-Ami T, Rozenman J, Yahav J, Sagy M, Barzilay Z. Computed tomography in children with esophageal and airway trauma. *J Pediatr Surg* 1988; **23**: 919–23.

27. Barlow B, Niemirska B, Ghandi RP. Stab wounds in children. *J Pediatr Surg* 1983; **18**: 926–9.

28. Ordog GJ, Prakash A, Wasserberger J, Balasubramaniam S. Pediatric gunshot wounds. *J Trauma* 1987; **27**: 1272–8.

Index

THE
SOCIETY OF
AUTHORS

Entered for the Society of Authors'

Medical Book Awards 1999

Sponsored by the Royal Society of Medicine

84 DRAYTON GARDENS, LONDON SW10 9SB

TELEPHONE 0171 373 6642   FACSIMILE 0171 373 5768

email: authorsoc@writers.org.uk